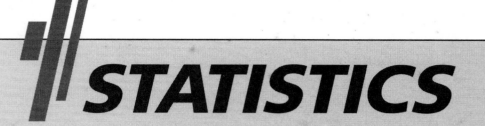

STATISTICS

A Health Sciences Orientation

Professor Charles M. Biles
Humboldt State University

WCB Wm. C. Brown Publishers
Dubuque, Iowa•Melbourne, Australia•Oxford, England

Dedication

To my dear wife, Carolyn,

and to our parents, Rose Rambousek Biles and Taylor York

Book Team

Editor *Paula-Christy Heighton*
Developmental Editor *Daryl Bruflodt*
Publishing Services Coordinator/Design *Barbara J. Hodgson*

Wm. C. Brown Publishers
A Division of Wm. C. Brown Communications, Inc.

Vice President and General Manager *Beverly Kolz*
Vice President, Publisher *Earl McPeek*
Vice President, Director of Sales and Marketing *Virginia S. Moffat*
Vice President, Director of Production *Colleen A. Yonda*
National Sales Manager *Douglas J. DiNardo*
Marketing Manager *Julie Joyce Keck*
Advertising Manager *Janelle Keeffer*
Production Editorial Manager *Renée Menne*
Publishing Services Manager *Karen J. Slaght*
Permissions/Records Manager *Connie Allendorf*

Wm. C. Brown Communications, Inc.

President and Chief Executive Officer *G. Franklin Lewis*
Corporate Senior Vice President, President of WCB Manufacturing *Roger Meyer*
Corporate Senior Vice President and Chief Financial Officer *Robert Chesterman*

Cover photos © Neil Zachary

Production/Design by Editorial Services of New England

Contents

**General
Features**

Statistics: A Health Sciences Orientation began seven years ago as a service course for undergraduate students majoring in nursing at Humboldt State University (HSU). The bachelor's degree in nursing at HSU requires the student to complete a course in statistics. This requirement was previously satisfied with a general education course, or a course in statistics for a social science. Although the requirement was satisfied, nursing students were not. They found little relevance in liberal arts and general statistics courses to their role as health care professionals.

My early courses introduced statistical topics by presenting a problem taken from a health sciences journal. As articles accumulated, in breadth and scope from a variety of journals, I abandoned textbooks on statistics for biological and health sciences, which students found too ponderous and mathematical, in favor of a Kinko's pack, which then evolved into this textbook.

Currently at HSU, statistics for the health sciences is a one-semester, three-unit course. The class meets twice a week for a 50-minute lecture and once a week for a 2-hour computer session using the statistical software package Minitab. The course prerequisite is intermediate algebra. The course is offered each semester to about 30 students. The student enrollment is about 85% undergraduates (mostly sophomores or juniors) majoring in nursing, nutrition, medical technology, premedicine, (predentistry, preveterinary, and pre–physical therapy) and 15% graduate students enrolled in the master's program in physical education. About one-third of the students own a home computer (PC or Macintosh) and purchase Minitab for their personal use.

At HSU, homework assignments, an integral part of the course, are collected during each class period and are read, evaluated, and returned the next class period. Accordingly, the text has been professor-, student-, reader-, and class-tested.

This textbook is designed as an *introductory* course in statistics for students in the health sciences. It is accessible to a broad range of students in a variety of health care disciplines. The key mathematical prerequisite is that the student have the following ability: given a formula and a list of numbers for the variables in the formula, he or she can substitute numbers for the letters and calculate the correct numerical answer using a calculator. No prior computer experience is assumed.

An introductory course in statistics for the health sciences is asked to do much: introduce descriptive statistics, probability, basic distributions, confidence intervals, basic tests of hypothesis, ANOVA, chisquared tests, and correlation/regression analysis, all with relevant applications, while developing a critical eye for the nuances of statistical design and proper interpretation of results. Covering such material is a considerable challenge.

This text addresses the task by exploiting the current literature. The primary journals used are *Heart and Lung*, the *Journal of the American Medical Association*, the *American Journal of Public Health*, and the *American Journal of Clinical Nutrition*. These journals were selected since they are carried by most academic libraries, most articles in them use statistics as a language to communicate results, and they cover a wide range of topics in their fields. In addition, articles from a broad spectrum of journals are included.

My general goal in writing this text is to provide a course in which students can learn to intelligently use the literature with a critical view toward what it means for patient (or client) care.

The text is organized in three major parts: Descriptive Statistics, Inferential Statistics, and Multifaceted Statistics. Each part is followed by a review section. Descriptive Statistics (Chapters 1–6) contains the basic material on how to present a raw data set, basic concepts of probability, and the basic distributions (binomial and normal). Inferential Statistics (Chapters 7–11) presents confidence intervals and tests of hypothesis. Specific details are provided for conducting one- and two-population tests for the proportion and an average. Multifaceted statistics (Chapters 12–14) presents an introduciton to ANOVA, chi-squared testing, and correlation/regression analysis. Throughout the text, concepts are introduced only as needed and motivated with both health science and statistical concerns. The material is presented to develop both understanding and confidence through practice.

Chapter 1 covers basic descriptive statistics. Section 1.1 introduces the basic vocabulary and motivation for statistics, and emphasizes the role of the frequency distribution table. The frequency distribution table is a good concept to launch into working with numbers and building student confidence. Section 1.2 introduces the concept of a random variable from a practical point of view, then focuses on calculating and interpreting the mean, median, range, and standard deviation for a numerical data set.

Chapter 2 further develops the condept of a random variable to fix the concept of numerical data and develop tools for exploring interval data sets. Section 2.1 presents a summary of common exploratory methods: dotplot, boxplot, stem-and-leaf, and histogram. Minitab is used to focus attention on the graphics and the story told by a data set, rather than tedious details of how to construct the graphic. Sections 2.2 and 2.3 are optional; these sections carefully go through step-by-step details needed to construct a histogram, with related tables and graphs, by hand. I sometimes include these sections, depending on the timing of the semester calendar. The beneficial effect of these sections is primarily building student confidence in working with numbers, tables, and graphs.

Chapter 3 introduces the basic concepts of probability needed for inferential statistics. Section 3.1 introduces the basic language and idea of probability and culminates with the Fundamental Principle of Counting. Section 3.2 is concerned with computational ideas. The section first introduces basic combinatorics (which later supports the formulation of the binomial random variable), then discusses some rules for computing a probability (especially the independence rule).

Chapter 4 applies the basic concepts of probability developed in Chapter 3 to diagnostic testing: sensitivity, specificity, and predictive value. The role of prevalence on predictive value is explored.

Chapter 5 introduces the concept of a discrete random variable. Section 5.1 discusses the role played by a discrete random variable when one is provided with a table of outcomes and associated probabilities. Stress is placed on how to read and apply the table. Section 5.2 details the most common discrete random variable, the binomial random variable.

Chapter 6 introduces the most common continuous random variable, one based on a normal distribution. Section 6.1 describes the details of a normal distribution and how to compute probabilities with the aid of a table of values for a standard normal distribution. Section 6.2 describes how to test a given data set of interval numbers to determine whether or not it is reasonable to assume that the data were drawn from a normal distribution. This section exploits the nscores and correlation test for normality in Minitab. The concept of test of hypothesis is presented in the specific setting of testing for normality. This introduction to test of hypothesis is pedagogically a valuable prelude to Chapter 9, which introduces hypothesis testing in general. The ability to test for normality is an important prerequisite for much of the remaining text.

Chapter 7 introduces the concept of a confidence interval. Section 7.1 discusses the notions of a point estimate and an interval estimate. The student is asked to construct a confidence interval for the mean when presented with either a raw data set or a data legend (sample size, mean, standard deviation). Both t-intervals and z-intervals are presented. The student must carefully check assumptions before constructing a confidence interval. When using a raw data set, an assumption of normality is checked using Minitab's nscores and correlation test developed in Section 6.2. Section 7.2 applies the skills developed in Section 7.1 to paired data. The utility of a paired-data confidence interval for the difference is stressed.

Chapter 8 further applies the confidence interval concept to a broader concept of an average value and to a proportion. Section 8.1 presents the sign interval for the median (Minitab-dependent). Guidance for selecting an appropriate confidence interval for a given situation is provided. Section 8.2 discusses confidence intervals for the proportion, including design features of sample size to obtain an interval estimate within a desired degree of accuracy.

Chapter 9 introduces the general concept of test of hypothesis. Section 9.1 stresses the formulation of the null and alternate hypotheses.

Chapter 10 details one-population tests of hypothesis for a proportion and an average value. Section 10.1 details test of hypothesis for a proportion. Testing of hypothesis begins with the proportion since this is the easiest to conduct. Section 10.2 covers tests of hypothesis for an average value. Necessary preliminaries are discussed and checked. Criteria for whether to use the mean or the median for the average are presented. Section 10.3 applies the material in Section 10.2 to paired data. The fundamental paired t-test is featured. Section 10.4 details the concept of the p-value.

Chapter 11 extends hypothesis testing to two populations. Section 11.1 compares a proportion between two populations. Section 11.2 compares a suitable average between two populations. The standard pooled t-test, large-samples z-test, Smith-Satterthwaite test, and Mann-Whitney test are presented. The student carefully checks assumptions in order to select the appropriate average (mean or median) and statistical test for comparing averages.

Chapter 12 is a basic introduction to ANOVA using Minitab. Section 12.1 applies one-way ANOVA when an appropriate raw data set is given. Section 12.2 applies one-way ANOVA when provided only with a summary legend (the sample size, mean, and standard deviation for each level). Section 12.3 provides an introduction to one-way repeated-measures ANOVA and to two-way ANOVA.

Chapter 13 is a basic introduction to chisquared tests. Section 13.1 presents a chisquared test for goodness of fit. Section 13.2 presents the chisquared test for independence of attributes.

Chapter 14 is a basic introduction to correlation and regression analysis. Section 14.1 presents correlation analysis for paired-interval data. A test of hypothesis for linear correlation is provided. Section 14.2 presents regression analysis.

The Computer

The personal teaching style and beliefs of the author permeate any textbook. One of my strong beliefs is that any statistics course should be accompanied with a hands-on computer experience. Students learn by doing. By using a computer, one not only spares the class from copious boring and tedious computations but covers much more material by focusing on concepts. I do not believe that students learn much by performing a great deal of hand calculations. For example, the main thing learned in taking a raw data set and carrying through all the calculations by hand for ANOVA is that one rarely gets the correct answer that way—there's simply too high a risk of making an arithmetic error. Use of a computer is natural in this day and age.

There are many statistical software packages available. My criteria for choice of statistical software in this course are the following:

- The package should be widely used.
- The package should be commonly available on most university systems to which students have access.
- The package should have a price tag *affordable to the general student*, available in both a PC and a Macintosh version.
- The package should use a reasonable amount of disk storage (under 10 megabytes) and be able to perform *well* with 4 MB RAM.
- Output should be available in a form that can be imported to common word processors such as Microsoft Word or WordPerfect.
- The package should be easy to learn.

I know of only two packages that meet my personal criteria: Systat and Minitab. Systat has an inexpensive student version (MyStat). Minitab has both an inexpensive student version marketed through Addison-Wesley and full version that is available at a student-affordable price through the university bookstore with a university site license.

From my own experience, for good teaching it is imperative that students who have their own home computer (PC or Macintosh) also have the opportunity to purchase the software for an affordable price for home use. Such students will study more and learn more. Professional heavy-duty packages such as SPPS, SAS, and BMDP, although wonderful packages for the professional statistician, are simply not appropriate for an introductory course in health sciences statistics. First, they are too hard to learn how to use. Second, and most important, there is no affordable version for student purchase. Further, students who do not have their own home computers need a software package that is easy to access and to learn how to use. Manuals that rival the New York telephone directory in size are too intimidating for any introductory statistics course.

Over the course of several years, I have found Minitab not only to be satisfactory but a product I can highly recommend (I have no financial interest in the company).

If someone would like to investigate other statistical computing packages, I recommend the review article "A Comparison of Five Student Versions of Statistics Packages" by Robin H. Lock published in *The American Statistician* 47, no. 1 (May 1993): 136–45. The article reviews five DOS platform packages.

In addition to a statistical package, one may be interested in the DOS platform computer-assisted instruction packages STATPRIM (Basic) by Mary R. Castles, Inc., St. Louis, and STAT^{2}tor (Intermediate/Advanced) by Yellow River Stationware, Inc., Monona, IA. These products are marketed by A.S.K. Data Systems, Inc., PO Box 766, Manchester, MO 63011, (800) 292-7211. STATPRIM is designed to aid students in nursing and allied health programs to understand an introductory statistics course. Instructors faced with students who have a very limited mathematics background and high math anxiety may be interested in investigating these programs.

Acknowledgments

I apologize for not being able to recognize in print everybody who in some way contributed to the preparation and production of this book. Some contributions were so great, however, that they must be acknowledged.

First and foremost, there is my wife, Carolyn, a practicing critical care nurse (BSRN, CCRN). Carolyn would patiently listen as I told her of my lecture in health sciences statistics. Frequently her critique was simply, "That's nice, but what does it mean for patient care?" Through her influence, and the response of the health science students in my classes, that question ("What does it mean for patient care?") has become the bottom line for most topics and examples presented in this text. I am also indebted to Carolyn for completely reading the manuscript through several stages of its evolution.

This manuscript began as a publishing venture with C. V. Mosby, Inc. I am particularly indebted to J. P. Lenney and Pattie Connors (both of whom have since moved on to other ventures) for the initial recruitment and development of this project. Continuous appreciation goes to Edie Podrazik at Mosby–Year Book for sending me articles of interest from the Year Book project. In addition, Gibson Kingren (AAPH, emeritus), John Machen, M.D., and Joe Carroll, M.D., supplied me with literature from their private collections. The project later moved to Wm. C. Brown Publishers in a reorganization within Times-Mirror, the parent firm to both companies. I appreciate the work of Jane Parrigin in launching the production phase of this text. Special thanks goes to John Fitzpatrick and his staff at Editorial Services of New England (Cambridge, Mass.), and to the folks at Publication Services, Inc. (Boston, Mass.) for the actual process of turning the manuscript into a textbook.

Several reviewers assisted at various stages of development. At the request of C.V. Mosby, the following reviewed premanuscript materials or reviewed early parts of the manuscript: Lothar Dohse, University of North Carolina Asheville; Harold Jacobs, East Stroudsburg University; William Gratzer, Iona College; Dennis O'Brien, University of Wisconsin at La Crosse; Keumhee Carriere, University of Iowa; Esther Haloburdo, St. Joseph College; Jeannine Raymond, California State University Fresno; H. R. Al-Khalidi, University of Illinois at Chicago Circle; Jorge G. Morel, University of South Florida; Willis Owen, University of Oklahoma; and Dana Quade, University of North Carolina. Elizabeth Low, University of Vermont, reviewed a later edition of the full manuscript. I appreciate the many fine suggestions and comments submitted by these reviewers. I feel especially appreciative of the thorough and professional review provided by Professor Dana Quade. I am also indebted to four anonymous reviewers who reviewed the manuscript near its final stage on behalf of Wm. C. Brown, Inc.

I am very indebted to my students from the past several years. They not only showed a great deal of patience while material was developed, but also eagerly critiqued and evaluated such material as this manuscript evolved.

Finally, my appreciation goes to the Department of Mathematics at Humboldt State University, my professional home since 1969. Particular thanks goes to the Department of Nursing who encouraged this project and to several professors in nutrition, physical education, and environmental engineering who regularly recommended my course.

Claimers and Disclaimers

Every effort was made to purge errors of all types from this manuscript. Any errors that have survived are, of course, my responsibility. In the spirit of accountability, I offer the following service to all adopters and purchasers of this text. Please feel free to communicate with me, either by post or by electronic mail. I will appreciate and acknowledge your calling any errors to my attention, or hearing any ideas or suggestions. All communications will be individually acknowledged to my best ability during the academic year at HSU (late August through mid-May). During the academic year I will maintain an email service whereby I can provide periodic updates for this text. My email address is

bilesc@axe.humboldt.edu

My postal address is

Professor Charles M. Biles
Department of Mathematics
Humboldt State University
Arcata, CA 95521-8922

In advance, thank you for your considerations.

Charles M. Biles

An Orientation to Descriptive Statistics

Statistics: A Health Sciences Orientation is a merger of statistics and health science. Both subjects play central roles in this book. Health care is the unifying *theme* for this text; statistics is the unifying *tool*.

Our subject matter is motivated by concerns of health care consumers, providers, and administrators.

> John was recently admitted to the cardiac intensive care unit. He had a heart attack and underwent coronary artery bypass graft surgery involving three coronary vessels. John's family is concerned. What are his chances for survival? Can he ever return to a normal life? What steps can John take to prevent a future occurrence?

Such questions of health care apply not only to John but to many other people like John. They apply to each of us personally: Can I take steps in my own life so this will not happen to me? Statistics is a tool that can help answer such questions. One begins by gathering and organizing data in such a way that a story can be told.

> John is 45 years old. He smokes a pack of cigarettes a day, is 20 pounds overweight, is stressed at work, and does not exercise.

Health care professionals note that John presents many risk factors. A risk factor is a recognized indicator of an increased likelihood of a health problem. People who present risk factors like John's are more likely to suffer a coronary event than those who do not. Generalities like risk factors and likelihoods are conclusions based on a statistical analysis of data from many patients like John. A major goal for this course is an understanding of the statistical procedures used to make these conclusions.

We will use statistical procedures in the same spirit that a skilled clinician uses diagnostic procedures. The clinician invokes diagnostic tests to better understand the condition of an individual patient. We will invoke statistical tests to better understand the condition of an entire population (group of people). There is a dynamic interplay between a population as a whole and the individuals making up that population. From this perspective, a respect for statistical procedures in the health sciences can help the student become a better health care provider at the individual level, as well as a better manager at the group level.

Before we can resolve questions of health care, we obviously must first formulate those questions. Part I of this text is devoted to gathering and organizing data in such a way that the presentation of the data suggests appropriate questions. Without such preparations, statistics is only a solution looking for a problem.

This is the first rule of applied statistics: Look at the data. Accordingly, we begin by developing basic skills for looking at data.

Introduction to Statistics

Most students in the health sciences enroll in a statistics course for one reason: Statistics is a requirement for the degree program. In Section 1.1, we look at part of the rationale behind this requirement.

Health science statistics is not a spectator sport. One cannot learn to critically read an article in *Heart and Lung* by listening to a lecture any more than one can learn to give intravenous medications by watching a demonstration. Of course, the demonstration is important to orient the novice practitioner. In order for professional development to proceed, however, one must gain confidence by *doing*.

The student begins "to do" statistics in Section 1.1 by constructing and presenting a basic frequency distribution table. This "hands-on" learning continues in Section 1.2, in which the student "boils down" a raw data set to its essentials.

The author hopes that the reader of Section 1.1 senses two positive feelings:

1. Hey, I can do this!
2. I learned something.

SECTION 1.1

Frequency Distribution Tables

OBJECTIVES　　This section will

1　Describe the science of statistics, including statistical design, descriptive statistics, and inferential statistics.

2　Describe why a course in statistics is important in a health science program.

3　Describe and define the terms: population, parameter, sample, statistic.

4　Determine the frequency and relative frequency of the characteristics in a given data set and present the results in (a) a frequency distribution table, (b) a bar graph, and (c) a pie chart.

The study of any subject begins with some general stage-setting vocabulary. The introductory words in this vocabulary are intended to describe the broad framework and orientation in which the study takes place. These words are appropriately introduced with descriptions rather than rigorous definitions. For example, biology is initially described as the science of living things. Biology has two main branches: botany (the study of plants) and zoology (the study of animals). It is neither implied nor necessary that the student have a rigorous definition of life, plant, and animal at this time, but that in general, at an intuitive level, one can distinguish between living and nonliving things, and between plants and animals.

We begin with an introductory description of statistics and present the main branches of this science. These should be understood and appreciated from a general, intuitive point of view.

The Science of Statistics

Statistics is the science that deals with methods of (1) collecting data, (2) presenting data, and (3) drawing valid conclusions from the data.

The branch of statistics that specializes in

- Collecting data is called **statistical design**
- Presenting data is called **descriptive statistics**
- Drawing valid conclusions from data is called **inferential statistics**

The goal of statistical design is to obtain data in the most efficient and economical manner for the purposes at hand. The goal of descriptive statistics is to describe a real-world situation through the organization and presentation of data. The goal of inferential statistics lies in explaining, forecasting, or managing events. This general overall view of statistics is displayed in Figure 1.1.1.

FIGURE **1.1.1**
The major branches of statistics are statistical design, descriptive statistics, and inferential statistics.

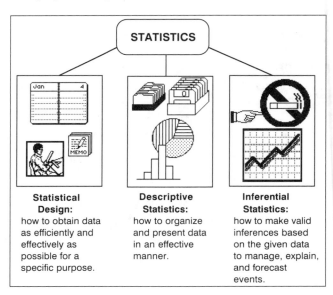

Statistical Design:
how to obtain data as efficiently and effectively as possible for a specific purpose.

Descriptive Statistics:
how to organize and present data in an effective manner.

Inferential Statistics:
how to make valid inferences based on the given data to manage, explain, and forecast events.

Statistics in the Health Sciences

A general knowledge of statistics is important for a health science practitioner (1) to read the health sciences literature with critical understanding and (2) to assess the status of a patient or client by taking measurements. A working knowledge of statistics is mandatory for research.

You will need a background in statistics to be a knowledgeable reader of most professional health science journals, such as the *New England Journal of Medicine*, *Lancet*, the *Journal of the American Medical Association*, *Heart and Lung*, the *American Journal of Nursing*, the *American Journal of Public Health*, *Pediatrics*, and the *American Journal of Clinical Nutrition*.

Statistics has become the international common language in which major problems in the health sciences are studied and the results are communicated. Emerson and Colditz tabulated the specific statistical skills used in articles published in the *New England Journal of Medicine* over a 3-year period. By learning the statistics in this course, you will have sufficient knowledge to be able to read critically about 80% of the statistical presentations published in articles in technical health science journals such as *Heart and Lung* or the *New England Journal of Medicine*.

Presentations of the results of research in health care (usually laden with statistics) are not just for researchers. Karin Kirchhoff argues that there needs to be greater coordination between educators, administrators, researchers, students, and staff. As Kirchhoff stresses: "The anticipated user of critical care research is the staff nurse at the bedside. He or she is expected to read research, evaluate a number of reports on a topic in nursing, make practical decisions, and then implement those changes." A general knowledge of statistics is important throughout the entire spectrum of health care professionals, from administrators and researchers to doctors and nurses.

Statistics is a valuable tool in both research and clinical practice. For example, only through statistics have we come to know that the most extensive health problems in the United States today are caused neither by communicable disease nor by genetics but rather result from poor decisions on the part of the patient: cigarette smoking, alcohol and drug abuse, and poor personal habits (especially nutritional and dental). Statistics is also a key tool in the evaluation and application of vaccination programs, drug effectiveness, public safety programs, and intervention therapies.

Such topics are important not only on an individual basis but also on a broad general level to health care administrators and managers concerned with large groups of people. The focus of attention in the health sciences can range from an individual (a patient or client) to small groups (a practice or research group) to large groups (an entire community). We now develop some basic concepts to fix the focus of attention.

Basic Concepts in Statistics

There are four fundamental statistical concepts that go together and should be learned as a team: population and sample, parameter and statistic.

The entire group of interest for some particular concern is known as a population. An initial step in any statistical study is to clearly identify the population of interest. The next step is to obtain relevant information about that population. How does one learn about an entire population? Usually it is immediately apparent that one cannot study all people (or objects) in the population as a whole. Resource constraints (money, time, personnel, material) alone usually prohibit a study of the entire population. With very rare exception, one must be content with studying a small piece of the population. The relatively small part of the population one actually studies is called a sample.

Population and Sample

The general group of interest and the actual group one gets to study are embodied in the terms population and sample.

DEFINITION ▮▮▮ Population

A **population** is a well-defined collection of objects.

A collection which is **well-defined** is one in which it is possible to distinguish between objects that belong to the collection of interest and objects that do not belong. In a health sciences study, one needs guidelines to determine whether or not a patient or client is a potential candidate for study. For example, the following populations are well defined:

1. All lung cancer patients so diagnosed by a licensed physician during the past 7 years
2. All cardiac patients in a coronary intensive care unit in the United States for whom cardiac output measurements are ordered
3. All adults age 18 or older who are currently or will be admitted over the next 5 years to an accredited hospital in California

In contrast, the following groups are not well defined: (1) all sick people, (2) all flu victims who need help, (3) all children who have a sore throat. The general terms "sick," "need help," and "child with a sore throat" are too vague and as such provide inadequate guidelines to determine whether a specific person is to be included.

A sample is the relatively small part of a population one actually studies to obtain information about that population.

DEFINITION ▮▮▮ Sample

A **sample** is a subset of a population obtained for the purpose of studying that population.

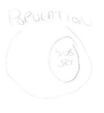

The following three examples represent samples drawn from each of the previous three populations:

1. A researcher at a major cancer center obtains the medical records of 30 patients admitted for treatment of lung cancer 5 years ago.
2. A researcher decides to obtain cardiac outputs on all cardiac patients admitted to the cardiac intensive care unit over the next 3 days.

3. A public health administrator selects five hospitals in various locations in California and will examine the records of the next 50 admissions at each hospital.

Parameter and Statistic

One makes a study about a population because one wants to know something about that population. The desired information is sometimes summarized as a single number measuring the status of the population. A conceptual measure of the general population of interest and the measurement one actually obtains from a sample are concepts embodied in the terms parameter and statistic.

DEFINITION **III Parameter**

A **parameter** is a measure of a population.

A parameter is a measure that describes the entire population. Parameters for the three previously presented populations include the following:

1. The fraction of lung cancer patients who survive at least 5 years (FRACTION)
2. Average cardiac output in liters per minute (RATE)
3. Average length of hospital stay in days (AVERAGE)

DEFINITION **III Statistic**

A **statistic** is a measure of a sample.

A statistic is a measure obtained from an actual sample. For example, based on the previous samples, researchers may find:

1. Eleven of thirty lung cancer patients admitted 5 years ago are still alive. Hence, in this sample, 11/30 of lung cancer patients survive at least 5 years.
2. The average cardiac output 24 hours after admission for the 29 patients admitted into the cardiac intensive care unit over the 3-day period was 4.5 liters per minute.
3. The average length of hospital stay for the next 250 patients admitted to 5 California hospitals was 3.7 days.

EXAMPLE 1.1.1 The medical records office at General Hospital has records on all 85,697 patients admitted and discharged since the hospital opened 20 years ago. An administrator is interested in the average length of patient stay at General Hospital. A programmer in the computer center reported that all records are computerized and that the average length of stay of all 85,697 patients is 4.8 days. Here the population of interest is all patients admitted and discharged from General Hospital; the parameter of interest is 4.8 days, the average length of hospital stay at General Hospital.

A clerk in medical records said that 76 patients had been discharged during the past week and that the average length of stay for those patients was 4.2 days.

Here the group of patients discharged last week is a sample from the population. This sample yielded a statistic of 4.2 days. Another clerk at a computer terminal called up patients records from 8 years ago in June for last names beginning with H to L and found the average length of stay of these 82 patients was 4.9 days. Here these 82 patients form another sample yielding a statistic of 4.9 days. This example for General Hospital is summarized in Figure 1.1.2.

In actual practice, a population parameter is rarely known. A major problem in statistics is how to get a handle on a population parameter when the information provided by a sample varies from sample to sample. One of the jobs of inferential statistics is to infer knowledge of a parameter for a population from a statistic provided by a sample.

A study begins by identifying a population of interest. To study a population one draws a sample and makes observations on each member in the sample. Sampling techniques are crucial since studying the entire population of interest is usually beyond the resource capabilities of the investigator. Even the U.S. Census, taken each decade, does not reach everybody. Even when possible, there are compelling reasons not to study every member in the population; a study of an entire population is frequently unethical and is simply impossible if it involves future projections.

Ethical considerations, by necessity, must play a major role in statistical design in the health sciences. For example, in determining safe and effective dosage levels for a chemotherapeutic drug, one cannot inject a cancer patient with the drug until a lethal amount is given. Many research institutions have an ethics committee to oversee and regulate projects from an ethical perspective.

Often a study is conducted for the purpose of forecasting into the future; for example, what is the most effective treatment to give patients admitted to a hospital for an apparent heart attack? Of course, one cannot yet treat future patients. However, hospital protocols are written to cover not just the current census but also future admissions. Frequently, a study of current or recent patients must suffice as a sample of a population needing future treatment. A major problem in research is to design a study for which one has a high level of confidence that the sampling strategy will obtain data reasonably representative of the population under study.

FIGURE **1.1.2**
General Hospital has served 85,697 patients in its history (patient population). The average length of hospital stay was 4.8 days (population parameter). The square windows show two samples drawn from this population. Each sample is accompanied by its statistic.

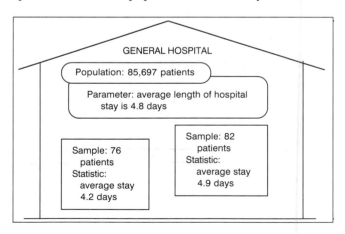

Summarizing Data

One obtains a raw data set by recording observations on each member in a sample drawn from a study population.

EXAMPLE 1.1.2   Jonsson et al studied the role played by tissue oxygenation in the healing process of surgical wounds. For each of 33 surgical patients the researchers recorded a perfusion score as a measure of tissue oxygenation. The raw data set was

```
0 1 1 1 2 1 1 2 3 3 2 3 3 2 3 2 1
3 3 3 2 3 3 3 3 3 3 3 3 3 3 3 2
```

Presentation of an unprocessed raw data set usually has a mind-boggling effect on the reader. An unorganized list of random observations can overwhelm anyone. The job now is to present the data in some efficient and comprehensible manner. One does this by presenting a numerical and pictorial summary of the raw data. Compare the raw data set given in Example 1.1.2 with the presentation in Figure 1.1.3.

Tables and graphs organize and compress raw data to give one a feel for the general distribution of the data. From Figure 1.1.3 we quickly see that most patients have a perfusion score of 3, some have scores of 1 and 2 (about equally divided), and it is unusual to have a perfusion score of 0.

Many authors summarize data by presenting both a frequency distribution table and an accompanying graphic. People differ regarding how they find presentations informative. Some people are more table-oriented; others, more picture-oriented. A presentation that offers both a tabular and a graphic display of a frequency distribution usually reaches a larger audience.

The frequency distribution table is an important tool for presenting data. The table gives one a feel for the distribution of the data in an organized way. Graphics such as pie charts and bar graphs are pictorial representations of the table. We now present guidelines for construction of such tables and graphs.

Frequency and Relative Frequency

A frequency distribution table is a common method of presenting data. Key ingredients to such a table are frequency and relative frequency (which may be expressed as a percentage).

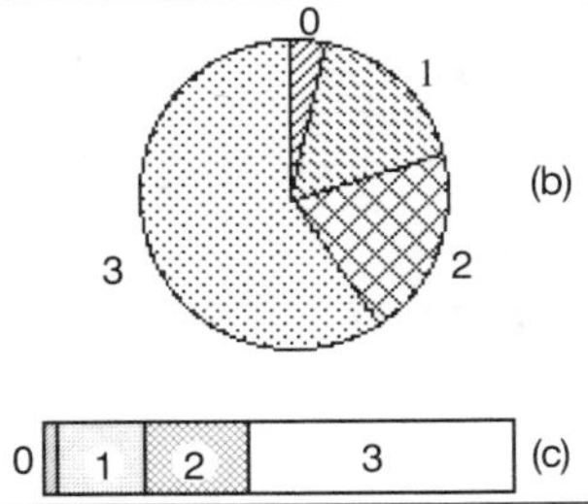

FIGURE **1.1.3**
Perfusion scores in surgery patients: (a) frequency distribution table, (b) pie chart, (c) bar graph.

Perfusion Score	Frequency	Percent
0	1	3
1	6	18
2	7	21
3	19	58
Total	33	100

(a)

Frequency

The **absolute frequency** is merely the number of times a given observation appears in a data set. The absolute frequency is usually just called the frequency of the observation. Since (absolute) frequency is just a count, frequency is *always* a whole number.

EXAMPLE 1.1.3 J. Sands gave the sex of patients in a research study as follows:

F M M F F M F M M M F F M M M

The frequency for females (F) in the group is 6; the frequency for males (M) is 9.

EXAMPLE 1.1.4 In the Jonsson et al surgical wound study (Example 1.1.2), there are 19 occurrences of a perfusion score of 3 in the sample data; hence, the frequency of a perfusion score of 3 is 19.

Relative Frequency

Merely providing the (absolute) frequency of an observation does not give one a sense of the size of this observation in relation to the whole data set. For example, suppose one reports that the frequency of a diagnosis of trauma is 10. Is trauma a frequent or rare occurrence? One does not know until one considers the frequency in the context of the whole. If trauma occurs 10 times in a data set of 11 observations, then trauma is the dominant diagnosis in the study. However, if trauma occurs 10 times in a data set of 1000, then trauma is a relatively small part of the whole diagnosis picture as far as frequency is concerned.

Accordingly, we define **relative frequency** of an observation as the fraction obtained by dividing the frequency of that observation by the size of the whole data set. A relative frequency is often denoted by p since it represents the proportion of the given observation in the whole data set. Formally, suppose we have a sample of size n, that is, a data set with n individual observations. A particular observation occurs x times in the data set. Then the (absolute) frequency is x, while the relative frequency p is given by $p = x/n$.

DEFINITION ▮▮▮ Relative Frequency

Relative frequency = (absolute frequency)/(sample size)

Let n = sample size
x = absolute frequency
p = relative frequency

Then, $p = \dfrac{x}{n}$

EXAMPLE 1.1.5 In Sands's study (Example 1.1.3) the relative frequency for females is 6/15 (= .40); for males, 9/15 (= .60).

EXAMPLE 1.1.6 In Jonsson's study (Example 1.1.2) the relative frequency for a perfusion score of 3 is 19/33 (= .58). The relative frequency for a perfusion score of 2 is 7/33 (= .21).

A relative frequency is often expressed as a percentage and as such is referred to as **percent relative frequency**, that is, relative frequency multiplied by 100. Hence,

$$\text{percent relative frequency} = \text{relative frequency} \times 100$$
$$= \left(\frac{x}{n}\right) \times 100$$

EXAMPLE 1.1.7 In the Sands study (Examples 1.1.3,5), 6 of the 15 patients are female. Hence, females make up 40% (6/15 = 0.40 = 40%) and males 60% of the patients in the sample.

EXAMPLE 1.1.8 In the Jonsson et al study (Examples 1.1.2,4,6), a perfusion score of 3 accounts for 58% (19/33 = .58 = 58%) of the sample.

How many places past the decimal point should one use to report a percentage or a relative frequency? We offer these guidelines adapted from Sumner:

■ Avoid unnecessary precision in presenting numbers. Reporting numbers with many places past the decimal point not only detracts from clarity but suggests an uncritical transfer from a calculator display or computer printout.

■ Percentages based on a sample size ≤ 100 should be presented as whole numbers (*percent* means "per hundred"). Percentages based on a sample size > 100 may be presented one place past the decimal point.

■ Relative frequencies are usually presented to two places past the decimal point when based on a sample size ≤ 100 and to three places past the decimal point when based on a larger sample size.

These guidelines are motivated by the purpose of descriptive statistics: to *inform* the reader. Hence, when presenting the final answer to a numerical computation, report using an appropriate number of decimal places. We caution, however, that numbers used in computations should not be rounded—only the *final answer* is rounded for presentation.

Frequency Distribution Tables

A good presentation of a frequency distribution table displays three columns:

Column 1 lists the characteristics of interest and carries a column heading suggestive of the general nature of those characteristics.
Column 2 displays the absolute frequency of each characteristic.
Column 3 displays the corresponding relative frequencies, which may be expressed as percent relative frequency.

Columns 2 and 3 should also display their respective totals. Since relative frequency and percent relative frequency are so closely related, it is unnecessary to present them both. In the health sciences literature, percent relative frequency is usually presented.

EXAMPLE 1.1.9 Simpson et al studied the recollections of several critical care patients within 24 to 48 hours after transfer from an intensive care experience. The patients in the study recalled various "Technical Care" actions as follows:

29 Medications
7 Specialized care (catheter sheath irrigation)
6 Fluids (IV)
6 Respiratory (gave oxygen)
4 Nursing care (changed dressing)
2 Surgery
7 Special procedure (angiograms)

First we note that the total number of individual observations is 61. This total is used as the basis for determining the relative frequencies. Using a calculator, the relative frequency for medications is $29/61 = 0.4754098361$ (Figure 1.1.4). One then rounds this calculator answer to 0.48 for ease of comprehension. Note that a relative frequency will always be a number between 0 and 1 since it is calculated as a part divided by the whole.

The complete frequency distribution table (Table 1.1.1) for the Simpson et al data set (Example 1.1.9) displays the technical care actions of interest, their (absolute) frequencies, and their relative frequencies. Although it is unnecessary to present both relative frequency and percent relative frequency, our early tables will carry both for the sake of illustration.

Comment By way of an important check, the relative frequency column should ideally add up to 1.00 and the percent relative frequency column to 100. As a result of round-off errors, one may obtain a relative frequency column that adds up to a

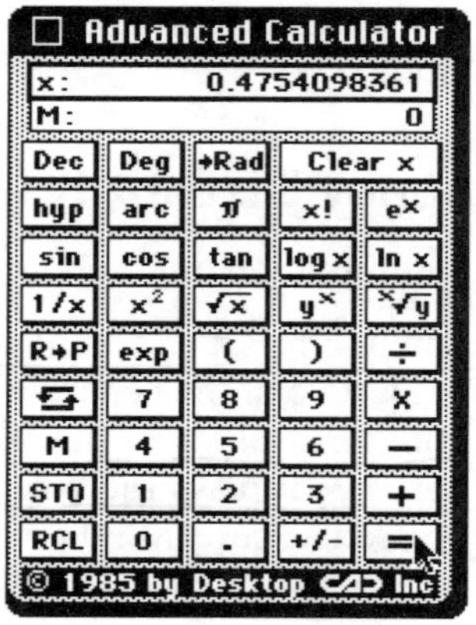

FIGURE **1.1.4**
A display of a calculator's answer for determining 29/61. One usually rounds the calculator answer down to just two or three places past the decimal point.

TABLE 1.1.1
Frequency distribution table for the Simpson et al technical care action data set.

Technical Care Action	Frequency	Relative Frequency	% Relative Frequency
Medication	29	0.48	48
Specialized care	7	0.11	11
Fluids	6	0.10	10
Respiratory	6	0.10	10
Nursing care	4	0.07	7
Surgery	2	0.03	3
Special procedure	7	0.11	11
Total	61	1.00	100

number very close to 1.00, such as 0.98 or 1.01. Such artifacts of computation, when they occur, are unavoidable consequences of round-off, although admittedly annoying. The only way to correct for such deviations from the ideal is to supply more precision by increasing the number of digits past the decimal point. This leads, however, to overwhelming rather than informing people. In descriptive statistics one must make occasional compromises between apparent numerical accuracy and ease of audience perception of the data presented. Hence, descriptive statistics is part science and part art, needing both scientific honesty and human consideration.

Graphics

A frequency distribution table usually is displayed graphically by either (1) a bar graph, (2) a broken bar graph, or (3) a pie chart. We illustrate each using the frequency distribution table constructed for Simpson's data (Example 1.1.9).

A **bar graph** is a graphic in which the whole is represented by a simple bar (rectangle). For convenience, construct a horizontal bar of length 100 mm and height 10 mm. Then each percentage point corresponds to 1 mm in the length of the bar; hence, each attribute listed in the frequency distribution table gets a piece of the bar with length in millimeters equal to the percent relative frequency (recall that the percent relative frequency column ideally adds up to 100%). Figure 1.1.5 presents a bar graph for the Simpson et al data (Example 1.1.9).

A **broken bar graph** (formally called a segmented bar graph) can be thought of as a regular bar graph that has been cut up with scissors. The resulting pieces of the bar are then stacked so that one can immediately see the comparative sizes of the various pieces. The stacking can be displayed either horizontally or vertically. Figure 1.1.6 displays broken bar graphs for the Simpson et al data (Example 1.1.9).

FIGURE 1.1.5
Bar graph for the Simpson et al technical care data.

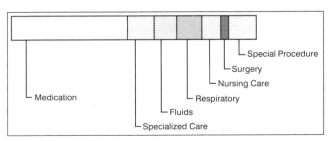

FIGURE **1.1.6**
The left graphic is a horizontally stacked broken bar graph for the Simpson et al data. The right graphic is a vertically stacked broken bar graph for the same data.

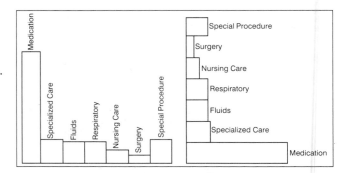

A **pie chart** is a graphic that uses a circle rather than a bar to represent the whole. First, use a compass (or some circular template) to construct a circle. Then, using a protractor, mark off a wedge for each attribute. The number of degrees for each wedge is computed by multiplying each relative frequency by 360:

wedge degrees = (relative frequency) × 360

Each wedge (piece of pie) corresponds to each attribute's share of the data. The results are displayed in Table 1.1.2.

TABLE **1.1.2**
Pie chart wedge calculations for the Simpson et al technical care data set.

Technical Care	Frequency	Degrees
Medication	29	171
Specialized care	7	41
Fluids	6	35
Respiratory	6	35
Nursing care	4	24
Surgery	2	12
Special procedure	7	41
Total	61	359

Comment To determine the number of degrees appropriate for each wedge (piece of pie), multiply each relative frequency by 360. Since relative frequency here is part of the calculation, do not round the relative frequency down to two decimal places. Such a rounding rule is to be applied only when presenting a relative frequency as a final answer. For example, the number of degrees for medication is determined by

degrees (medication)
= (relative frequency for medication) × 360
= (29/61) × 360
= 171.1475410   (calculator answer)
= 171 degrees   (displayed final answer)

Comment The degree column in Table 1.1.2 sums to 359 rather than the ideal 360 (the number of degrees in a circle). This is an unavoidable artifact of rounding off to the nearest degree. It is acceptable in graphics to give the extra degree to an arbitrary piece of the pie, preferably either to the largest wedge or to the wedge with the

FIGURE **1.1.7**
Pie chart for the
Simpson et al technical
care data.

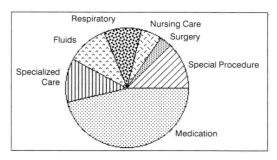

greatest decimal degree part under 0.5 (if the wedge had a decimal degree part 0.5 or more, it has already been rounded up). The pie chart in Figure 1.1.7 gives the extra degree to the largest slice, medication.

EXERCISES 1.1

Warm-ups 1.1

Jacobs et al recorded the follow-up condition of patients with optic neuritis. They determined whether the optic neuritis status of the patient was improved (I), unchanged (U), or worse (W) from the time of first documented diagnosis. They reported their observation as a clinical outcome. The data were as follows:

| I | U | I | I | W | I | W | W | W | I | I | I | I | I | I | W | I | I | I | W | I | I | I | I |
| W | W | I | I | I | I | I | U | I | U | I | W | I | I | U | I | I | I | I | I | I | W | I | U |

1. In this research study the population of interest is "patients with a definite isolated idiopathic optic neuritis." The researchers cannot study all such patients, so they concentrate on a study group of patients who have the condition of interest: isolated idiopathic optic neuritis. The group of patients the researchers actually study is called a (select one of the following): population, parameter, sample, statistic, graphic.

2. The sample size is the number of subjects in the given study. The sample size is often denoted by n. Here, n = _____.

3. List the individual characteristics in the clinical outcome category: _____, _____, _____.

4. The frequency of characteristic I (improved) is the number of times I occurs in the data set. Here the frequency for I is ____. The frequency for U is ____. The frequency for W is ____.

5. The sum of the three frequencies in (4) is ____. Is this sum equal to the sample size n?

6. The relative frequency of a characteristic is equal to the frequency of that characteristic divided by the sample size; that is, relative frequency = frequency/size. The resulting calculation should be rounded and reported to two places past the decimal point.

   The frequency for I (improved) is ____.
   The sample size is ____.
   The relative frequency for I = ____/____ = ____.

7. The relative frequency for U = ____/____ = ____.

8. The relative frequency for W = ____/____ = ____.

9. Ideally, the sum of the relative frequencies is 1.00. Do the relative frequencies for I, U, and W add up to 1.00?

10. Percent relative frequency is the relative frequency multiplied by 100.

    The percent relative frequency for I = ____ × 100 = ____

    The percent relative frequency for U = ____ × 100 = ____

    The percent relative frequency for W = ____ × 100 = ____

11. Ideally, the percent relative frequencies add up to ____ %.

12. A frequency distribution table should contain three columns: a *category* column, a *frequency* column, and a *relative frequency* column (one may report the relative frequency as percent relative frequency). The totals for the frequency and (percent) relative frequency should also be included in the table. Complete the frequency distribution table shown in Table 1.1.3.

TABLE **1.1.3** Frequency distribution table.

Clinical Outcome	Frequency	Relative Frequency
Improved (I) Unchanged (U) Worse (W)		
Total		

Problems **1.1**

1. Gift et al presented the frequency data shown in Table 1.1.4.

TABLE **1.1.4** Frequency data from Gift et al.

Sensation	Number reporting	Relative Frequency	Percent Relative Frequency
Burning	15		
Pain or hurting	13		
Pulling or yanking	9		
Pressure	5		
Other	3		
Total			

a. Complete the frequency distribution table.

b. Construct (1) a bar graph, (2) a broken bar graph, and (3) a pie chart illustrating your frequency distribution table.

2. A research article by Cooper et al contained the following results: "Of the total of 2521 responders, 1962 made the diagnosis of SVT, 542 diagnosed VT, and 17 did not commit themselves to either diagnosis. Of the 542 responders who correctly diagnosed VT, only 14 cited all three morphologic clues, 46 listed two of the three clues, 98 based their diagnosis on one clue, and 384 gave no basis for their diagnosis." Construct a frequency distribution table and accompanying bar graph corresponding to each of the preceding sentences.

3. The research article by Mitchell et al carried information shown in Table 1.1.5. Determine the frequency for each hospital size. Be sure to account for all $n = 2412$ hospitals in the survey. Also remember that a frequency is always a whole number.

TABLE **1.1.5** Data from Mitchell et al.

No. of beds	AACN hospital survey* ($n = 2412$)
<50	9.0
50–099	19.0
100–199	28.0
200–299	17.0
300–399	10.0
400 +	17.0

*Values are expressed as percentages.

4. The study by Simpson et al (Example 1.1.9) on the recollections of critical care patients also contained the information in Table 1.1.6 for the category of alleviation of concerns. Make a frequency distribution table for the research factor of alleviation of concerns. Construct a bar graph, a broken bar graph, and a pie chart illustrating the frequency distribution table.

TABLE **1.1.6** Data from Simpson et al for alleviation of concerns.

Frequency	Action	Exemplary Statement
24	Attentive	Gave me good attention
13	Provide information	Instructions about catheterization
13	Empathetic	Nurses were cheerful and indicated competence; they knew how to handle a cardiac patient
5	Reduce anxiety	Always reassuring me

5. Shively studied the effect of position change on mixed venous oxygen saturation in coronary artery bypass patients. She obtained demographic and clinical data on each patient in her sample, including sex and the number of grafts.

Patient	1	2	3	4	5	6	7	8	9	10
Sex	M	M	F	F	M	M	M	M	F	M
Grafts	3	4	3	3	5	3	2	3	4	2

Patient	11	12	13	14	15	16	17	18	19	20
Sex	F	F	M	M	M	M	M	M	M	M
Grafts	3	3	3	2	4	5	2	3	4	3

Patient	21	22	23	24	25	26	27	28	29	30
Sex	M	M	M	M	F	M	F	M	M	M
Grafts	2	3	4	3	4	2	2	2	3	3

a. Construct a frequency distribution table and percent relative frequency bar graph for sex.

b. Construct a frequency distribution table and percent relative frequency bar graph for grafts.

c. For each sex individually, construct a frequency distribution table for the number of grafts. Contrast and compare the result with a suitable graphic.

6. In research one frequently compares two different groups with respect to the same set of attributes. One draws a sample and constructs a corresponding (relative) frequency bar graph for each group. Figure 1.1.8 displays three common techniques for visually comparing these bar graphs for the two groups. ·

Mitchell et al presented the information shown in Table 1.1.7 comparing the source of primary system failure in patients in the demonstration sample ($n = 192$) with that in 13 U.S. hospitals ($n = 5030$) from another study.

Construct a frequency distribution table for both the demonstration group and the group of 13 U.S. hospitals. Graphically compare the two groups using the three methods described.

*TABLE **1.1.7*** Data from Mitchell et al.

Primary System Failure	Demonstration Sample	13 U.S. Hospitals
Cardiovascular	103	1710
Respiratory	40	907
Gastrointestinal	21	496
Neurologic	19	951
Other	9	966

7. Pierce et al studied two chest tube clearance protocols called (1) milking and (2) stripping. The number of manipulation episodes for each patient was recorded as shown in Figure 1.1.9. A manipulation episode occurred when the attending nurse needed to apply the clearance protocol to clear the chest tube line during the 8½-hour research period. The authors reported their result by displaying the following merged broken bar graphs (see Problem 6).

a. Construct a frequency distribution table for the number of manipulation episodes for the milking protocol.

*FIGURE **1.1.8***
Three basic bar graph displays for comparing two groups of data.

a. Side by Side. Place the two bar graphs near each other in parallel.

b. Directional Broken Bar Graphs. Construct a vertically stacked broken bar graph for each group, using a vertical line as a common backbone for both groups. Draw the broken bar extending to the right for one group and to the left for the other group.

c. Merged Broken Bar Graphs. This technique starts with the broken bar graph for each group. The pieces for each attribute are placed adjacent to each other with spacing to separate attributes.

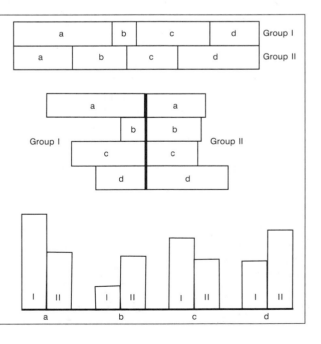

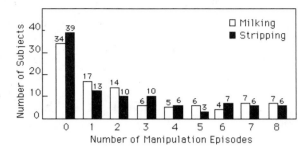

b. Construct a frequency distribution table for the number of manipulation episodes for the stripping protocol.

c. What do you think? Based on the graph and tables, do you feel that one protocol appears to do a better job in reducing the number of tube clearance interventions?

8. A 1988 preliminary report on invasive cancer frequency contained the information about Del Norte, Humboldt, and Lake counties in California shown in Table 1.1.8.

a. Construct a frequency distribution table for cancer primary site for Del-Norte County.

b. Construct a frequency distribution table for cancer primary site for Humboldt County.

c. Construct a frequency distribution table for cancer primary site for Lake County.

d. Consider the frequency distribution table you constructed in part (a). The relative frequency for each cancer type represents the proportion of that cancer type among all cancers in a given county. For example, 32.3% of all cancers reported for Del Norte County were cancers of the digestive system. Although informative, the

table has limitations. In addition to the types of cancer, a public health worker is also concerned about *incidence* of cancer, that is, the annual rate at which cancer appears in the population at large. The incidence rate per 100,000 (I) is determined by dividing the number of cancers (C) by the county population (P) and then multiplying by 100,000:

$$I \text{ (incidence rate)} = \frac{C \text{ (number of cancers)}}{P \text{ (population of the county)}} \times 100,000$$

Complete Table 1.1.9.

TABLE *1.1.9*
Cancer incidence for three northern California counties.

County	Population	Total Cancers	Incidence
Del Norte	21,200		
Humboldt	131,500		
Lake	81,800		

9. J. Isner reported on 31 patients who suffered a catastrophic (death or limb amputation) complication from balloon aortic valvuloplasty. The main causes of the fatalities were reported as ventricular perforation (9), severe aortic regurgitation (4), fatal cardiac arrest (13), and fatal cerebrovascular accident (2). There were 3 amputations. Construct (1) a frequency distribution table, (2) a bar graph, and (3) a pie chart describing these catastrophic complications.

10. (Hard) A research abstract by Kirby et al is provided in Figure 1.1.10. The abstract describes research investigating the presence of drugs or alcohol among patients admitted to a trauma center from the emergency room.

a. The first table presented in the abstract concerns results of drug screens. Critique the table.

TABLE *1.1.8*
Cancer data for three northern California counties.

Primary Site	Del Norte	Humboldt	Lake
Digestive System	20	118	48
Respiratory	24	102	84
Breast	6	68	28
Genitals	8	88	54
Urinary Tract	2	56	26
Other	2	106	52

FIGURE **1.1.10**   Research abstract from Kirby et al.

ALCOHOL AND DRUG USE AMONG TRAUMA PATIENTS ADMITTED TO AN INTENSIVE CARE UNIT. Jackie M. Kirby, RN, MSN, CCRN, Blaine L Enderson, MD, Kimball I Maull, MD, FACS, University of Tennessee Medical Center, Knoxville, Tenn.

Introduction. Alcohol abuse is known to be an aggravating factor in trauma and injury severity, but little is known about the effects of other drugs. The odor of alcohol on the breath suggests intoxication but most drugs offer few clinical signs to alert critical care practitioners. The behavioral and physical sequelae of alcohol and drug use are well described and often create patient care problems. Impairment can disguise injuries, alter the neurological examination, contribute to airway management difficulties, and alter the patient's response to pain and pain medications. This study was designed to describe the incidence of alcohol and drug use among trauma patients admitted to an intensive care unit (ICU).

Method. During the 5-month period beginning March 1, 1988, blood alcohol concentrations (BACs) and urine drug screens were obtained in the emergency department from patients admitted to a level 1 trauma center by the trauma service. Urine samples were screened for THC, benzodiazepine, cocaine, barbiturates, PCP, opiates, and amphetamine. Pre-hospital records were reviewed to determine if drugs were administered prior to the patient's arrival. Data were analyzed using descriptive statistics and chi-square.

Results. During the study period 496 patients were admitted by the adult trauma service, with 270 (54%) admitted to one of five ICUs. Of this number, both BACs and urine drug screens were obtained from 212 (81%) patients. The majority of patients were male (71%) and 35 years of age or younger (67%). The mean length of stay in an ICU was 3.3 days, with a mean hospital stay of 13 days. Over half (58%) of the patients were positive for drugs and/or alcohol. The data are illustrated in the tables below.

Results of drug screens	
Marijuana	75 (34%)
Benzodiazepine	34 (15%)
Cocaine	13 (6%)
Opiates	13 (6%)
Barbiturates	6 (3%)
Amphetamines	6 (3%)
PCP	0 (0%)

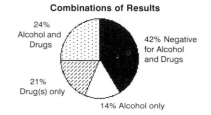

Combinations of Results

24% Alcohol and Drugs

42% Negative for Alcohol and Drugs

21% Drug(s) only

14% Alcohol only

Positive results by age	Drugs	Alcohol	Either
14–35 years	55%	40%	65%
36 +	22%	27%	44%

Positive results by sex	Drugs	Alcohol	Either
Male	49%	44%	65%
Female	33%	16%	40%

Conclusions. Alcohol and drug use among injured patients admitted to an ICU was comparable in this study, suggesting that the drug problem may be greater than previously recognized, especially among young males. Over half of the patients who were positive for alcohol were also positive for drugs. This association suggests the need for further study of synergistic effects.

b. The second table in the abstract intends to describe positive results of drug and alcohol screening by age. The age factor has two attributes: 14–35 and 36 +. The second factor of drugs and alcohol screening results does not have an attribute list that is exhaustive and mutually exclusive. An alternative choice for a list of attributes for the second factor is drugs only, alcohol only, both drugs and alcohol, neither drugs nor alcohol. Construct a frequency distribution table using the alternative attributes for each of the two age-groups. Graphically display the results using the methods of Problem 6.

c. Redo the last table (positive results by sex), using the guidelines stated in (b).

d. Construct a frequency distribution table to accompany the pie chart for combinations of results given in the abstract.

Problems 11–20 are based on research by Donnelly et al about adult respiratory distress syndrome (ARDS). They reported data shown in Table 1.1.10 for three groups of patients at risk for developing ARDS: those with trauma (T), pancreatitis (P), and perforated bowel (PB).

11. What proportion of the study patients is in the trauma (T) group?

12. What proportion of the study patients is in the pancreatic (P) group?

13. What proportion of the study patients is in the perforated bowel (PB) group?

14. What proportion developed ARDS?

15. What proportion of patients died while being treated in the hospital?

16. Construct a frequency distribution table and graphic for the risk category.

17. Construct a frequency distribution table and graphic for the developed ARDS category.

18. Construct a frequency distribution table and graphic for hospital outcomes.

19. Construct a frequency distribution table and bar graph for risk among the patients who developed ARDS.

20. Construct a frequency distribution table and bar graph for risk among the non-ARDS patients.

TABLE **1.1.10**
Data from Donnelly et al.

Patient Number	Risk Group	Developed ARDS	Hospital Outcome
1	T	yes	lived
2	T	yes	died
3	T	yes	lived
4	T	yes	lived
5	PB	yes	died
6	PB	yes	lived
7	P	yes	died
8	T	no	lived
9	T	no	died
10	T	no	died
11	T	no	died
12	T	no	lived
13	T	no	lived
14	T	no	lived
15	T	no	died
16	T	no	lived
17	T	no	lived
18	T	no	lived
19	T	no	lived
20	T	no	lived
21	P	no	lived
22	P	no	lived
23	P	no	lived
24	P	no	lived
25	P	no	lived
26	PB	no	lived
27	PB	no	lived
28	PB	no	lived
29	PB	no	died

Problems 21–24 are based on research by Nordstöm et al, who reported on infant mortality in Sweden. There were 355,601 live singleton births in Sweden during 1983 to 1986. Of these, 2012 died during their first year. Of the 2012 infant deaths, "congenital conditions were the main cause, reported for 778 deaths. Immaturity-related conditions and sudden infant death syndrome (SIDS) accounted for 427 and 324 deaths, respectively. Asphyxia-related conditions caused 214 deaths, and 157 deaths were caused by infections. All remaining causes formed a group of 112 deaths."

21. What proportion of live singleton births die during their first year?

22. Construct a frequency distribution table for the main causes of infant death.

23. What proportion of infant deaths are due mainly to congenital conditions?

24. Construct a suitable graphic to accompany the frequency distribution table constructed in Problem 22 in the form of a bar graph or a pie chart.

25. *Parade Magazine* is an insert in the Sunday edition of several newspapers. "Ask Marilyn" is a popular regular column in *Parade Magazine*. A reader asked Marilyn: "If a population is plagued by four ailments, and the percentage having each are 80%, 75%, 70%, and 70%, at least what percentage has all four?"

a. Consider a group of 20 people. Call the four ailments A, B, C, and D. Show by example that the group may have 80% with ailment A, 75% with B, 70% with C, and 70% with D, but that no member in the group has all four ailments.

b. Using the example you constructed in (a), make a frequency distribution table describing the "number of ailments" for people in the group (how many in your group have three ailments? two ailments?, etc.).

c. What proportion of people in your group has three ailments? Marilyn said at least 95% have three ailments. Is your answer consistent with Marilyn's claim?

SECTION 1.2

Descriptive Statistics

OBJECTIVES   This section will

1   Describe the term random variable, distinguishing between a categorical random variable and a quantitative random variable.

2   Describe and calculate measures of central tendency, including the mean and the median.

3   Describe and calculate measures of variation, including the range and standard deviation. The description of the standard deviation includes the Empirical Rule and Chebyshev's Theorem.

Why include statistics in any health science? Statistics is interesting and necessary in a health science context to the degree that the study of variability is interesting and necessary. An obvious fact is that not all people are alike. Different patients have different health care problems. The same condition in two patients calls for different treatments due to differences in age, health status, allergies, place of residence, and so forth. Clients presenting themselves to a weight control specialist need different regimens of diet and exercise. Communities need different health education programs and management programs due to differences in race, ethnic characteristics, age structure, and economics. This variability is a major source of both interest and problems in any health science. Statistics is a basic tool for studying variation.

Variation

The first step in any research program is to determine the population of interest. The next step is to determine what we want to know about the individuals in that population. Consider approaching an individual from the population of interest. What question(s) do we want to ask; that is, what precisely do we want to know about this individual? On a professional (rather than personal) level, we do not want to know everything about the individual. Gathering and recording information is expensive. Selecting the right question(s) to ask is an important part of statistical design.

For example, consider the case of health care professionals interested in the population of cardiac patients admitted to the hospital for a heart attack. Some important determinations to make about an individual in this population are gender, age, weight, pulse rate, serum cholesterol level, and smoking history. Each determination is made by formulating a specific question and then applying an appropriate procedure to obtain the answer. The appropriate procedure may be to make a simple observation (gender), conduct an interview (age), read an instrument (weight), apply a procedure (pulse rate), or order laboratory work (serum cholesterol).

Smoking history is a general category that needs further refinement. The question "What is your smoking history?" is too vague. Perhaps we only want to know whether the patient smokes (yes or no). Perhaps we need to know more extensive information (never smoked, former smoker, current smoker), coupled with further details for smokers (how long or how much?).

The reason that questions must be carefully and precisely formulated is that different people give different responses. The key problem that one is faced with is **variation**: the simple fact that individuals in the population are different from each other. Variation is a major source of interest and problems in any health science. Statistics is the tool we need to cope with this variation.

We now focus on a population where we may ask an individual a well-formulated question. Examples include:

What is your gender? (male, female)
What is your age? ___years
What is your weight? ___kilograms
What is your pulse rate? ___beats per minute
What is your serum cholesterol level? ___mg/dL
Do you smoke? (never, former smoker, current smoker)

The construction of well-formulated questions is a key part of statistical design. The idea of the well-formulated question is formally embodied in a statistical concept called the random variable.

Florence Nightingale

Florence Nightingale, the "passionate" statistician, was born May 12, 1820, in Florence, Italy (after which she was named), to upper-class English parents and died August 13, 1910. She received excellent early preparation in mathematics from her father and a favorite aunt. She was tutored by mathematician James Sylvester (who developed the theory of invariants with Arthur Cayley), and she was reputed to be his most distinguished pupil. She was also influenced by the work of Adolphe Quetelet, a Belgian scientist who applied statistical methods to data from several fields, including "moral" statistics (social sciences).

In response to a "call from God," Nightingale decided to pursue nursing as a career. She received clinical education from the Fliedners at Kaiserwerth and Maison de la Providence in Paris. In 1854 she was named by Lord Sidney Herbert (England's secretary at war) to be a nursing administrator ("Superintendent of the Female Nursing Establishment of the English General Hospitals in Turkey") for a group of 40 nurses in Scutari during the Crimean War. No woman had ever been so distinguished before. Nightingale was an innovator in the collection, tabulation, interpretation, and graphical display of descriptive social statistics. Her "Notes on Matters Affecting the Health, Efficiency, and Hospital Administration of the British Army" showed that, among other things, the number of soldiers killed by disease was more than seven times greater than those felled in battle. She made an urgent plea for keeping standardized medical statistics and advocated establishment of a Statistical Department of the Army. Her reports were regularly read by Queen Victoria, who awarded her the St. George's Cross.

She was a pioneer in the graphic illustration of statistics and used polar area charts ("coxcombs") to display mortality figures. She compared observed numbers of deaths in the British Army with expected numbers of deaths among civilians to show that mortality from disease among British soldiers was about twice that of civilians. She wrote, "Our soldiers enlist to death in the barracks." She wanted "revenge for reform" (Woodham-Smith 1951).

She became a Fellow of the Royal Statistical Society in 1858. She advocated recording health and housing information in the 1861 census. She introduced (along with a statistical colleague, William Farr) standard data-collection forms, which were used by hospitals to record vital statistics, and she drew up a program (Sanitary Statistics) for the 1860 International Statistical Congress. The forms were published in the *Journal of the Royal Statistics Society* in 1862.

She became an honorary member of the American Statistical Association (ASA) in 1874. She sent ASA an acceptance letter along with the "Annual Sanitary Report of the India Office" and *Life or Death in India* as "a small contribution to (ASA's) library."

Nightingale zealously pursued establishment of an Oxford professorship in applied statistics. This would have been the first university teaching of statistics ("social physics"). There was much correspondence between Francis Galton and her on this subject. For a variety of reasons (financial, and the fact that the subject was not covered in university examinations) the project was eventually abandoned.

Karl Pearson acknowledged her as a "prophetess" in the development of applied statistics. In 1857, the year of Pearson's birth, she was already using tables of observed and expected mortality counts for British soldiers.

Statistics, she proclaimed, was the most important science in the whole world, for upon it depends the practical appreciation of every other [science] and of every art; the one science essential to all political and social administration, all education, for it only gives exact results of our experience. To understand God's thoughts, we must study statistics, for these are the measure of his purpose (Walker, 1929).

The study of statistics was, for her, a religious duty. (Contributed by Loveday Conquest.)

References

Anderson, R.L., Monroe, R.J., and Nelson, L.A. (1979), "Gertrude M. Cox—A Modern Pioneer in Statistics" in Biometrics, 35, 3–7.

Cohen, B. (1984), "Florence Nightingale," in *Scientific American*, 250, 128–137.

Walker, H. (1929), Studies in the History of Statistical Method, Baltimore: Williams and Wilkins.

Woodham-Smith, C. (1951), Florence Nightingale 1820–1910, New York: McGraw-Hill.

Random Variables

An observation that can differ from object to object is called a **random variable** (denoted RV). The variable is called "random" because there is no way to predict what one will see until one makes the observation. In the design of any study, a researcher must initially decide on both the population and the RVs of interest. The population defines *who* the research is about. A random variable defines *what* about them is of interest.

There are two main types of random variables: categorical (also called qualitative) and quantitative. When presented with a random variable, the first task is to ascertain its type.

Categorical Random Variable

A **categorical random variable** classifies an object by assigning to the object precisely one option from a given list of possibilities. A categorical RV may appear on a patient's or client's history chart by listing the options; one usually just circles or checks the applicable response. Examples of categorical RVs are:

Gender: male, female
Cigarette smoker: yes, no
Smoking history: nonsmoker, former smoker, current smoker
Exercise level: sedentary, light, active
Pain level: none, low, moderate, severe

An option on the list of possibilities is formally called an **attribute**. Hence, a categorical RV is presented by displaying its list of attributes. We now note two technical details concerning the list of attributes accompanying a given categorical RV.

In order to define a categorical RV, the given list of attributes must be mutually exclusive and exhaustive. A list of attributes is **mutually exclusive** if only one attribute from the list may be assigned to any given individual. A list of attributes is **exhaustive** if it is large enough to accommodate all possibilities. When an individual from the population of interest is presented, the categorical RV assigns precisely one attribute to that individual; hence, the individual is categorized from the viewpoint of the given RV.

The following attribute list does not describe a categorical RV:

Symptom: fever, chills, headache, nausea, insomnia

This list of symptoms is not mutually exclusive since a given patient may present several of these symptoms simultaneously. The list is not exhaustive since a patient may present none of the given symptoms but may have a symptom not on the list, such as vomiting or diarrhea. This list, however, may be thought of as a list of categorical RVs, each having the attributes present or absent;

Fever: present, absent
Chills: present, absent
Headache: present, absent

Quantitative Random Variable

A **quantitative random variable** measures or counts with a number. Examples include height, weight, serum cholesterol level, systolic blood pressure, number of children, age, and so forth. The essential distinction between a categorical and a quantitative random variable is that a categorical RV is nonnumerical in nature while a quantitative RV yields numbers that count or measure something.

One decides on how to organize and present data by first deciding on the type of RV that underlies the data. A *categorical* data set is nicely displayed by means of a frequency distribution table as presented in Section 1.1. There are two major general descriptive methods for displaying a *quantitative* data set: the describe method (presented in this section) and the table method (presented in Chapter 2). Both of these "summarize and display" techniques are very common in the literature; only rarely are the raw data given.

In the **describe method** (also called "simple descriptive statistics"), one boils down an entire quantitative data set to a representative number accompanied by some measure of variation. In the health sciences literature, a data set is often compressed and simply reported as "the mean plus or minus the standard deviation." The key facet of the describe method is that it first deals with variation by attempting to eliminate it. What would everybody look like if everybody were the same? What would be an adult's weight if all adults weighed the same? For a quantitative RV, this idealized common value, assuming no variation, is commonly called an "average" and formally called a "measure of central tendency."

Measures of Central Tendency

The describe method only applies to a quantitative data set. Let $\{x_1, x_2, \ldots, x_n\}$ denote a data set of numerical observations that either count or measure something. The generic notation $\{x_1, x_2, \ldots, x_n\}$ means that we have available n numerical observations where x_1 denotes the first number, x_2 the second number, and so forth.

EXAMPLE 1.2.1 To illustrate each of the computations for determining measures of central tendency, we will utilize a data set from Brandstetter et al. The data represent the Pao_2 (partial pressure of arterial oxygen, a blood gas measurement for the amount of oxygen in arterial blood) levels measured in mm Hg of 11 patients 30 minutes after initiation of feeding through a nasogastric tube:

62　85　85　50　84　93　58　99　77　88　82

Here, $x_1 = 62$, $x_2 = 85$, $x_3 = 85$, $x_4 = 50$, . . . , $x_{11} = 82$.

In order to boil down such a data set to some representative meaningful number, we report a typical value and a measure of variation. This typical value is commonly called an "average" and technically called a **measure of central tendency**. There are two common measures of central tendency in the health sciences: the mean and the median.

Mean

The **mean** of a numerical data set (technically called the *sample* mean) is computed using the formula

$$\text{MEAN} = (x_1 + x_2 + \ldots + x_n)/n$$

This formula directs one to first add up all the numerical entries in a data set, then to divide this sum by the number of entries.

The somewhat cumbersome expression $(x_1 + x_2 + \ldots + x_n)$ means to add up all the x's (entries) in the data set. This expression is often abbreviated "Σx." The symbol Σ (sigma) denotes a Greek S (for "sum"); hence, this is called "sigma notation" or "summation notation." The notation "Σx" may be read as "sum up all the x's," or simply "sigma x." Accordingly,

$$\text{MEAN} = \Sigma x/n$$

The mean is the average value in that it represents each object's "fair share"; that is, think of each measurement as a value to be thrown into a pot with the accumulated pot redistributed equally among all the objects.

There is a standard notation for the mean. When one is referring to the mean of an entire population, then one denotes the mean by μ (Greek m). It is standard practice in statistics to denote a population parameter with a Greek letter (see the Appendix for a table of the Greek alphabet). When one is referring to a sample mean, one usually denotes the mean by $\bar{x}$ (read x bar). Accordingly, for a sample of size n,

$$\bar{x} = \Sigma x/n$$

EXAMPLE 1.2.2 The mean for the Brandstetter et al data set (Example 1.2.1) is computed as follows:

$$\Sigma x = 62 + 85 + 85 + 50 + 84 + 93 + 58 + 99 + 77 + 88 + 82$$
$$= 863$$

$$n = 11$$

So $\bar{x} = (\Sigma x)/n$

$$= 863/11$$

$$= 78.45454545 \text{ (calculator answer)}$$

$$= 78.5 \text{ (round to one more place than data)}$$

Hence, the sample mean patient Pao_2 is 78.5 mm Hg.

In computing the mean for a given data set, a natural question is "How many decimal places should I use in reporting the answer?" We recommend reporting the mean to one more place than used in reporting the original data. In Example 1.2.2, a calculator yields $863/11 = 78.45454545$. Reporting the full calculator answer has two problems. First, all those decimal places are mind-boggling rather than informative. Second, reporting all the decimal places implies a precision of measurement far beyond the scope of the study. Because collecting data is expensive, one wants to report what information one can. However, one needs to report in an honest fashion. Hence, we report the sample mean in Example 1.2.2 as $\bar{x} = 78.5$. Verbally, the mean PaO_2 of the 11 patients in the Brandstetter et al study is 78.5 mm Hg.

The essentials about the mean are summarized in the following definition:

DEFINITION ▮▮▮ (Sample) Mean

Background   Let $x_1, x_2, \ldots, x_n$ be a numerical sample of size n.

Description   The mean is calculated by

$$\text{mean} = \frac{\text{sum of all the sample numbers}}{\text{sample size}}$$

Formula   Let n = sample size
Σx = sum of the numbers in the sample
$\bar{x}$ = sample mean
Then $\bar{x} = \dfrac{\Sigma x}{n}$

Round-off Rule   Report the sample mean rounded to one more decimal place than the original data.

Median

First, sort the data set into an increasing array of numbers in order from smallest to largest. The **median** is the midway point in the sorted array. Half the data lies above the median, and half lies below.

EXAMPLE 1.2.3   Sorting the Brandstetter et al data set (Example 1.2.1), we obtain

50   58   62   77   82   84   85   85   88   93   99

The midpoint observation is 84; that is, there are five sample entries lower than 84 and five entries higher than 84. Hence, the median is 84.

If the sample contains an odd number of entries, there is always a middle number in the ordered array. The median is then this middle number. If the data set has an even number of entries, however, the middle is occupied by a pair of numbers. The median in this case is obtained by taking the mean of these two middle numbers, which is always halfway between them. For example, the median of

1   4   9   12   17   94

is the mean of 9 and 12, which is 10.5.

The notation for the median follows the same general spirit as the notation for the mean. Since the word *median* begins with m and the Greek m (μ) has been preempted by the mean, we choose to denote the *population* median by η (Greek eta) since η looks a lot like an n, the letter following m. The usual symbol for a *sample* median is $\tilde{x}$. The standard notations for the mean and median are summarized in Table 1.2.1.

	Population	Sample
Mean	μ	$\bar{x}$
Median	η	$\tilde{x}$

TABLE *1.2.1*
Standard notations for mean and median.

The contrast between the mean and median is portrayed in Figure 1.2.1 for the Brandstetter et al data set (Example 1.2.1). Recall that the mean may be thought of as the "fair share" amount; the median, a "halfway" value. From a physical viewpoint, the mean acts as a balance point. In Figure 1.2.1, think of the horizontal number line as a seesaw. Now consider each data point to represent a child, where all the children weigh the same. Then the seesaw will balance perfectly at the mean.

When the distribution of the data is symmetrical in that the distribution of the lower half of the data mirrors the distribution for the upper half, then the mean and median tend to be the same. The farther apart the mean and median, the more unbalanced is the data set.

FIGURE *1.2.1*   The mean and the median for the Brandstetter et al data are displayed. The **median** separates the data set so that half of the data lies below the median and the other half lies above the median. The **mean** acts as a balance point. If the number line represented a seesaw and each data point represented a child of equal weight, then the seesaw would balance at the mean.

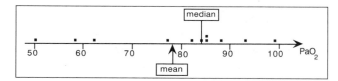

The essentials about the median are contained in the following definition:

DEFINITION III Median	
Background	Let $x_1, x_2, \ldots, x_n$ be a numerical sample of size n.
Description	First, sort the data set by arranging the numbers in order from the smallest to the largest. The median is the midway point in the sorted data set.

Measures of Variation

A **measure of variation** is a measure of the spread of the data. It is important to have both a measure of central tendency and a measure of variation. Two data sets can have the same mean but have vastly different distributions if one data set is much more spread out. For example, consider the following two groups of numbers.

Group 1:   99   100   100   100   101
Group 2:   0   50   100   150   200

Both groups have a mean (and median) of 100; that is, they both have the same measure of central tendency. However, the spread of the numbers is clearly different. The numbers in Group 1 are much more compact, while the numbers in Group 2 are much more spread out.

There are two common measures of variation: the range and the standard deviation.

Range

The **range** simply measures the full spread of the data. The (statistical) range is the arithmetic difference between the largest (maximum) and smallest (minimum) values in the data set.

DEFINITION ▌▌▌ Range

$$\text{Range} = \text{Maximum} - \text{Minimum}$$

In the literature the range is often reported by merely stating the minimum and maximum without actually carrying out the subtraction (e.g., range: 50–99, indicating the data ranged from 50 to 99).

EXAMPLE 1.2.4 The range of the Brandstetter et al data (Example 1.2.3) is computed by

$$\text{range} = \text{maximum} - \text{minimum}$$
$$= 99 - 50$$
$$= 49$$

This range of 49 is the length of the interval from 50 to 99 when plotted on the number line. Figure 1.2.2 displays the range of the Brandstetter et al data set.

Variance and the Standard Deviation

The most common measure of variation is the standard deviation. Its meaning is not as clear and simple as the range. The meaning of the standard deviation is intimately tied to the concept of distribution of the data. The standard deviation for a numerical data set is called the **sample standard deviation**.

Comment Many concepts in statistics (e.g., the mean, median, and range) are intuitively understandable. Their commonsense components can be conveniently exploited to develop their technical side, easing the student into calculations and formal properties. Other concepts in statistics, like the standard deviation, defy an initial intuitive understanding. We adopt a two-step approach for such concepts, whose essence is really rooted in abstract mathematics. The first step is to mechanically focus on the calculation: here is the formula, here are some data, plug the numbers into the formula, calculate the answer. The second step is to exploit that number to guide an explanation leading to understanding. Using this approach, most

FIGURE **1.2.2**
The range of the
Brandstetter et al data set.

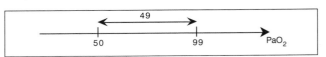

students find the first step basically quick and easy (although often tedious). The second step takes more patience and study. Most students are surprised (many even pleasantly so) to find that the math (step 1) is really the easy part! We adopt this two-step approach in developing the standard deviation. First just focus on calculating the standard deviation. Afterward we explain what the standard deviation is using the Empirical Rule and Chebyshev's Theorem.

The definitions for the sample variance and sample standard deviation are as follows:

DEFINITION ▮▮▮ Variance and Standard Deviation

n = sample size

$\bar{x}$ = sample mean

s^2 = sample variance

s = sample standard deviation

Sample Variance $\quad s^2 = \dfrac{\Sigma(x - \bar{x})^2}{n - 1}$

Sample Standard Deviation $\quad s = \sqrt{\text{sample variance}}$

To compute the sample standard deviation, first compute the sample variance and then take the (positive) square root of the sample variance. When using pencil, paper, and calculator, the following equivalent formula for the sample variance is easier to use:

$$s^2 \text{ (sample variance)} = \frac{n\Sigma x^2 - (\Sigma x)^2}{n(n - 1)}$$

EXAMPLE 1.2.5 We illustrate the use of the previous formula to compute the sample variance and standard deviation for the Brandstetter et al data (Example 1.2.1).

$n \quad = 11$

$\Sigma x \quad = 863 \quad$ (from Example 1.2.2)

$\Sigma x^2 \quad = 62^2 + 85^2 + 85^2 + 50^2 + 84^2 + 93^2 + 58^2 + 99^2 + 77^2$
$\quad + 88^2 + 82^2 = 70061$

So, $s^2 = \dfrac{n\Sigma x^2 - (\Sigma x)^2}{n(n - 1)}$

$\quad = \dfrac{11(70061) - (863)^2}{11(10)}$

$\quad = 235.4727273$ (calculator value for the sample variance)

Hence, $s = \sqrt{\text{sample variance}}$

$\quad = \sqrt{235.4727273}$

$\quad = 15.34512063$ (calculator value for the sample standard deviation)

$\quad = 15.3$

Comment It is acceptable to round off in reporting the variance; however, do not round on your calculator before taking the square root to obtain the standard deviation. No rounding should occur until you report your final answer. Both the mean and standard deviation should be reported to one decimal place further than the data.

The most common way in the literature of describing quantitative data is just to report mean $\pm$ standard deviation. For example, the Brandstetter et al data set (Example 1.2.1) could simply be reported by: the sample PaO_2 was 78.5 ± 15.3 mm Hg. Of course the original raw data are lost, but we do have a measure of central tendency and a measure of variation; that is, we have a summarized version of the data.

For small data sets, a statistical calculator is invaluable. Because of the tediousness of computations, calculating the mean and sample standard deviation is easiest by computer, especially for larger data sets. Computer output obtained by Minitab showing the descriptive statistics for the Brandstetter et al data is displayed in Figure 1.2.3.

The Empirical Rule

For simplicity, we will refer to the sample standard deviation simply as the standard deviation from now on. The standard deviation is usually denoted by s or SD in the literature. Accordingly, mean $\pm$ standard deviation is denoted by $\bar{x} \pm$ s or $\bar{x} \pm$ SD. However, there is no accepted rule; personal taste and context guide whether to use s or SD for the standard deviation. Sometimes both notations are useful, as the following discussion of the Empirical Rule illustrates.

What is the sample standard deviation? Technically, the standard deviation is a measure of variation in the sample data, a guide to the spread of a data set. To understand how the standard deviation measures variation in a sample, we impose "windows" upon a data set.

Center the window at the data mean ($\bar{x}$) and, from that point, open the window one standard deviation (s) in each direction. One thereby obtains the 1SD window view of the data extending from $\bar{x} -$ s to $\bar{x} +$ s (Figure 1.2.4a). Normally, about 68% of the data is exposed in the 1SD window.

The 2SD window extends two standard deviations on each side of the mean, from $\bar{x} - 2s$ to $\bar{x} + 2s$ (Figure 1.2.4b). Normally, about 95% of the data is exposed in the 2SD window. Similarly the 3SD window extends three standard deviation units on each side of the mean, from $\bar{x} - 3s$ to $\bar{x} + 3s$ (Figure 1.2.4c). Normally, about 99.7% of the data is exposed in the 3SD window.

In practice, one normally sees a good majority of the data in the 1SD window, most of the data in the 2SD window, and (virtually) all of the data in the 3SD window. These results occur so often in practice that collectively they are referred to as the **Empirical Rule**, the rule of "what one normally sees in practice" (Table 1.2.2).

Chebyshev's Theorem

The Empirical Rule describes the distribution of data in normal practice. Of course, there are aberrations; a given situation does not have to be "normal." Accordingly, one wonders whether there is some floor or baseline that can act as a guarantee; that

FIGURE 1.2.3
Minitab output for the
Brandstetter et al data
set (Example 1.2.1).

```
MTB > NOTE Enter the data, print, and check for accuracy:
MTB > NAME C1 'DATA SET'
MTB > SET C1
DATA> 62 85 85 50 84
DATA> 93 58 99 77 88 82
DATA> END OF DATA
MTB > PRINT C1

DATA SET
    62   85   85   50   84   93   58   99   77   88   82

MTB > NOTE Measures of CENTRAL TENDENCY:
MTB >
MTB > MEAN C1
    MEAN = 78.455
MTB >
MTB > MEDIAN C1
    MEDIAN = 84.000
MTB >
MTB > NOTE Measures of VARIATION:
MTB >
MTB > RANGE C1
    RANGE = 49.000
MTB >
MTB > STANDARD DEVIATION C1
    ST.DEV. = 15.345
MTB >
MTB > NOTE You can have it all with the DESCRIBE command.
MTB >
MTB > DESCRIBE C1

              N    MEAN   MEDIAN  TRMEAN   STDEV   SEMEAN
DATA SET     11   78.45    84.00   79.33   15.35     4.63

                 MIN     MAX      Q1      Q3
DATA SET       50.00   99.00   62.00   88.00

MTB > NOTE For details concerning the output, type HELP DESCRIBE
```

FIGURE 1.2.4
The (a) 1SD, (b) 2SD,
and (c) 3SD windows
are displayed.

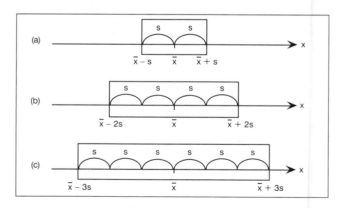

is, how much of a data set *must* appear in a given window? Although normally there is about 68% of the data in the 1SD window, there is no guarantee that this must occur. In extreme cases the 1SD window may in fact contain no data. However, the 2SD window must always contain at least 3/4 (75%) of the data. The 3SD window

TABLE **1.2.2**
The Empirical Rule states that in normal practice quantitative data are approximately distributed as follows.

Standard Deviation Window	Proportion of the Data in View
1SD	About 68%
2SD	About 95%
3SD	About 99.7%

must always contain at least 8/9 (88.9%) of the data. In general, for any number $k \geq 1$, at most $1/k^2$ of the data can lie outside of the kSD window. This baseline guarantee is formally known as **Chebyshev's Theorem.**

Chebyshev's Theorem

Let $\bar{x}$, s be the mean and standard deviation of $x_1, x_2, \ldots, x_n$. Let $k \geq 1$. Then the proportion of the data that falls outside the interval $(\bar{x} - ks, \bar{x} + ks)$ is at most $1/k^2$. Further, at least $1 - 1/k^2$ of the data falls between the numbers $\bar{x} - ks$ and $\bar{x} + ks$.

Note that we have been referring to the interval $(\bar{x} - ks, \bar{x} + ks)$ as the kSD window. Chebyshev's Theorem may be thought of as "Chebyshev's Guarantee" since the theorem guarantees that a given window must contain at least a certain proportion of the data. The practical impact is summarized in Table 1.2.3.

TABLE **1.2.3**
Chebyshev's Theorem for $k = 1, 2, 3, 4, 5$.

k	Interval	Outside: At Most $1/k^2$	Inside: At Least $(1 - 1/k^2)$
1	$(\bar{x} - s, \bar{x} + s)$	$1/1^2 = 1$	0
2	$(\bar{x} - 2s, \bar{x} + 2s)$	$1/2^2 = 1/4 = .250$	.750
3	$(\bar{x} - 3s, \bar{x} + 3s)$	$1/3^2 = 1/9 = .111$	.889
4	$(\bar{x} - 4s, \bar{x} + 4s)$	$1/4^2 = 1/16 = .062$	.938
5	$(\bar{x} - 5s, \bar{x} + 5s)$	$1/5^2 = 1/25 = .040$	.960

EXAMPLE 1.2.6 Suppose a data set has a mean of 14. If the standard deviation is 2, then at least 75% of the data must fall between 10 and 18 (the 2SD window). If the standard deviation is 4, then at least 75% of the data must fall between 6 and 22.

EXAMPLE 1.2.7 Using the Brandstetter et al data (Example 1.2.1), $\bar{x} = 78.5$ and $s = 15.3$. Figure 1.2.5 displays the 1SD and 2SD windows. The 1SD window is the interval (63.2, 93.8). Note that the 1SD window contains $7/11 = 0.64$ (64%) of the data. The 2SD window (47.7, 109.1) contains all of the data. The Brandstetter data set is typical of the kind of small data set obtained in normal practice.

Chebyshev's Theorem is very conservative in practice. It merely guarantees that at least 75% of the data will be found within the 2SD window centered at the mean and that at most 25% of the data will fall outside this window. In the Brandstetter et al data, a good majority of the data is exposed inside the 1SD window, and all of the data lies inside the 2SD window.

FIGURE **1.2.5** The Brandstetter et al data are displayed on the number line with the 1SD and 2SD windows superimposed on the data. The inside dashed-line window is the 1SD window, and the outside solid-line window is the 2SD window.

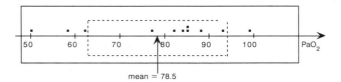

mean = 78.5

In normal practice the standard deviation may be conveniently thought of as a measure of the size of the window we need to construct about the mean in order to see a good majority of the data. The 2SD window usually allows one to view almost all of the data. A data point outside the 2SD window, often called an **outlier,** is considered an unusual or rare observation.

An Application: Time Series Graphs

Bodai et al evaluated the use of a catheter system that allows oxygen insufflation during suctioning procedures in a variety of clinical settings. An underlying goal was to identify a procedure without harmful side effects to prevent suction-induced hypoxemia. Endotracheal suctioning is important in the respiratory care of patients requiring ventilatory support. One known risk of suctioning is hypoxemia, determined by depressed PaO_2.

The data in Table 1.2.4 are PaO_2 readings for six patients (data set 4, group 2, routine suctioning). PaO_2 measurements were taken for each of the six patients at four successive times: (1) just before (start), (2) just after (end), (3) 1 minute after, and (4) 5 minutes after suctioning. The suctioning session from start to end lasted 1 minute. The time after suctioning from end to 5 minutes is the recovery period from the suctioning episode.

TABLE **1.2.4**
PaO_2 data from Bodai et al.

Patient	Start	End	1 min	5 min
1	90	67	73	122
2	78	86	82	78
3	90	57	63	83
4	69	40	54	59
5	70	59	100	130
6	84	114	74	73

A table that condenses raw numerical data by displaying the sample size, mean, and standard deviation is called the sample **legend**. Table 1.2.5 gives the legend for the Bodai et al PaO_2 raw data set (Table 1.2.4).

We portray these results graphically by constructing a **time series graph**, a two-dimensional graphic in which time is plotted along the horizontal and the measurement of interest (here, PaO_2) is plotted along the vertical. In the time series graph we plot not only the mean value at each time but also the accompanying 1SD window.

TABLE 1.2.5
The sample legend for the Bodai et al Pa_{O_2} data set. The legend condenses a sample to the sample size, mean, and SD.

	Start	End	1 min	5 min
Size	6	6	6	6
Mean	80.2	70.5	74.3	90.8
SD	9.4	26.0	15.9	28.5

TABLE 1.2.6
The endpoints for the 1SD window at each of the four times for the Bodai et al Pa_{O_2} data set. Each interval is centered at the mean.

	$\bar{x} - SD$	$\bar{x}$	$\bar{x} + SD$
Start	70.8	80.2	89.6
End	44.5	70.5	96.5
1 min	58.5	74.3	90.2
5 min	62.3	90.8	119.3

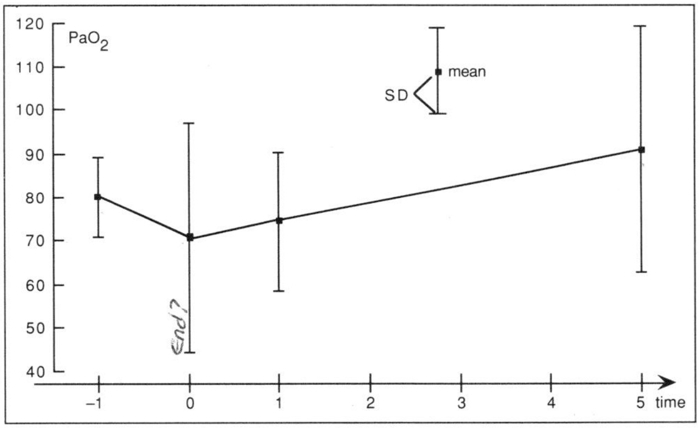

FIGURE 1.2.6
Pa_{O_2} (mm Hg) from start to 5 minutes after suctioning (mean ± SD) for the routine method (time in minutes).

The 1SD window is displayed as an interval from $\bar{x} - $ SD to $\bar{x} + $ SD. The mean is displayed as a point plotted at the center of the interval. The mean and 1SD interval endpoints for the Bodai et al Pa_{O_2} data are given in Table 1.2.6.

The resulting time series graph is displayed in Figure 1.2.6. The time series graph is informative about the effect of suctioning on the sample group as a whole. A typical course is followed by the line connecting the means. The 1SD window displays the context of typical individual variation.

EXERCISES 1.2

Warm-ups 1.2

Shipley et al gave the fat-free mass (FFM) measured in kg of 5 septic patients in their study as follows:

$$47.0 \quad 38.7 \quad 44.7 \quad 41.8 \quad 42.2$$

The researchers reported that the septic patients in the study were hospital inpatients being treated in part with parenteral nutrition in a surgical nutrition unit. None of the subjects were receiving steroids or drugs known to affect metabolic rates.

1. What is the population of interest in the Shipley et al study?

2. The RV of interest here is FFM. Is FFM a categorical or a quantitative random variable?

Section 1.2   Descriptive Statistics / **35**

3. The size of the given sample is n = ____.

4. Complete Table 1.2.7.

TABLE **1.2.7** Calculation of x^2.

x	x^2
47.0	
38.7	
44.7	
41.8	
42.2	
Sum	

5. The sample mean is denoted by (indicate one): $\bar{x}$, μ, s, n, $\tilde{x}$, η.

6. The sum of the sample numbers is denoted by Σx. Here, $\Sigma x = $ ____.

7. The sample mean is computed by $\bar{x} = \Sigma x/n = $ ____ /____ = ____ (report $\bar{x}$ to one more decimal place than the numbers in the given data set).

8. The standard deviation is the (positive) square root of the (indicate one): mean, sample, range, variance, median.

9. When using a hand calculator, the sample variance, s^2, is conveniently computed by applying the formula

$$\text{variance} = \frac{n\Sigma x^2 - (\Sigma x)^2}{n(n-1)}$$

Here, $n = $ ____ , $\Sigma x = $ ____ , $(\Sigma x)^2 = $ ____ , $\Sigma x^2 = $ ____ .

So, variance $= \dfrac{5(\Sigma x^2) - (\Sigma x)^2}{20} = \dfrac{5(\underline{}) - (\underline{})}{20}$ = ____ .

Note: Do not round your calculator answer.

10. The standard deviation (SD) is simply the square root of the variance. Hence,

$SD = \sqrt{\text{variance}}$

$= \sqrt{\underline{}}$

$= \underline{}$.

Note: Report the SD to one decimal place farther than the data.

11. The usual way of summarizing a numerical data set is simply mean ± SD. Here the summary report is ____ ± ____ .

12. The 1SD window is the interval mean ± SD. Here,
mean = ____
SD = ____
mean − SD = ____
mean + SD = ____
Thus, the 1SD window is the interval from ____ to ____ .

13. The number of observations in the data set that fall inside the 1SD window is ____. This is ____% of the size of the data set.

14. The 2SD window is the interval $\bar{x}$ ± 2SD. Here,

$\bar{x} - 2SD = $ ____ $\bar{x} + 2SD = $ ____ .

Hence, the 2SD window is the interval that goes from ____ to ____ . The number of observations in the data set that fall inside the 2SD window is ____ . This is ____% of the size of the data set.

15. The sorted data set is the data set presented in increasing order from smallest to largest. Here the sorted data set is

38.7 ____ ____ ____ 47.0

16. The sample median is denoted by (indicate one): $\bar{x}$, μ, s, n, $\tilde{x}$, η.

17. The sample median is the middle number in a sorted data set. Here, $\tilde{x} = $ ____ .

18. The range of a numerical data set is calculated by

range = maximum − minimum

Here, maximum = ____ , minimum = ____ .
Hence, range = ____ .

Problems 1.2

1. In a study of cardiac patients, Stone et al reported the hematocrit for eight patients:

39.2 36.4 38.3 36.8 42.9 37.0 39.1 41.2

   a. Determine the mean, median, range, and standard deviation for this data set.

   b. Plot the data on the number line. Display the 1SD, 2SD, and 3SD windows.

   c. What proportion of the data lies in the 1SD, 2SD, and 3SD windows? Compare with the Empirical Rule and Chebyshev's Theorem.

2. Papadakis et al reported the temperatures in degrees Celsius of eight patients as follows:

36.9 35.9 36.5 36.4 38.2 36.8 37.0 39.1

  a. Determine the mean, median, range, and standard deviation for this data set.

  b. Plot the data on the number line. Display the 1SD, 2SD, and 3SD windows.

  c. What proportion of the data lies in the 1SD, 2SD, and 3SD windows? Compare with the Empirical Rule and Chebyshev's Theorem.

3. Consider the Shively data set (data set 5, appendix). For both group 1 and group 2 at baseline,

  a. Determine the mean, median, range, and standard deviation.

  b. Plot the data on the number line. Display the 1SD, 2SD, and 3SD windows.

  c. What proportion of the data lies in the 1SD, 2SD, and 3SD windows? Compare with the Empirical Rule and Chebyshev's Theorem.

  d. Do you think that, in general, the baseline $S_{V}O_2$ for the two groups is basically the same? Explain your answer.

4. Sands reported on the incidence of pulmonary aspiration in intubated patients receiving enteral nutrition through wide- and narrow-bore nasogastric feeding tubes. The ages of the patients in the narrow-bore group were:

16 25 26 50 51 55 62 63 67 78

  a. Determine the mean, median, range, and standard deviation of the ages of the patients in Sands's study.

  b. What proportion of the sample data lies in the $\bar{x} \pm s$ window?

  c. How does the proportion in (b) compare with the Empirical Rule and Chebyshev's Theorem?

5. The Brandstetter et al article studies the effect of nasogastric feeding on arterial oxygen tension by measuring PaO_2 just before feeding and 30 minutes later. The full data set for the 11 patients in the study group is given in Table 1.2.8.

  a. Calculate the mean, median, range, and standard deviation of the first PaO_2 measurements.

TABLE **1.2.8** The Brandstetter et al PaO_2 data set.

Patient	1st PaO_2	2nd PaO_2	Change
1	60	62	−2
2	83	85	−2
3	87	85	2
4	52	50	2
5	86	84	2
6	95	93	2
7	59	58	1
8	101	99	2
9	80	77	3
10	91	88	3
11	89	82	7

  b. Calculate the mean, median, range, and standard deviation of the second PaO_2 measurements.

  c. The motivation for the study was a concern that meal-induced hypoxemia may occur in asymptomatic patients with chronic obstructive pulmonary disease. Hypoxemia is indicated if, in a given patient, PaO_2 decreases as a result of feeding. Hence, the RV of real interest is the change, where

$$\text{change} = \text{1st } PaO_2 - \text{2nd } PaO_2$$

  i. Determine the mean, median, range, and standard deviation of the change in PaO_2 level as a result of feeding.

  ii. Construct a 1SD, 2SD, and 3SD window on the Change data set. Compare with the Empirical Rule and Chebyshev's Theorem.

  d. Describe verbally what you feel is the general course of PaO_2 in a patient as a result of nasogastric feeding.

6. Stone et al reported time series data for PaO_2 blood levels before and after administration of five different lung hyperinflation volumes (Table 1.2.9). The data show the mean $\pm$ SD for PaO_2 of the patient sample at several times. The "control" time indicates start of the hyperinflation protocol, which lasted for 2 minutes. Then PaO_2 was measured immediately after hyperinflation (time 0) and several times afterward in order to monitor PaO_2 recovery within 5 minutes (300 seconds). The column headings in the table give time after suctioning in seconds (hence, "control" is at time −120 seconds).

TABLE 1.2.9 The Stone et al Pao$_2$ time series data.

Time	Control	0	30 sec	60 sec	120	180	300
V$_T$	133 ± 27.7	195 ± 54.8	146 ± 30.4	140 ± 23.8	138 ± 27.9	135 ± 29.4	133 ± 29.1
12 cc/kg	131 ± 30.5	214 ± 58.3	147 ± 33.0	142 ± 34.2	137 ± 30.8	137 ± 31.5	129 ± 30.3
14 cc/kg	130 ± 30.0	233 ± 81.4	153 ± 40.0	144 ± 33.0	140 ± 36.1	139 ± 37.2	138 ± 34.8
16 cc/kg	132 ± 27.5	243 ± 71.6	177 ± 3.2	154 ± 17.7	149 ± 18.3	142 ± 21.4	137 ± 20.9
18 cc/kg	135 ± 23.3	249 ± 31.5	176 ± 17.4	160 ± 17.6	154 ± 22.8	146 ± 24.2	139 ± 24.3

(handwritten margin note: 7 vert. line, get mean on each, plot SD)

Construct a time series graph for the Volumes designated by

a. V$_T$ **b.** 12 cc/kg   **c.** 16 cc/kg   **d.** 18 cc/kg

Each graph should plot the mean for each specified time and display the 1SD window at each plotted point. The axes should be labeled and accurately scaled (use graph paper or a metric ruler). Finally, adjacent plotted points should be joined by a straight line. Figure 1.2.7 displays the time series graph for the volume 14 cc/kg.

FIGURE 1.2.7
A time series graph for the volume 14 cc/kg for the Stone et al data given in Problem 1.2.6. Each interval represents the mean ± SD. The mean points are joined by a straight line.

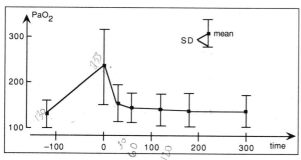

7. A patient's charted cardiac output obtained by a thermodilution method is the mean of three separate successive measurements. The cardiac output session is considered acceptable if all three measurements are within 0.5 L/minute of each other (i.e., range ≤ 0.5). A room temperature thermodilution cardiac output session yields the results of 4.1, 4.3, and 4.1 L/minute on three successive trials.

   a. What is the range of the data set?

   b. Is this an acceptable cardiac output session?

   c. What cardiac output is charted for the patient?

Problems 8 and 9 are based on research by Donovan et al, who studied the effect of eating on the nitrogen content of milk and plasma of nursing mothers. The study was carefully controlled. Each of five mothers was given a controlled breakfast at 8 A.M. (no eating or drinking ≥ 3 hours prior). The researchers noted that human milk is unique in that some 18% to 30% of the total nitrogen is nonprotein. In particular, the researchers wanted to test the idea that postmeal changes in plasma levels of non protein nitrogen are reflected in the mother's milk. A major component of nonprotein nitrogen is urea, a product of metabolism. The urea nitrogen concentrations for postmeal plasma and milk are given at the start (just before the meal), and postmeal at 15 minutes, 30 minutes, 1 hour, 1.5 hours, 2 hours, and 3 hours.

8. The data for urea nonprotein nitrogen in milk are shown in Table 1.2.10.

   a. Determine the mean urea nitrogen concentration in milk for each of the seven times (start, 15 minutes, 30 minutes, 1 hour, 1.5 hours, 2 hours, 3 hours) in the Donovan et al study.

   b. Determine the standard deviation for nitrogen concentration in milk for each of the seven times.

   c. Construct a sample legend (see Table 1.2.5) for the data presented in Table 1.2.10.

   d. Display the endpoints for the 1SD window at each time (see Table 1.2.6).

   e. Construct a time series graph depicting the course of urea nitrogen concentration in milk (see Figure 1.2.6).

   f. Describe verbally the general course of the time series constructed in (e).

9. The data for urea nitrogen concentration in plasma are given in Table 1.2.11.

TABLE **1.2.10** Urea nitrogen concentration in milk (mmol/L).

Subject	Start	15 min	30 min	1 hour	1.5 hour	2 hours	3 hours
1	6.2	6.4	6.8	6.2	6.8	6.5	7.2
2	5.2	5.5	5.7	5.5	6.2	5.7	6.5
3	5.0	6.7	5.1	5.3	6.2	5.6	5.5
4	3.8	6.1	3.5	3.9	3.8	3.3	5.0
5	4.6	4.2	4.6	4.3	7.7	3.4	4.2

TABLE **1.2.11** Urea nitrogen concentration in plasma (mmol/L).

Subject	Start	15 min	30 min	1 hour	1.5 hour	2 hours	3 hours
1	2.9	4.6	4.2	5.7	5.9	5.6	5.4
2	3.6	4.2	4.2	6.0	4.8	4.2	4.1
3	4.6	7.2	6.6	6.2	6.1	4.8	5.0
4	2.7	3.9	3.6	3.6	3.5	3.8	6.6
5	3.5	3.7	4.2	4.3	5.4	3.6	4.6

a. Determine the mean urea nitrogen concentration in plasma for each of the seven times (start, 15 minutes, 30 minutes, 1 hour, 1.5 hours, 2 hours, 3 hours) in the Donovan et al study.

b. Determine the standard deviation for nitrogen concentration in plasma for each of the seven times.

c. Construct a sample legend (see Table 1.2.5) for the data presented in Table 1.2.11.

d. Display the endpoints for the 1SD window at each time (see Table 1.2.6).

e. Construct a time series graph depicting the course of urea nitrogen concentration in plasma (see Figure 1.2.6).

f. Describe verbally the general course of the time series constructed in (e).

10. Gueco et al studied treatment of kidney transplant patients. Serum creatinine is an end product in the metabolism of the enzyme creatine found in muscle and skeletal tissue. One of the functions of the kidneys is to eliminate creatinine from serum.

Accordingly, an elevated creatinine level indicates renal (kidney) dysfunction. Normal serum creatinine range is 0.8 to 1.4 mg/dL. Gueco et al presented the following data on 12 patients in a study group of kidney transplant patients (mg/dL):

0.8 1.0 1.1 1.2 1.3 1.4 1.5 1.5 1.5 1.5 1.6 1.6

For these data, $\Sigma x = 16.0$ and $\Sigma x^2 = 22.06$.

a. What is the sample mean?

b. What is the sample median?

c. What is the sample standard deviation?

d. What is the 1SD window for these data?

e. What proportion of the sample lies within the 1 standard deviation window?

f. What is the 2SD window for these data?

g. What proportion of the sample lies within the 2SD window?

h. Display the data with the 1SD and 2SD windows on the number line (see Figure 1.2.5).

i. Using the display in (h), compare with the Empirical Rule and Chebychev's Theorem.

CHAPTER **1** OVERVIEW

Summary

The major activities in **statistics** are obtaining data, presenting data, and interpreting data. These activities motivate the major branches of statistics: statistical design, descriptive statistics, and inferential statistics. In the health sciences, a knowledge of statistics is necessary to utilize the literature and conduct research.

Applied statistics works with data. One obtains data by drawing a **sample** from a **population** and making an observation regarding each member in the sample. In the real world, resource constraints require that we view a population based on knowledge obtained from a sample. A measure of interest about the population as a whole is called a **parameter**. The corresponding measure for a sample is a **statistic**.

The most common method for presenting basic data is the **frequency distribution table**. A frequency distribution table has three columns: characteristics, **frequency**, and **relative frequency**. Relative frequency may be expressed as **percent relative frequency**. A frequency distribution table should be accompanied by an illustrative graphic such as a **bar graph**, **broken bar graph**, or **pie chart**.

Variation (individual differences) is the main factor behind the need for statistics. In any statistical study, the main ingredients that need to be specified initially are a **population** and a **random variable** of interest. The two main kinds of random variables are categorical and quantitative.

A **categorical random variable** is defined by an **exhaustive** and **mutually exclusive** list of **attributes**. Each member in the population has precisely one attribute from the given list. A **quantitative random variable** is defined by a number that either counts or measures something.

How one should organize data depends on the nature of the underlying random variable. A categorical data set is presented with a **frequency distribution table**. A quantitative data set is presented using the **describe method** or the **table method**.

The describe method presents a quantitative data set with a **measure of central tendency** and a **measure of variation**. The most common measures of central tendency are the **mean** and the **median**. The most common measures of variation are the **range** and the **standard deviation**.

In the literature, the usual way of describing quantitative data is **mean ± SD**. The **Empirical Rule** and **Chebyshev's Theorem** provide insights into the nature of the standard deviation as a measure of variation. A **time series graph** applies the mean ± SD summary for quantitative data to display the course of an activity in time.

Keywords

Chebyshev's Theorem	measure of variation
Empirical Rule	range
frequency	standard deviation
absolute frequency	population and parameter

relative frequency
percent relative frequency
frequency distribution table
graphic
bar graph
broken bar graph
pie chart
measure of central tendency
mean
median

random variable
categorical random variable
quantitative random variable
sample and statistic
statistical design
statistics
descriptive statistics
inferential statistics
time series graph
variation

References

Arnold J et al: Lipid infusion increases oxygen consumption similarly in septic and nonseptic patients. *Am J Clin Nutr* 53, no. 1 (January 1991): 143.

Bodai B et al: A clinical evaluation of an oxygen insufflation/suction catheter. *Heart Lung* 16, no. 2 (January 1987): 39.

Brandstetter R: Effect of nasogastric feedings on arterial oxygen tension in patients with symptomatic chronic obstructive pulmonary disease. *Heart Lung* 17, no. 2 (March 1988): 170.

Cooper J et al: Why are so many critical care nurses unable to recognize ventricular tachycardia in the 12-lead electrocardiogram? *Heart Lung* 18, no. 3 (May 1989): 243.

Donnelly S et al: Interleukin-8 and development of adult respiratory distress syndrome in at-risk patient groups. *Lancet* 341, no. 8846 (13 March 1993): 643.

Donovan et al: Postprandial changes in the content and composition of nonprotein nitrogen in human milk. *Am J Clin Nutr* 54, no. 1 (December 1991): 1017.

Emerson J and Colditz G: Statistics in practice. *N Engl J Med* 309, no. 12 (22 September 1983): 709.

Gift A et al: Sensations during chest tube removal. *Heart Lung* 20, no. 2 (March 1991): 131.

Gueco I et al: Ketoconazole in posttransplant triple therapy: Comparison of costs and outcomes. *Transplant Proc* 24, no. 5 (October 1992): 1709.

Isner J: Acute catastrophic complications of balloon aortic valvuloplasty, *J Am Coll Cardiol* 17, no. 6 (May 1991): 1436.

Jacobs L et al: Clinical and magnetic resonance imaging in optic neuritis. *Neurology* 41, no. 1 (January 1991): 15.

Jonsson K et al: Tissue oxygenation, anemia, and perfusion in relation to wound healing in surgical patients. *Ann Surg* 214, no. 5 (November 1991): 605.

Kirby J et al: Alcohol and drug use among trauma patients admitted to an intensive care unit. *Heart Lung* 18, no. 3 (May 1989): 297–98.

Kirchhoff K: Who is responsible for research utilization? *Heart Lung* 20, no. 3 (May 1991): 308.

Mitchell P et al: American Association of Critical-Care Nurses Demonstration Project: Profile of excellence in critical care nursing. *Heart Lung* 18, no. 3 (May 1989): 219.

Nordström M et al: Social differences in Swedish infant mortality by cause of death, 1983 to 1986. *Am J Public Health* 83, no. 1 (January 1993): 26.

Papadakis M et al: Treatable abdominal pathologic conditions and unsuspected malignant neoplasms at autopsy in veterans who received mechanical ventilation. *JAMA* 265, no. 7 (20 February 1991): 885.

Pierce J et al: Effects of two chest tube clearance protocols on drainage in patients after myocardial revascularization surgery. *Heart Lung* 20, no. 2 (March 1991): 125.

Sands J: Incidence of pulmonary aspiration in intubated-patients receiving enteral nutrition through wide- and narrow-bore nasogastric feeding tubes. *Heart Lung* 20, no. 1 (January 1991): 75.

Shively M: Effect of position change on mixed venous oxygen saturation in coronary artery bypass surgery patients. *Heart Lung* 17, no. 1 (January 1988): 51.

Simpson T et al: American Association of Critical-Care Nurses Demonstration Project: Patients' recollections of critical care. *Heart Lung* 18, no. 4 (July 1989): 325.

Stone K et al: Effects of lung hyperinflation on mean arterial pressure and postsuctioning hypoxemia. *Heart Lung* 18, no. 4 (July 1989), 377.

Sumner D: Lies, damned lies—or statistics? *J Hypertens* 10 (1992): 3.

CHAPTER 2

Quantitative Data

In Chapter 1 we introduced the frequency distribution table as an effective tool for describing categorical data. This chapter examines methods for describing quantitative data. Section 2.1 surveys several common graphic techniques used for exploring a data set. Sections 2.2 and 2.3 detail the construction of a frequency distribution table with accompanying graphics for quantitative data.

Throughout this textbook we illustrate statistical concepts useful for approaching real problems in the health sciences by working with real data obtained from recent health sciences literature. A collection of data sets is given in the Appendix. Data Set 1 was reported by Daily and Mersch from their research on determining cardiac output. We use this data set repeatedly throughout the text; it is one of our "running examples." We excerpt from the introduction by Daily and Mersch:

> Measurement of cardiac output by the thermodilution method has become an integral part of the management of the critically ill patient. Even in hemodynamically stable patients, however, cardiac output values can vary considerably. These variations may be due to (1) technical errors in the performance of thermodilution measurement, (2) actual physiologic alterations that are occurring within the patient, and (3) errors in signal production and processing as a result of cyclic alterations in the temperature of the blood in the pulmonary artery that normally occur during the respiratory cycle.
>
> Based on the belief that precise cardiac output determinations depend on a maximum injectate/blood temperature difference, some critical care units routinely use iced injectate as the indicator. Preparation of the iced injectate, however, has several drawbacks. If room temperature (RT) injectate provides equally accurate and reproducible cardiac output values, the potential for contamination could be reduced as could nursing time and patient cost. On the other hand, if iced injectate values correlated more closely with the Fick method of determining cardiac output (i.e., the standard), time and cost would be justified and additional effort should be directed toward solving the problem of contamination.

At this point we invite the student to turn to Data Set 1 and just look at the numbers. Note that each patient has cardiac output measured by three different methods. Do the three methods yield the same cardiac output for all practical purposes? We emphasize, as Daily and Mersch noted in their opening paragraph, that *variation* is a key source of interest and problems. When variation is a source of problems, statistics is a necessary tool for problem solving, leading to providing better care.

The first rule of applied statistics is to look at the data. This involves more than just staring at numbers. Just as a microscope, magnifying glass, telescope, and even ordinary eyeglasses are useful for viewing aspects of the real world, statistics provides useful tools for assisting one in viewing and exploring data.

SECTION 2.1 *Graphical Descriptive Statistics*	**OBJECTIVES** This section will **1** Describe and determine the basic contexts of a data set: nominal, ordinal, and interval. **2** Describe and determine (using Minitab) the basic graphics in the descriptive statistics of interval data: sort and dotplot, boxplot, stem-and-leaf, and histogram.

Chapter 1 introduced the frequency distribution table, which was illustrated graphically with a bar graph or pie chart. Both the table and the graphic serve as effective methods for describing categorical data. This chapter focuses on a *quantitative* data set. The individual entries in a quantitative data set are *numbers*. However, the *context* of any number is as important as the number itself. Assessing the context of the entries in a data set is crucial since the methods of presentation and analysis of the data depend on that context.

Basic Data Contexts

In statistics there are three basic contexts for data: nominal, ordinal, and interval. The following example uses all three of these contexts.

EXAMPLE 2.1.1   John is patient number 71 in a study of cardiac patients. In college John graduated 71st in his class of 171. Last month John made 71 sales for Acme Products. John weighs 71 kg.

Patient number 71 gives John an identification label in a research study. John's rank in his graduating class tells us something about his relative position but does not tell us much about the quality of his work. John's sales record of 71 gives us the count of the number of sales he made last month. And John's weight of 71 kg is a measure of his biomass. Not all numbers are created equal. A number in a data set also imparts a great deal about the context of the information recorded by that number.

Nominal Data

A **nominal data set** consists of names or labels that identify a subject in the study or a characteristic of that subject. Nominal data are also called "categorical data" since their function is to serve as names or labels (i.e., categories).

In identifying a subject in a study, we can use a name (John) or an identification number (patient 71, or a Social Security number). In either case, the sole purpose is to identify the subject (patient) studied. An identification number is useful in preserving confidentiality.

In identifying a characteristic of a subject in a study, we can use the name of that characteristic or identify it by some code number. Code numbers are useful labels for computer encoding of data. For example,

Gender: male = 1, female = 2
State of residence: Alabama = 1, Alaska = 2, . . . , Wyoming = 50
Physician in charge: 1 = Dr. Kildare, 2 = Dr. Casey, 3 = Dr. Seuss, 4 = Dr. Spock
Hair color: 0 = bald, 1 = brown, 2 = black, 3 = blond, 4 = red, 5 = gray, 6 = other

Note that the category of gender, for example, could just as well be coded as female = 1, male = 2.

A **nominal number** merely acts as a name or identifying label (John is patient number 71). A nominal number is arbitrary in the sense that the number does not count or measure anything; it merely identifies something. It makes no sense to obtain descriptive statistics such as the mean or standard deviation for a data set of nominal numbers. For example, if the study size is $n = 141$, then 71 would be the average of the patient numbers from 1 to 141. This certainly does not imply that John is an average patient!

Ordinal Data

An **ordinal data set** consists of labels or numbers that imply some sort of ranking. The necessary ingredient for ordinal data is a system for ranking an observation. Examples abound in the real world.

Grades: A, B, C, D, F
Mobil Travel Guide: *, **, ***, ****, *****
Survey: disagree, neutral, agree
Cost: free, inexpensive, moderate, expensive
Military: private, corporal, sergeant, . . . , general
Horse race: win, place, show, also ran
Bureaucracy: staff, manager, president
Apgar score: 0, 1, 2, 3, 4, 5, 6, 7, 8, 9, 10

These rankings place things in an order without measuring the distance between ranks; in fact, distance between ranks usually has no precise meaning. In a ranking system, one just wants to indicate that one option is better than another without measuring how much better.

An **ordinal number** is a number used as a rank (e.g., John graduated 71st in his class). Ordinal numbers are useful for coding ranked responses. For example, a survey may ask one to give a ranked response to the following statement: "My insurance coverage is adequate." The responder is asked to circle one of the following:

Strongly Disagree	Disagree	Neutral	Agree	Strongly Agree
0	1	2	3	4

Note that the responses could just as well be coded from 1 through 5, or -2, -1, 0, 1, 2. The important thing is that an *ordered* set of numbers is used to indicate the ranks.

Interval Data ~size implied~ ~intervals must be consistant~

An **interval number** is a number that counts or measures something. An **interval data set** consists of interval numbers. Interval numbers carry an inherent notion of size, allowing us to calculate a meaningful difference between two given numbers. For example, the difference between 80 and 75 kg is exactly the same as the difference between 70 and 65 kg (in both cases the difference is 5 kg). Of course, this does not imply the same clinical significance to those differences. A weight loss of 5 kg may be clinically much more significant to one person than another. However, the *amount* of weight loss is determined by the weight before and the weight after.

An interval number that reports a count is necessarily a whole number (e.g., John made 71 sales last month). An interval number that reports a measure is based on some ruler or scale (e.g., John weighs 71 kg) and by nature is a decimal number (even if rounded to a whole number). Hence, an interval data set must consist of numbers.

Interval data that report measurements naturally occur as decimal numbers. The number of places past the decimal point one reports depends on the precision of the instrument(s) one uses for measurement. To measure time, we can use a time scale based on years (John is 45 years old), or one could use an atomic clock. Reporting time in nanoseconds can be important to a computer electrical engineer but is not important in recording the age of a patient. One basically should use common sense in deciding how many significant figures to use in recording interval numbers. We recommend that all data in an interval data set be recorded to the same number of places past the decimal point. Examples of interval data include

Age (in years): 71, 45, 25, 39, . . .
Weight (in kg): 65, 71, 68, 75, . . .
Height (cm): 193, 180, 186, 183, . . .
Cardiac output (liters/minute): 2.60, 5.16, 6.18, 3.22, . . .
Body mass index (kg/m^2): 10.1, 19.4, 42.3, 23.3, . . .

Any research study begins by identifying a population and random variable of interest (i.e., who and what to study). One gathers data by obtaining a sample from the population and applying the random variable to each member in the sample. The relationship between the random variable of interest and the context of the data produced by a sample is illustrated in Figure 2.1.1.

FIGURE **2.1.1**
The relationship between a random variable and a data set. There are two major kinds of random variables: categorical (nonnumerical) and quantitative (numerical). Each kind may produce a nominal or ordinal data set. Only a quantitative random variable can produce an interval data set.

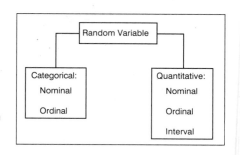

If there are just a few basic whole numbers that repeat throughout a data set (e.g., perfusion scores data set in Example 1.1.2.), the table and graph methods presented in Chapter 1 are adequate descriptive methods. Consequently, Chapter 1 contains the basic tools needed for presenting nominal or ordinal data. However, one needs other tools when dealing with a data set made up of decimal numbers or with many different whole numbers. In this event one needs to present the data set in a way that illustrates the *distribution* of the data. Study that focuses on obtaining insights into the nature of the distribution of the data is called exploratory data analysis.

Exploratory Data Analysis

Exploratory data analysis (EDA) is the process of examining a raw data set in order to uncover special features about the nature of the distribution of the data. Are the data uniformly spread throughout the range? Do the data seem to occur in "clumps"? Does there seem to be a particular pattern to the data? EDA is especially useful in comparing two sets of data.

Several tools have been developed to assist in EDA. These tools include the sort, the dotplot, the boxplot, the stem-and-leaf diagram, and the histogram. Since their construction can be technical and tedious, a computer is invaluable. We will illustrate each of these tools by applying Minitab to the room temperature cardiac output data set (Appendix, Data Set 1). This data set is displayed in Figure 2.1.2.

Sort and Dotplot

The data set in Figure 2.1.2 presents raw data from a single quantitative random variable, room temperature cardiac output. In presenting such a data set, from the human side it helps to **sort** the data (arrange the data from smallest to largest). The sorted room temperature cardiac output data set is presented in Figure 2.1.3. From

FIGURE **2.1.2**
The raw room temperature cardiac output data set from Daily and Mersch (Data Set 1).

2.60	5.16	6.18	3.22	4.99	3.62	3.31	4.11
5.24	4.27	3.42	4.70	5.42	5.36	2.63	3.70
5.39	5.44	3.86	6.68	5.35	3.26	4.06	2.64
5.40	5.93	5.90	4.11	4.44			

FIGURE 2.1.3
The sorted Daily and
Mersh room temperature
cardiac output data set.

2.60	2.63	2.64	3.22	3.26	3.31	3.42	3.62
3.70	3.86	4.06	4.11	4.11	4.27	4.44	4.70
4.99	5.16	5.24	5.35	5.36	5.39	5.40	5.42
5.44	5.90	5.93	6.18	6.68			

the sorting, one immediately sees that the data range from a minimum of 2.60 to a maximum of 6.68. There are no obvious clumps of data.

The **dotplot** is a visual graphic of the sorted data set. The dotplot is a graphic obtained by plotting each data point on the number line with a "dot." The dot is plotted just above the number line. If a number in the data set occurs more than once, than the dots are stacked, one over the other. The sort and dotplot are easily done in Minitab. Figure 2.1.4 displays Minitab's sort and dotplot for the Daily and Mersch room temperature cardiac output data.

Note that the original data are given to the hundredths position (second place past the decimal point). The distance from one number to its potential neighbor is 0.01. This distance, called the **unit of measurement,** indicates the size of a step as one proceeds down the number line to plot data points. Here, there are 3 steps from 2.60 to 2.63, 1 step from 2.63 to 2.64, but 58 steps from 2.64 to 3.22 as one proceeds down the number line. To encompass the range of the data set, one needs 408 steps, where each step measures 0.01.

FIGURE 2.1.4
Minitab output for
constructing a sort
and dotplot for the
Daily and Mersch
room temperature
cardiac output data
set.

```
MTB > NOTE    Enter and display the data.
MTB > SET C1
DATA> 2.60  5.16  6.18  3.22  4.99
DATA> 3.62  3.31  4.11  5.24  4.27
DATA> 3.42  4.70  5.42  5.36  2.63
DATA> 3.70  5.39  5.44  3.86  6.68
DATA> 5.35  3.26  4.06  2.64  5.40
DATA> 5.93  5.90  4.11  4.44
DATA> END OF DATA
MTB > NAME C1 'Raw Data'
MTB > OW 70     #Set output width to 70 characters.
MTB > PRINT C1

Raw Data
   2.60    5.16    6.18    3.22    4.99    3.62    3.31    4.11    5.24    4.27
   3.42    4.70    5.42    5.36    2.63    3.70    5.39    5.44    3.86    6.68
   5.35    3.26    4.06    2.64    5.40    5.93    5.90    4.11    4.44

MTB > NAME C5 'SortData'
MTB > SORT C1 INTO C5
MTB > PRINT C5

SortData
   2.60    2.63    2.64    3.22    3.26    3.31    3.42    3.62    3.70    3.86
   4.06    4.11    4.11    4.27    4.44    4.70    4.99    5.16    5.24    5.35
   5.36    5.39    5.40    5.42    5.44    5.90    5.93    6.18    6.68

MTB > DOTPLOT C1

                                           .
             .            .            :
         :     .:. .. . : ..  .  . :.:   :  .    .
        -----+---------+---------+---------+---------+-Raw Data
           3.0       4.0       5.0       6.0       7.0
```

A printer, however, can print only a limited number of characters across the page. To account for the width of the page (80 characters) and margins, Minitab's dotplot uses 66 characters (steps). A 66-step dotplot clearly is not wide enough to accommodate a data set of 408 steps. Hence, Minitab rounds the data set until accommodation is reached. Rounding the Daily and Mersch room temperature cardiac output data set to the nearest tenth produces a data set that ranges from 2.6 to 6.7. The unit of measurement for the rounded data set is 0.1. In this rounded context, the data set has 41 steps (each individual step has a length of 0.1). Now the rounded data set can be fit on the dotplot as displayed in Figure 2.1.4.

This process is much like taking a photograph. One must back off a sufficient distance so that the scene to be photographed is within the view scope of the camera. The view scope of the dotplot is 66 steps. One must back off from a data set (round) until the data set is encompassed within the view scope of the dotplot. Fortunately, Minitab does all this automatically.

Boxplot

Minitab's output displaying the boxplot for the Daily and Mersch room temperature cardiac output data is presented in Figure 2.1.5. If the computer you are working on has graphics capabilities, the GBOXPLOT command yields a graphics boxplot, that is, one that can be sent to a graphics package or to a laser printer (the *G* in GBOXPLOT stands for "graphics").

The **boxplot** is a nice exploratory graphic for previewing the distribution of numerical data. The middle half of the data set is displayed by presenting a "box." The reference crosspoint in the box is located at the median. The upper and lower quarter of the data set are portrayed by "whiskers" extending from the right and left of the box, respectively. Outliers (when present) are plotted as individual points.

The boxplot in Figure 2.1.5 indicates that the room temperature cardiac output data set is basically symmetrical. The + in the middle of the box (located at the median) is centered, and both "whiskers" (lines extending from the right and left ends of the box) are about the same length. There are no outliers.

FIGURE *2.1.5*
Minitab's boxplot for the Daily and Mersch room temperature cardiac output data.

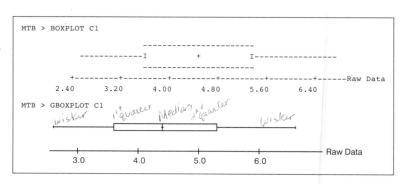

FIGURE **2.1.6**
The rounded raw room
temperature cardiac output data
set from Daily and Mersch (Data
Set 1).

2.6	5.2	6.2	3.2	5.0	3.6	3.3	4.1
5.2	4.3	3.4	4.7	5.4	5.4	2.6	3.7
5.4	5.4	3.9	6.7	5.4	3.3	4.1	2.6
5.4	5.9	5.9	4.1	4.4			

Stem-and-Leaf Diagram

In our discussion of the dotplot for the Daily and Mersch cardiac output data set, we noted that the unit of measurement was 0.01 (i.e., the data are reported to the second place past the decimal point). Using this unit of measurement as a basic step size for the data, one needs 408 steps to encompass the range of the data set from 2.60 to 6.68. From this point of view, a dotplot of the data would be quite sparse. The dotplot would show a panorama of 408 steps with only 28 actual points being occupied by data (note that $n = 29$, but 4.11 occurs twice). To give a fuller body to the view of the data, we "group" the data simply by rounding to the next decimal position. The rounded raw data set is given in Figure 2.1.6.

Each number in the data set has two natural components. The left part of the number (which for these data is the whole-number part) is called the **stem**. The last digit of the number (which for these data is the decimal part) is called the **leaf**. We now construct a graphic that lines up the stems (here: 2, 3, 4, 5, 6) down the first column (Figure 2.1.7a). We then attach the leaves to each stem. Figure 2.1.7b attaches the leaves for the first five data entries. (Here the first five data entries are 2.6, 5.2, 6.2, 3.2, and 5.0. The first entry, 2.6, has a stem of 2 and a leaf of 6; the second entry, 5.2, has a stem of 5 and a leaf of 2; the third entry, 6.2, has a stem of 6 and a leaf of 2; the fourth entry, 3.2, has a stem of 3 and a leaf of 2; the fifth entry, 5.0, has a stem of 5 and a leaf of 0.) Note that there are no spaces separating the leaves. Figure 2.1.7c shows the completed stem-and-leaf diagram drawn by hand. Figure 2.1.7d sorts the leaves.

Minitab's **stem-and-leaf** diagram for the Daily and Mersch room temperature cardiac output data set is displayed in Figure 2.1.8. Although the essence of our hand-drawn stem-and-leaf diagram is displayed in Minitab's output, there are some obvious differences.

In the first line of output Minitab informs us of the size of the data set ($N = 29$). In the second line Minitab states Leaf Unit = 0.10. This means that Minitab took the data set to just the first place past the decimal point; anything beyond the first place past the decimal point was simply ignored. The graphic itself presents three columns

FIGURE **2.1.7**
Stem-and-leaf diagram for
the Daily and Mersch raw
data set. (a) The data stems;
(b) data stems with leaves for
2.6, 3.2, 5.2, 5.0, and 6.2;
(c) the completed stem-
and-leaf diagram for the raw
data set; (d) the leaves on
each stem are sorted.

(a)	(b)	(c)	(d)
2	2 6	2 666	2 666
3	3 2	3 2634793	3 2334679
4	4	4 137114	4 111347
5	5 20	5 20244444499	5 02244444499
6	6 2	6 27	6 27

FIGURE **2.1.8**
Minitab's stem-and-leaf
diagram for the Daily and
Mersch room temperature
cardiac output data.

```
MTB > STEM-AND-LEAF C1

Stem-and-leaf of Raw Data   N  = 29
Leaf Unit = 0.10

    3     2  666
    7     3  2234
   10     3  678
   (5)    4  01124
   14     4  79
   12     5  12333444
    4     5  99
    2     6  1
    1     6  6
```

of numbers. The numbers in the first column cumulate the frequencies from the ends (start and finish) of the data. Reading down the first column, the first data class has three entries. The next class picks up four more entries, accounting for seven altogether. The next class picks up three more entries, accounting for ten altogether. The number in the first column enclosed in parentheses indicates the median group; that is, the median occurs within this branch of the diagram, and there are five entries in this group. Minitab's diagram also uses more branches (here, nine) than our hand-drawn diagram in Figure 2.1.7.

Histograms

The histogram is perhaps the most common graphic used for describing an interval data set. The **histogram** is a bar graph type of graphic in which the numbers in the data set have been grouped into classes.

The frequency distribution table method of Section 1.1 is not helpful in presenting the room temperature cardiac output data set. Each member of this data set occurs only once, except 4.11, which occurs twice. A listing of the 28 distinct numbers in the data set with an accompanying frequency of 1 (2 for 4.11) is not illuminating. It is desirable to group the data in some fashion (is 2.63 really much different from 2.60 or 2.64?). An advantage of grouping is that we can keep track of just a few groups (e.g., low, low normal, normal, high normal, high).

Minitab permits one to easily obtain a quick histogram. Figure 2.1.9 displays a basic quick histogram for the cardiac output data set. Both the line printer version and the graphics version are displayed. In the line printer histogram each data point in the class is plotted with a *. In the graphics histogram each class is represented by a rectangle. The graphics version draws the rectangles if the computer one is using has this capability. In both cases, Minitab displays the midpoint for each data class and the class frequency (count).

Comment Minitab selects the midpoint of each of the classes to be "nice" numbers, that is, nice from a people standpoint. The user may specify the number of classes by utilizing Minitab's subcommand structure for the main HISTOGRAM command. However, the user must specify the location of the midpoint for the first class

FIGURE **2.1.9**
Minitab's histogram
for the Daily and
Mersch room
temperature cardiac
output data. The first
histogram is the
"regular" version; the
second, the
"graphics" version.

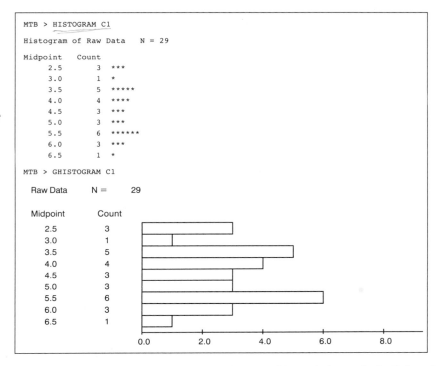

and the width of a given class. For this one will need the technicalities given in the remainder of this chapter. Minitab's HISTOGRAM command is perfectly adequate for a quick "thumbnail" sketch of the data.

EXERCISES 2.1

Warm-ups
2.1

Table 2.1.1 presents a profile of patients adapted from data presented by Jacobs et al. Jacobs et al studied relationships between optic neuritis and brain lesions shown on magnetic resonance imaging. The patients were followed through 4 years of follow-up. The table presents five items for each patient in the Jacobs et al study: patient number, gender, the eye affected by optic neuritis, age, and the general follow-up condition of the patient at follow-up compared with condition at time of entry in the study.

1. What are the three different contexts for the entries making up a data set?

2. What data context basically
   a. Labels an observation?
   b. Orders an observation?
   c. Measures an observation?

3. The Jacobs et al data shown in Table 2.1.1 presents five columns: patient, gender, eye, age, and outcome. Identify the context of the entries in each column; that is, are the entries nominal, ordinal, or interval?

4. A quantitative data set is a data set consisting of

_____ .

5. What is the function of the numbers in the patient column in Table 2.1.1?

6. The outcome column in Table 2.1.1 describes an ordinal data set. The key feature of ordinal data is an implied ranking scheme. What ranking scheme is implied by this data set?

TABLE **2.1.1**
Data set adapted from
Jacobs et al.

Patient	Gender	Eye	Age	Outcome
1	M	Right	28	Improved
2	F	Right	30	Unchanged
3	F	Right	23	Improved
4	F	Right	31	Improved
5	M	Right	33	Worse
6	M	Right	17	Improved
7	F	Right	41	Worse
8	M	Right	21	Worse
9	F	Left	49	Improved
10	F	Right	29	Improved
11	F	Left	35	Improved
12	M	Right	61	Improved
13	F	Left	49	Improved
14	F	Left	21	Improved
15	F	Left	32	Improved
16	F	Left	22	Worse
17	M	Left	50	Improved
18	F	Right	37	Improved
19	M	Left	28	Improved
20	F	Right	25	Worse
21	M	Left	40	Improved
22	F	Left	55	Improved
23	F	Right	12	Improved
24	F	Right	20	Worse
25	F	Right	20	Worse
26	F	Right	28	Worse
27	M	Right	40	Improved
28	M	Left	47	Improved
29	F	Left	30	Improved
30	F	Left	18	Improved
31	M	Left	35	Improved
32	F	Left	52	Unchanged
33	M	Right	19	Improved
34	F	Right	33	Unchanged
35	F	Right	24	Improved
36	F	Left	31	Worse
37	M	Right	30	Improved
38	F	Right	41	Improved
39	F	Right	22	Unchanged
40	M	Left	43	Improved
41	F	Right	38	Improved
42	F	Left	21	Improved
43	M	Right	56	Improved
44	F	Left	25	Improved
45	M	Right	27	Improved
46	F	Left	36	Worse
47	F	Left	31	Improved
48	F	Left	32	Unchanged

7. The age column describes an interval data set. A display that arranges the ages from smallest to largest is called a _____ of the data.

8. Construct a stem-and-leaf diagram by hand for the age data using the following stems: 1, 2, 3, 4, 5, 6.

Figure 2.1.10 contains five graphics constructed in Minitab describing the age data.

9. Which graphic (a, b, c, d, or e) is a dotplot?

10. Which graphic is a boxplot?

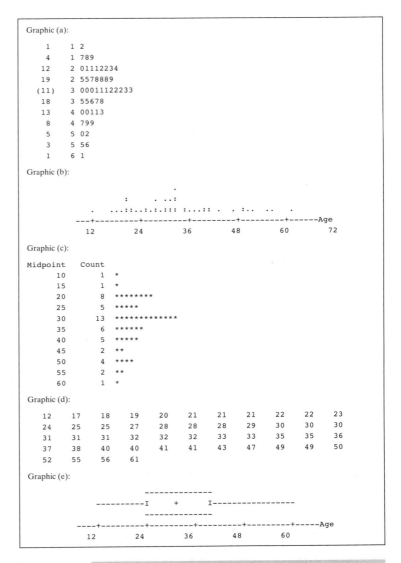

FIGURE **2.1.10**
Five graphics constructed in Minitab describing the age data set.

Graphic (a):

```
   1     1 2
   4     1 789
  12     2 01112234
  19     2 5578889
 (11)    3 00011122233
  18     3 55678
  13     4 00113
   8     4 799
   5     5 02
   3     5 56
   1     6 1
```

Graphic (b):

```
                                   .
                    :      . ..:
           .  ...::...:.:.::: :...:: . . .:.. ..   .
        ---+---------+---------+---------+---------+------Age
          12        24        36        48        60        72
```

Graphic (c):

```
Midpoint    Count
      10       1   *
      15       1   *
      20       8   ********
      25       5   *****
      30      13   *************
      35       6   ******
      40       5   *****
      45       2   **
      50       4   ****
      55       2   **
      60       1   *
```

Graphic (d):

```
   12    17    18    19    20    21    21    21    22    22    23
   24    25    25    27    28    28    28    29    30    30    30
   31    31    31    32    32    32    33    33    35    35    36
   37    38    40    40    41    41    43    47    49    49    50
   52    55    56    61
```

Graphic (e):

```
                          --------------
                ---------I      +      I-----------------
                          --------------
           ----+---------+---------+---------+---------+-----Age
              12        24        36        48        60
```

11. Which graphic is a stem-and-leaf diagram?

12. Which graphic is a histogram?

13. Which graphic is a sort?

14. Provide a verbal description for the distribution of the age data.

15. What is the study of a data set for general clues to the nature of the distribution of the data called?

Problems 2.1

1. Identify each of the following data sets as nominal, ordinal, or interval:
   a. The Jonsson et al data set given in Example 1.1.2
   b. The Sands data set given in Example 1.1.3
   c. The Simpson et al data set given in Example 1.1.9
   d. The Mitchell et al data set given in Problem 1.1.3

e. The Shively data sets given in Problem 1.1.5:
  i. Patient
  ii. Sex
  iii. Grafts
f. The Brandstetter et al data set in Example 1.2.1
g. The Stone et al data set in Problem 1.2.1
h. The Papadakis et al data set in Problem 1.2.2
i. The five columns in the Clark and Hoffer data (Appendix, Data Set 6)

2. Construct a stem-and-leaf diagram for the Daily and Mersch ITCO data set (Appendix, Data Set 1).

Problems 3–7 apply to the Barcelona et al data set (Appendix, Data Set 2).

3. Construct a stem-and-leaf diagram by hand for both the iced and the room temperature cardiac outputs, prefilled syringes. Contrast and compare the two distributions based on your diagrams.

4. A key motivation for the study was to see whether room and iced temperature injectates gave comparable cardiac output readings. We focus on the prefilled syringes in this problem. Construct a new column of data by taking the difference D = iced − room for each patient in the study. For the first and second patients, $D = 3.8 - 3.7 = 0.1$; for the third patient, $D = 3.2 - 3.2 = 0.0$. Now construct a stem-and-leaf diagram for the column D of differences. Does the stem-and-leaf diagram appear to be centered about 0? Or does the diagram appear more heavily weighted toward the positive or the negative?

Comment Note that if in general there is no difference in cardiac output measurement between these two methods, then iced = room; that is, D = iced − room = 0. If, in general, the Iced method yields the higher measurement, then iced > room; i.e., D = iced − room > 0. Finally, if in general the Iced method yields the lower measurement, then iced < room; i.e., D = iced − room < 0. Hence, one can get a good feel for how these two methods compare by examining an EDA graphic for the *difference* between the two methods.

5. Using Minitab, for the prefilled syringes, iced data set, construct the following:
  a. Sorted data set
  b. Dotplot

c. Boxplot
d. Stem-and-leaf diagram
e. Histogram
f. Graphics histogram

6. Using Minitab, for the prefilled syringes, room data set, construct the following:
  a. Sorted data set
  b. Dotplot
  c. Boxplot
  d. Stem-and-leaf diagram
  e. Histogram
  f. Graphics histogram

7. Using Minitab, obtain the following graphics for the Co-Set data: BY HAND.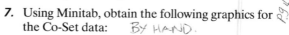
  a. Construct a dotplot for the iced data set.
  b. Construct a dotplot for the room data set.
  c. Contrast and compare the iced and room distributions.
  d. One difficulty in contrasting and comparing as requested in (c) is that the scales for the two graphics from (a) and (b) are different; that is, the graphics start at different locations on the number line. To contrast and compare, it would help considerably if the two dotplots were placed on the SAME scale. To accomplish this, assuming that the iced and room data are in columns C3 and C4, respectively,

```
MTB > DOTPLOT C3 C4;
SUBC> SAME.
```

  Contrast and compare the results.

Problems 8–11 apply to the Clark and Hoffer data set (Appendix, Data Set 6).

8. Construct a stem-and-leaf diagram by hand for the weight data set.

9. Using Minitab, for the weight data set, construct the following:
  a. Sorted data set
  b. Dotplot
  c. Boxplot
  d. Stem-and-leaf diagram
  e. Histogram
  f. Graphics histogram

10. Using Minitab, for the body mass index data set, construct the following:

   a. Sorted data set

   b. Dotplot

   c. Boxplot

   d. Stem-and-leaf diagram

   e. Histogram

   f. Graphics histogram

11. Construct a stem-and-leaf diagram by hand for the body mass index data set. Do you find this graphic very informative or illustrative? Explain.

12. Sütsch et al reported the following data on the aortic diameter of 54 patients with type A dissection (aortic diameter measured in centimeters using transthoracic echocardiography).

6.5	5.4	4.9	6.3	6.3	6.2	4.5	6.5	6.7	5.3
5.4	3.7	5.2	4.8	4.4	6.2	4.1	6.5	6.0	7.8
6.9	4.7	4.3	5.0	9.0	5.7	7.1	5.5	5.9	6.1
8.1	5.8	6.6	6.0	5.5	5.0	5.5	6.0	4.7	6.0
6.5	6.6	7.6	5.5	6.2	5.9	6.4	6.2	7.0	5.5
11.0	7.1	5.1	4.0						

   a. Determine the mean, median, range, and standard deviation.

   b. Determine the 1SD, 2SD, and 3SD windows. What proportion of the data lies in each window? Compare with the Empirical Rule.

   c. Display the sorted data set and dotplot.

   d. Display a boxplot. Based on the boxplot, what items would appear to be outliers?

   e. Display a stem-and-leaf diagram.
   Comment In Minitab, contrast the following two diagrams:

```
MTB > STEM-AND-LEAF C1
MTB > STEM-AND-LEAF C1;
SUBC> INCREMENT 1.
```

   The increment subcommand allows you to control the size of the leaves. For further explanation, `MTB > HELP STEM-AND-LEAF INCREMENT`.

   f. Display a histogram.

   g. Verbally describe the distribution of aortic diameter for the given patient population.

SECTION 2.2
Class Limits

OBJECTIVES   This section will

1 Determine a set of class limits for a given numerical data set. The number of classes should conform to Sturges's Rule unless otherwise specified.

2 Construct a frequency distribution table for grouped data based on a given set of class limits.

3 Construct a bar graph and polygon from a given frequency distribution table.

A data set consisting of interval numbers may be presented in a variety of ways. One may condense the data using the describe method presented in Section 1.2. One may sort and display the data using the graphic tools given in Section 2.1: dotplot, boxplot, stem-and-leaf, or histogram. This section presents the table method for summarizing and displaying a data set of interval numbers. The strength of this method is that it allows an investigator to explore and present data using both tables and graphs that highlight the distribution of the data. The key activity in the table method is to group the data.

The Rationale for Grouping

The foundation work in the table method is to reasonably *group the data into classes*. Although this grouping conceivably could be done haphazardly, we present a step-wise procedure that will yield good results for the study and presentation of data.

To illustrate each step of the grouping procedure, we continue to use the room temperature cardiac outputs from Daily and Mersch (already displayed in Figure 2.1.2). Two preliminary comments are in order. First, in presenting a raw data set, from the human side it helps considerably just to sort the data as displayed in Figure 2.1.3. Second, as already discussed in Section 2.1, the frequency distribution table method of Section 1.1 is unenlightening since each individual number basically occurs only once. This suggests grouping the data in some fashion.

Although it seems desirable to group interval data, how should the grouping be done? Initially one is tempted by personal convenience and quite naturally may construct the frequency distribution table with accompanying graph as shown in Figure 2.2.1.

For presentation to lay audiences, such an approach is acceptable, perhaps even preferable. However, cardiac outputs are unaware of the convenience humans see in the base 10 system of enumeration. Cardiac output, as any random variable (RV), has its own distribution in the population of interest. Hence, to maximize what we can learn about the distribution, we now proceed with a method of grouping that is more natural to the RV being studied rather than to the foibles of human convenience.

Class Limits

The purpose of the grouping procedure is to maximize one's feeling for the *distribution* of the RV in the population as a whole based on the data supplied by the sample. Our grouping procedure is a bit tedious and involves nine steps, each of which has been formulated to contain only one feature. At this stage of development in health sciences statistics, it is better to do many simple steps rather than a few involved ones.

We now proceed with the nine-step grouping procedure. Each step is illustrated by example using the Daily and Mersch data set of room temperature cardiac outputs.

1. Obtain the **sorted raw data set**.

Example: We will use the room temperature injectate cardiac output data from Daily and Mersch to illustrate each step.

FIGURE 2.2.1
An intuitive grouped frequency distribution table and accompanying bar graph for the room temperature cardiac output data.

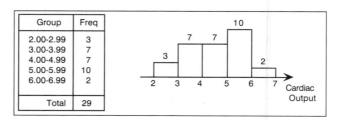

Group	Freq
2.00-2.99	3
3.00-3.99	7
4.00-4.99	7
5.00-5.99	10
6.00-6.99	2
Total	29

2.60	2.63	2.64	3.22	3.26	3.31	3.42	3.62
3.70	3.86	4.06	4.11	4.11	4.27	4.44	4.70
4.99	5.16	5.24	5.35	5.36	5.39	5.40	5.42
5.44	5.90	5.93	6.18	6.68			

2. Determine the **sample size** (n). *Count data* [*unit size = 0.01*]
   Example: $n = 29$.

3. Determine the **number of classes** (k) for grouping the data. [*5*]

The number of classes can be obtained from Table 2.2.1.

TABLE 2.2.1
The number of classes to use is determined by the sample size. This table is derived from Sturges's Rule.

Sample Size	Number of Classes
4–7	3
8–15	4
16–31	5
32–63	6
64–127	7
128–255	8
256–511	9
512–1024	10

Table 2.2.1 is derived from **Sturges's Rule**. You may preempt the use of this rule if there is some obvious convenience factor suggested by the background or presentation of the data; otherwise, Sturges's Rule provides an acceptable guide for the number of classes to use in grouping the data. Throughout this text we use Sturges's Rule unless otherwise indicated.

Example: $n = 29$, so $k = 5$ by Sturges's Rule. Note that a sample size of 16 to 31 justifies five classes; one needs a sample size of 32 to 63 to justify six classes.

We now proceed to break up the data set into k exhaustive and mutually exclusive classes (in our example, $k = 5$).

4. Determine the **unit of measurement** (u) for the data set. [*0.01*]

We illustrate the concept of unit of measurement by example.

EXAMPLE 2.2.1 Table 2.2.2 displays four specific data sets: A, B, C, and D.

TABLE 2.2.2
Four data set samples (A, B, C, D).

Data Set	Data	u
A	5.135, 6.938, 7.230, 4.002	0.001 — *all the same no. places*
B	3.94, 4.00, 19.63, 14.86	0.01
C	2.7, 9.6, 3.0, 4.8, 19.3	0.1
D	57, 96, 33, 20, 16, 9, 73	1

Note that in data set A, all the numbers go out to the third place past the decimal point; so, $u = 0.001$. In data set B, all the numbers go out to the second place past the decimal point; so, $u = 0.01$. In data set C, all the numbers go out to the first place past the decimal point; so, $u = 0.1$. All the numbers in data set D are whole numbers; so $u = 1$.

Example: In the Daily and Mersch cardiac output study, the numbers all go to the second place past the decimal point; so, $u = 0.01$.

5. Compute the **unit extended range** (*uer*) of the data set.

In general, **_uer_ = maximum − minimum + _u_**; that is, the unit extended range is the range extended by u, the unit of measurement.

Example: $uer = \text{maxi} - \text{mini} + u$
$$= 6.68 - 2.60 + 0.01$$
$$= 4.09$$

6. Determine the **class width** (*w*).

In general, **_w_ = (_uer_)/_k_** rounded *upward* at the unit of measurement's decimal position. Hence, the class width is determined by dividing the unit extended range (*uer*) by the number of classes (*k*). If the division is not exact by the unit of measurement's decimal position, round up at that decimal place.

Example: $w = (uer)/k$
$$= 4.09/5$$
$$= 0.818 +$$
$$= 0.82 \text{ (rounded up at the hundredths position)}$$
Hence, $w = 0.82$.

7. Determine the **adjusted range** (*ar*).

In general, the adjusted range is k times w; that is, **_ar_ = _k_ × _w_**.

Example: $ar = k \times w = (5) \times (0.82) = 4.10$

The relationship between the range, unit extended range, and adjusted range is depicted in Figure 2.2.2.

8. Select the **(adjusted) minimum** (*m*).

The minimum data value may be adjusted downward by an amount not exceeding the quantity $ar - uer$. The (adjusted) minimum tells us where to start the first class; that

FIGURE **2.2.2**   The data range from 2.60 to 6.68 (range = 4.08). The unit extended range) (*uer*) extends the range by a unit of measurement (here, $u = 0.01$). The adjusted range (*ar*) covers the *uer* and is evenly divisible by the number of classes. The adjusted range is a length that will be subdivided into five pieces of equal length. The adjusted range is the shortest length, evenly divisible by 5, that encompasses the entire data set.

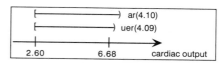

is, the (adjusted) minimum is the lower limit for the first class. The purpose of the adjustment is to center the graphic over the data. Without this adjustment our graphic would always start at the data minimum and leave an "overhang" of $ar - uer$ on the right-hand side of the graphic. The overhang, an artifact of creating a uniform graphic (the classes all have the same width), does not contain any data.

Example: The data minimum is 2.60. Since

$$ar - uer = 4.10 - 4.09 = 0.01$$

we may adjust down one unit of measurement step to 2.59. Hence, we have a choice for starting our first class at 2.60 (the actual minimum) or 2.59 (an adjusted minimum). Since 2.60 is a more convenient number than 2.59, we choose to start at 2.60 (here, no adjustment to the data minimum is needed). ~Because of class of 5

9. Determine the classes by specifying the **lower and upper class limit** for each class.

In general, let k = number of classes
m = (adjusted) minimum
w = class width
u = unit of measurement

The general directions for constructing the **class limits** are provided in Table 2.2.3. Using these directions, one obtains the class limits for the Daily and Mersch room temperature cardiac output as shown in Table 2.2.4.

TABLE **2.2.3**
The class limits are constructed according to the given guide-lines. It is easiest to calculate the column of lower class limits, then the column of upper class limits.

	Class Limits	
Class	Lower	Upper
1	m	$m + w - u$
2	$m + w$	$m + 2w - u$
3	$m + 2w$	$m + 3w - u$
. . .	. . .	. . .
k	$m + (k - 1)w$	$m + kw - u$

Example: We use $k = 5, m = 2.60, w = 0.82$, and $u = 0.01$.

TABLE **2.2.4**
Class limits for the Daily and Mersch room temperature cardiac output data.

	Class Limits	
Class	Lower	Upper
1	2.60	3.41
2	3.42	4.23
3	4.24	5.05
4	5.06	5.87
5	5.88	6.69

We now summarize and display our work for constructing the class limits for the room temperature cardiac output data.

1. The sorted data set:

   2.60 2.63 2.64 3.22 3.26 3.31 3.42 3.62 3.70 3.86
   4.06 4.11 4.11 4.27 4.44 4.70 4.99 5.16 5.24 5.35
   5.36 5.39 5.40 5.42 5.44 5.90 5.93 6.18 6.68

2. The sample size: $n = 29$.
3. The number of classes: $k = 5$ (Sturges's Rule).
4. The unit of measurement: $u = 0.01$.
5. The unit extended range: $uer = 4.09$
6. The class width: $w = 0.82$.
7. The adjusted range: $ar = 4.10$
8. The (adjusted) minimum: $m = 2.60$ (options: 2.60, 2.59).
9. The class limits (Table 2.2.5).

TABLE **2.2.5**
The class limits.

Class Limits	
Lower	Upper
2.60	3.41
3.42	4.23
4.24	5.05
5.06	5.87
5.88	6.69

Comment Make sure that the minimum number in the data set falls in the first class and that the maximum number falls in the last class. If one makes an arithmetic error, it frequently can be caught by noting that the last class is too small to accept the data maximum.

Frequency Distribution Table

Once we have the class limits, the foundation work has been completed. To finish the project of constructing the frequency distribution table, we proceed now as in Section 1.1, treating each class like a category for the data. Note that the classes are mutually exclusive (a measurement value can fit into only one class) and exhaustive (each value must fit into a class). The class frequencies are easy to obtain from the sorted data set; then (percent) relative frequencies are computed. For example, Table 2.2.6 displays the frequency distribution table for the room temperature cardiac output data set.

TABLE **2.2.6**
Frequency distribution data for the Daily and Mersch room temperature cardiac output data.

Class	Frequency	% Relative Frequency
2.60–3.41	6	4/29 = .206 21
3.42–4.23	7	24
4.24–5.05	4	14
5.06–5.87	8	28
5.88–6.69	4	14
Totals	29	101*

*Deviation from 100% due to round-off error.

PUT THAT IF >100

Graphics

Once a frequency distribution table has been constructed, one should construct an accompanying graphic. The graphic serves two purposes. First, one purpose of descriptive statistics is to give an organized presentation of a given data set. Some people are table-oriented; others, graph-oriented. Hence, a presentation that provides both a table and an accompanying graph (or vice versa) reaches a larger audience. Second, a major reason for doing descriptive statistics is exploratory data analysis, that is, a more intense look at the data for clues to the nature of the distribution of the underlying random variable in the population. The two main types of graphs for a frequency distribution table for grouped data are bar graphs and polygons.

Bar Graphs

Three kinds of bar graphs can be constructed based on a frequency distribution table for grouped data; namely, a frequency bar graph, a relative frequency bar graph, or a percent relative frequency bar graph.

The **frequency bar graph** corresponding to the frequency distribution table for the room temperature cardiac output data (Table 2.2.6) is displayed in Figure 2.2.3.

There are several features that go into the presentation of a good frequency bar graph. The graph is presented vertically. Each class is represented by a rectangle (bar). The base of the rectangle corresponds to the class limits and is labeled at the class mark. The **class mark** is the midpoint of the class and is obtained by taking the mean of the class limits, that is,

Class mark = (lower class limit + upper class limit)/2

The height of a rectangle in a frequency bar graph corresponds to the class frequency. Each class frequency should be indicated directly or by supplying a vertical scale. Finally, the axes are labeled and the graph is captioned. Note that there is a gap of one measurement unit between the bars.

Similarly, one constructs a (percent) **relative frequency bar graph** by constructing a bar graph in which the height of a rectangle corresponds to the class (percent) relative frequency. For example, the percent relative frequency bar graph for the room temperature cardiac output data is shown in Figure 2.2.4.

FIGURE *2.2.3*
Frequency bar graph for the Daily and Mersch room temperature cardiac output set based on the frequency distribution table displayed in Table 2.2.6.

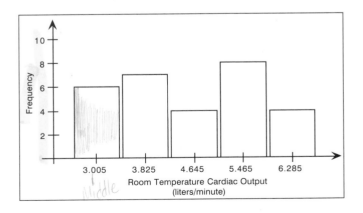

FIGURE **2.2.4**
Percent relative frequency bar graph for the Daily and Mersch room temperature cardiac output data set based on the frequency distribution table displayed in Table 2.2.6.

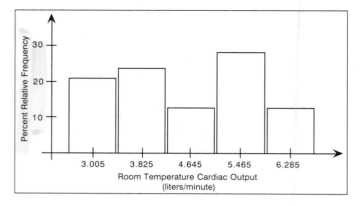

FIGURE **2.2.5**
Percent relative frequency polygon for the Daily and Mersch room temperature cardiac output data set based on the frequency distribution table displayed in Table 2.2.6.

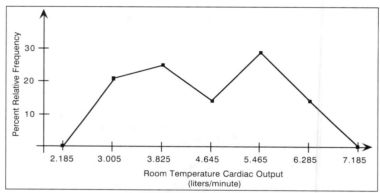

Polygons

Corresponding to each of the three kinds of bar graphs, one can construct a **polygon**. For illustration, the percent relative frequency polygon for the room temperature cardiac output data is shown in Figure 2.2.5.

A polygon depicts the same information as a bar graph, but with a slightly varied graphic. Instead of using the rectangle (bar) to represent a class, a polygon simply plots a point at the appropriate height above the class mark. In addition, an imaginary class is included to both the left and the right, with a zero point plotted at the respective marks. After the points are plotted they are joined by straight line segments (i.e., connect the dots); hence, the polygon. The purpose of the imaginary classes with their zero points is to anchor the polygon to the horizontal axis; without them, the polygon appears to be levitating above the axis.

Warm-ups 2.2

In this warm-up we construct a frequency distribution table for the Barcelona et al cardiac output data, prefilled syringes, iced temperature injectates (Appendix, Data Set 2). The first rule of applied statistics is to look at the data. The ordered data set is

```
2.2  2.4  2.7  2.7  2.8  2.9  3.0  3.1  3.2  3.2  3.3
3.4  3.4  3.4  3.4  3.5  3.5  3.5  3.5  3.7  3.7  3.8
3.8  3.8  3.8  3.8  3.8  3.9  4.0  4.0  4.2  4.5  4.6
4.7  4.8  5.0  5.3  5.7  6.2  6.7  7.2
```

1. The size of this data set is $n = \underline{41}$.

2. Using Sturges's Rule, the number of classes $k = \underline{6}$.

3. Sturges's Rule is (select the best response):
   a. Mandatory for good statistical practice
   b. The most common method for grouping data
   (c.) An arbitrary rule of convenience
   d. The most reliable method for grouping data

4. The purpose of Sturges's Rule is to assist in deciding
   a. How many observations are in the data set
   (b.) How many classes to break the data up into
   c. Whether one should analyze the data set
   d. What the mean and standard deviation should be
   e. What the range of the data set is

5. The unit of measurement for these data is $u = \underline{.1}$.

6. The unit extended range is calculated by $uer = max - min + u$.
   Here, maximum $= \underline{7.2}$
   Minimum $= \underline{2.2}$
   $u = \underline{.1}$
   So, $uer = $ maximum $-$ minimum $+ u$
   $= \underline{7.2} - \underline{2.2} + \underline{.1}$
   $= \underline{5.1}$.

7. The class width (w), is obtained by dividing the *uer* by the number of classes (k). If the division is not exact at the unit of measurement's position, then one rounds *up* at the unit of measurement's position. Here,
   $uer = \underline{5.1}$ and $k = \underline{6}$.
   So, $uer/k = \underline{5.1} / \underline{6} = \underline{.85}$.
   Hence, $w = \underline{.9}$.

8. The adjusted range (ar) is calculated by $k \times w$. Here,

$ar = k \times w = \underline{.9} \times \underline{6} = \underline{5.4}$.

9. To determine the best place to start the frequency distribution table, we need to determine the lower limit for the first class. In order to consider our options, we calculate the quantity

$ar - uer = \underline{5.4} - \underline{5.1} = \underline{.3}$. $.3 = 3 \text{ steps}$
   $.1 = 1 \text{ step}$

How many unit of measurement steps are represented by this quantity? $\underline{3}$

10. We now create a full list of suitable options for the lower limit for the first class. We start at the minimum and then decrease this number stepwise by the number of steps allowed (warm-up 9). Here, the data minimum is $\underline{2.2}$.

Starting from the data minimum and decreasing three unit of measurements, one unit at a time, we obtain our list of options:

$m = \underline{2.2, 2.1, 2.0, 1.9}$.

To center the bar graph, we choose an option in the middle. The middle options are 2.1 and 2.0. For "humanitarian" reasons we choose 2.0 as the lower limit of the first class.

11. The lower class limits are obtained by repeatedly adding the class width (here, $w = .9$) to 2.0. Complete Table 2.2.7 for the lower class limits.

TABLE **2.2.7** The lower class limits.

Class	Lower Class Limit
1	.9 2.0 2.0
2	2.9
3	3.8
4	
5	
6	

12. For the upper class limits, each class ends just before the next one begins. Since the second class begins at 2.9, the first class ends at 2.8. Complete Table 2.2.8 for the class limits.

TABLE **2.2.8** The class limits.

| Class | Class Limits | |
	Lower	Upper
1	2.0	2.8
2	2.9	
3		
4		
5		
6		

13. Once the class limits are determined, construction of the frequency distribution table from the sorted data set is a matter of counting and simple computations. Complete the following frequency distribution table, Table 2.2.9.

TABLE **2.2.9** The frequency distribution table.

| Class Limits | | Frequency | Relative Frequency |
Lower	Upper		
2.0	2.8		
2.9			
Total			

Comment Notice how most of the detail work is focused on obtaining the lower limit of the first class. Once one has the lower limit of the first class, the class width, and the sorted data set, one has all the tools needed to construct the frequency distribution table. The detail work in obtaining the lower limit of the first class is needed to obtain a bar graph that is "centered" over the data and for which the bars are all of the same width.

Problems 2.2

For each data set specified in problems 1–12,

a. Construct a frequency distribution table. In showing your work, display the sorted data set, *n* (sample size), *k* (number of classes using Sturges's Rule), *u* (unit of measurement), *uer* (unit extended range), *w* (class width), *ar* (adjusted range), *m* (include a list of all options for the adjusted minimum and indicate your choice), and the frequency distribution table.

b. Using your frequency distribution table from (a), construct
   i. a frequency bar graph and polygon
   ii. a relative frequency bar graph and polygon
   iii. a percent relative frequency bar graph and polygon

1. The Daily and Mersch cardiac output study, iced temperature injectates (see Appendix, Data Set 1).

2. The Daily and Mersch cardiac output study, Fick method (see Appendix, Data Set 1).

3. The Barcelona et al cardiac output study (see Appendix, Data Set 2) for the Co-set system, iced injectate (Co-set column).

4. The Barcelona et al cardiac output study (see Appendix, Data Set 2) for the Co-set system, room temperature injectate.

5. The Daily and Mersch cardiac output study (see Appendix, Data Set 1) for the difference, room − Fick.

6. The Daily and Mersch cardiac output study (see Appendix, Data Set 1) for the difference, iced − Fick.

7. The Barcelona et al cardiac output study (see Appendix, Data Set 2), prefilled syringes, room temperature injectates.

8. The Barcelona et al cardiac output study (see Appendix, Data Set 2), prefilled syringes, for the difference, iced − room.

9. The Clark and Hoffer metabolism study (see Appendix, Data Set 6) for age.

10. The Clark and Hoffer metabolism study (see Appendix, Data Set 6) for height.

11. The Clark and Hoffer metabolism study (see Appendix, Data Set 6) for weight.

12. The Clark and Hoffer metabolism study (see Appendix, Data Set 6) for body mass index.

13. Macey and Bouman reported data for the age distribution of 51 patients in their study as displayed in Table 2.2.10.

TABLE 2.2.10 The Macey and Bouman age distribution data set.

Age (years)	n
21–30	18
31–40	11
41–50	12
51–60	6
61–70	3
71–80	1

a. Is the number of classes justified by Sturges's Rule?

b. Are the class limits consistent with good statistical practice?

c. Complete the frequency distribution table by adjoining a column of relative frequencies.

d. Construct (i) a frequency bar graph and polygon and (ii) a relative frequency bar graph and polygon.

14. Jacobs et al reported the ages of 48 patients in their study:

```
28  30  23  31  33  17  41  21  49  29  35  61
49  21  32  22  50  37  28  25  40  55  12  32
20  28  40  47  30  18  35  52  19  33  24  31
30  41  22  43  38  21  56  25  27  36  31  32
```

a. Determine the mean, median, range, and standard deviation.

b. What proportion of the data falls in the 1SD window? 2SD window? 3SD window? Compare with the Empirical Rule.

c. Construct a frequency distribution table.

d. Construct a frequency bar graph and polygon.

e. Construct a relative frequency bar graph and polygon.

SECTION 2.3

Class Boundaries

OBJECTIVES   This section will

1 Determine a set of class boundaries for a given data set.

2 Construct a frequency distribution table for grouped data based on a given set of class boundaries.

3 Construct a histogram and ogive from a given frequency distribution table that is based on class boundaries.

The first job in grouping a set of interval data is to construct the class limits. Based on the class limits, one can then construct a frequency distribution table and an accompanying bar graph. Looking at the bar graph, one observes gaps between the bars (for example, see Figure 2.2.3). This gap has a width of u, the unit of measurement. The gap is not real but is an artifact of the precision with which human beings can make measurements; that is, there are members of the population that reside in the gaps, but human limitation in measurement leads to round-off, which places a member in one of the classes. The goal of this section is to remove the gaps.

Class Boundaries

To close the gaps between the classes in a fair and unbiased manner, extend each class limit by $u/2$, half a unit of measurement. Each lower limit is decreased by $u/2$, and each upper limit is increased by $u/2$. An extended class limit is called a **class boundary**. To construct the class boundaries, first construct the class limits, then extend each limit by $u/2$.

$$\text{Class boundary} = \text{class limit} \pm u/2$$

For example, the class boundaries for the Daily and Mersch room temperature cardiac output data (see Figure 2.1.2) are displayed in Table 2.3.1.

TABLE **2.3.1**
Class limits, boundaries, and marks for the Daily and Mersch room temperature cardiac output data set.

Class	Limits		Boundaries		Class Mark
	Lower	Upper	Lower	Upper	
1	2.60	3.41	2.595	3.415	3.005
2	3.42	4.23	3.415	4.235	3.825
3	4.24	5.05	4.235	5.055	4.645
4	5.06	5.87	5.055	5.875	5.465
5	5.88	6.69	5.875	6.695	6.285

Comment By utilizing boundaries instead of limits, the classes are still exhaustive and mutually exclusive. From a practical point of view, the classes are still exhaustive and mutually exclusive using boundaries since none of the sample data actually lies in a gap. From a technical point of view, only the lower boundary belongs to the class; a class extends from the lower boundary (inclusively) to the upper boundary (exclusively). Using boundaries is advantageous because the gaps are closed and the length of a class corresponds to the class width; that is,

$$\text{Class width} = \text{upper class boundary} - \text{lower class boundary}$$

The only disadvantage to class boundaries over class limits is the human inconvenience of needing one more place past the decimal point in identifying a class.

Frequency Distribution Table

A frequency distribution table based on class boundaries is exactly the same as it was for class limits with the single exception that one uses boundaries rather than limits to identify a class.

Table 2.3.2 displays the frequency distribution table based on class boundaries for the Daily and Mersch room temperature cardiac output data. The classes are defined by the boundaries given in the cardiac output column. The first class extends from 2.595 (inclusively) to 3.415 (exclusively).

In addition to the frequency distribution table, one can also construct a **cumulative frequency distribution table**. In a cumulative table one adds (cumulates) the class frequencies as one moves down the table. Table 2.3.3 displays the cumulative frequency distribution table for the Daily and Mersch cardiac output data. For the sake of illustration, for each class the table displays the class boundaries, frequency, cumulative frequency, cumulative relative frequency, and cumulative percent relative frequency.

TABLE 2.3.2

Frequency distribution table for the Daily and Mersch room temperature cardiac data set. The classes are defined by the class boundaries.

Cardiac Output (liters/minute)	Frequency	Relative Frequency
2.595–3.415	6	.21
3.415–4.235	7	.24
4.235–5.055	4	.14
5.055–5.875	8	.28
5.875–6.695	4	.14
Total	29	1.01*

*Deviation from 1.00 due to round-off error.

TABLE 2.3.3 Cumulative frequency distribution table for the Daily and Mersch room temperature cardiac output data set.

Cardiac Output (liters/minute)	Frequency	Cumulative Frequency	Cumulative Relative Frequency	Cumulative % Relative Frequency
2.595–3.415	6	6	.207	20.7
3.415–4.235	7	13	.448	44.8
4.235–5.055	4	17	.586	58.6
5.055–5.875	8	25	.862	86.2
5.875–6.695	4	29	1.000	100.0

Graphics

The term **histogram** usually applies to any bar graph constructed from a frequency distribution table based on class boundaries. Accordingly, one may construct a frequency, relative frequency, or percent relative frequency histogram. An **ogive** is a graphic that plots the cumulative frequency at each class boundary and then connects the dots with straight line segments. One may also construct a frequency, relative frequency, or percent relative frequency ogive.

Like the bar graphs constructed from a frequency distribution table (based on class limits), histograms are also presented vertically, captioned with labeled axes, with each class identified at the class mark. Figure 2.3.1 displays a percent relative frequency histogram for the Daily and Mersch cardiac output data.

An ogive is a graphic that displays the *cumulative* frequencies. The graph is constructed by plotting a point of the accumulated frequency over each class boundary. The first class boundary is plotted with a frequency of zero in order to anchor the graphic to the horizontal. The last class boundary must account for all of the data. Adjacent points are then joined by a straight line segment. The percent relative frequency ogive for the Daily and Mersch cardiac output data is displayed in Figure 2.3.2.

Note that an ogive is a curve that is *increasing* from left to right. The median can be estimated graphically by determining the horizontal value that corresponds to 50% relative frequency (about 4.5 for the cardiac output example).

FIGURE **2.3.1**
Percent relative frequency histogram for the Daily and Mersch room temperature cardiac output data set based on the class boundaries shown in the frequency distribution table displayed in Table 2.3.2.

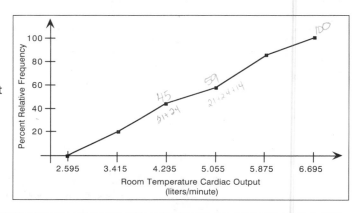

FIGURE **2.3.2**
Percent relative frequency ogive for the Daily and Mersch room temperature cardiac output data set based on the frequency distribution table displayed in Table 2.3.3.

We continue from Warm-ups 2.2. The final frequency distribution table for the Barcelona et al cardiac output data, prefilled syringes, iced temperature injectates, is displayed in Table 2.3.4.

TABLE **2.3.4** Frequency distribution table for the Barcelona et al cardiac output data, prefilled syringes, iced temperature injectates.

Class Limits		Frequency	Relative Frequency
Lower	Upper		
2.0	2.8	5	
2.9	3.7	16	
3.8	4.6	12	
4.7	5.5	4	
5.6	6.4	2	
6.5	7.3	2	
Total		41	

1. Fill in the relative frequency column.

2. The unit of measurement (u) for the sample data is
$u =$ _____.

3. To obtain the class boundaries, we extend each class limit by $u/2$. Here,

$u/2 =$ _____$/2 =$ _____.

4. The lower class boundaries are obtained by subtracting $u/2$ from each lower limit. The upper class boundaries are obtained by adding $u/2$ to each upper class limit. Complete Table 2.3.5.

TABLE 2.3.5 The class boundaries.

| Lower Class Boundary | Class Limits | | Upper Class Boundary |
	Lower	Upper	
1.95	2.0	2.8	2.85
2.85	2.9	3.7	3.75
	3.8	4.6	
	4.7	5.5	
	5.6	6.4	
	6.5	7.3	

5. Complete the frequency distribution table based on class boundaries as shown in Table 2.3.6.

TABLE 2.3.6 The frequency distribution table based on class boundaries.

| Class Boundaries | | Frequency | Relative Frequency |
Lower	Upper		
1.95	2.85		
2.85	3.75		
3.75			
4.65			
5.55			
6.45			
Total		41	

6. A bar graph depicting the frequency distribution table based on class boundaries rather than class limits has which one of the following features?

   a. It is more accurate.

   b. It is easier to understand.

   (c.) There are no gaps between classes.

   d. It is much easier to draw.

   e. The calculations are reduced.

7. In this text a bar graph depicting a frequency distribution table based on class boundaries is called:

   a. An ogive

   b. A polygon

   c. A class mark

   d. A chart

   (e.) A histogram

8. A histogram is a graphic depicting a frequency distribution table based on class boundaries. Each class is represented by a rectangle. The base of the rectangle is centered at the

   a. Lower class limit

   b. Upper class limit

   (c.) Class mark

   d. Lower class boundary

   e. Upper class boundary

9. In constructing a histogram, the base of each rectangle is labeled at the class mark, which is halfway between the class boundaries. The class mark is calculated by

Class mark = (lower class boundary + upper class boundary)/2

Hence, the class marks are calculated by

Class 1 mark = $(1.95 + 2.85)/2 = 4.80/2 = 2.40$

Class 2 mark = (____ + ____)/2 = ____/2 = ____

Class 3 mark = (____ + ____)/2 = ____/2 = ____

Class 4 mark = (____ + ____)/2 = ____/2 = ____

Class 5 mark = (____ + ____)/2 = ____/2 = ____

Class 6 mark = (____ + ____)/2 = ____/2 = ____

10. In constructing a histogram, the height of each rectangle corresponds to the class

   a. Frequency

   b. Relative frequency

   c. Percent relative frequency

   d. Any of the above

   e. None of the above

11. Label the tic marks on the horizontal and vertical axes for the percent relative frequency histogram displayed in Figure 2.3.3.

12. A cumulative frequency distribution table is obtained by adding (cumulating) the frequencies as one moves through the classes. Complete Table 2.3.7.

TABLE **2.3.7** Cumulative frequency distribution table.

Class Boundary		Frequency	Cumulative Frequency	Relative Frequency	Cumulative Relative Frequency	% Relative Frequency	Cumulative % Relative Frequency
Lower	Upper						
		5	5	.12	.12		12
		16	21	.39			
		12	33	.29			
		4	37	.10			
		2	39	.05			
		2	41	.05	1.00		100

FIGURE **2.3.3** Percent relative frequency histogram for the Barcelona et al cardiac output data.

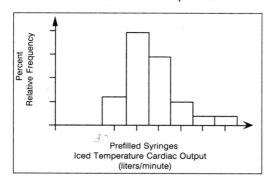

Prefilled Syringes
Iced Temperature Cardiac Output
(liters/minute)

13. The graphic obtained by plotting the cumulative frequency at each class boundary (from the lower boundary of the first class to the upper boundary of the last class) and joining adjacent points with a straight line is called

   a. An ogive

   b. A histogram

   c. A frequency polygon

   d. A bar graph

   e. A pie chart

14. The cumulative frequency at the lower boundary of the first class is always

   a. 0

   b. The class frequency

   c. The class relative frequency

   d. 100

   e. 1

15. The cumulative relative frequency at the upper boundary of the last class is always (use the same options as in Warm-up 14).

Problems 2.3

Problems 2.3.1–14 are continuations of Problems 2.2.1–14. For each of the following data sets, construct

   a. **A frequency distribution table based on class boundaries**

   b. **The corresponding frequency or percent relative frequency histogram**

   c. **The corresponding cumulative frequency table**

   d. **A percent relative frequency ogive**

1. The Daily and Mersch cardiac output study, iced temperature injectates (see Appendix, Data Set 1).

2. The Daily and Mersch cardiac output study, Fick method (see Appendix, Data Set 1).

3. The Barcelona et al cardiac output study (see Appendix, Data Set 2) for the Co-set system, Iced injectate (Co-Set column).

4. The Barcelona et al cardiac output study (see Appendix, Data Set 2) for the Co-set system, room temperature injectate.

5. The Daily and Mersch cardiac output study (see Appendix, Data Set 1) for the difference, room − Fick.

6. The Daily and Mersch cardiac output study (see Appendix, Data Set 1) for the difference, iced − Fick.

7. The Barcelona et al cardiac output study (see Appendix, Data Set 2), prefilled syringes, room temperature injectates.

8. The Barcelona et al cardiac output study (see Appendix, Data Set 2), prefilled syringes, for the difference, iced − room.

9. The Clark and Hoffer metabolism study (see Appendix, Data Set 6) for age.

10. The Clark and Hoffer metabolism study (see Appendix, Data Set 6) for height.

11. The Clark and Hoffer metabolism study (see Appendix, Data Set 6) for weight.

12. The Clark and Hoffer metabolism study (see Appendix, Data Set 6) for body mass index.

13. The Macey and Bouman age distribution data set (Table 2.2.10).

14. Jacobs et al reported the ages of 48 patients in their study:

```
28  30  23  31  33  17  41  21  49  29  35  61
49  21  32  22  50  37  28  25  40  55  12  32
20  28  40  47  30  18  35  52  19  33  24  31
30  41  22  43  38  21  56  25  27  36  31  32
```

CHAPTER 2 OVERVIEW

Summary

Statistical presentation and analysis of numerical data are driven by the context of the numbers making up a data set. There are three basic number contexts: nominal, ordinal, and interval. A **nominal** number names, an **ordinal** number ranks, and an **interval** number counts or measures.

Data sets made up of nominal and ordinal numbers basically are presented using the tools presented in Chapter 1. A presentation of an interval data set requires techniques that can illustrate the distribution of the data. A preliminary study of a data set focused on the distribution of the data is called **exploratory data analysis** (EDA). Some useful tools for EDA are **sort** and **dotplot, boxplot, stem-and-leaf** diagram, and **histogram**.

The **table method** describes a *quantitative* data set consisting of *interval* data. The key feature in this method is to **group** the data. Grouping should be done on an intuitive and commonsense level when making a presentation to a nontechnical audience. For a more technical audience, one should use a grouping method in keeping with the nature of the data. A good initial guide is to apply **Sturges's Rule** to determine the number of classes to be used in the grouping scheme.

The grouping protocol is guided by the desire to construct classes of equal width that span the given data set. A class begins at its lower **class limit** and ends at its upper class limit. The classes are exhaustive and mutually exclusive. One can then easily construct a frequency distribution table based on the class limits. To accompany the frequency distribution table, one may construct a frequency (relative frequency, percent relative frequency) **bar graph** or **polygon**.

Descriptive statistics for a quantitative data set consisting of interval numbers involves a fair amount of work.

The **distribution** of the data is a key factor to illustrate in presenting the data. To present the data, one displays a **frequency distribution table**. The essential ingredient in constructing the table is to **group** the data. One first groups the data by determining the **class limits**. The frequency distribution table based on class limits is really only an intermediate step. One finalizes the table by extending each class limit to a **class boundary**. The class boundaries serve to eliminate the gaps between classes and thus smoothes the presentation of the data.

Once one has constructed a frequency distribution table based on class boundaries, one constructs an accompanying graphic. The most common such graphics are the **histogram** and the **ogive**.

Keywords

adjusted minimum
adjusted range
bar graph
   frequency bar graph
   percent relative
      frequency bar graph
   relative frequency bar
     graph
boundary
   upper class boundary
   lower class boundary
boxplot
class
class limit
   lower class limit
   upper class limit
class mark
cumulative frequency

median
numbers
   interval
   nominal
   ordinal
ogive
polygon
   frequency polygon
   percent relative
     frequency polygon
   relative frequency
     polygon
quantitative data
range
raw data
sample size
sort
stem-and-leaf diagram

data set
distribution
exploratory data analysis
 (EDA)
frequency distribution
 table
histogram

Sturges's Rule
unit extended range
unit of measurement
width
limit
 lower class limit
 upper class limit

References

Barcelona M et al: Cardiac output determined by the thermodilution method: Comparison of ice temperature injectates versus room temperature injectates contained in prefilled syringes or a closed injectate delivery system. *Heart Lung* 14, no. 3 (May 1985): 232.

Clark H and Hoffer L: Reappraisal of the resting metabolic rate of normal young men. *Am J Clin Nutr* 53 (1991): 21.

Daily E and Mersch J: Thermodilution cardiac outputs using room and ice temperature injectate: Comparison with the Fick method. *Heart Lung* 16, no. 3 (May 1987): 294.

Jacobs L et al: Clinical and magnetic resonance imaging in optic neuritis. *Neurology* 41, no. 1 (January 1991): 15.

Macey B and Bouman C: An evaluation of validity, reliability, and readability of the Critical Care Family Needs Inventory. *Heart Lung* 20, no. 4 (July 1991): 398.

Sütsch G et al: Predictability of aortic dissection as a function of aortic diameter. *Eur Heart J* 12, no. 12 (December 1991): 1247.

Sturges H: The choice of a class interval, *J Am Stat Assoc* 21 (1926): 65.

Probability

In order to study a problem, one first defines a population and selects a random variable of interest. Study of the whole population is usually impossible due to time and resource constraints. Hence, one confines a study to a sample from the population. One studies the sample by collecting data about the random variable of interest from each member of the sample. Once the data are obtained, one presents the data in some informative way. The usual method for presenting data is the frequency distribution table.

The (percent) relative frequency column of a frequency distribution table deserves further attention. A relative frequency can be looked at from two points of view. From an initial descriptive point of view, a relative frequency describes how much of a given data set is attributable to a certain category or class. From a subsequent inferential point of view, a relative frequency acts as a probability in estimating the chance that a member from the population presented at random will have a certain characteristic or will fall in a certain class.

The initial motivation for constructing a frequency distribution table is to describe a given data set. Subsequently, one may apply the table to make administrative or forecasting decisions. These decisions are based on the relative frequencies viewed as probabilities. For example, Table 2.3.2 displays the frequency distribution table we constructed to describe the Daily and Mersch room temperature cardiac output data.

From an inferential point of view, a manager may view the relative frequencies to apply not just to the sample but to the population at large. One may order supplies or arrange staffing on the assumption that the distribution of patient acuity is reasonably approximated by the frequency distribution table. Reading the first two rows of Table 2.3.2, a manager may conjecture that about 45% of the patients in the coronary care unit have a cardiac output less than 4.2 and need more intensive surveillance.

Probability is the bridge that connects descriptive to inferential statistics. Probability is the foundation that supports our ability to draw valid and practical conclusions from a data set. Section 3.1 develops the basic orientation for probability, including basic vocabulary and a key computational rule (Fundamental Principle of Counting). Section 3.2 continues our development of the computational aspects of probability.

OBJECTIVES   This section will

1   Describe the three contexts of probability: theoretical, empirical, and subjective.

2   Describe the following terms: experiment, sample space, event.

3   Describe the following terms: probability (including the three formal properties of probability) and equiprobable space.

4   State and apply the Fundamental Principle of Counting to determine the size of the sample space of a multistage experiment.

The term *probability* covers a spectrum of meanings from the common and intuitive to the technical. We begin our orientation to probability with an intuitive description of the various contexts in which this term is used. Everyone has a day-to-day intuitive idea of probability learned from childhood games of chance (playing cards or rolling dice in a game of Monopoly) and from daily weather reports. The motivation behind the concept of probability is to be able to deal with chance *variation*.

Contexts of Probability

On an intuitive level, probability is a generic term that covers three contexts: theoretical (also called classical), empirical, and subjective.

Theoretical Probability

In general, a **theoretical probability** is computed on the basis of "theory," usually some intuitive idea of fairness. For example, we can assert that the chance of a heads showing on a toss of a fair coin is "50-50." This means that we are intuitively assigning the probability of heads showing on a toss of a fair coin as 50% (.5 in decimal form). This probability assignment is made from "common sense," even if a person has never flipped a coin.

EXAMPLE 3.1.1   For convenience, denote the probability of a certain occurrence by P[occurrence].

a. In a flip of a fair coin, P[heads] $= 1/2 = 0.5$ and P[tails] $= 1/2 = .5$.

b. In a random roll of a fair die, $P[2] = 1/6 = .17$.

c. In a random roll of a fair die, P[even] $=$ no. (even)/no. (die faces) $= 3/6 = .5$.

d. In drawing a card from a well-shuffled deck, P[spade] $=$ no. (spades)/no. (deck) $= 13/52 = .25$.

Empirical Probability

An **empirical probability** is based on data. The data are collected and summarized in the form of a frequency distribution table. The corresponding relative frequencies describe the proportions of the various observations in the study. When applied to the entire population of interest, a relative frequency may be viewed as an estimate of the probability that an individual selected at random will present a given attribute. An empirical probability is thus based on a relative frequency obtained as a result of a study.

EXAMPLE 3.1.2 Each of the following presents a set of empirical probabilities:

a. There are four ABO blood types: A, B, AB, and O. The ABO blood type of a U.S. resident drawn at random is given by:

$$P[A] = .41 \quad P[AB] = .04$$
$$P[B] = .09 \quad P[O] = .46$$

b. There are two Rh blood types: Rh+ and Rh−. The Rh blood type of a U.S. resident drawn at random is given by:

$$P[Rh+] = .85 \text{ and } P[Rh-] = .15$$

c. Table 3.1.1 displays a frequency distribution table for room temperature cardiac outputs based on the Daily and Mersch study.

TABLE **3.1.1**
Room temperature cardiac output.

Cardiac Output (liters/minute)	Frequency	Relative Frequency
2.60–3.41	6	.21
3.42–4.23	7	.24
4.24–5.05	4	.14
5.06–5.87	8	.28
5.88–6.69	4	.14
Total	29	1.01*

*Deviation from 1.00 due to round-off error.

Hence, based on this study, the probability that a randomly selected cardiac patient has a cardiac output between 3.4 and 4.2 liters per minute is about 24%.

A frequency distribution table plays the important role of acting as a bridge from which the results of a research study may be transported to the population at large. Inferential statistics (covered later) will allow us to assess how much confidence we can place in such transport.

Subjective Probability

A **subjective probability** is based on a person's guess (sometimes educated). A subjective probability may be issued as a way to describe how a person feels about something. Evidence in support of a subjective probability often is only circumstantial.

EXAMPLE 3.1.3 A subjective probability is a personal assessment of an individual opinion about some matter.

    a. $P[$nuclear war by 2000$] = .03 = 3\%$.

    b. A nurse or doctor may need to exhibit a subjective probability in dealing with a seriously injured person (or the family) in critical or emergency settings. A common question is, What are my chances of survival (or recovery)? The answer to such a question is often a subjective probability based on a mixture of a feeling for the situation and the practitioner's own personal experience. In such situations, a probability is often offered in a general verbal sense like "good" or "critical," rather than being given as a specific number.

In the future, we will not consider subjective probabilities, but only consider theoretical or empirical probabilities.

Basic Vocabulary

We continue our orientation to probability with a presentation of the basic vocabulary of the subject. The concepts of experiment, sample space, and event are central for our general understanding. These concepts should be learned together as an integrated package.

Experiment and Sample Space

An **experiment** is a procedure that produces an outcome. The **sample space** of a given experiment is the list of all possible outcomes for the experiment. What makes an experiment interesting from a statistical perspective is not only that does one not know the outcome in advance but that the outcome can vary as the experiment is repeated. Again, *variation* is the key source of interest and problems.

EXAMPLE 3.1.4 Each of the following illustrations describes an experiment and displays its sample space, the set of all possible outcomes to the experiment.

    a. Experiment: toss a coin
        Sample space: heads, tails

    b. Experiment: roll a die
        Sample space: 1, 2, 3, 4, 5, 6

    c. Experiment: obtain a patient's ABO blood type
        Sample space: A, AB, B, O

d. Experiment: obtain a patient's Rh blood type
Sample space: Rh+ , Rh−

e. Experiment: have three children
Sample space: GGG, GGB, GBG, BGG, GBB, BGB, BBG, BBB

In studying the illustrations in Example 3.1.4, one senses that there is something more complex about Example 3.1.4e in comparison with Example 3.1.4a–d. Example 3.1.4e, the experiment of having three children, is an example of a multistage experiment. A **multi-stage experiment** may be considered as a sequence of component experiments. A component in a multistage experiment is called a **stage**.

A **simple experiment** (also called a **trial**) is an experiment that cannot be broken down any further into a sequence of other experiments. One is reminded here of the analogy between molecules and atoms in chemistry (multistage is to simple as molecule is to atom). Example 3.1.4a–d illustrates simple experiments.

EXAMPLE 3.1.5 The experiment of having three children is formalized as a multistage experiment as follows. We first note that the experiment may be considered as a sequence of three stages, where each stage is the simple experiment of having one child. The simple experiment is formally defined by

Simple experiment: have one child
Sample space: girl, boy

The multistage experiment of having three children is now easily visualized as an experiment consisting of a sequence of three successive simple experiments. Hence, the experiment of having three children may be viewed as a three-stage experiment.

One illustrates the sample space of a multistage experiment with a **tree diagram**, which portrays the outcome for each stage separately as a branch on a tree. A tree diagram for the experiment of having three children is displayed in Figure 3.1.1.

At the "Start:" the tree has a branch for each option in the first stage of the multistage experiment (here, G = girl and B = boy). For each possible outcome in the first stage, the tree branches again to display the possible outcomes for the second stage, and so forth. By tracing through a branch of the tree, one obtains one of the possible outcomes for the multistage experiment. By tracing through all possible

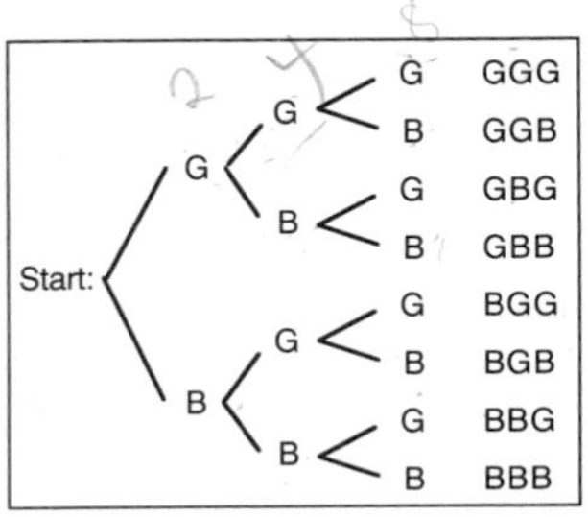

FIGURE 3.1.1
Tree diagram representing the experiment of having three children. Each branching stage represents the simple experiment of having one child. At the "Start:" the first child could be either a girl (G) or a boy (B). Similarly, the second child could be either one of the same two options, G or B; then the third child. Tracing through each possible branch produces the sample space with its eight possibilities for the makeup of a family with three children.

```
                              G    GGG
                        G  <
                   G  <      B    GGB
                        B  <  G    GBG
                              B    GBB
Start: <
                        G  <  G    BGG
                   B  <       B    BGB
                        B  <  G    BBG
                              B    BBB
```

branches, one obtains the sample space (the complete list of outcomes) for the multistage experiment. In Figure 3.1.1 the sample space consisting of the eight outcomes for the makeup of a family with three children is listed to the right of the tree.

Event

An **event** is a subset of a sample space. Frequently, an event is obtained merely by inspection. One obtains the sample space for some experiment of interest. Then, from the outcomes in the sample space, one makes a list of those outcomes meeting some criterion of interest.

EXAMPLE 3.1.6 This example depicts three events for having a family of three children.

The event E of having at least one girl in a family of three children:

E = {GGG, GGB, GBG, GBB, BGG, BGB, BBG}.

The event F of having at least two boys in a family of three children:

F = {GBB, BGB, BBG, BBB}.

The event H of having at least two girls in a family of three children:

H = {GGG, GGB, GBG, BGG}.

Two events are **mutually exclusive** if none of the outcomes in one event occur in the other event. For example, in drawing a card from a deck, the events ace and face card are mutually exclusive. In Example 3.1.6 the events F and H are mutually exclusive; however, events E and F are not mutually exclusive (GBB is an outcome in common to both E and F).

The **complement** of an event is the set of all outcomes that do not occur in it. For example, the complement of the event face card is the set of all cards that are not face cards. The complement of an event E is denoted by E'.

EXAMPLE 3.1.7 Using the events E, F, and H from Example 3.1.6,

E' = {BBB}
F' = {GGG, GGB, GBG, BGG}
H' = {GBB, BGB, BBG, BBB}

Note that given any event A, an outcome must either belong to A or not belong to A. If the outcome does not belong to A, then it belongs to the complement of A. Hence, A and A' form an exhaustive and mutually exclusive list of events for the outcomes in the experiment. In general, if a list of events is **exhaustive**, any given outcome from the sample space must belong to at least one of the events on the list.

Formal Probability

At the beginning of this section we presented the three general contexts for probability. In addition to these intuitive ideas, probability is a formal subject in its own right. At first the technical definition of formal probability does not seem promising. However, it will help when we get to the computational aspects of probability.

Let S be a sample space of a given experiment. Formally, a **probability** is a rule that assigns a number to the events in S in such a way that the following three properties hold:

1. $P[S] = 1$, (100% or 1)
2. $0 \leq P[E] \leq 1$ for any event E in S,
3. $P[A \text{ or } B] = P[A] + P[B]$ for any mutually exclusive events A and B of S.

Note that the formal definition of a probability only gives three *properties* that a probability must have. The definition does not explain how to determine the probabilities; that is, it does not spell out how numbers (probabilities) are to be assigned to events. Despite this apparent shortcoming, this definition is informative.

Formal probability may be thought of as a ruler that measures the likelihood of an event (Figure 3.1.2). The probability of an event is always a number between 0 and 1 (rule 2). An event with probability 0 is said to be impossible since it will not occur. An event with probability 1 is said to be a sure event because it will occur (rule 1). If a probability is less than .5, it is more unlikely to occur than it is likely to occur. An event with a probability greater than .5 is more likely than unlikely to occur. An event with a probability of .5 is just as likely to occur as not. An event with a probability of .9 is likely; with probability .1, unlikely.

The simplest situation in which the assignment of probabilities can be made is an experiment that results in an equiprobable space. The sample space of a given experiment is an **equiprobable space** if each outcome in the sample space has an equal chance of occurring. Hence, if the sample space is of size n, then the probability of any particular outcome is $1/n$; that is,

$P[x] = \frac{1}{n}$ for each outcome x

Further, if A is any event (set of outcomes) in an equiprobable space S, then $P[A]$ = no. A/no. S; that is,

$$P[A] = \frac{\text{number of outcomes in the event A}}{\text{number of outcomes in the sample space } S}$$

EXAMPLE 3.1.8 Draw a card at random from a well-shuffled standard deck of 52 cards. Each card has an equal chance of being drawn. The deck is an equiprobable space.

$P[\text{7 of diamonds}] = 1/52 = .019$
$P[\text{ace}] = 4/52 = .077$
$P[\text{face card}] = 12/52 = .231$
$P[\text{spade}] = 13/52 = .25$

FIGURE **3.1.2**
A formal probability ruler.

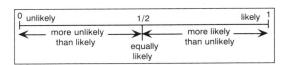

EXAMPLE 3.1.9 Cystic fibrosis (CF) is an example of a genetically inherited double recessive disease. At a given gene locus, an individual may have a dominant gene A or a recessive gene a. A person with a genetic makeup of AA is healthy (with respect to CF) and is not a carrier. A person with a genetic makeup of Aa or aA is physically healthy (no CF) but is a carrier for the disease. A person of genetic makeup aa develops CF. Suppose that two healthy, but carrier, parents have a child. They are interested in the probability of having a healthy child. The experiment here is having a child. This experiment may be viewed as a two-stage experiment with

> Stage 1: inherit a gene from mother
> Stage 2: inherit a gene from father

The sample space for this two-stage experiment consists of all possible genotypes for the child. To determine the sample space, we construct a tree diagram as shown in Figure 3.1.3.

The laws of Mendelian genetics infer that the tree shown in Figure 3.1.3 depicts an equiprobable space; that is, each genotype has an equal probability of being selected. Hence,

P[healthy child] $= 3/4 = .75$ AA, Aa, aA, aa
P[cystic fibrosis child] $= 1/4 = .25$
P[healthy, noncarrier child] $= 1/4 = .25$
P[healthy, carrier child] $= 2/4 = .5$

The Fundamental Principle of Counting

As the size of a multistage experiment increases, constructing a tree becomes more complex. If the number of stages is beyond three or the number of stage options is large, then the tree can have so many branches that the informative nature of the display is lost. However, we will still need to know at least how many branches there are in the tree (i.e., the size of the sample space). Fortunately, the **Fundamental Principle of Counting** lets us determine the size of a multistage experiment in an easy fashion.

FIGURE 3.1.3
Tree diagram for the genetic makeup of a child whose parents are healthy but carry cystic fibrosis. The dominant healthy gene is denoted by A. The recessive cystic fibrosis gene is denoted by a.

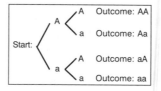

Fundamental Principle of Counting

Suppose an experiment is conducted in k stages. Suppose stage 1 can occur in n_1 ways; stage 2 in n_2 ways; . . . ; stage k in n_k ways. Then the number N of possible outcomes for the multistage experiment is given by

$$N = n_1 \times n_2 \times \ldots \times n_k$$

Situations that show the utility of the Fundamental Principle of Counting include computing the size of the sample space of: automobile license plates, codons (see Problem 3.1.4) making up the genetic triplet code, flip one coin and roll one die, roll two dice, have three children. Of course, one can obtain the size of the sample space for a multistage experiment by constructing a tree. But if the experiment has many stages, or the stages have a large number of options, a tree not only is unwieldy but may be mind-boggling rather than informative. The Fundamental Principle of Counting lets us count the number of outcomes in the sample space without having to make a list of the outcomes.

To apply the Fundamental Principle of Counting, we first must recognize the multistage experiment. Accordingly, portray the experiment by drawing a set of blank lines, one short line for each stage in the multistage experiment:

$$\text{Stage } \overline{}_{1} \ \overline{}_{2} \ \overline{}_{3} \cdots \overline{}_{k}$$

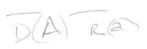

We now envision the experiment being completed stage by stage. First count the number n_1 of ways that stage 1 can be completed, then count the number n_2 of ways that stage 2 can be completed, and so forth; finally, count the number of ways n_k that stage k can be completed. One then computes the size of the sample space for the full k-stage experiment by applying the Fundamental Principle of Counting:

$$N = n_1 \times n_2 \times \ldots \times n_k$$

EXAMPLE 3.1.10 We reconsider the experiment of a couple having a family of three children. To obtain the size of the sample space without constructing the tree, we first portray the three-stage experiment:

$$\overline{\text{child 1}} \ \ \overline{\text{child 2}} \ \ \overline{\text{child 3}}$$

Now in each blank enter the number of different genders that each child can assume (obviously two in each case, either girl or boy):

$$\underset{\text{child 1}}{2} \ \ \underset{\text{child 2}}{2} \ \ \underset{\text{child 3}}{2}$$

Applying the Fundamental Principle of Counting yields $N = 2 \times 2 \times 2 = 8$. Hence, the size of the sample space is 8.

EXAMPLE 3.1.11 Consider the experiment of rolling one die and flipping one coin. How many possible outcomes are there? That is, what is the size of the sample space for this two-stage experiment? First indicate the two stages:

$$\overline{\text{die}} \ \overline{\text{coin}}$$

Now enter the number of outcomes for each stage:

$$\frac{6}{\text{die}} \ \frac{2}{\text{coin}}$$

Applying the Fundamental Principle of Counting yields $N = 6 \times 2 = 12$.

EXAMPLE 3.1.12 At a certain university there are 184 health science students in which there are 63 premajors, 12 freshman majors, 27 sophomore majors, 44 junior majors, and 38 senior majors. A committee of the Student Health Sciences Association is to be made up of one student from each group. How many possibilities are there? Note that this is a five-stage experiment.

$$\overline{\text{premajor}} \ \overline{\text{freshman}} \ \overline{\text{sophomore}} \ \overline{\text{junior}} \ \overline{\text{senior}}$$

Now enter the number of choices for each stage:

$$\frac{63}{\text{premajor}} \ \frac{12}{\text{freshman}} \ \frac{27}{\text{sophomore}} \ \frac{44}{\text{junior}} \ \frac{38}{\text{senior}}$$

Applying the Fundamental Principle of Counting,

$$N = 63 \times 12 \times 27 \times 44 \times 38 = 34,128,864$$

No wonder group representation can be quite complex!

Comment The previous Example 3.1.12 generalizes as follows: Suppose that S is a set that contains n elements. In S, there are n_1 objects of type 1, n_2 objects of type 2, . . . , and n_k objects of type k. Now suppose that you want to select exactly one member of each type in S. In how many ways can this be done? Imitating the solution displayed in Example 3.1.12 yields $N = n_1 \times n_2 \times \ldots \times n_k$.

EXERCISES 3.1

Warm-ups 3.1

1. The probability that a head will show up on a toss of a fair coin is 50%. This is an example of

   a. A subjective probability

   b. An empirical probability

   c. A theoretical probability

   d. A relative frequency

   e. A sample space

2. Based on the Daily and Mersch room temperature data, about 65% of cardiac patients have a cardiac output less than 5 liters/minute. Based on this study, one estimates that the probability that the next admitted patient has a cardiac output under 5 liters/ minute is about 65%. This is an example of (use the same options as in Warm-up 1).

3. An experiment is a procedure that produces an outcome. The list of all possible outcomes that can be produced by the experiment is called

   a. An event
   b. A probability
   c. A tree diagram
   d. The sample space
   e. The Fundamental Principle of Counting

4. An example of a multistage experiment is

   a. Blood type five patients
   b. Assess the alertness status (awake, disoriented, asleep, comatose) of 3 patients
   c. Determine the immunization of 20 elderly patients given a flu shot
   d. Determine the discharge status (remain, to home, another care facility) of 4 patients
   e. All of the above

Warm-ups 5–10 relate to the graphic shown in Figure 3.1.4.

5. The graphic depicts the immunization status of three patients who are given a flu shot. As a result of the shot, the patient was successfully immunized (V, for vaccination) against the flu or failed (F) to become immunized. The graphic depicting the experiment is called

   a. A tree diagram
   b. A histogram
   c. A line diagram
   d. A boxplot
   e. A polygon

FIGURE **3.1.4**
Graphic for Warm-ups 3.1.5–10.

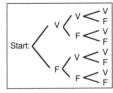

6. One purpose of a tree is that one can construct the sample space for a given multistage experiment. List the eight outcomes in the sample space generated by the tree.

7. A list of outcomes (i.e., a subset) taken from a sample space is called

   a. A complement
   b. An event
   c. A probability
   d. Combinatorics
   e. A tree diagram

8. List the outcomes in each of the following events:

   a. Everyone is immunized: ____
   b. No one is immunized: ____
   c. At least two people are immunized: ____, ____, ____, ____
   d. At most two people are immunized: ____, ____, ____, ____, ____, ____, ____
   e. Exactly two people are immunized: ____, ____, ____

9. The event E "exactly one person is immunized" is given by E = {VFF, FVF, FFV}. The complement (E′) of E is given by

   E′ = {____, ____, ____, ____, ____}

10. The size of the sample space can be computed by using the following scheme (pt means patient):

    $$\frac{2}{1^{st}\ pt} \times \frac{2}{1^{st}\ pt} \times \frac{2}{1^{st}\ pt}\ .$$

    So, $N = 2 \times 2 \times 2 = 8$.

    This is an illustration of

    a. A tree diagram
    b. The Fundamental Principle of Counting
    c. An event
    d. A probability
    e. Descriptive statistics

11. What would be the size of the sample space if you wanted to determine the immunization status of five patients who are given a flu shot?

    $N = 5.$
    $\overline{2}$

Problems 3.1

1. In General Hospital there are 26 medical-surgical nurses, 12 intensive care nurses, 16 emergency room nurses, and 43 floor care nurses. A committee is to be formed that consists of four nurses, one from each of these areas. How many such committees are possible?

2. A family has four children.

   a. Identifying each child by gender only, construct a tree displaying the birth order of the children. Display the sample space.

   b. List the sample points in each of the following events.

   A: The first child is a girl.
   B: The oldest and youngest children are girls.
   C: Exactly two of the four children are girls.
   D: Exactly one of the four children is a girl.
   E: Two are boys and three are girls.
   F: All of the children are girls.

   c. Determine the size of the sample space by applying the Fundamental Principle of Counting.

   d. Assuming that each gender is equiprobable, determine the probability of each event listed in (b).

3. Suppose we define a blood profile as a report that states both the ABO and Rh blood types.

   a. Construct a tree that displays all the various blood profiles. The tree should be based on the ABO phenotypes A, B, AB, and O, and on the Rh phenotypes Rh+ and Rh−. Exhibit the sample space.

   b. Compute the number of profiles by applying the Fundamental Principle of Counting.

4. In the RNA genetic code, a codon is a three-letter "word" written from the four-letter RNA "alphabet." Each letter represents one of the four ribonucleotides: U (uracil), A (adenine), G (guanine), and C (cytosine). Each codon represents one of the 20 amino acids or "stop." For example, ACG is the codon for the amino acid threonine; UUU, phenylalanine; UAG, stop. Protein synthesis begins by linking a series of these proteins together until a stop is encountered.

   a. How many RNA codons are there?

   b. Of the possible RNA codons, 61 are known to code for the 20 amino acids; the others code for stop. How many codons code for stop?

   c. A codon codes for the amino acid valine if and only if the codon starts with GU. How many equivalent codons are there for valine?

   d. There are six synonyms for arginine, six for leucine, four for valine, three for isoleucine, and two for lysine. How many different but equivalent ways can one code the chain "arginine–leucine–valine–isoleucine–lysine"?

   e. Suppose that the four ribonucleotides are equally abundant and that the placement of a given ribonucleotide is random and equally likely.

      i. What is the probability that a randomly formed codon will begin with G or U and end with A or C?

      ii. What is the probability that a randomly formed codon will begin with U, end with C, and have no repetitions?

      iii. Construct a tree diagram representing all codons that can be formed beginning with A or C and ending with U. Give the sample points of all codons in this event. What is the probability that such a codon will be formed?

   f. How many codons contain three different letters?

   g. How many codons contain at least two identical letters?

5. Isner reported on 492 patients enrolled in the Mansfield Scientific Aortic Valvuloplasty Registry who underwent balloon aortic valvuloplasty. The procedure was uncomplicated in 391 patients; complications occurred in 101 patients. The complications were catastrophic (resulting in death or leg amputation) in 31 patients. Based on the given data,

   a. What is the probability that a patient who undergoes balloon aortic valvuloplasty

      i. Will suffer a complication?
      ii. Will suffer a catastrophic complication?

   b. What is the probability that a complication will be catastrophic?

6. Consider the cystic fibrosis example (Example 3.1.9). Suppose a healthy noncarrier (AA) woman has a child with a healthy carrier (Aa) man. What is the probability that the child will

a. Have cystic fibrosis?

b. Carry cystic fibrosis?

c. Not have cystic fibrosis but carry the disease?

d. Not carry cystic fibrosis?

e. Not have cystic fibrosis?

7. The regular hospital patient menu lists choices as follows (patients just circle their choices). A patient selects exactly one item from each food category:

Beverage: none, coffee, tea, milk, juice
Salad: none, lettuce, fruit cup
Entree: none, chicken, beef, fish
Potato: none, baked, mashed
Vegetable: none, carrots, beans
Dessert: none, ice cream, cake, pie

How many different patient meals can be served based on these choices?

SECTION 3.2	OBJECTIVES	This section will describe and apply the
Combinatorics	**1**	Subset Rule
	2	Complement Rule
	3	Multiplication Rule when given a probability tree diagram or a frequency distribution tree diagram
	4	Independence Rule

Section 3.1 introduced the Fundamental Principle of Counting, which is useful for determining the size of a multistage experiment and eliminates the drudgery of having to make a tree diagram for a large multistage experiment. This section is devoted to some further computational aspects of counting and probability.

In Objective 1 we introduce a counting rule for solving a subset problem. As a preliminary, we first review the factorial concept, a computational notation from algebra. The formal study of counting procedures is called **combinatorics**.

Objectives 2–4 introduce computational aspects of complex probability. Complex here does not mean difficult. A complex event is an event composed of simpler parts. If one knows the probability for simple events, then one should be able to exploit those known probabilities to determine the probability of an event made up of those simple parts. In that spirit we present the Complement Rule, the Multiplication Rule, and the Independence Rule.

Prerequisite Skills

Combinatorics is the formal study of counting procedures. Combinatorics contain timesaving devices for calculating the size of a sample space in several common situations. One device is factorial, which appears on several scientific calculators as the $x!$ button. This device is used in another calculation called a combination (the

Cn,x or nCx button on a scientific calculator). We now present the factorial and combination concepts.

Factorial

As a preview to the concept of factorial, consider the calculations applied in the following example.

EXAMPLE 3.2.1 Consider a psychiatric ward in which there are five patients who need one-on-one care. On a given day, five staff are called for this duty. In how may ways can the staff assignment be made? To answer this question, we view the situation in terms of the Fundamental Principle of Counting. We first draw a line for each patient:

$$\underline{\hspace{1.5cm}}\quad\underline{\hspace{1.5cm}}\quad\underline{\hspace{1.5cm}}\quad\underline{\hspace{1.5cm}}\quad\underline{\hspace{1.5cm}}$$
patient 1 patient 2 patient 3 patient 4 patient 5

We view the staff assignment for an individual patient as a stage. The Fundamental Principle of Counting directs us to count the number of ways we can accomplish each individual stage. The first stage is to assign a staff member to patient 1. This can be done in five ways. Next, we have four staff left from which we can make the assignment for patient 2. Continuing, the staff assignment for each patient, stage by stage, is counted by

$$\underbrace{5}_{\text{patient 1}}\quad\underbrace{4}_{\text{patient 2}}\quad\underbrace{3}_{\text{patient 3}}\quad\underbrace{2}_{\text{patient 4}}\quad\underbrace{1}_{\text{patient 5}}$$

Applying the Fundamental Principle of Counting, the total number N of ways the patient assignment could be made is

$$N = 5 \times 4 \times 3 \times 2 \times 1 = 120$$

A problem like Example 3.2.1 occurs whenever we have n objects for which we want to make a one-to-one assignment. Applying the Fundamental Principle of Counting, the assignments can be visualized in stages as follows:

$$\underbrace{n}_{\text{object 1}}\quad\underbrace{n-1}_{\text{object 2}}\quad\underbrace{n-2}_{\text{object 3}}\cdots\underbrace{1}_{\text{object } n}$$

Hence, the number of ways the assignment can be made is $N = n \times (n - 1) \times \ldots \times 2 \times 1$.

This calculation is performed sufficiently often that it is formalized as the **factorial**: n-factorial is the product obtained by multiplying the whole numbers from n down to 1. The number n-factorial is denoted by $n!$.

DEFINITION ▌▌▌ Factorial

$n! = n \times (n - 1) \times \ldots \times 2 \times 1$ for any natural number n
$0! = 1$
The symbol $n!$ is read "n-factorial."

EXAMPLE 3.2.2 We illustrate some factorial computations:

   a. $5! = 5 \times 4 \times 3 \times 2 \times 1 = 120$

   b. $4! = 4 \times 3 \times 2 \times 1 = 24$

   c. $3! = 3 \times 2 \times 1 = 6$

   d. $2! = 2 \times 1 = 2$

   e. $1! = 1$

   f. $0! = 1$ (by definition)

Comment If you have a scientific calculator, locate the $x!$ button. Enter 5, then depress the $x!$ button. The display window will show 120.

Note that for any natural number $n, n! = n \times (n-1)!$. This property of factorial is particularly useful for calculating factorials involving large numbers. We will colloquially refer to this property of factorial as "unraveling." Applying it is much like peeling an onion one layer at a time.

EXAMPLE 3.2.3 We illustrate the property $n! = n \times (n-1)!$ by "unraveling" 52! one step at a time for three steps.

$$52! = 52 \times 51!$$
$$= 52 \times 51 \times 50!$$
$$= 52 \times 51 \times 50 \times 49! \text{ etc.}$$

Combination

The factorial tool is used in defining another computational device called the **combination** of n and k and formally defined as follows.

DEFINITION ▮▮▮ Combination

Suppose n and k are whole numbers where $k \leq n$.

Then, $C(n,k) = \dfrac{n!}{k! \times (n-k)!}$

The symbol $C(n,k)$ is called the combination of n and k.

At this time it is totally unclear why any sane person would want to perform such a calculation. For the moment we ask the reader's indulgence and merely focus on the skill of calculating the combination. We will apply this skill soon, however, in solving the fundamental subset problem.

EXAMPLE 3.2.4 We illustrate the combination formula. The illustration shows how to calculate a combination by hand using the "unravel" technique displayed in Example 3.2.3.

   a. $C(8,5) = \dfrac{8!}{5! \times (8-5)!}$ applying the definition of combination

   $\quad\quad\quad = \dfrac{8!}{5! \times 3!}$ simplifying: $8 - 5 = 3$

$$= \frac{8 \times 7 \times 6 \times 5!}{5! \times 3!}$$

"unravel" the numerator factorial until it matches, the larger factorial in the denominator The 5! in the numerator cancels the 5! in the denominator. Then write out the factors in 3!.

$$= \frac{8 \times 7 \times 6}{3 \times 2 \times 1}$$

cancel common factors

$$= 8 \times 7$$

$$= 56$$

b. $C(52,5) = \frac{52!}{5! \times 47!}$

$$= \frac{52 \times 51 \times 50 \times 49 \times 48 \times 47!}{5! \times 47!}$$

$$= \frac{52 \times 51 \times 50 \times 49 \times 48}{5 \times 4 \times 3 \times 2 \times 1}$$

$$= 52 \times 51 \times 10 \times 49 \times 2$$

$$= 2{,}598{,}960$$

c. $C(5,0) = \frac{5!}{0! \times 5!} = \frac{5!}{1 \times 5!} = \frac{5!}{5!} = 1$

Comment By applying "unravel and cancel" (as illustrated in Example 3.2.4a and b), the denominator in the original combination fraction will always completely cancel out. Hence, the answer to a combination calculation will always be a whole number. Also note that by canceling you avoid a great deal of unnecessary arithmetic.

In order to calculate by hand a combination involving a large number, apply the unravel and cancel technique. This technique minimizes the arithmetic one must perform. In Example 3.2.4b we were spared the frightening task of determining 52! by hand (now, that's a relief).

For convenience, Table 1 (Appendix) gives values of $C(n, k)$ for $n = 2$ through $n = 20$ and $k = 2$ through $k = 10$. If $n > 20$, you either will need a calculator having a combination button (often keyed Cn, x or nCx; some calculators use y instead of n) or will need to be able to calculate the quantity by hand with the unravel and cancel technique.

The Subset Problem

We now have all the computational tools needed to solve an important type of counting problem called the subset problem. Examples of the subset problem include the following:

How many poker hands are there?
How many possibilities are there for California 6/49 Lotto?
How many committees of four people can I appoint from a staff of 12 volunteers?
How many ways can I assign three patients from a ward of eight to a staff nurse?

The two key ingredients in each of these questions are (1) an original pool of a certain number of objects and (2) a need to withdraw a given number of members from the pool. The common question throughout is, In how many ways can I accomplish the task? We reformulate the previous four questions to indicate the subset problem by explicitly indicating the two key ingredients.

In how many ways can I extract a hand of 5 cards from a standard deck of 52 cards?

In how many ways can I pick 6 different numbers from a list of 49 whole numbers (the list contains the numbers from 1 to 49, inclusive)?

In how many ways can I appoint 4 people from a staff of 12 volunteers?

In how many ways can I select 3 patients from a ward of 8 patients?

In general, the subset problem asks, In how many ways can I select a subset of k objects from a given pool of n objects? The answer is simply $C(n, k)$, the combination of n and k. Our concern will be with *applying* this fact, not in mathematically deriving it.

The Subset Problem

Problem In how many ways can I select a subset of k objects from a given pool of n objects?

Solution $C(n,k) = \frac{n!}{k! \times (n-k)!}$

EXAMPLE 3.2.5 How many distinct poker hands can be dealt from a standard deck of 52 cards? The solution is $C(52, 5)$. From Example 3.2.4b, this calculates to 2,598,960. With all these possibilities, no wonder poker is a game of chance.

EXAMPLE 3.2.6 How many possibilities are there for California 6/49 Lotto? The solution is $C(49, 6) = 13,983,816$ (we leave the computational details as an exercise). Hence, your chances of winning the grand prize by picking the single correct six number combination in 6/49 Lotto is 1 in 13,983,816. We recommend you save your money, unless you want to purchase a dollar's worth of fantasy.

EXAMPLE 3.2.7 How many committees of four can I pick from a staff of 12 volunteers? Solution: $C(12,4) = 495$ (Appendix, Table 1, $n = 12$, $k = 4$).

EXAMPLE 3.2.8 How many ways can I assign three patients in a ward of eight patients to a staff nurse? Solution: $C(8,3) = 56$ (Appendix, Table 1, $n = 8$, $k = 3$).

The Complement Rule

The Complement Rule merely says that once we know the probability of an event happening, we also know (by a simple calculation) the probability of that event not happening. If there is a 30% chance of rain tomorrow, then there is a 70% chance of it not raining. Everyone has applied this rule in ordinary life. The only thing we are really adding here is a formal name for the rule.

EXAMPLE 3.2.9 Suppose we assess the probability that a patient will survive a surgical procedure as 80%. Along with this comes the implied assessment that the probability the patient will not survive the surgery is 20%.

Recall that an event E is merely a subset of the sample space. Hence, an event is a list of outcomes of interest from some point of view. A natural accompaniment to any list of outcomes is the companion list of outcomes that are not on the original list. The list of outcomes not specified in an event E is called the **complement** of E. Hence, any sample space splits into two pieces: the outcomes in the given event E and the outcomes E' not in the given event E.

The **Complement Rule** formally says that if the probability of an event is known, then the probability of the complement event is calculated by

$$P[\text{complement of an event}] = 1 - P[\text{event}]$$

EXAMPLE 3.2.10

$$
\begin{aligned}
P[\text{not face card}] &= 1 - P[\text{face card}] \\
&= 1 - 12/52 \\
&= 40/52 \\
&= .77 \text{ or } 77\%
\end{aligned}
$$

The essentials of the Complement Rule are summarized in the following box:

The Complement Rule

Description The probability of the complement of an event is 1 minus the probability of the event.

Formula Let E' be the complement of the event E.
Then, $P[E'] = 1 - P[E]$

Multiplication Rule for Probability

The multiplication rule for probability is the tool needed to compute a probability for an outcome to a multistage experiment. For illustration, we consider the following "Let's Make a Deal" two-stage game. Three prizes are shown to a contestant: a new car (C), a new mountain bike (B), and a jewelry box (J). Each prize is locked. In the first stage of the game, one draws a ticket from a prize box containing six tickets: C, B, B, J, J, and J. In the second stage of the game, the contestant chooses one from among five keys on a panel next to the prize. On the key panel for the car, only one key opens the car while the other four keys are duds. On the bike panel, two keys will open the bike lock while the other three keys are duds. On the jewelry box panel, three keys will open the box while the other two keys are duds. A contestant wins the prize if the key chosen opens the prize. We inquire, What are the chances of winning a prize? What is the probability of winning the car?

To answer questions about the probability for a multistage experiment, first construct a tree diagram for the experiment. The individual outcomes for the multistage experiment are obtained by tracing through the possible branches of the tree from the "Start:". Hence, the tree diagram is useful for displaying the sample space for the experiment. The tree diagram for Let's Make a Deal is displayed in Figure 3.2.1.

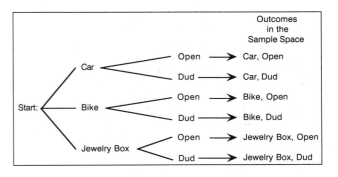

FIGURE **3.2.1**
Tree diagram and
sample space for Let's
Make a Deal.

We now consider the project of assigning probabilities to each outcome in the sample space. To complete the project, we need to develop the tree diagram further. We enhance the tree diagram by displaying the probability for each outcome at each stage. In Let's Make a Deal, we first draw a ticket from the prize box containing six tickets: C, B, B, J, J, and J. The three possible prizes (outcomes) are the car (C), bike (B), and jewelry box (J). The probability that we draw the car ticket is 1/6; a bike ticket, 2/6; and a jewelry box ticket, 3/6. Enter these first-stage probabilities on the tree diagram (Figure 3.2.2).

Once the first-stage probabilities are entered onto the tree diagram, compute and enter the second-stage probabilities. To enter the second-stage probabilities, consider each first-stage outcome, one at a time.

If we drew the car ticket, we then choose one key from among the five keys on the car key panel. Only one of these five keys opens the car. So the probability of drawing the key that opens the car is 1/5; the probability of a dud is 4/5.

If we drew the bike ticket, we then choose a key from the bike key panel. The probability of choosing a key that opens the bike lock is 2/5; the probability of a dud is 3/5.

If we drew the jewelry box ticket, we then choose a key from the jewelry box key panel. The probability of choosing a key that opens the jewelry box is 3/5; the probability of a dud is 2/5.

Figure 3.2.3 displays the completed probability tree diagram for Let's Make a Deal. A **probability tree diagram** for a multistage experiment displays on each branch of the tree the probability for each outcome at each stage.

FIGURE **3.2.2**
Tree diagram and
sample space for Let's
Make a Deal. The
first-stage probabilities
are placed on the
branches of the tree
from the "Start:".

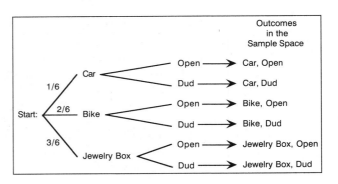

FIGURE **3.2.3**
Tree diagram and sample space for Let's Make a Deal. The probability for each outcome at each stage is displayed on the corresponding branch of the tree diagram.

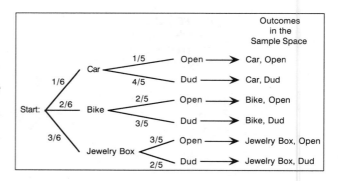

Once the probability tree diagram for a multistage experiment is constructed, one can easily compute the probability for each outcome. To obtain the probability for an outcome in a multistage experiment, one simply multiplies the probabilities along each branch of the route in the tree diagram that produces the outcome. The probabilities for the outcomes in the sample space for Let's Make a Deal are calculated as follows:

$$P[\text{car,open}] = \tfrac{1}{6} \times \tfrac{1}{5} = \tfrac{1}{30} \qquad P[\text{car,dud}] = \tfrac{1}{6} \times \tfrac{4}{5} = \tfrac{4}{30}$$

$$P[\text{bike,open}] = \tfrac{2}{6} \times \tfrac{2}{5} = \tfrac{4}{30} \qquad P[\text{bike,dud}] = \tfrac{2}{6} \times \tfrac{3}{5} = \tfrac{6}{30}$$

$$P[\text{box,open}] = \tfrac{3}{6} \times \tfrac{3}{5} = \tfrac{9}{30} \qquad P[\text{box,dud}] = \tfrac{3}{6} \times \tfrac{2}{5} = \tfrac{6}{30}$$

Using these probabilities, one can now assess the probability of interesting events.

EXAMPLE 3.2.11 $P[\text{win the car}] = P[\text{car,open}]$

$$= \tfrac{1}{30}(= .03 \text{ or } 3\%)$$

$P[\text{win a prize}] = P[\text{win car or win bike or win box}]$

$$= P[\text{win car}] + P[\text{win bike}] + P[\text{win box}]$$

$$= P[\text{car,open}] + P[\text{bike,open}] + P[\text{box,open}]$$

$$= \tfrac{1}{30} + \tfrac{4}{30} + \tfrac{9}{30}$$

$$= \tfrac{14}{30}(= .47 \text{ or } 47\%)$$

$P[\text{no prize}] = 1 - P[\text{prize}] \text{ (Complement Rule)}$

$$= 1 - \tfrac{14}{30}$$

$$= \tfrac{16}{30}(= .53 \text{ or } 53\%)$$

A probability tree diagram first displays the tree diagram for the multistage experiment. The tree diagram is then enhanced by displaying the probability for each outcome at each stage along the corresponding branch of the tree. An outcome in the sample space is displayed by tracing a route from "Start:" through the tree diagram. The probability for an outcome is calculated by multiplying the probabilities displayed on the branches along the route that produces the outcome. This procedure for calculating the probabilities for an outcome to a multistage experiment is called the **Multiplication Rule**.

Recall that a probability can be thought of in a theoretical or an empirical context. The probabilities displayed in Let's Make a Deal are theoretical. Many probabilities in the health sciences, however, are determined on the basis of data. A probability based on data is an empirical probability. To emphasize the *empirical* aspect of a study involving a multistage experiment, researchers sometimes present their data in the form of a frequency distribution tree diagram. A **frequency distribution tree diagram** is a tree diagram for a multistage experiment enhanced with the (absolute) frequencies from data collected in a study. These frequencies may be converted to relative frequencies. These relative frequencies are the empirical probabilities.

EXAMPLE 3.2.12 Ryan et al studied smoking behaviors in a large sample of postal service applicants in Boston. They reported data concerning race and smoking status as shown in Table 3.2.1.

TABLE *3.2.1*
Data from Ryan et al about race and smoking habits.

Smoking Status	White	Black	Asian
Smoker	757	53	15
Nonsmoker	1521	107	84
Totals	2278	160	99

Figure 3.2.4 displays a frequency distribution tree diagram for the data shown in Table 3.2.1.

The relative frequency distribution tree diagram is based on the computations shown in Tables 3.2.2 and 3.2.3. Table 3.2.2 is a frequency distribution table for the race data collected by Ryan et al. Table 3.2.3 displays a frequency distribution for the smoking status for each of the three races reported in the Ryan et al study.

TABLE *3.2.2*
Frequency distribution table for the race data collected by Ryan et al.

Race	Frequency	Relative Frequency
White	2278	.898
Black	160	.063
Asian	99	.039
Total	2537	1.000

The frequency tree diagram shown in Figure 3.2.4 can be converted to a relative frequency tree diagram as shown in Figure 3.2.5. Note that the relative frequencies (empirical probabilities) are read one stage at a time. For example, in the

FIGURE *3.2.4*
A frequency distribution tree for the race and smoking status data collected by Ryan et al.

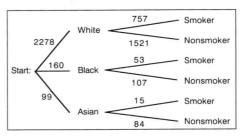

3.2.3 Frequency distribution table for the smoking status for each of the three races reported by Ryan et al.

Smoking Status	White		Black		Asian	
	Frequency	Relative Frequency	Frequency	Relative Frequency	Frequency	Relative Frequency
Smoker	757	.332	53	.331	15	.152
Nonsmoker	1521	.668	107	.669	84	.848
Totals	2278	1.000	160	1.000	99	1.000

study of postal applicants in Boston, .898 are white. Of these white applicants, .668 are nonsmokers. Applying the multiplication rule, we conclude that .898 × .668 = .600 are white nonsmokers.

One implication of this study is that smoking habits of postal applicants in Boston appear to differ between races. Clearly, the proportion of smokers is about the same between blacks and whites; however, the proportion of smokers among Asians appears significantly smaller. In technical language, we say that race and smoking status are **dependent**; that is, the relative frequency of smoking differs among the races studied.

Independence Rule

Figure 3.2.6 illustrates two simple experiments where each experiment has known outcomes and probabilities.

Now consider the two-stage experiment obtained by performing the two given simple experiments in sequence. Two stages are said to be **independent** if the outcomes and probabilities in one stage apply the same way to each outcome in the other stage. For example, gender and Rh factor are independent (biologically, gender and Rh factor are independent since each genetic trait is located on a different chromosome; i.e., a person's gender is unaffected by the Rh factor and vice versa). In particular, the distribution of the Rh factor (.85 positive and .15 negative) is the same among females as among males.

To further illustrate the concept of independence, consider the following situations. ABO blood type is independent of the Rh factor (their genes are on different chromosomes). If you flip two unattached fair coins, say a penny and a dime, the

FIGURE 3.2.5
A relative frequency distribution tree for the race and smoking status data collected by Ryan et al.

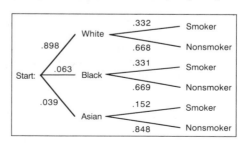

FIGURE *3.2.6*
Two simple experiments where the outcomes and their probabilities are known.

Experiment 1 Gender of a US newborn.		Experiment 2 Rh factor of a US newborn.	
Gender	Probability	Rh Factor	Probability
Female	.5	+	.85
Male	.5	−	.15

outcome for the penny is independent of the outcome for the dime. In contrast, the presence of hemophilia and gender are dependent since hemophilia occurs only in males. An obvious case of dependence is gender and ovarian cancer.

Independent stages allow one to quickly compute probabilities for multistage outcomes without the necessity of constructing a probability tree. One merely applies the multiplication rule directly, as the following examples illustrate:

EXAMPLE 3.2.13
$P[\text{Rh}+ \text{ female}] = P[\text{Rh}+] \times P[\text{female}]$
$= .85 \times .5$
$= .425 \ (42.5\%)$

EXAMPLE 3.2.14 ABO blood type and Rh factor are independent outcomes. Hence,

a. $P[\text{A}+] = P[\text{type A}] \times P[\text{Rh}+]$
$= .41 \times .85$
$= 0.3485$

b. $P[\text{B}-] = P[\text{type B}] \times P[\text{Rh}-]$
$= .09 \times .15$
$= .0135$

EXAMPLE 3.2.15 ABO blood type, Rh factor, and gender are all independent. Hence,

a. $P[\text{A}+ \text{ female}] = P[\text{A}]P[\text{Rh}+]P[\text{female}]$
$= .41 \times .85 \times .50$
$= .174 \ (17.4\% \text{ or } 174 \text{ out of } 1000)$

b. $P[\text{B}- \text{ male}] = P[\text{B}]P[\text{Rh}-]P[\text{male}]$
$= .09 \times .15 \times .50$
$= .007 \ (.7\% \text{ or } 7 \text{ out of } 1000)$

The Independence Rule, a special multiplication rule for independent outcomes, is summarized in the following box:

The Independence Rule

Suppose *x* is an outcome in stage 1 and *y* is an outcome in stage 2, where stage 1 and stage 2 are independent stages. Then

$$P[x \text{ and } y] = P[x] \times P[y]$$

Warm-ups
3.2

1. A formal study of counting procedures is called
   a. Descriptive statistics
   b. Factorial
   c. Combinatorics
   d. Distributions

2. For any natural number n, $n! =$ **a.** $n \times (n - 1)$
   b. $n \times (n - 1)!$
   c. $n \times n$
   d. n

3. $6! = 6 \times 5 \times 4 \times 3 \times 2 \times 1 = 720$.
   Hence, $7! = 7 \times 6! = 7 \times$ ____ = ____.

4. $0! =$ **a.** 0
   b. 1
   c. There is no such thing
   d. $0 \times (-1)!$

5. For any natural number n, $C(n, 0) = 1$
   $$C(n, 1) = n$$
   $$C(n, n - 1) = n$$
   $$C(n, n) = 1$$
   Hence,

   $C(7, 6) =$ ____ $C(7, 0) =$ ____
   $C(7, 7) =$ ____ $C(7, 1) =$ ____

6. In how many ways can one choose 3 members from a staff of 8? This question is an example of
   a. Independence
   b. A factorial
   c. A probability
   d. A subset problem

7. The number of ways one can choose 3 members from a staff of 8 is denoted by
   a. $C(8, 3)$ **b.** $C(3, 8)$ **c.** $3!$ **d.** $8!$

8. From Appendix Table 1, $C(8, 3) =$ ____. Hence, the number of ways one can choose 3 members from a staff of 8 is ____.

9. The Independence Rule states that the probability $P[A$ and $B]$ for independent outcomes A and B is computed by
   a. $P[A] + P[B]$
   b. $P[A] - P[B]$
   c. $P[A] \times P[B]$
   d. $C(A, B)$

10. Suppose that $P[\text{type A blood}] = .41$ and $P[\text{Rh}-] = .15$. Then $P[A-] =$
    a. $.41 + .15 = .56$
    b. $.41 - .15 = .26$
    c. $.41 \times .15 = .0615$
    d. $.41/.15 = 2.73$
    e. $C(.41, .15) = .41!/.15! = 6.343$

11. The probability that a person does not have A− blood is
    a. .44 **b.** 0 **c.** .9385 **d.** .74

12. The answer to Warm-up 11 illustrates
    a. The subset problem
    b. The Multiplication Rule
    c. The Independence Rule
    d. The Complement Rule

Problems 3.2

1. Evaluate each of the following:
   a. $C(7, 5)$ **b.** $C(10, 3)$ **c.** $C(5, 0)$ **d.** $C(6, 6)$
   e. $C(9, 8)$ **f.** $C(9, 1)$

2. ABO blood type and Rh blood type are independent of each other. Applying the probabilities given in Example 3.1.2 for ABO and Rh blood types, what is the probability that a random U.S. resident
   a. Will be $AB-$? **b.** Is not $AB-$?
   c. Is an $AB-$ female? **d.** Is an $O+$ male?

3. Suppose we define a blood profile as a report that states both the ABO and Rh blood types (these blood types are independent). The sample space of blood profiles is not an equiprobable space. Determine the probability of each outcome in the sample space by applying the probabilities for the individual blood types given in Example 3.1.2. Present your results in a table with the blood profiles entered in the first column and the corresponding probabilities in the second column.

4. In General Hospital's intensive care unit on a certain day, there are 8 patients and 3 nurses, of which 2 are staff nurses and 1 is the charge nurse. The patient assignment is to be made so that each staff nurse has 3 patients and the charge nurse has 2 patients. In how many ways can the patient assignment be made?

5. There are 18 staff nurses working on a given floor who want to attend a clinical workshop. The hospital, for staffing reasons, can allow only 6 to attend the workshop. To be "fair," the administration selects the attendees in a random drawing. In how many ways can 6 staff nurses be selected from the pool of 18 applicants?

6. A group of 12 patients is available for use in a study. Seven are to be selected at random and receive an experimental treatment. The other 5 are to receive the standard treatment and serve as controls.
   a. In how many ways can this be done?
   b. One of the patients, C. Nyle, has made some wisecracks about serving as a guinea pig. What is the probability that Mr. Nyle will be chosen for the experimental group?

7. In a cardiac intensive care unit, there are 6 patients who need one-on-one nursing care. Correspondingly, there are 6 cardiac nurses who are scheduled. In how many ways can the one-on-one patient assignment be made in which the 6 nurses are assigned to the 6 patients?

8. California 6/49 Lotto later became 6/52 Lotto. In how many ways can 6 numbers be drawn at random from a pool of numbers 1 through 52 inclusive? Is there much of a difference in the chances of winning "the big one" in 6/49 Lotto compared with 6/52 Lotto?

9. Sickle cell anemia is a dominant recessive genetic blood disorder peculiar to blacks. The gene for sickle cell is located on a different chromosome than the gene for cystic fibrosis; hence, the two conditions are independent of each other. Suppose that each member of a couple planning a child is physically healthy with respect to both sickle cell anemia and cystic fibrosis; however, both are genetic carriers of both diseases. Thus, the genetic makeup of both parents is SsAa with respect to sickle cell and cystic fibrosis.
   a. What is the probability that their child will be free of both sickle cell anemia and cystic fibrosis?
   b. What is the probability that their child will carry neither condition?
   c. What is the probability that the child will contract cystic fibrosis but not sickle cell anemia?
   d. What is the probability that the child will contract sickle cell anemia but not cystic fibrosis?
   e. What is the probability that the child will contract both sickle cell anemia and cystic fibrosis?

10. Jain et al conducted a study to determine the outcome of apparently stillborn infants who received cardiopulmonary resuscitation (CPR). They noted the difficulties an apparent stillborn presents to the attending physician. A nonaggressive approach may deny an infant a chance of normal life. On the other hand, resuscitative efforts may result, at best, in delayed death or survival of a severely handicapped infant.

    Jain et al studied 81,243 mother-infant pairs (deliveries) at 13 Illinois hospitals during 1982–86. Of the 81,243 deliveries, 613 infants registered a zero Apgar score at 1 minute of age (i.e., apparently stillborn).

    Of these 613 infants who registered a zero Apgar score at 1 minute of age, 520 had showed no prebirth sign of life at the time of hospital admission. These cases were determined to be fetal death, and no CPR was administered to attempt resuscitation. The other 93 of these 613 infants were given CPR. The attempt at resuscitation was made since the infant showed prebirth signs of life after hospital admission for delivery.

    Of the 93 infants for whom CPR resuscitation efforts were made, 31 did not respond; 62 were resuscitated and transferred to the neonatal intensive care unit (NICU).

Of the 62 transfers to the NICU, 26 died while in the NICU; 36 were eventually discharged to home. Of those discharged to home, 3 subsequently died shortly as infants; 33 survived to follow-up.

a. Construct a frequency distribution tree that traces the various events of the original 81,242 deliveries; that is, construct a tree that displays the various events described by Jain et al, along with the observed frequency for that event.

b. Construct a probability tree that traces the various events of the 81,243 deliveries in the Jain et al study.

c. Based on the Jain et al data, what is the probability that a newborn will have a zero Apgar score at 1 minute of age?

d. Based on the Jain et al data, what is the probability that a newborn showing prebirth signs of life but having a zero Apgar score at 1 minute
   i. Will be resuscitated by CPR?
   ii. Will be discharged to home?
   iii. Will be discharged to home and survives to follow-up?

11. Garrard et al studied 5752 patient records from 60 western nursing homes. Of these 5752 patients, 996 were taking neuroleptic (i.e., antipsychotic) drugs (NEs) at the time of admission to the nursing home. The study period lasted 3 years. A patient was followed for the three-year study period, or up to time of discharge if the patient was discharged during the study period.

Of the 996 patients taking NEs at the time of nursing home admission, only 509 were eligible for NE therapy according to federal Heath Care Financing Administration (HCFA) guidelines. The other 487 patients on NEs were not eligible for that therapy according to HCFA guidelines.

Of the 509 patients eligible for NE therapy at the time of nursing home admission, 164 had NE therapy discontinued in the nursing home; 345 were continued on NE therapy during the study period. Of these 345 patients, 46 were ineligible for such therapy at the end of the study period (or at discharge) according to HCFA guidelines; the other 299 were still eligible.

Of the 487 patients on NE therapy and HCFA-ineligible, 306 were continued on NE therapy after nursing home admission, while 181 had their NE

therapy discontinued during the study period. Of these 306 patients who were continued on NE therapy, 275 were ineligible for NE therapy at the end of the study period (or at discharge); the other 31 patients became eligible for NE therapy during their nursing home stay.

Of the 4756 patients not taking NEs at the time of nursing home admission, 4407 were not taking NEs at the end of study or at time of discharge. The other 349 patients had NE therapy initiated while in the nursing home. Of these, 150 were eligible for the therapy according to HCFA guidelines, while 199 were ineligible.

a. Construct a frequency distribution tree for the data reported by Garrard et al. The tree should display the events described by the study and state the observed frequencies for these events.

b. Construct a probability tree for the data. The tree should display the events and their probabilities. The probabilities are calculated based on the observed frequencies.

Based on the given study, what is the probability that a randomly selected patient is

c. Taking NEs at the time of admission to a nursing home?

d. Taking NEs at the time of admission but is ineligible for NE therapy?

e. Taking NEs at the time of admission to the nursing home, although ineligible, but continued NE therapy at the nursing home?

f. Taking NEs at the time of admission, although ineligible, but continued NE therapy while in the nursing home although still ineligible at the end of the study period or at the time of discharge?

The scenarios in Problems 12–14 are adapted from Schneiderman and Kaplan. These researchers compared students' fear of accidental exposure to the blood of hepatitis B compared with their fear of accidental exposure to the HIV virus.

12. You just became stranded in an isolated place. If you stay put, you will die of exposure within 48 hours. There are only two routes to safety, both of which expose you to danger. The first route sends you through infested terrain where the probability of being bitten along the way by a poisonous insect is 25%. The probability that one dies from the bite

is 5%. The second route sends you through a less infested area (only 1% chance of being stung), but a sting is lethal (probability of death from the insect is 100%).

a. Which route would you take: first or second?

b. Apply the Multiplication Rule to determine the probability of death for the first route.

c. Apply the Multiplication Rule to determine the probability of death for the second route.

d. Does knowing the probability of death from the two routes affect your choice?

e. In a study of university health science students in southern California, 58 of 91 students chose the first route. What proportion of students chose the first route? Does this surprise you? What explanation might you offer for this result?

13. You just became stranded in an isolated place. If you stay put, you will die of exposure within 48 hours. There are only two routes to safety, both of which expose you to danger. The first route sends you through infested terrain where it is certain (probability 100%) that you will be bitten along the way by a poisonous insect; however, the probability that one dies from the bite is only 1%. The second route sends you through a much less infested area (only 5% chance of being stung), but the chance of dying from the sting is 25%.

a. Which route would you take: first or second?

b. Apply the Multiplication Rule to determine the probability of death for the first route.

c. Apply the Multiplication Rule to determine the probability of death for the second route.

d. Does knowing the probability of death from the two routes affect your choice?

e. In a study of university health science students in southern California, 28 of 90 students chose the second route. What proportion of students chose the second route? Does this surprise you? What explanation might you offer for this result?

14. One danger facing a clinical health care worker is an accidental needle stick. An accidental needle stick is dangerous since it may expose the caretaker to infection, such as hepatitis B or AIDS. The risk of contracting hepatitis B from an infected patient through an accidental needle stick is about 25%. Hepatitis B carries a 5% mortality (i.e., there is a

5% chance of dying as a result of contracting hepatitis B). The risk of contracting AIDS from an infected patient through an accidental needle stick is about 1%; however, the mortality rate is 100%. Suppose that you have volunteered for health care work in an isolated poor country, in which hepatitis B and AIDS are equally prevalent. The local government is short on supplies and offers you one protective immunization.

a. Which vaccine do you choose (you may choose a vaccine either for hepatitis B or for AIDS)? Both vaccines are equally effective (assume 100% effectiveness). Explain your choice.

b. What is the probability of an unvaccinated person dying of hepatitis B?

c. What is the probability of an unvaccinated person dying of AIDS?

d. Does knowing the probability of death from the two alternatives affect your choice?

e. In a study of university health science students in southern California, 56 of 83 students chose the hepatitis B vaccine. What proportion of students chose the hepatitis B vaccine? Does this surprise you? What explanation might you offer for this result?

15. Keno is a popular gambling game in casinos. Some state lotteries also feature Keno. In a game of Keno, the casino randomly picks 20 numbers from 1 to 80. To play, you pick up a Keno game card, which displays numbers from 1 to 80 (see Figure 3.2.7). You select 1 or more numbers on the card (the maximum number you can select depends on the house rules). At a later time, the casino displays its 20 picks on the screen. You win if enough of your picks matches the casino's picks.

a. How many Keno displays are possible (i.e., in how many ways can you randomly select 20 numbers from 1 through 80 inclusive)?

b. One Spot Keno is played by marking just one number on the Keno card. If your number is displayed on the casino screen, you win. What is the probability that you will win in One Spot Keno?

c. Two Spot Keno is played by marking two spots on a Keno game card (i.e., pick two numbers from 1 to 80).

    i. In how many ways can you play Two Spot Keno?

FIGURE **3.2.7**
A Keno game
card.

1	2	3	4	5	6	7	8	9	10
11	12	13	14	15	16	17	18	19	20
21	22	23	24	25	26	27	28	29	30
31	32	33	34	35	36	37	38	39	40
41	42	43	44	45	46	47	48	49	50
51	52	53	54	55	56	57	58	59	60
61	62	63	64	65	66	67	68	69	70
71	72	73	74	75	76	77	78	79	80

ii. In Two Spot Keno, what is the probability that exactly one of your picks matches those of the casino? (Hint: Think of picking Keno numbers as a two-stage experiment where stage 1 is picking from among winning numbers and stage 2 is picking from among losing numbers. You will need to apply the Subset Rule at each stage, then apply the Multiplication Rule for a two-stage experiment. This procedure will allow you to count the number of ways that you can pick exactly one winning number and one losing number.)

iii. To win Two Spot Keno in the California lottery, both of your picks must match. What is the probability of winning in Two Spot Keno in the California lottery?

d. In Four Spot Keno you mark four spots on the Keno game card (i.e., pick four numbers from 1 to 80).

   i. In how many ways can you play Four Spot Keno?

   ii. What is the probability that exactly one of your picks will match?

   iii. What is the probability that exactly two of your picks will match?

   iv. What is the probability that exactly three of your picks will match?

   v. What is the probability that exactly four of your picks will match?

   vi. To win a prize in Four Spot Keno in the California lottery, you must have two or more matches. What is the probability of winning a prize playing Four Spot Keno in the California lottery?

CHAPTER **3** *OVERVIEW*

Summary

The three contexts for probability are theoretical, empirical, and subjective. A **theoretical probability** often is based on an intuitive notion of fairness. An **empirical probability** is based on data. A **subjective probability** is based on personal opinion.

Basic concepts supporting probability include experiment, sample space, and event. An **experiment** is a procedure that produces a (variable) outcome. The **sample space** of an experiment is a list of all possible outcomes that can be produced by the given experiment. An **event** is a subset of the sample space.

The simplest situation for computing probabilities involves an equiprobable space. An **equiprobable space** is a sample space for which each outcome is equally likely to occur when the experiment is performed.

An experiment may be simple or multistage. A **multistage experiment** may be viewed as a sequence of other experiments. A **simple experiment** can not be broken down further into a sequence of simpler experiments. A multistage experiment can be displayed by a **tree diagram**.

Combinatorics is the study of counting procedures, including the Fundamental Principle of Counting and the Subset Rule. The **Fundamental Principle of Counting** allows one to quickly compute the number of outcomes in a multistage experiment by multiplying the number of separate outcomes for each individual stage. The **Subset Rule** specifies that the number of subsets with k elements that can be extracted from a set of n elements is $C(n,k)$, the **combination** of n and k.

The **Complement**, **Multiplication**, and **Independence** rules allow one to compute a complex probability from knowledge of its component parts. The Multiplication Rule is applied in tandem with a **probability tree diagram**.

Keywords

combination C(n,k)
combinatorics
complement of an event
Complement Rule
equiprobable space
event
   exhaustive events
   mutually exclusive events
experiment
   multistage experiment
   simple experiment
factorial $n!$
Fundamental Principle of
   Counting
independent events
Independence Rule

Multiplication Rule
outcome
probability
   empirical probability
   subjective probability
   theoretical probability
relative frequency
sample space
stage
Subset Rule
tree diagram
   frequency tree diagram
   probability tree diagram
   relative frequency tree
     diagram

References

Daily E and Mersch J: Thermodilution cardiac outputs using room and ice temperature injectate: Comparison with the Fick method. *Heart Lung* 16, no, 3 (May 1987): 294.

Garrard J et al: Evaluation of neuroleptic drug use by nursing home elderly under proposed Medicare and Medicaid regulations. *JAMA* 265, no. 4 (January 1991): 463.

Isner J: Acute catastrophic complications of balloon aortic valvuloplasty. *J Am Coll Cardiol* 17, no. 6 (May 1991): 1436.

Jain L et al: Cardiopulmonary resuscitation of apparently stillborn infants: Survival and long-term outcome. *J Pediatr* 118, no 5 (May 1991):778.

Ryan J et al: Occupational risks associated with cigarette smoking: A prospective study. *Am J Pub Health* 82, no. 1 (January 1992): 29.

Schneiderman J and Kaplan R: Fear of dying and HIV infection vs hepatitis B infection. *Am J Public Health* 82, no. 4 (April 1992): 584.

Applications

We pause in our development of statistical concepts to present an essential application in the health sciences: diagnostic testing. Again, the key concern is patient care, and a valuable tool is statistical reasoning. The student will see how the ideas developed thus far—frequency, summary presentation of data, and probability—are indispensable toward developing insight and appreciation of the role that diagnostics play in patient management. Also note that, once again, individual variation is the source of interest and problems.

Diagnostics are much more complex than the naive idea of "run a test to see if the patient has this or that condition." The interested reader can explore the topic in more depth in the following references:

1. Dorothy Nelkin and Laurence Tancredi. *Dangerous Diagnostics*. New York: Basic Books, 1989.

   This book describes the dangers and dilemmas of applying social or psychological diagnostic tests to pigeonhole people into behavioral categories.
2. P. Chang. Evaluating imaging test performance: An introduction to Bayesian analysis for urologists. *Monographs in Urology* 12, no. 2 (1991): 18–34.

   This monograph is full of friendly advice to practicing clinicians about the application of diagnostic testing. We examine some of Dr. Chang's advice in Exercise 4.1.8.

SECTION 4.1	**OBJECTIVES** This section will
Diagnostic Testing	**1** Describe the terms sensitivity, false-negative rate, specificity, false-positive rate, predictive values, and accuracy of a diagnostic test.
	2 Determine the sensitivity, false-negative rate, specificity, false-positive rate, predictive values, and accuracy of a diagnostic test when provided with a two-factor frequency distribution table for test result versus presence of condition.
	3 Describe why prevalence of a condition is important in the design of a diagnostic testing program.

> **4** Construct a two-factor frequency distribution table for test result versus presence of condition when provided with appropriate data. The table should be accompanied by a statement describing the population of interest, the condition of interest, and the prevalence of the condition in the population.

A diagnostic test is an indirect procedure used to determine the status of a person or the cause of a condition in a patient. For example, Jill wonders whether she is pregnant. She purchases an early pregnancy test (EPT) kit from a drugstore to determine her status with regard to pregnancy. John was just admitted to the emergency room at General Hospital for chest pain, diaphoresis (sweating), shortness of breath, and a pain in his arm. The physician suspects a heart attack is the cause of John's condition. The physician orders laboratory tests to confirm his suspicions about the cause of John's distress. The key in both Jill's and John's cases is that a direct observation of their concern is not possible; hence, an indirect diagnostic test is called for as a tool to assess the condition of interest.

The Diagnostic Test

Often a direct observation of a condition of concern is impossible or impractical; hence, an indirect observation is made. Examples include a drugstore EPT test for pregnancy, Pap smear for cervical cancer, and treadmill S-T segment depression analysis for coronary artery disease. A young fetus cannot be seen directly, but a change in urine chemistry due to a change in body chemistry due to pregnancy may be observable by a color change in a home EPT kit. Direct observation of cervical cancer would involve a biopsy, but abnormal cells sloughed off by a malignancy may be readily swabbed, stained, and seen under a microscope. Direct observation of a clogged artery would involve angiography, but change in the S-T segment of the cardiac cycle due to an altered cardiac rhythm due to the clogged artery may be seen on an electrocardiogram strip.

A diagnostic test is called for when a condition of interest cannot be observed directly. Since diagnostic tests rely on an indirect observation of a condition, they are not perfect. In this section we discuss how to evaluate the effectiveness of a diagnostic test. Consider now a set of people and a condition of interest. Suppose that the condition is difficult to observe directly (such as early pregnancy, early cancer, asymptomatic coronary artery disease). The problem is to distinguish between those who have the condition and those who do not. Since the condition is difficult to observe directly, an indirect diagnostic test is advised.

An ideal diagnostic test must perform two distinct jobs:

1. The test must give a "positive" result (i.e., condition present) to those people who have the condition.
2. The test must give a "negative" result (i.e., condition absent) to those people who do not have the condition.

The problem is that there is *no such thing as an ideal diagnostic test*. No diagnostic test does both of these jobs perfectly. Usually, the better a test does on one job, the worse it does on the other.

An example of how difficult it can be to make precise definitions of "condition present" and "condition absent" with appropriate tests is the case of death. The issue is central in the topic of organ procurement. This topic is important not only in medicine but has serious social and legal implications with ethical overtones. For example, the California Transplant Donor Network recommends that health care personnel identify a patient as dead when network criteria for brain death are met. The network's guidelines for determination of brain death involve six major criteria. The network recommends that a patient's family be notified that the patient is dead (not just brain-dead), even though there may be circulatory function. In fact, intact circulation is an organ donor criterion.

Sensitivity and False-Negative Rate

In order to appreciate the utility of a diagnostic test, several concepts are needed. Recall the two jobs that an ideal diagnostic test needs to perform. The first is to identify those people in the population who have the condition of interest. When the test is given to a person with condition, the test result may be either a (true) positive or a (false) negative. The **sensitivity** (denoted Sn) of the test is the probability that a person with condition tests positive. The **false-negative rate** $(F - R)$ is the probability that a person with condition tests negative. For example, suppose a study is conducted in which the diagnostic test is applied to 100 with-condition people, of whom 92 test positive ($+$) and 8 test negative ($-$). Then, according to the study,

> Sn (sensitivity)
> = (number of true positives)/(number with condition)
> = 92/100
> = .92 or 92%

and

> F $-$ R (false-negative rate)
> = (number of false negatives)/(number with condition)
> = 8/100
> = .08 or 8%

Note that the terms Sn and F $-$ R go together. They apply *only to the population with condition*. Since any person with condition tests either $+$ or $-$ (ambiguous cases are treated as $-$), then

> $(Sn) + (F - R) = 1.00$ or 100%

Specificity and False-Positive Rate

The second job of a diagnostic test is to identify those people in the population who are condition-free. When the test is given to a condition-free person, the test result may be either a (false) positive or a (true) negative. The **specificity** (Sp) of the test is the probability that a condition-free person will test negative. The **false-positive rate** (F + R) is the probability that a condition-free person will test positive. For example, suppose a study is conducted in which the diagnostic test is applied to 100 condition-free people, of whom 87 test − and 13 test +. Then, according to the study,

Sp (specificity)
= (number of true negatives)/(number condition-free)
= 87/100
= .87 or 87%

and

F + R (false-positive rate)
= (number of false positives)/(number condition-free)
= 13/100
= 0.13 or 13%

Note that the terms Sp and F + R go together. They apply *only to the condition-free population*. Since any condition-free person tests either + or − (ambiguous cases are treated as −), then

(Sp) + (F + R) = 1.00 or 100%

Predictive Value

When a health science practitioner is presented with a patient or client for assessment, diagnostic tests may be ordered. Of course, if the practitioner can observe directly the presence or absence of the condition of interest, no diagnostic test is needed. When a condition cannot be observed directly, the practitioner orders a test (usually several tests). What good are the results of a test? Upon receipt of the test results, the practitioner then knows the results of the test; the key information, however, remains the status of the patient. In an ideal diagnostic test, the test result correlates perfectly with the status of the patient: A + test result corresponds to condition present, a − test result to condition absent. Again, however, *there is no such thing as an ideal diagnostic test*. In order to apply a test result back to the patient, we need the predictive value of the test.

The **predictive value of a positive test** (PV +) is the probability that a person with a positive test result actually has the condition of interest. The **predictive value of a negative test** (PV −) is the probability that a person with a negative test result actually is condition-free. For example, suppose 100 people are tested for a condition using a certain diagnostic test in which 53 people tested + and 47 tested −. By direct observation it was determined that of the 53 people who tested positive, 49 actually had the condition; of the 47 who tested negative, 46 were actually condition-free. Then,

PV+ (predictive value of a positive test)
= (number with condition)/(+ test result)
= 49/53
= .92 or 92%

and

PV− (predictive value of a negative test)
= (number condition-free)/(− test result)
= 46/47
= .98 or 98%

The **accuracy** of a test is the probability that a given test result is correct (corresponds to the actual status of the condition in the patient). Using the previous example, 49 of 53 positive tests were correct and 46 of 47 negative results were correct. Hence,

Accuracy
= (number of correct test results)/(number of tests)
= 95/100
= .95 or 95%

Summarizing, the key facets of a diagnostic test are the following:

Sn: the probability that a person with condition gets a + test result
F − R: the probability that a person with condition gets a − test result
Sp: the probability that a condition-free person gets a − test result
F + R: the probability that a condition-free person gets a + test result
PV+: the probability that a person who gets a + test result actually has the condition
PV−: the probability that a person who gets a − test result is actually condition-free
Accuracy: the probability that a diagnostic test yields a result consistent with the status of the patient being tested.

Computational Aspects of Diagnostics

Thus far we have presented the basic concepts of diagnostic testing. In a given health science situation, the practitioner needs to know the specific values of those concepts for a given test in order to assess whether or not the test may provide any useful information.

The key facets of a diagnostic test are estimated by calculating them from the results of a research study as follows:

$$Sn = \text{(number of + tests among conditions)/(number with condition)}$$
$$F - R = \text{(number of - tests among conditions)/(number with condition)}$$
$$Sp = \text{(number of - tests among condition-free)/(number condition-free)}$$
$$F + R = \text{(number of + tests among condition-free)/(number condition-free)}$$
$$PV+ = \text{(number with condition among + tests)/(number of + tests)}$$
$$PV- = \text{(number condition-free among - tests)/(number of - tests)}$$
$$Accuracy = \text{(number of correct test results)/(number of tests given)}$$

To facilitate computations, the raw research data are summarized in the form of a **two-factor frequency distribution table**. The two factors with attributes of interest are

Condition status: present, absent
Test result: positive, negative

The general framework for the frequency distribution table is a two-column, two-row table in which the columns occupy the condition factor and the rows the test factor as displayed in Table 4.1.1.

TABLE **4.1.1**
The general framework for the two-factor frequency distribution table diagnostic concepts.

		CONDITION		
		Present	Absent	Total
TEST	+	(a)	(b)	(e)
RESULT	—	(c)	(d)	(f)
	Total	(g)	(h)	(n)

Cells (a)(b)(c)(d) are occupied by the respective **two-factor frequencies**; (e)(f)(g)(h) are called **marginal totals** and represent single-factor frequencies; (n) contains the **grand total** of the size of the study group.

EXAMPLE **4.1.1** Roberts et al studied the use of fever (temperature greater than or equal to 38°C) as a diagnostic indicator for postoperative atelectasis as evidenced by X-ray observation. Table 4.1.2 displays the data in a two-factor frequency distribution table.

TABLE **4.1.2**
Two-factor frequency distribution table for the Roberts et al data.

		X-RAY FILM EVIDENCE OF ATELECTASIS		
		Yes	No	Total
FEVER	Yes	72 (a)	37 (b)	109 (e)
≥38°C	No	82 (c)	79 (d)	161 (f)
	Total	154 (g)	116 (h)	270 (n)

The diagnostic quantities are computed as follows:

$$Sn = \frac{\text{number of + tests among patients with atelectasis}}{\text{number of patients with atelectasis}}$$

$$= \frac{(a)}{(g)} = \frac{72}{154} = .468 \text{ or } 46.8\%$$

$$F - R = \frac{\text{number of - tests among patients with atelectasis}}{\text{number of patients with atelectasis}}$$

$$= \frac{(c)}{(g)} = \frac{82}{154} = .532 \text{ or } 53.2\%$$

$$Sp = \frac{\text{number of - tests among patients without atelectasis}}{\text{number of patients without atelectasis}}$$

$$= \frac{(d)}{(h)} = \frac{79}{116} = .681 \text{ or } 68.1\%$$

$$F + R = \frac{\text{number of + tests among patients without atelectasis}}{\text{number of patients without atelectasis}}$$

$$= \frac{(b)}{(h)} = \frac{37}{116} = .319 \text{ or } 31.9\%$$

$$PV+ = \frac{\text{number of patients with atelectasis}}{\text{total number of + tests}}$$

$$= \frac{(a)}{(e)} = \frac{72}{109} = .661 \text{ or } 66.1\%$$

$$PV- = \frac{\text{number of patients without atelectasis}}{\text{total number of - tests}}$$

$$= \frac{(d)}{(f)} = \frac{79}{161} = .491 \text{ or } 49.1\%$$

$$Accuracy = \frac{\text{number of correct test results}}{\text{total number of tests}}$$

$$= \frac{(a+d)}{(n)} = \frac{(72+79)}{270} = .559 \text{ or } 55.9\%$$

The Role of Prevalence

Before ordering a diagnostic test, a health science practitioner needs to know that the test result will be useful in some way. The basic quantities assessing the usefulness of a test are its predictive values. In particular, PV+ measures the probability that a person who tests positive actually has the condition tested for; PV−, the probability that a person who tests negative is actually condition-free. The PV of a test, however, is a function of the prevalence of the condition in the population.

The **prevalence** of a condition is the proportion in the population of interest who actually have the condition. For example, if in a town of 10,000 there are 500 people stricken with the flu, the prevalence for flu in the town is 500/10,000, that is, .05 or 5%.

EXAMPLE 4.1.2 Consider the Roberts et al study referred to in Example 4.1.1. The sample in the study consisted of 270 patients who had undergone elective intra-abdominal surgery. In the sample of 270 patients, 109 displayed fever; hence, the sample prevalence of fever among such patients is 109/270 = .404 or 40.4%. The prevalence of atelectasis as evidenced by X-ray was 154/270 = .570 or 57.0%.

The predictive values of a given diagnostic test ultimately will be determined by the prevalence of the condition being tested for. We illustrate by applying a diagnostic test for which Sn = .90 and Sp = .95 to a population of 100,000 where the prevalence is (1) 10%, (2) 1%, and (3) 0.1%.

Case 1: Prevalence Is 10%

With a prevalence of 10%, 10,000 (100,000 × .10 = 10,000) people in the population have the condition and 90,000 are condition-free. Of the 10,000 people with condition, we can expect 9,000 to get a + test result (Sn = .9, and 10,000 × .9 = 9,000) and 1,000 to get a − test result. Of the 90,000 condition-free people, we can expect 85,500 (Sp = .95, and 90,000 × .95 = 85,500) to get a − test result and 4,500 to get a + test result. These results are summarized in the two-factor frequency distribution Table 4.1.3.

TABLE 4.1.3
Two-factor frequency distribution table for case 1, 10% prevalence.

		CONDITION		
		Present	Absent	Total
TEST	+	9,000	4,500	13,500
	−	1,000	85,500	86,500
	Total	10,000	90,000	100,000

Hence, PV+ = (number with condition)/(number of + tests)
= 9,000/13,500 = .667 or 66.7%

and

PV− = (number condition-free)/(number of − tests)
= 85,500/86,500 = .988 or 98.8%

We see that a person who tests negative here has a very high probability of being condition-free. A negative test result may be viewed as a "clean bill of health" with occasional exceptions. However, a positive test result is not definitive for the condition; in fact, one out of every three people with a positive test result is actually condition-free. This test, however, is still clinically useful. A negative result gives strong evidence to rule out the condition. Note that while the prevalence for the condition in the initial population was only 1/10, the prevalence for the condition among those who test positive is 2/3. Hence, a + test result may be useful as a screen for further testing.

Case 2: Prevalence Is 1%

With 1% prevalence, 1,000 people have the condition and 99,000 are condition-free. The expected results of the testing program on the population are displayed in Table 4.1.4.

Hence, PV+ = 900/5,850 = .154 or 15.4%

and

PV− = 94,050/94,150 = .9989 or 99.89%

TABLE 4.1.4
Two-factor frequency distribution table for case 2, 1% prevalence.

		CONDITION		
		Present	Absent	Total
TEST	+	900	4,950	5,850
	−	100	94,050	94,150
	Total	1,000	99,000	100,000

With the prevalence down to 1%, although a − test result provides strong evidence for condition-free, a + result seems useless as a diagnostic indicator.

Comment PV− was computed to four digits for comparison purposes (see Table 4.1.6).

Case 3: Prevalence Is .1%

With a prevalence of .1%, only 100 people actually have the condition and 99,900 are condition-free. The expected results of the testing program are displayed in Table 4.1.5.

TABLE 4.1.5
Two-factor frequency distribution table for case 3, 0.1% prevalence.

		CONDITION		
		Present	Absent	Total
TEST	+	90	4,995	5,085
	−	10	94,905	94,915
	Total	100	99,900	100,000

Hence, $PV+ = 90/5{,}085 = .018$ or 1.8%

and

$PV- = 94{,}905/94{,}915 = .99989$ or 99.989%

Although a negative test result is quite convincing for condition-free, a positive test result does not mean much; fewer than 2% of those testing + actually have the condition.

Summarizing the results of these three cases, the role of prevalence to predictive value is indicated in the Table 4.1.6.

TABLE 4.1.6
The effect of prevalence on predictive value is illustrated for the three cases.

Prevalence	PV+	PV−
10.0%	.667	.988
1.0%	.154	.9989
0.1%	.018	.99989

EXAMPLE 4.1.3 Pantaleo et al studied the use of thallium scintigraphy as a noninvasive diagnostic tool for coronary artery disease (CAD). In the study, 190 patients with suspected CAD underwent coronary arteriography and exercise thallium-201 myocardial imaging. Of the 148 patients with CAD, 115 had positive thallium-201 scintigrams. Of the 42 patients with normal coronary arteriograms, 37 were predicted correctly as normal by the thallium-201 scintigraphy.

In order to analyze the results of this study, we first construct a two-factor frequency distribution table. The condition of interest is CAD. The two factors are the disease factor (CAD or no CAD) and the test factor (+ scintigram or − scintigram). The resulting frequency distribution table is displayed in Table 4.1.7.

TABLE **4.1.7**
Two-factor frequency distribution table for the Pantaleo et al data.

		DISEASE		
		CAD	no CAD	Total
TEST	+	115	5	120
	−	33	37	70
	Total	148	42	190

Hence, Sn = 115/148 = .78 = 78%

F − R = 33/148 = .22 = 22%

Sp = 37/42 = .88 = 88%

F + R = 5/42 = .12 = 12%

PV+ = 115/120 = .96 = 96%

PV− = 37/70 = .53 = 53%

Accuracy = 152/190 = .80 = 80%

Prevalence = 148/190 = .78 = 78%

The high prevalence (78%) of CAD in the study group is indicative that the study was made on coronary patients. Hence, the primary usefulness of the research would be to see if scintigraphy can act as a screen for those who should undergo arteriography. At the time of the research study, the protocol was that all such patients would undergo arteriography (a method of direct observation for coronary artery obstruction). The research was conducted with the intention of seeing whether a positive scintigram could act as a diagnostic screen to assist in eliminating unnecessary arteriograms. In this regard, the PV+ is sufficiently high (95.8%) that those patients with + scintigrams should undergo arteriography. Unfortunately, a patient with a − scintigram still has a 52.9% probability of having CAD. Although it is clear that a patient with a + scintigram should undergo arteriography, it is unclear what to do with a − test result. The negative scintigram makes it more difficult than before to test these patients since the prevalence of CAD is lower in the − scintigram group than in the original group of patients.

In health science diagnostics, which is preferable: highest Sn, Sp, or PV + ? One cannot have it all (i.e., 100% on all counts). In practice, the following general guidelines are followed.

Highest Sn (preferably 100%) is desired when the disease is serious and should not be missed, when the disease is treatable, and when false positives do not lead to serious economic or psychological trauma. Examples include the Pap smear for cervical cancer, venereal disease, and phenylketonuria.

Highest Sp (preferably 100%) is desired when the disease is serious but is not treatable, when knowledge of absence of the disease is of value, and when false negatives can lead to serious economic or psychological trauma. Examples include multiple sclerosis and social drug testing (e.g., for athletes).

Highest PV + (preferably 100%) is desired when treatment of a false positive has serious consequences. Examples include cancers that require surgery and/or radiation treatments.

EXERCISES 4.1

Warm-ups 4.1

Student's crud (SC) is a common condition on college campuses. It may be described as flulike, with a general feeling of tiredness and lack of energy, accompanied by a great desire for the world to stand still for a while.

A study was conducted to obtain a simple diagnostic test to identify SC. A cootie test was devised in which the back of the throat was swabbed with a cotton swab, then the tip was thoroughly wiped on the circle of a specially prepared microscope slide. The preparation on the slide contained a staining agent that stained the cooties believed to be responsible for SC. The slide was placed under a microscope, and the stained cooties in the circle were counted. A cootie count (CC) in excess of five was considered diagnostic for SC. The study obtained the data displayed in Table 4.1.8 about the cootie test for SC.

TABLE **4.1.8**
Data for the cootie test for student's crud.

		DISEASE STATUS		
		SC Present	SC Absent	
COOTIE	CC > 5	63	2	
TEST	CC ≤ 5	7	78	

1. Table 4.1.8 displays a two-factor frequency distribution table. What are the two factors involved?

2. Looking at the disease status factor, a student either has SC or does not have SC. The total number of students in the study who have SC is obtained by adding the SC present column. The total number of students with SC present is ___; the total number of students with SC absent is ___.

3. Looking at the cootie test factor, a student has either a CC > 5 or a CC ≤ 5. The total number of

students in the study who have a CC > 5 is ___; the total number of students with a CC ≤ 5 is ___.

4. The sensitivity (Sn) of a diagnostic test is defined as the probability that a sick person will be detected by the test. Based on the given cootie test data,

$$Sn = \frac{\text{number with CC} > 5 \text{ among SC present}}{\text{number with SC present}} = \frac{63}{70} =$$

5. The false-negative rate (F − R) is the probability that a sick person will be missed by the test. Based on the given cootie test data,

$$F - R = \frac{\text{number with CC} \leq 5 \text{ among SC present}}{\text{number with SC present}} = \frac{7}{70} =$$

6. The specificity (Sp) of a test is the probability that a healthy (i.e., free of SC) student will obtain a negative test result. Here,

$$Sp = \frac{\text{number with CC} \leq 5 \text{ among SC absent}}{\text{number with SC absent}} = \underline{\quad} =$$

7. The false-positive rate (F + R) is the probability that a healthy student (i.e., free of SC) will be misdiagnosed as having SC. Here,

$$F + R = \frac{\text{number with CC} > 5 \text{ among} \underline{\quad}}{\text{number with} \underline{\quad}} = \underline{\quad} =$$

8. The predictive value of a positive test result (PV +) is the probability that a person with a positive test for SC (i.e., CC > 5) actually has SC. Here,

$$PV+ = \frac{\text{number SC present with CC} > 5}{\text{number with CC} > 5} = \underline{\quad} =$$

9. The predictive value of a negative test result (PV −) is the probability that a person with a negative test for SC (i.e., CC ≤ 5) is actually free of SC. Here,

$$PV- = \frac{\text{number SC absent with CC} \underline{\quad}}{\text{number with CC} \leq 5} = \underline{\quad} =$$

10. The accuracy of a test is the probability that a given student will be diagnosed correctly by the test. Here,

$$\text{Accuracy} = \frac{\text{number of correct results}}{\text{number of tests}} = \frac{141}{150} =$$

11. The prevalence of the disease in a study is the proportion of those in the study who have the disease. Here,

$$\text{Prevalence of SC} = \frac{\text{number with SC}}{\text{total number in study}} = \underline{\quad} =$$

12. Summarizing the results of the cootie test study,

Prevalence of SC is ___%

Sn = ___%   F − R = ___%
Note that (Sn) + (F − R) = ___%

Sp = ___%   F + R = ___%
Note that (Sp) + (F + R) = ___%

PV + = ___%   PV − = ___%

13. The Pap smear, used primarily as a diagnostic indicator for cervical cancer, tests for the presence of abnormal cells. The PV + for a Pap smear for cervical cancer is about 50%. This means that

a. A woman who has a Pap smear has a 50% chance of getting cervical cancer.

b. A woman who has cervical cancer has a 50% chance of having a positive Pap smear result.

c. A woman who has cervical cancer has a 50% chance of surviving.

d. A woman who has a positive Pap smear has a 50% chance of having cervical cancer.

e. A woman who has a Pap smear has a 50% chance that the smear correctly indicates her condition.

Problems 4.1

1. Roberts et al, in an attempt to increase the sensitivity of fever as a diagnostic indicator of postoperative pulmonary complications after abdominal surgery, further analyzed their data by redefining fever as a temperature greater than or equal to 37.7°C. They reported the data shown in Table 4.1.9.

TABLE **4.1.9** Data reported by Roberts et al.

		X-RAY FILM EVIDENCE OF ATELECTASIS		
		Yes	No	Total
FEVER	Yes	105	61	166
≥37.7°C	No	49	55	104
	Total	154	116	270

a. Determine the Sn, F − R, Sp, F + R, PV+, PV −, and accuracy of the test.

b. What is the prevalence of fever in the study sample? What is the prevalence of atelectasis in the study sample?

c. Does a redefinition of fever from greater than or equal to 38°C to 37.7°C improve the diagnostic ability of fever as an indicator for atelectasis in these patients?

2. Every nurse's dreaded fear in caring for a post–myocardial infarction (MI) patient is a lethal arrhythmia. The presentation of six premature ventricular contractions per minute, for example, by many hospital protocols, allows the nurse to intervene immediately (a doctor need not be present). Sudden cardiac death is a major health care problem in the United States (up to 1000 cardiac arrests occur every day). In the majority of patients, coronary artery disease is the underlying abnormality. Sudden death after MI most often is caused by ventricular tachycardia (VT). Determining which post-MI patients are prone to VT currently is done through electrophysiology studies. These procedures are invasive, costly, and inefficient for large-volume screening purposes. A noninvasive method to screen for post-MI patients prone to VT is very desirable.

Lynn M. Lansdowne recently reported on signal-averaged electrocardiograms (ECGs). She reported on a study of 66 post-MI patients who were without bundle branch blocks, had normal sinus rhythm during recording, and were not receiving antiarrhythmic medications (the majority of post-MI patients). In this study group, 39 of the patients had repeated episodes of VT (hence, were prone to VT). The other 27 patients who had no history of VT served as the control group.

A diagnostic test was devised that observed the QRS duration of a signal-averaged ECG. Among the 39 patients in the prone-to-VT study group, 36 had a reading of less than 25 microvolts during the last 40 milliseconds of the QRS waveform; the other 3 had a reading of at least 25 microvolts during the last 40 milliseconds. In 25 of the 27 control patients, the reading was at least 25 microvolts during the last 40 milliseconds of the QRS waveform. Hence, we define the diagnostic test "less than 25 microvolts during the last 40 milliseconds duration of the QRS waveform" as a positive indicator for the condition "prone to VT."

a. Construct a two-factor frequency distribution table that displays the prone-to-VT condition against the test condition of "less than 25 microvolts in the last 40 milliseconds of the QRS waveform."

b. For this research,
   i. Describe the population of interest.
   ii. Describe the condition of interest.
   iii. Determine the prevalence of the condition of interest in the sample.

c. Determine the Sn, F − R, Sp, F + R, accuracy, PV + , and PV − for the diagnostic test.

d. What do you think? Based on your analysis, does this new noninvasive diagnostic test seem clinically useful?

3. Copin et al were interested in developing a noninvasive procedure to rule out a diagnosis of pulmonary embolism (PE) during acute respiratory failure (ARF) of chronic obstructive pulmonary disease (COPD) patients. Utilizing a reading from a capnograph (a device that reads and records various ventilatory measurements) and a blood gas measurement, the researchers devised a quantity they called "R."

There were 34 patients in the research study, of which 17 presented PE and 17 had no indication of PE (established by pulmonary angiography, an invasive procedure). All 17 PE patients had R > 5. Of the 17 patients without PE, 6 had R > 5 and 11 had R < 5. These results are summarized in Table 4.1.10.

TABLE **4.1.10** Two-factor frequency distribution table showing the data from Copin et al.

	CONDITION	
	PE	No PE
R > 5	17	6
R < 5	0	11

The researchers considered using R > 5 as a positive diagnostic indicator for PE in a COPD patient with ARF.

a. Determine the prevalence for PE among COPD patients with ARF in the study group.

b. Determine the Sn, F − R, Sp, F + R, accuracy, PV + , and PV − for this diagnostic test.

c. Does this diagnostic procedure seem useful to rule out a diagnosis of PE during ARF of COPD patients? Explain.

4. An editorial in *Chance* discussed the topic of random testing for AIDS. The editorial was motivated by an announcement by then-secretary of the Department of Health and Human Services, Otis Bowen, that the agency take blood samples from a random sample of 45,000 U.S. citizens and test the blood for the presence of HIV antibodies. The editor illustrated his argument with a test that was .999 sensitive and .990 specific using an estimated prevalence of .006 for AIDS in the general population. Determine the $F + R, F - R, PV+, PV-$ and accuracy of such a test. Do you think such a screening test would be desirable as public policy?

For Problems 5–7, determine each of the following:

a. What is the disease or condition of interest?

b. What is the proposed diagnostic procedure? How does it compare with the current or standard procedure?

c. Is the prevalence of the condition of interest in the general population given in the article? What is the prevalence of the condition of interest in the study?

d. Construct an appropriate two-factor frequency distribution table showing the condition factor versus the test factor. On the basis of your table, determine the Sn, $F - R$, Sp, $F + R$, $PV+$, $PV-$, and accuracy for the proposed diagnostic procedure.

e. What do you think? Does the new diagnostic procedure seem to be useful?

5. A newspaper article heralded a new test developed to detect the spread of bladder cancer. The article stated that 46,000 Americans develop bladder cancer each year. Most current methods for detecting bladder cancer involve hospitalization and invasive biopsy. The article described a new test developed by the National Cancer Institute (NCI). The new test is a relatively simple urine test for autocrine motility factor (AMF), a substance secreted by cancer cells. In the accompanying research study, the NCI tested urine from 22 patients with bladder cancer and 27 controls (patients with noncancerous conditions of the urinary tract). Among these 49 test subjects, there were 2

false positives and no false negatives for the condition of bladder cancer.

6. A newspaper article reported on a new diagnostic breakthrough for detection of colon cancer. The article noted that colon cancer strikes 140,000 Americans annually. Of these, 60,000 die, making colon cancer second only to lung cancer for the annual incidence of cancer mortality. Current diagnostic procedure consists of a digital examination and stool analysis for blood. The new procedure is a chemical test of a rectal smear obtained with a glove. In the research study to determine the effectiveness of this simple new procedure, 12 patients with known colon cancer were all diagnosed correctly. Five of 59 controls (patients with no detectable cancer) tested positive.

7. Squires and Ellison reported on a newly developed "scorecard" system for assessing the condition of beta-strep throat in school-age children. The usual method for diagnosing beta-strep throat is a throat culture. However, it takes several days to get the results of the test. The researchers were concerned with elementary school children who present pharyngitis. Usually, pharyngitis is not a problem unless beta-strep is involved, in which case the untreated child can develop serious complications like rheumatic fever. Further, beta-strep is contagious. A scorecard assessment was developed with the hope that the school nurse could make a useful on-the-spot diagnosis and indicate whether a child should be kept home from school. A study was done on 285 elementary school children. The authors reported that 19% of the throat cultures were positive. The scorecard predicted nonstrep pharyngitis with 83% accuracy. The scorecard predicted strep infections with 29% accuracy.

8. The predictive value of a positive test result ($PV+$) is related to prevalence, sensitivity (Sn), and specificity (Sp), by the formula

$$PV+ = \frac{Sn \times Prevalence}{(Sn \times prevalence) + [(1 - Sp) \times (1 - prevalence)]}$$

Apply this formula to determine $PV+$ for each of the following scenarios adapted from Chang (reference given in the introduction to this chapter). The standard test for syphilis is called VDRL. Suppose Sn = .90 and Sp = .85. Explain whether the VDRL test would provide any clinically useful information.

a. A young woman self-presents at a gynecology clinic. She indicates her concern that she might have syphilis. A quick verbal history indicates that she has been sexually active with multiple partners over the past 8 months. She has a past history of multiple episodes of pelvic inflammatory disease. Needle marks on her arm indicate that she may be an intravenous drug abuser. On the basis of her presenting history, you assess a prior probability (prevalence) of about 75%; that is, in your clinical experience, about 75% of patients presenting similar circumstances have syphilis.

b. A young woman self-presents at a gynecology clinic. She indicates her concern that she might have syphilis. Oral history reveals that the woman is a virgin living in a convent studying to be a nun. She is guilt-ridden over "impure, immoral thoughts" and is afraid that she may have contracted syphilis as punishment for her sins. Although you are not very experienced with such cases, you assign her a prior probability (prevalence) of .1%, believing that this is probably too high.

c. What is the point that Dr. Chang is making with such examples?

Problems 9–15 are based on research by Jonsbu et al. The researchers studied emergency room (ER) patients suspected of having a myocardial infarction (MI). In particular, Jonsbu et al were interested in defining elements in case histories that might reliably discriminate between MI and non-MI patients in the ER. Such elements would assist in defining a hospital protocol for deciding whether to send an ER patient to the coronary care unit (CCU) or to the general care ward. After a preliminary analysis of 76 elements, the researchers further considered five of the elements: substernal pain, chest oppression, severe pain (requiring morphine or similar painkiller for relief of pain), nausea and/or vomiting, and perspiration. The data concerning the ability of each of these five elements to act as a diagnostic indicator for MI are given in Exercises 9–13. The researchers studied 200 consecutive ER admissions for chest pain and suspected MI. Of these, 73 had an MI and 127 did not. Note that the job at hand is to be able to distinguish reasonably between MI and non-MI patients from basically simple criteria.

For each element described in Problems 9–13,

a. Complete the given two-factor frequency distribution table.

b. Determine the Sn, F − R, Sp, F + R, PV+, PV−, and accuracy of the element as a diagnostic indicator of MI.

9. A partial two-factor frequency distribution table for the element substernal pain is given in Table 4.1.11.

TABLE **4.1.11** Substernal pain.

		SUBSTERNAL PAIN		
		Yes	No	Total
MI	Yes	68		73
	No		25	127
	Total	170		200

10. A partial two-factor frequency distribution table for the element chest oppression is given in Table 4.1.12.

TABLE **4.1.12** Chest oppression.

		CHEST OPPRESSION		
		Yes	No	Total
MI	Yes	60		73
	No		40	127
	Total	147		200

11. A partial two-factor frequency distribution table for the element severe pain is given in Table 4.1.13.

TABLE **4.1.13** Severe pain.

		SEVERE PAIN		
		Yes	No	Total
MI	Yes	54		73
	No		92	127
	Total	89		200

12. A partial two-factor frequency distribution table for the element nausea and/or vomiting is given in Table 4.1.14.

TABLE **4.1.14** Nausea and/or vomiting.

		NAUSEA/VOMITING		
		Yes	No	Total
MI	Yes	33		73
	No		103	127
	Total	57		200

13. A partial two-factor frequency distribution table for the element perspiration is given in Table 4.1.15.

TABLE **4.1.15** Perspiration.

		PERSPIRATION		
		Yes	No	Total
MI	Yes	41		73
	No		105	127
	Total	63		200

14. Based on their research, Jonsbu et al constructed a set of criteria for CCU referral from the ER for MI. The criterion was based on the five elements: substernal pain, chest oppression, severe pain, nausea and/or vomiting, and perspiration. The basically simple criterion for referral to the CCU from the ER is that the patient present at least three of the five elements, including at least two from among the first three elements; otherwise the patient is referred to the general care ward. Using this criterion, a study of 950 admissions to the ER at a major hospital facility in Norway resulted in referrals shown in Table 4.1.16.

TABLE **4.1.16** Jonsbu criterion referrals.

		REFERRED TO		
		CCU	Ward	Total
MI	Yes	400		422
	No		366	528
	Total	562		950

Hence, 422 of the 950 ER patients were eventually confirmed as MI patients. Of these 422 MI patients, the Jonsbu criterion correctly referred 400 to the CCU and incorrectly referred 22 to the general care ward. Of the 528 patients not requiring CCU observation, the Jonsbu criterion correctly sent 366 patients to the general care ward.

a. Complete the two-factor frequency distribution in Table 4.1.16.

b. Determine the Sn, F − R, Sp, F + R, PV+, PV −, and accuracy of the Jonsbu criterion for diagnosing MI patients needing CCU observation.

15. (Continued from 14) Regular hospital practice resulted in referrals shown in Table 4.1.17 for the 950 patients portrayed in Exercise 14.1.14.

TABLE **4.1.17** Regular hospital practice referrals.

		REFERRED TO		
		CCU	Ward	Total
MI	Yes	375		422
	No		230	528
	Total	673		950

a. Complete the two-factor frequency distribution in Table 4.1.17.

b. Determine the Sn, F − R, Sp, F + R, PV+, PV −, and accuracy of regular hospital practice for diagnosing MI patients needing CCU observation.

c. Do you think that the Jonsbu criterion is an improvement over regular hospital practice for determining whether to send an ER patient to the CCU or the general care ward?

Problems 16–19 are based on research by Neinaber et al, who studied four noninvasive imaging procedures to diagnose dissection of the thoracic aorta in patients suspected of having the condition. The four methods were magnetic resonance imaging (MRI), transesophageal echocardiography (TEE), transthoracic echocardiography (TEE), and computerized tomography (CT). For each method described in Problems 16–19, determine the Sn, F − R, Sp, F + R, PV+, PV−, and accuracy.

16. The data for MRI are given in Table 4.1.18. For MRI, Yes means that dissection of the thoracic aorta is indicated; No means that dissection is contraindicated.

TABLE **4.1.18** Data for magnetic resonance imaging.

	DISSECTION PRESENT		
	Yes	No	Total
Yes	58	1	59
No	1	45	46
Total	59	46	105

17. The data for TEE are given in Table 4.1.19. For TEE, Yes means that dissection of the thoracic aorta is indicated; No means that dissection is contraindicated.

TABLE **4.1.19** Data for Transesophageal echocardiography.

	DISSECTION PRESENT		
	Yes	No	Total
Yes	43	6	49
No	1	20	21
Total	44	26	70

18. The data for CT are given in Table 4.1.20. For CT, Yes means that dissection of the thoracic aorta is indicated; No means that dissection is contraindicated.

TABLE **4.1.20** Data for computerized tomography.

	DISSECTION PRESENT		
	Yes	No	Total
Yes	45	4	49
No	3	27	30
Total	48	31	79

19. The data for TTE are given in Table 4.1.21. For TTE, Yes means that dissection of the thoracic aorta is indicated; No means that dissection is contraindicated.

TABLE **4.1.21** Data for transthoracic echocardiography.

	DISSECTION PRESENT		
	Yes	No	Total
Yes	37	8	45
No	25	40	65
Total	62	48	110

20. "Ask Marilyn" is a feature in *Parade Magazine,* a common supplement in Sunday newspapers. One reader asked Marilyn to consider a testing situation in which the prevalence of a condition was 5% in the general population. The diagnostic test used was 95% sensitive and 95% specific. Suppose a person is selected at random from the general population and tests positive. The reader inquired what such a result suggests; in particular, would one conclude that the individual is likely to have the condition? Marilyn answered that the chances are only 50–50. Explain whether this answer is correct.

CHAPTER **4** OVERVIEW

Summary

An appreciation of **diagnostic testing** involves several applications of basic **probability**. Probability is a necessary tool in understanding diagnostic testing since there is no such thing as a perfect diagnostic test. Some of the fundamental concepts needed to apply diagnostic testing are sensitivity and **false-positive rate**, **specificity** and **false-negative rate**, **predictive value**, and **accuracy**. A key determinant in whether a diagnostic test is actually useful is the **prevalence** of the condition in which the test is applied. Each of these key ingredients for understanding diagnostic testing is rooted in probability.

Keywords

accuracy	probability
diagnostic test	sensitivity (Sn)
false-negative rate (F − R)	specificity (Sp)
false-positive rate (F + R)	true positive
predictive value	true negative
(PV +, PV −)	two-factor frequency
prevalence	distribution table

References

The Editors: Random testing for AIDS? *Chance* 1, no. 1 (Winter 1988): 9.

Chang P: Evaluating imaging test performance: An introduction to Bayesian analysis for urologists. *Monogr Urol* 12, no. 2 (1991): 18.

Chopin C et al: Use of capnography in diagnosis of pulmonary embolism during acute respiratory failure of chronic obstructive pulmonary disease. *Crit Care Med* 18, no. 4 (April 1990): 353.

Diagnostic breakthrough noted: New rapid test can detect colon cancer accurately, early. *Eureka Times-Standard*, 10 March 1987, 13.

Jonsbu J et al: Rapid and correct diagnosis of myocardial infarction: Standardized case history and clinical examination provide important information for correct referral to monitored beds. *J Intern Med* 229 (1991): 143.

Lansdowne L: Signal-averaged electrocardiograms. *Heart Lung* 19, no. 4 (July 1990): 329.

New test developed to detect spread of bladder cancer. *Eureka Times-Standard,* 5 October 1988, 10.

Nienabor C et al: The diagnosis of thoracic aortic dissection by noninvasive imaging procedures. *N Engl J Med* 328, no. 1 (7 January 1993): 1.

Pantaleo N et al: Thallium myocardial scintigraphy and its use in the assessment of CAD. *Heart Lung* 10, no. 1 (January 1981): 61.

Roberts J et al: Diagnostic accuracy of fever as a measure of postoperative pulmonary complications. *Heart Lung* 17, no. 2 (March 1988): 166.

Squires R and Ellison G: Prediction of streptococcal pharyngitis: an option for school nurses? *J Sch Health* 56, no. 6 (August 1986): 218.

vos Savant M: Ask Marilyn. *Parade Magazine*, 6 September 1992, 22.

CHAPTER 5

Discrete Distributions

In Chapters 5 and 6 we take a deeper look at the concept of a random variable. In particular, we focus on the properties of an interval random variable. There are two types of interval random variables: discrete and continuous. Chapter 5 focuses on discrete random variables; Chapter 6, continuous.

In this chapter we shift our viewpoint from the "past" to the "future." The past focused on what we have already observed (in a sample). The future focuses on what we will see or, more precisely, on what we probably will see. We do know we will encounter *variation*. To understand variation we will need a model for the random variable of interest. Two basic probability models are used to explain chance variation: the coin-flip model for a simple categorical random variable and the normal distribution model for a continuous random variable. We will need a firm grasp of these models before we launch into inferential statistics. Hence, Chapters 5 and 6 form an interlude in which we develop these statistical models needed for inferential statistics in Chapters 7–14.

Section 5.1 introduces the key features of a discrete random variable. In Section 5.2 we study the most common discrete random variable, the binomial random variable. In particular, we talk about coin flips as if that were important. It is. Many situations are best explained using a coin flip model. A patient is either sick (heads) or OK (tails). A diagnostic test will either detect (heads) or not detect (tails) a medical condition of concern. A genetic trait may be dominant (heads) or recessive (tails). The genetic makeup of a child whose parents are heterozygous carriers of a genetic condition is the result of Mother Nature's coin flip. So is the gender of the child. The "luck of the draw" is often explained by the flip of a coin.

SECTION 5.1	**OBJECTIVES** This section will
Discrete Random Variables	**1** Describe an interval random variable, distinguishing between a discrete and continuous random variable.
	2 Describe the coin-flip model.
	3 Describe and apply a probability density function for a given discrete random variable.
	4 Determine the mean and standard deviation for a given discrete random variable when provided with its probability density function.

The genetics of the inherited disease cystic fibrosis (CF) was introduced in Example 3.1.9. The probability that a child born to CF carrier parents will develop CF is one out of four. Botkin and Alemagno point out major concerns regarding CF:

- CF is the most common lethal genetic disease among Caucasians.
- About 1 out of every 25 Caucasians is a carrier for CF.
- The incidence of CF among Caucasians is 1 case per 2500 births.
- CF carrier screening is now promising since the gene for CF has been identified.

EXAMPLE 5.1.1 Jack and Jill are planning a family. They are concerned since each is a carrier for cystic fibrosis (CF). They realize that there are risks involved, so they consult a genetics counselor, who tells them there is no way to guarantee the genetic makeup of a child. The counselor shows the couple Table 5.1.1, which displays the probability of CF among children of CF carrier parents.

TABLE **5.1.1**
Distribution tables for the number of CF children in a family.

	(a)			(b)			(c)	
	1 child			*2 children*			*3 children*	
No. CF	*Prob*	*C Prob*	*No. CF*	*Prob*	*C Prob*	*No. CF*	*Prob*	*C Prob*
0	.75	.75	0 w(f	.56	.56	0	.42	.42
1	.25	1.00	1 w CF	.38	.94	1	.42	.84
			2	.06	1.00	2	.14	.98
						3	.02	1.00

No. CF = number of children in the family with cystic fibrosis.
Prob = probability.
C Prob = cumulative probability. – alway be 1

Table 5.1.1 contains a great deal of information. First, one cannot tell Jack and Jill specifically what will happen to them (will a child have CF?). One can only explain the possibilities with their likelihoods. In the background is a particular random variable X of interest:

X = number of children in the family with cystic fibrosis

Most questions of interest about X can be answered using the information in these tables. This is the case for any random variable like X; that is, one can construct a distribution table and apply the table to address concerns. The details about how to do this form the subject matter for this section. We begin by reviewing and further developing the concept of a random variable, the concept behind these informative tables.

Random Variables

A research team begins by first designing a program of study.

- A population of interest is defined, specifying *who* is of interest in the study.

- A random variable is defined, specifying *what* about the individuals in the population is of interest.
- A sampling strategy is selected in order to obtain an unbiased sample from the population.
- Data are gathered by applying the random variable to each member of the sample.

Once data are gathered, one then processes them in order to obtain the story they tell. The processing begins with descriptive statistics, an organized presentation of the data. The tools one applies to describe data effectively depend on the nature of the random variable that describes the data.

The term random variable (RV) was introduced in Chapter 1. There, we distinguished between a categorical (nonnumerical) and a quantitative (numerical) RV. The distinction is useful in guiding descriptive statistics. A data set gathered for a categorical RV is effectively described by means of a frequency distribution table (ungrouped) with accompanying graphics in the form of a bar graph or pie chart, as in Section 1.1.

A data set gathered for a quantitative RV consists of numbers. In order to describe a numerical data set, one must first assess the context of the numbers: nominal, ordinal, or interval. Nominal and ordinal data, although numerical, are often categorical in nature. Such data sets are best described by methods applied to categorical data. Interval data consist of numbers that behave like "real" numbers; that is, they carry an intrinsic notion of size. Interval numbers count or measure. One may choose from an assortment of tools to describe an interval data set.

- The describe method (Section 1.2) boils down a data set to a representative or typical number.
- Exploratory data analysis (EDA; Section 2.1) focuses on illustrating the general distribution of the data.
- The table method (Sections 2.2 and 3) condenses the data into a grouped format.

In this section we first take a closer look at a quantitative RV that yields an interval data set.

Interval Random Variables

An **interval random variable** is a quantitative RV that yields a data set of interval numbers. An interval number carries with it an intrinsic notion of size. The key feature is that one can subtract two interval numbers and obtain a meaningful difference between them. For example, if Jack weighs 72 kg and Jill weighs 60 kg, then Jack weighs 12 kg more than Jill. Here, $72 - 60 = 12$ yields a meaningful difference.

This "meaningful difference" feature of interval numbers does not exist for nominal (naming) or ordinal (ranking) numbers. For example, consider encoding hair color with the nominal scheme

$0 =$ bald, $1 =$ brown, $2 =$ black, $3 =$ blond, $4 =$ red, $5 =$ gray, $6 =$ other

The data set {1, 1, 6, 0, 6, 3, 3, 4}, although quantitative since it consists of numbers, is not an interval data set. The numbers do not count or measure anything. The numbers are only arbitrary synonyms for hair categories. Interval descriptive statistics (e.g., mean, standard deviation) is a nonsense activity for this data set. Jack has brown hair (hair category 1) and Jill is a redhead (hair category 4). However, the numerical difference, $4 - 1 = 3$, does not determine any *amount* of difference between Jack's and Jill's hair, just that they are different. In fact, taking the difference $4 - 1$ here makes as much sense as taking the difference "red − brown"!

An interval number is obtained by performing a *count* or a *measurement*. A count yields a *whole number* (0, 1, 2, 3, 4, 5, . . .). A measurement yields a *decimal number* (even though the decimal number might be rounded up to a whole number). Consequently, we distinguish between two kinds of interval RVs: discrete and continuous.

Discrete Random Variables

A **discrete random variable** is an interval RV that is specified by counting something. The key feature of a discrete RV is that *all possible values can be listed* (enumerated).

EXAMPLE 5.1.2 An RV is usually denoted by a capital letter. A generic value a discrete RV may assume is denoted by the corresponding lowercase letter. The following examples describe discrete RVs:

COUNTS.

A = number of admissions to General Hospital in a day
a = 0, 1, 2, 3, 4, 5, . . .

B = number of grafts in coronary artery bypass graft surgery
b = 1, 2, 3, 4

C = number of children in a family
c = 0, 1, 2, 3, 4, 5, . . .

G = number of girls in a family with five children
g = 0, 1, 2, 3, 4, 5

P = number of days in a week one has headache pain
p = 0, 1, 2, 3, 4, 5, 6, 7

Continuous Random Variables

A **continuous random variable** is an interval RV that is specified by a measurement.

EXAMPLE 5.1.3 The following are examples of continuous RVs:

W = weight of a person (kg)
C = serum cholesterol level (mg/dl)
L = length of intravenous therapy (hours)
BMI = body mass index (kg/m^2)
T = temperature (°C)
CO = cardiac output (liters/minute)
H = height of a person (cm)

The key feature of a continuous RV is that *all* numbers between any two possibilities are also possible; that is, a continuous RV presents an unbroken, continuous spectrum of possibilities. For example, if one person weighs 60 kg and another 72 kg, then all numbers between 60 and 72 are also possible (i.e., reasonable numbers for weight). If one person has a cardiac output of 4.36 liters/minute and another 5.81 liters/minute, then all the numbers between 4.36 and 5.81 are also possible cardiac output values.

This "in-between" property is the distinguishing feature between a continuous RV and a discrete RV. A discrete RV cannot attain in-between values. For example, the number of girls in a family of four children can only take on the values 0, 1, 2, 3, or 4. In-between values like 1.7 or 3.648 are impossible.

The in-between feature is possible for a continuous RV because a continuous RV is specified by a measurement. A measurement is by nature a *decimal* number. In practice, the full decimal number (all places past the decimal point) is unknown. What gets measured and recorded is a rounded-off version of the actual number. In practice, one even frequently rounds to a whole number. For example, John weighs 71 kg. This does not mean that John's weight is mathematically exactly 71 kg. The number of places one can report in a decimal measurement is limited in practice by the precision of the instrument used to make the measurement. The hospital scale says John weighs 71 kg; the Space Agency has a more precise scale that can report John's weight as 71.273 kg.

The number of decimal places one needs to record measurements is an important consideration in statistical design. Increased precision is always expensive. Excessive precision is not only costly but foolish since it lends nothing of interest to the research design. For example, consider taking a history of an adult patient. Recording the patient's age in years is totally adequate. One can be more precise by knowing the number of weeks, days, hours, or even minutes; however, such finery is unnecessary.

Classification of Random Variables

Thus far in this text, we have carefully introduced concepts and accompanying terminology to classify the nature of a given RV. This is pivotal because the methods used to describe a corresponding data set and the methods used to analyze that data depend on the nature of the RV that describes the data. Our first key concept was that of the **random variable** itself. We then distinguished between categorical and quantitative RVs (names versus numbers). Among quantitative RVs, we distinguished between nominal, ordinal, and interval variables (names, ranks, and "real" numbers). Now, among interval RVs, we further distinguished between discrete (counting) and continuous (measuring) variables. The complete set of guidelines for determining the nature of an RV is shown in Figure 5.1.1.

We need these distinctions involving an RV in order to deal with a key problem in the health sciences: **variation**—people are different. One way to cope with variation, instead of considering each individual in the group, is to *consider the group as an individual*. We applied this approach in descriptive statistics (Chapters 1 and 2), for example, in boiling down a set of interval numbers to simply mean ± standard deviation.

FIGURE **5.1.1**
The various kinds of
random variables.

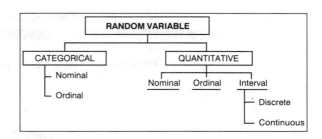

From the science viewpoint in the health sciences, one gets a handle on variation by understanding the nature of the **distribution** of the underlying RV of interest. What values can the RV take on? Which possibilities are more frequent or more rare? An understanding of the distribution is obtained in two ways. One method is *empirical*: Obtain *data* and apply EDA (exploratory data analysis with appropriate tables and graphs). The other method is *theoretical*: Postulate a *model* for the RV of interest and obtain a frequency distribution based upon the model.

Once one knows the distribution for the RV of interest (whether empirically or theoretically), one may apply this knowledge to the future: What can I expect for my next observation (or group of observations)? The distribution will not tell us what we will see but what we probably will see. The distribution displays possibilities and probabilities.

In preparation for inferential statistics (Chapters 7–14), we will need two probability models. The purpose of such a model is to explain the distribution of an RV of interest. In Chapter 6 we develop the normal distribution model, the most common and important model describing a continuous RV. In this chapter we develop the binomial model (Section 5.2) based on the theory of coin flips. The binomial model is the most common and important model describing a discrete RV. The utility of a probability model was introduced in Example 5.1.1. If Jack and Jill proceed with their plans to have children, the actual number of CF children they will have is the result of the luck of the draw—the result of Mother Nature's coin flips. The coin-flip model is the most basic conceptual model for explaining the distribution of chance variation.

The Coin-Flip Model

Consider tossing a fair coin. The coin toss describes an experiment. The random outcomes to the experiment are heads (H) and tails (T). The definition of a "fair" coin is that each outcome is equiprobable. This idealized coin can be depicted using a probability tree diagram and a probability table, as shown in Figure 5.1.2.

FIGURE **5.1.2**
(a) Probability tree
diagram; (b) table for the
toss of a fair coin.

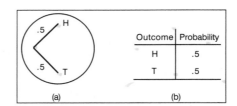

Figure 5.1.2 shows a **model** of a fair coin. A model is an idealization of a way one perceives some facet of reality; accordingly, a model is a theoretical tool. The coin-flip model is the simplest model possible that can display variation. In order to have variation, there must be at least two possible alternatives (hence, the "coin flip").

Now consider the experiment of flipping three fair coins independently (the outcome for one coin does not affect the outcome of another coin). We will be interested in the number of heads that shows up. Notice that the appropriate response to the question "How many heads show on a toss of three independent fair coins?" is a number: 0, 1, 2, 3. We recognize that the question describes a discrete RV, since the answer is obtained by *counting* something. Figure 5.1.3 displays a model for the three-coin-toss experiment.

Figures 5.1.2 and 5.1.3 both display a model for a coin-tossing experiment. Both figures start with (a), a diagram portraying the experiment. The purpose of the diagram is to visualize the presentation of (b), a table that lists all possibilities along with their respective probabilites for the RV of interest. Such a table, called a "probability density function," is precisely what is needed to answer questions of interest about a discrete RV.

Probability Density Function

We can model the three-coin-toss experiment by displaying a probability tree diagram (Figure 5.1.3a) or a summary table (Figure 5.1.3b). The summary table has two columns. The first column displays all the possibilities; the second column displays the corresponding probabilities. A model for a discrete RV that displays each possibility along with the corresponding probability is called a **probability density function (PDF).** Hence, our summary table represents a PDF for the three-coin-toss experiment.

We emphasize that the PDF for a discrete random variable is a *theoretical* tool. It describes what we "should" see. The PDF serves as a theoretical model about how one views a population at large. Note that we did not really flip any coins to obtain the probability tree diagram or the table in Figure 5.1.3.

How do real coins behave? That is another matter! A researcher would design an experiment to conduct the appropriate activity: Obtain three fair coins, put them in a cup, shake well, roll them, and count the number of heads. When one repeats this

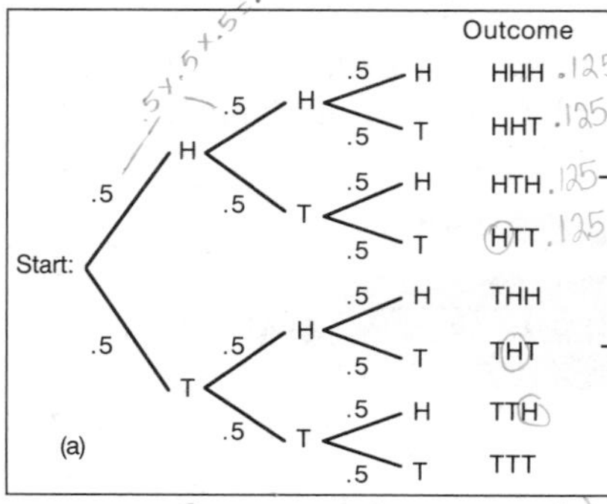

FIGURE **5.1.3**
(a) Probability tree
diagram; (b) table
for the independent
toss of three fair
coins.

activity over and over, one notices *variation* in the number of heads. The number of heads is not the same from toss to toss but instead varies randomly. After many repetitions the researcher would summarize the observed results in a (relative) frequency distribution table. One now inquires whether the observed variation is reasonably explained by the coin-flip model. Do the observed relative frequencies reasonably match the probabilities in the coin-toss PDF? (This specific question will be taken up later in Section 13.1.) These questions capture the main motivation for statistics: How can I explain the variation that I see? The purpose of the PDF for a discrete RV is to serve as a model to explain variation.

The PDF is a valuable tool that can be used for a variety of chores, such as assessing the probability of a particular value for the RV. For example, in the three-coin-toss experiment (Figure 5.1.3), the probability that no heads will show is .125. The probability that exactly two heads will show is .375. The implication is that if we were to perform the three-coin-toss experiment many times, we would expect about 12.5% of the tosses to show no heads; about 37.5%, two heads.

EXAMPLE 5.1.4 We can now recognize that Table 5.1.1 shown to Jack and Jill in Example 5.1.1 is a collection of three PDFs. For example, Table 5.1.1(c) is the PDF describing the number of CF cases in a planned family of three children where both parents are CF carriers. From this PDF, Jack and Jill see that the probability that all three children will be physically free of CF is 42%. Although it is possible that all three children could have CF, they feel this is highly unlikely since the associated probability is only 2%. They are concerned that there is a 42% chance that exactly one child will have CF. And they are particularly concerned that there is a 58% chance that at least one child in three will develop cystic fibrosis.

In addition to being able to compute the probability for events of interest, the PDF has other uses, such as computing an average and a measure of variation.

In order to be able to utilize the PDF for these additional chores, we need to introduce some generic notation so that we can talk about various aspects of a PDF in general. We have already mentioned that an RV is often named with a capital letter, say X. A generic value that X can take on is denoted by the corresponding lowercase letter (here, x). The first thing that one can read from a PDF for X is the probability that X takes on the value x in a given experiment; that is, we can read Prob$[X = x]$ from the table. For brevity and convenience, this probability is denoted by $f(x)$; that is,

$$f(x) = \text{Prob}[X = x]$$

This equation reads that the probability that the RV X takes on the value x in any experiment is $f(x)$. In a PDF the values for x are written in the first column in increasing order. The corresponding probabilities, $f(x)$, are placed in the second column. Note that the sum of the $f(x)$, column must be 1 since the first column must list all possible values the RV can take on. When an experiment is run, the RV must have one of the values shown in the first column. Since the first column accounts for all possibilities, the probability that an experiment will show a value in the first column is a certainty.

EXAMPLE 5.1.5 A public health worker conducts a study of families with four children in a large urban area. The researcher is interested in family dynamics caused by culture and gender makeup. In a given family of four children, the researcher obtains the number of girls in the family. We note that the number of girls in a family of four children defines a discrete RV. The possible values are 0, 1, 2, 3, and 4. We formalize this RV as follows:

X = number of girls in a family with four children
x = 0, 1, 2, 3, 4

The PDF for this discrete RV is displayed in Table 5.1.2.

TABLE **5.1.2**
PDF for the discrete random variable X = number of girls in a family with four children. The x column displays the possible values for X. The $f(x)$ column displays the corresponding probabilities.

x	f(x)
0	.0625
1	.2500
2	.3750
3	.2500
4	.0625

In Section 5.2 we will detail how to obtain the probabilities displayed in the $f(x)$ column. The curious reader who cannot wait to know where the probabilities in the $f(x)$ column in Table 5.1.2 came from is invited to construct a probability tree diagram like that in Figure 5.1.3. In the remainder of this section, we show how to read and apply the PDF table. We will use Example 5.1.5 and Table 5.1.2 to illustrate the various computations shown in the rest of this section.

The first job now is just to get comfortable with reading a PDF. From the PDF table shown in Table 5.1.2, $f(3)$ = .2500; that is, the probability that a random family of four children has exactly three girls is .2500 (25%). What is the probability that a family of four childdren has all boys? In that case the number of girls is zero. From the PDF, $f(0)$ = .0625. Hence, the probability that the family has all boys is about 6%. The probability that the family has all girls is obtained by noting that the number of girls is four (i.e., x = 4); hence, from the PDF, $f(4)$ = .0625. What is the probability that the family has an equal number of boys and girls? In that case, x = 2. From the PDF, $f(2)$ = .3750. So the probability for an equal number of boys and girls is 37.5%.

Note that the sum of the $f(x)$ column is 1.0000. This reflects the fact that the first column lists *all* possible values for X. Values not occurring in the x column are impossible. An outcome that is impossible has probability 0. Hence, $f(-2)$ = 0, $f(7)$ = 0, $f(2.6)$ = 0; and $f(3.792)$ = 0.

Applying a PDF, one can compute the probability for a variety of interesting events.

EXAMPLE 5.1.6 What is the probability that a family of four children all have the same gender?

P[same gender]
= P[all girls or all boys]
= P[all girls] + P[all boys]   (mutually exclusive rule)
= $f(4)$ + $f(0)$
=   .0625   +   .0625
= .1250

Hence, the probability that all four children in the family have the same gender is .1250; that is, about one family in eight (1/8 = .125) with four children should have their children all of the same gender.

EXAMPLE 5.1.7 What is the probability that the family has more girls than boys?

$$P[\text{more girls than boys}]$$
$$= P[X = 3 \text{ or } X = 4]$$
$$= P[X = 3] + P[X = 4]$$
$$= f(3) + f(4)$$
$$= .2500 + .0625$$
$$= .3125$$

Almost one-third of the families with four children will have more girls than boys.

EXAMPLE 5.1.8 What is the probability that the number of girls in a family of four children is between one inclusively and four exclusively? First, note that X is the RV that counts the number of girl children. Thus, the question asks for the probability that $1 \le X < 4$.

$$P[1 \le X < 4]$$
$$= P[X = 1 \text{ or } X = 2 \text{ or } X = 3]$$
$$= P[X = 1] + P[X = 2] + P[X = 3]$$
$$= f(1) + f(2) + f(3)$$
$$= .2500 + .3750 + .2500$$
$$= .8750$$

[handwritten: 1 or more than 1 but less than 4
1. 2500
2. 3750
3 + 2500]

Hence, the probability that the number of girls in a family of four children is between one inclusively and four exclusively is .8750 (87.5%).

Cumulative Density Function

In addition to the PDF, sometimes a cumulative version known as the **cumulative density function (CDF),** is presented. The cumulative density at x, denoted by $F(x)$, is the probability that the RV X will take on a value up to and including but not exceeding x. Continuing with the earlier example, the CDF for X, the number of girls in a family with four children, is displayed in Table 5.1.3.

TABLE **5.1.3**
CDF for X, the number of girls in a family with four children.

x	F(x)
0	.0625
1	.3125
2	.6875
3	.9375
4	1.0000

From the CDF Table 5.1.3, $F(2) = .6875$; that is, the probability that a family of four children has ≤ 2 girls (either 0, 1, or 2 girls inclusively) is .6875 (68.75%). Also, $F(-3) = 0$ since $x \leq -3$ is impossible; $F(6) = 1$ since $x \leq 6$ for all possible values of x.

Formally, $F(x)$ is the probability that the RV X takes on a value less than or equal to x; that is,

$$F(x) = \text{Prob}[X \leq x]$$

In a CDF table the last entry must be 1 since all possible values for X are then accounted for. The CDF is constructed from a PDF in the same way that a cumulative relative frequency table is constructed from a relative frequency table (Section 2.3).

The PDF and CDF tables are interchangeable from the viewpoint that either one can be constructed from the other. For example,

$$\begin{aligned} f(2) &= F(2) - F(1) \\ &= .6875 - .3125 \\ &= .3750 \end{aligned}$$

When the number of possible values for a discrete RV is small, one may combine the PDF and CDF into a single table. For the family of four (Example 5.1.5), the combined PDF and CDF table is shown in Table 5.1.4.

TABLE **5.1.4**
Combined PDF and CDF for X, the number of girls in a family with four children.

x	f(x)	F(x)
0	.0625	.0625
1	.2500	.3125
2	.3750	.6875
3	.2500	.9375
4	.0625	1.0000

How does one obtain a PDF for a given RV? The probabilities in a PDF may be either theoretical or empirical. In Section 5.2 we show how to determine the PDF for a discrete RV that theoretically is based on a coin-flip model. Many practical discrete RVs, however, are not based on theory. One must conduct a research study to estimate the PDF as it applies to the population at large. The research study produces a frequency distribution table that one uses as an estimate for the PDF. For example, Figure 1.1.3 displays the results for the Jonsson et al perfusion score study. Using that table we estimate that about 60% of patients with a surgical wound have a perfusion score of 3.

In addition to being able to use a PDF (or CDF) to calculate the probability of an event of interest, one can use the PDF to determine two other key quantities concerning the discrete RV of interest: the mean and the standard deviation.

The Mean of a Discrete Random Variable

Suppose that X denotes a discrete RV. The **mean** for a discrete RV X is a measure of central tendency for X, just like the mean for a quantitative data set is a measure of central tendency for a data set. However, the mean for an RV is a more abstract concept than the mean for a data set. We will first focus on merely calculating the mean for an RV. After we know how to calculate it, we will focus on explaining what it "means" (this is the approach we used for the standard deviation for a data set). We follow this procedure for more abstract ideas because the calculation is the easy part! An appreciation for the mean of an RV must evolve.

The mean for the RV X is denoted by μ_X (μ for mean and the subscript of X to denote the RV). Actually, the mean of a discrete RV is easy to calculate from its PDF. To facilitate the computation, construct a worksheet with three columns: x, $f(x)$, and $xf(x)$. The first two columns, x and $f(x)$, come from the PDF for X; the third column must be calculated. The third column is calculated by multiplying each possibility x by its associated probability $f(x)$, thereby obtaining the product $xf(x)$. The sum of the $xf(x)$ column yields μ_X, the mean of X.

EXAMPLE 5.1.9 The computations for the mean for the number of girls in a family of four children are shown in Table 5.1.5. First, multiply each possibility in column x by its corresponding probability in column $f(x)$, and place the answer in the $xf(x)$ column. Then, add up the $xf(x)$ column. The sum of the $xf(x)$ column is 2.00; hence, $\mu_X = 2.00$ (or simply, $\mu_X = 2$).

TABLE **5.1.5**
Calculations for determining the mean number of girls in a family of four children based on the PDF displayed in Table 5.1.2. Here, $\mu_X = 2$.

x	f(x)	xf(x)
0	.0625	.00
1	.2500	.25
2	.3750	.75
3	.2500	.75
4	.0625	.25
		2.00

According to the computations displayed in Example 5.1.9, the mean number of girls in a family of four children is two. The simple interpretation is that *on average* a family with four children will have two girls.

The mean for a discrete RV is often called its **expected value**. Recall that the PDF for the RV that counts the number of girls in a family of four children (Table 5.1.4) comes from the coin-flip model. It assumes that Mother Nature flips an equiprobable (male, female) coin in assigning a gender to a child. Based on this coin-flip model, the PDF presents the theoretical probabilities of a family of four children having 0, 1, 2, 3, or 4 girls. The actual number of girls in a family, according to this model, is a chance result that is the luck of the draw. So much for theoretical models. What about real families?

In a study of real families, a researcher would survey many families with four children. The researcher then obtains a real data set. If the coin-flip model is appropriate, then the researcher anticipates that the observed data set mean $\bar{x}$ is close to the "expected" $\mu_X = 2$. Hence, the mean of the RV, μ_X, predicts what a researcher can expect for a data set mean, *if* the researcher were to actually go out into the field and collect data. Accordingly, a theoretical discrete RV with its companion PDF can be a valuable conceptual tool in statistical design, guiding a researcher as to what can be expected based on certain assumptions. Research can be designed to test those assumptions.

Because of this expected value interpretation for μ_X, the mean for the RV X, some researchers prefer and use an alternate notation, $E[X]$ ($E[X]$ is read "expected value of X"). Note that "mean value of X" and "expected value of X" are alternative expressions for the same concept. It is a matter of personal preference which one to use.

The computations for the mean of X (as displayed in Example 5.1.9) are nicely summarized by the following formula:

$$\mu_X = \Sigma x f(x)$$

Alternatively, $E[X] = \Sigma x f(x)$. Either way, the formula directs us to sum up (Σ) the products ($x f(x)$) obtained by multiplying each possibility (x) by its probability ($f(x)$). Finally, when the RV X is understood, for convenience, one may drop the subscript X in μ_X for denoting the mean; that is, the mean μ of the RV X is given by

$$\mu = \Sigma x f(x)$$

The Standard Deviation

As with data, the **standard deviation of a random variable** X, denoted by σ_X, is the square root of the variance. Hence, almost all the work in determining the standard deviation is done by calculating the variance of X. Because the standard deviation is not an immediately intuitive concept, we focus first on computing it (the easy part), then on explaining it.

The **variance** of X (denoted by $V[X]$, $Var[X]$, or σ^2) is defined by statisticians as

$$V[X] = \Sigma(x - \mu)^2 f(x)$$

For the sake of computation; however, use the equivalent formula

$$V[X] = \Sigma x^2 f(x) - \mu^2$$

The advantage of this alternate formula is that the variance is obtained in the fewest possible computational steps. When computing the variance for a discrete RV by hand from a PDF, we will always use this alternate formula.

Actually, the standard deviation of a discrete RV is easy to calculate from its PDF (it's a bit more tedious than calculating the mean). To facilitate computing the variance, construct a worksheet with five columns: x, $f(x)$, $x f(x)$, x^2, and $x^2 f(x)$. The first two columns, x and $f(x)$, come from the PDF for X; the third, fourth, and fifth columns must be calculated. Note that the first three columns are already in place from calculating the mean. Hence, to Table 5.1.5 in Example 5.1.9, we append two new columns, x^2 and $x^2 f(x)$. To obtain the variance of X, find the sum of the $x^2 f(x)$ column and then subtract μ^2. We illustrate using the example of the family of four children.

EXAMPLE 5.1.10 Calculation of the variance and standard deviation for X = the number of girls in a family with four children.

TABLE **5.1.6**
Calculation worksheet for obtaining the variance of X.

x	$f(x)$	$xf(x)$	x^2	$x^2f(x)$
0	.0625	.00	0	.00
1	.2500	.25	1	.25
2	.3750	.75	4	1.50
3	.2500	.75	9	2.25
4	.0625	.25	16	1.00
		2.00		5.00

To obtain the x^2 column, square each entry in the x column (fortunately, a quick and easy task). To obtain the $x^2f(x)$ column, multiply each entry in the x^2 column by the corresponding entry in the $f(x)$ column (a calculator usually is handy). Now, add up the $xf(x)$ and $x^2f(x)$ columns.

Here, $\Sigma xf(x)$ = Sum of $xf(x)$ column = 2.00
$\Sigma x^2f(x)$ = Sum of $x^2f(x)$ column = 5.00

Hence, $\mu = \Sigma xf(x) = 2.00$

and

$$V[X] = \Sigma x^2f(x) - \mu^2$$
$$= 5.00 - (2.00)^2$$
$$= 5 - 4$$
$$= 1$$

So $\sigma = \sqrt{V[X]} = \sqrt{1} = 1$

What does it all mean? We first note that the number of girls in a family of four children is not constant but may vary from family to family. This *variation* is the source of both interest and problems. For our example, we can say that a "typical" family of four children has 2 ± 1 girls; that is, between one and three girls. In general, the "typical" value taken on by a discrete RV X is usually given by its mean (μ) plus or minus the standard deviation (σ); that is, $\mu \pm \sigma$.

Computing the Mean and Standard Deviation

Sometimes students miscalculate the mean for a discrete random variable by confusing it with the mean for a data set. These two versions of the mean need to be kept distinct since they are computed differently. The data mean is computed from a set of numbers in a sample. The RV mean is computed from a PDF. When asked to compute the mean, one must first determine whether one wants the mean for a data set or the mean for an RV.

In the sequel, we now present a summary of the formulas needed to compute the mean and standard deviation for a data set and an RV. When a data set is given, it may be presented in the form of raw, unprocessed data or in a condensed summary form like a frequency distribution table (ungrouped).

Raw Data Set

The data are presented as a raw data set $\{x_1, x_2, x_3, \ldots, x_n\}$. Then

mean: $\bar{x} = \Sigma x/n$

variance: $s^2 = \dfrac{n(\Sigma x^2) - (\Sigma x)^2}{n(n-1)}$

EXAMPLE 5.1.11 Data set = $\{1,3,2,5,3\}$

Here, n (size of data set) = 5

Σx (sum of data) = $1 + 3 + 2 + 5 + 3 = 14$

Σx^2 (sum of squares) = $1^2 + 3^2 + 2^2 + 5^2 + 3^2$
$= 1 + 9 + 4 + 25 + 9$
$= 48$

Hence,

mean: $\bar{x} = \Sigma x/n = 14/5 = 2.8$

variance: $s^2 = \dfrac{n(\Sigma x^2) - (\Sigma x)^2}{n(n-1)}$

$= \dfrac{5(48) - (14)^2}{5(4)} = 2.2$

standard deviation: $s = \sqrt{\text{variance}} = \sqrt{2.2} = 1.5$

Data Set: Frequency Distribution Table

Here, the raw data has been processed for presentation; that is, the data are given in the condensed form of a frequency distribution table (ungrouped) as shown in Table 5.1.7.

TABLE **5.1.7**
The general form for a frequency distribution table. The various observations are listed down the first (x) column. The respective frequencies (f) are listed in the second column.

Observation (x)	Frequency (f)
x_1	f_1
x_2	f_2
x_3	f_3
...	...
x_k	f_k

In Table 5.1.7, f stands for *frequency* for a given observation. The total sample size N is the sum of the individual frequencies; that is, $N = \Sigma f$.

Then   mean: $\bar{x} = (\Sigma xf)/N$

variance: $s^2 = \dfrac{N(\Sigma x^2 f) - (\Sigma xf)^2}{N(N-1)}$

EXAMPLE 5.1.12 Suppose a data set is given by means of the frequency distribution table (columns x and f in Table 5.1.8). For ease in calculating the mean and standard deviation, add three more columns: xf, x^2 and x^2f.

The xf column is obtained by multiplying each observation x by its corresponding frequency f.

The x^2 column is obtained by squaring each observation in the x column.

The x^2f column is obtained by multiplying each x^2 by its corresponding frequency.

TABLE 5.1.8
Worksheet for computing the mean and standard deviation from a frequency distribution table.

x	f	xf	x^2	x^2f
1	4	4	1	4
2	6	12	4	24
3	1	3	9	9
5	3	15	25	75
	14	34		112

We first obtain the sums (Σ) for the f, xf, and x^2f columns:

$$N = \Sigma f = 4 + 6 + 1 + 3 = 14 \text{ (total sample size)}$$
$$\Sigma xf = 34$$
$$\Sigma x^2f = 112$$

Then, mean: $\bar{x} = \dfrac{\Sigma xf}{N} = \dfrac{34}{14} = 2.4$

Variance: $s^2 = \dfrac{N(\Sigma x^2f) - (\Sigma xf)^2}{N(N-1)}$

$$= \frac{14(112) - (34)^2}{14(13)}$$

$$= 2.26 \text{ (2.263736264 calculator unrounded)}$$

Standard deviation:

$$s = \sqrt{\text{variance}}$$
$$= \sqrt{2.263736264} \text{ (use unrounded variance)}$$
$$= 1.5 \text{ (round the final answer)}$$

Random Variable

The general form for a PDF is provided as shown in Table 5.1.9.

TABLE 5.1.9
The general form for a PDF.

x	$f(x)$
x_1	p_1
x_2	p_2
...	...
x_k	p_k
	1.00

Then, mean: $\mu = E[X] = \Sigma xf(x)$

variance: $\sigma^2 = V[X] = (\Sigma x^2f(x)) - \mu^2$

EXAMPLE 5.1.13 A PDF is given in Table 5.1.10. Table 5.1.11 expands the original PDF by adding on three additional columns for ease in computing the mean and the variance. One recognizes that Table 5.1.10 is a PDF since the entries in the second column are decimals (probabilities) that add up to 1.

TABLE **5.1.10**
A PDF.

x	f(x)
1	.4
2	.1
3	.5
	1.0

TABLE **5.1.11**
The PDF with three columns added on for computing the mean and standard deviation.

x	f(x)	xf(x)	x²	x²f(x)
1	.4	.4	1	.4
2	.1	.2	4	.4
3	.5	1.5	9	4.5
	1.00	2.1		5.3

Hence,   mean: $\mu_X = \Sigma xf(x) = 2.1$

variance: $V[X] = (\Sigma x^2 f(x)) - \mu^2$

$= 5.3 - (2.1)^2$

$= 0.89$

standard deviation: $\sigma_X = \sqrt{V[X]} = \sqrt{0.89} = 0.9$

EXERCISES 5.1

Warm-ups
5.1

1. In a well-designed study, one must first clearly define the population of interest, that is, specify *who* is to be studied. Second, one determines *what* about each individual in the population is of interest in the context of the study. Formally, this "what" is called a
    a. Question
    b. Random variable
    c. Parameter
    d. PDF
    e. Variance

2. The two major kinds of RVs are
    a. Descriptive and inferential
    b. Mean and variance
    c. Mean and standard deviation
    d. Categorical and quantitative
    e. Describe and table

3. The two major kinds of interval RVs are
    a. Discrete and continuous
    b. Categorical and numerical

c. PDF and CDF

d. Mean and variance

e. Describe and table

4. Which of the following are discrete RVs? For a given cardiac patient,

   a. Number of grafts in a bypass surgery

   b. Number of intravenous lines

   c. Number of visitors on a given day

   d. Number of D5W bags hung on a given day

   e. All of the above

5. A fundamental tool for working with a discrete RV is the probability density function (PDF). Let X = number of grafts in a coronary artery bypass graft (CABG) surgery. Table 5.1.12 displays the data from a large research study. What does each column in the table represent?

TABLE 5.1.12
The distribution for X, the number of grafts in CABG.

x	f(x)
1	.32
2	.48
3	.14
4	.06
	1.00

6. What does $f(3)$ denote?

   a. How many CABG patients had three grafts

   b. The probability a CABG patient has exactly three grafts

   c. The probability a CABG patient has at least three grafts

   d. The probability a CABG patient has at most three grafts

   e. The number of times a three occurs

7. The probability that a CABG patient has two grafts is
   a. .32 b. .48 c. .14 d. .06 e. .70

8. $P[1 \le X < 4] =$
   a. .32 b. .06 c. 1.00 d. .94 e. .68

9. The CDF associated with the PDF for CABG patients is shown in Table 5.1.13.
   What does $F(3)$ denote? Use the same options as in Warm-up 6.

10. Fill in the blank columns in Table 5.1.14.

TABLE 5.1.13 A combined PDF and CDF for the number of grafts in patients undergoing CABG surgery.

x	f(x)	F(x)
1	.32	.32
2	.48	.80
3	.14	.94
4	.06	1.00

TABLE 5.1.14 A computational spreadsheet to accompany the PDF for the number of grafts in patients undergoing CABG surgery.

x	f(x)	xf(x)	x^2	$x^2 f(x)$
1	.32			
2	.48			
3	.14			
4	.06			
	1.00			

11. The formula for the expected value of X is given by $E[X] = \Sigma x f(x)$. Hence, $E[X] =$
    a. 10 b. 1.00 c. 1.94 d. 30 e. 4.46

12. The formula for the variance of X is given by
    $$V[X] = \Sigma x^2 f(x) - \mu_X^2$$
    $$= \underline{\quad} - (\underline{\quad})^2$$
    $$= \underline{\quad}$$

13. The standard deviation for X is $\sigma_X = \sqrt{V[X]}$. Here,
    $$\sigma_X = \sqrt{\underline{\quad}} = \underline{\quad}$$

14. Consider the PDF given in Table 5.1.15.

TABLE 5.1.15
A PDF.

x	f(x)
0	.12
1	.21
2	.27
3	.19
4	.10
5	.04
6	.07
	1.00

a. $P[X = 3] = \underline{\quad}$ b. $P[X \le 3] = \underline{\quad}$

c. $P[X < 3] = \underline{\quad}$ d. $P[X > 3] = \underline{\quad}$

e. $P[X \ge 3] = \underline{\quad}$

15. Using the PDF in Warm-up 14, the probability that X is

   a. Exactly 2 is ____

   b. At most 2 is ____

   c. At least 2 is ____

   d. Fewer than 2 is ____

   e. More than 2 is ____

Problems 5.1

1. State whether each of the following RVs is categorical or quantitative. If the RV is quantitative, state whether it is discrete or continuous.

   a. Temperature of a patient

   b. Number of bypasses performed in cardiac surgery

   c. Volume of blood products administered during surgery

   d. Number of correct answers obtained on a 16-question continuing education examination

   e. Number of nurses on the hospital code team

   f. Gender

   g. Number of limbs covered by thermal blankets for a postoperative patient

   h. Number of leads for an electrocardiogram

   i. Site of catheter insertion

   j. Brand of stethoscope

   k. Body surface area

   l. Religious preference of the patient

2. The PDF displayed in Table 5.1.16 describes the RV X, the number of emergency room admissions due to trauma at General Hospital during the night shift.

TABLE 5.1.16
A PDF for the number of night shift emergency room admissions due to trauma at General Hospital.

x	f(x)
0	.13
1	.36
2	.24
3	.10
4	?
5	.07

   a. $f(0) =$

   b. $f(1) =$

   c. $f(5) =$

   d. What must the $f(x)$ column add up to?

   e. $f(4) =$

   f. Construct the CDF.

   g. $F(0) =$

   h. $F(1) =$

   i. $F(4) =$

   j. $f(-3) =$

   k. $f(7) =$

   l. $F(7) =$

   m. $P[1 \le X \le 3] =$

   n. $P[1 \le X < 3] =$

   o. $P[1 < X \le 3] =$

   p. $P[1 < X < 3] =$

   q. $E[X] =$

   r. $\mu_X =$

   s. $V[X] =$

   t. $\sigma_X =$

3. Table 5.1.17 describes a PDF for the RV G, the number of girls in a family of five children.

TABLE 5.1.17
A PDF for the number of girls in a family of five children.

g	f(g)	F(g)
0	.03125	
1	.15625	
2	.31250	
3	.31250	
4	.15625	
5	.03125	

   a. Construct the CDF; that is, fill in the $F(g)$ column.

   b. What is the probability the family will have

      i. All girls?

      ii. All boys?

      iii. At least one girl?

      iv. At least one boy?

      v. A majority of girls?

      vi. A majority of boys?

   c. Determine the expected value, variance, and standard deviation of G.

4. A computer simulation of 100 families, each having five children, was performed. The number of girls among the five children was counted for each family. The tabulated sample results are displayed in Table 5.1.18.

TABLE 5.1.18
A frequency distribution table for a computer simulation of 100 families, each of which has five children.

Number of girls	Frequency
0	3
1	22
2	31
3	32
4	10
5	2

Hence, of the 100 families surveyed, 3 families had no girls, 22 families had one girl, and so forth.

a. Determine the sample mean (i.e., the average number of girls in a family of five children in the above sample of 100 families).

b. Determine the sample variance and sample standard deviation.

c. In the simulation, how many families had
   i. All girls?
   ii. All boys?
   iii. At least one girl?
   iv. At least one boy?
   v. A majority of girls?
   vi. A majority of boys?

5. Alspach made a study of critical care orientation programs. Survey participants were asked to indicate how many critical care unit (CCU) instructors were assigned to their particular CCU. The reported number of instructors per CCU ranged from none to four. In her report, Alspach presented the information displayed in Table 5.1.19 for the number of CCU instructors in a CCU.

TABLE 5.1.19
A frequency distribution table for the Alspach data.

Number of CCU Instructors	Frequency	Percent
0	49	33
1	75	51
2	16	11
3	5	3
4	3	2
Total	148	100

a. Let X denote the number of CCU instructors assigned to a CCU. Is X a categorical or numerical RV? If numerical, is X discrete or continuous?

b. Determine the mean number of CCU instructors per CCU.

c. Determine the variance and standard deviation for the number of CCU instructors per CCU.

Determine the appropriate mean and standard deviation for each situation described in Problems 6–8.

6. A researcher measured the PaO_2 level for six patients:
   60   62   80   73   83   86

7. A researcher was interested in studying the effects of a certain counseling and education program. The researcher studied 56 groups of four clients each. The distribution for the number of clients in the group of four helped by the program is shown in Table 5.1.20.

TABLE 5.1.20
A frequency distribution table for the number of clients in each group of four helped by a counseling program.

Number in Group Helped	Frequency
0	4
1	5
2	14
3	25
4	8

For example, among the 56 counseling groups, 25 of the groups had three out of the four clients in the group helped by the program.

8. The researcher in Problem 5.1.7 noted that an earlier study reported the success rate of a similar counseling and education program as shown in Table 5.1.21.

TABLE 5.1.21
Relative frequency distribution table for the number of clients in a group of four helped by a counseling program.

Number in Group Helped	Relative Frequency
0	.10
1	.15
2	.25
3	.35
4	.15

Problems 9–11 further consider Jack and Jill's situation in Example 5.1.1. Let X denote the RV that counts the number of children in the given family who develop cystic fibrosis (CF).

9. Consider the PDF described by Table 5.1.1(a). This table addresses the appropriate possibilities with probabilities if Jack and Jill decide to have one child.

a. What is the probability that the child will develop CF? Will be free (physically) of CF?

b. Determine the expected value of X.

c. Determine the standard deviation for X.

d. Provide a verbal interpretation for the values calculated in (b) and (c).

10. Consider the PDF described by Table 5.1.1(b). This table addresses the appropriate possibilities if Jack and Jill decide to plan on a family of two children.

a. What is the probability that none of the children will develop CF?

b. What is the probability that exactly one child will develop CF?

c. What is the probability that both children will develop CF?

d. What is the probability that at least one child will develop CF?

e. Determine the expected value of X.

f. Determine the standard deviation of X.

g. Provide a verbal interpretation for the values calculated in (e) and (f).

11. Consider the PDF described by Table 5.1.1(c). This table addresses the appropriate possibilities if Jack and Jill decide to plan on a family of three children.

a. Determine the expected value of X.

b. Determine the standard deviation of X.

c. Provide a verbal interpretation for the values calculated in (a) and (b).

12. Constine et al studied the effects of cranial radiotherapy on brain tumors in children. The distribution of hormonal abnormalities in such children is displayed in Table 5.1.22.

TABLE **5.1.22**
Distribution of the number of hormonal abnormalities in children undergoing radiotherapy for brain tumors.

Number of Abnormalies	Relative Frequency
0	.10
1	.28
2	.25
3	.25
4	.12

a. What proportion of these children present no hormonal abnormality?

b. What proportion of these children present
  i. One hormonal abnormality?
  ii. At least one hormonal abnormality?
  iii. At most one hormonal abnormality?

c. What proportion of these children present
  i. Exactly two hormonal abnormalities?
  ii. More than two hormonal abnormalities?
  iii. At least two hormonal abnormalities?
  iv. At most two hormonal abnormalities?

d. What is the expected (average, mean) number of hormonal abnormalities presented by such a child?

e. What is the standard deviation in the number of hormonal abnormalities presented by such a child?

13. (A diversion) A magazine sponsored a multimillion-dollar promotional sweepstakes in which a person could win a variety of cash prizes. The game card indicated the cash prizes with odds of winning as shown in Table 5.1.23.

TABLE **5.1.23**
Cash prizes and odds of winning the prize.

Prize	Odds of Winning
$20	1 to 3,496
$100	1 to 367,080
$500	1 to 1,468,320
$1,000	1 to 7,341,600
$5,000	1 to 24,472,000
$10,000	1 to 73,416,000
$100,000	1 to 73,416,000
$2,000,000	1 to 73,416,000

Let the RV X be the amount won as a result of entering the contest. Our goal here is to compute $E[X]$, the expected value of winnings for entering the contest. In order to compute $E[X]$, we will need to transform the odds chart into a PDF. In order to do so, we first note that a "prize" of $0 is certainly possible; however, note that the odds of entering the contest and not winning anything are not listed. We can circumvent that problem with the Complement Rule; that is, we compute the probability of winning a cash prize and subtract that from 1. Second, we must convert odds to probabilities. Suppose the odds for outcome x are listed as "a to b" (or a out of b, a to b, or $a:b$). Then the probability for x is computed by $f(x) = a/(a + b)$; that is, in general, there are a winners and b losers. For example, if the odds of winning are listed as 5 to 7, then the probability of winning is 5/12, which is

.417 or 41.7%. In this game, the odds for winning $20 are 1 to 3496; hence, the probability that an entrant wins $20 is 1/3497 = .000286.

a. Show that $f(0) = .999710$.

b. Construct a PDF for X.

c. Compute the expected value of X. Compare E[X] against the cost of a postage stamp.

d. Obtain a commercial game card that lists the prizes and odds of winning. Utilizing the dollar value of the prizes, construct a PDF for the game and determine the expected winnings for entering the game.

SECTION 5.2

Binomial Random Variables

OBJECTIVES   This section will

1 Describe the terms Bernoulli trial, binomial experiment, and binomial random variable.

2 Determine the mean, variance, and standard deviation for a given binomial random variable.

3 Construct a probability density function for a given binomial random variable.

In Section 5.1 we studied the concept of a probability density function (PDF) for a discrete RV. Table 5.1.1 displays PDFs for the number of cystic fibrosis (CF) cases in a family of one, two, or three children from CF carrier parents. Table 5.1.2 shows a PDF for the number of girls in a family of four children. The PDF was used (1) to obtain the probability of an interesting event and (2) to calculate the mean and standard deviation. In this section we focus on constructing the PDF (i.e., just how do we obtain the individual probabilities shown in a PDF?) for the binomial RV.

The binomial RV is the most fundamental and common discrete RV. The binomial is fundamental in being an important research tool. It is common in serving as a model for many ordinary real-world situations (Tables 5.1.1 and 5.1.2 are PDFs for binomial RVs). The binomial RV is also easy to demonstrate physically. The basic component of the binomial RV is the coin flip, formally called a "Bernoulli trial."

Bernoulli Trial

A **2-trial** is an experiment with exactly two outcomes. Hence, a 2-trial is the simplest experiment that can display variation. The two outcomes of a 2-trial are generically called **success** and **failure**. In statistics these designations are arbitrary and carry no evaluative or psychological content. They are motivated by the general nature of a categorical RV. Suppose a researcher has in mind some particular attribute of interest. When a sample unit is drawn, the researcher either succeeds or fails to observe the attribute of interest. Hence, the essential spirit of a 2-trial is "Either you see it or you don't."

A **Bernoulli trial** is a 2-trial in which the probability of success does not change when the experiment is repeated. It is customary to denote the probability of success (S) by p and failure (F) by q. Since S and F are the only possible outcomes in a Bernoulli trial, then

p (probability of success) $+ q$ (probability of failure) $= 1$

A Bernoulli trial can be portrayed nicely by a tree diagram as shown in Figure 5.2.1.

A common model for a Bernoulli trial is a coin flip (Figure 5.2.2). By definition, a fair coin is one for which the probability of heads (H) and the probability of tails (T) are both .5. A loaded or biased coin is a coin that is not fair.

In this section we will discuss coin flips as if they were important. They are. A good model for a Bernoulli trial with probability of success p is simply a coin for which the probability of heads (success) showing up on any given toss is p.

EXAMPLE 5.2.1 The following are examples of Bernoulli trials:

a. Experiment: Flip a fair coin.
Outcomes: heads ($p = .5$), tails ($q = .5$)

b. Experiment: Have a child.
Outcomes: girl ($p = .5$), boy ($q = .5$)

c. Experiment: Draw a card from a well-shuffled deck.
Outcomes: club ($p = .25$), nonclub ($q = .75$)

d. Experiment: Pick a letter at random from the alphabet.
Outcomes: vowel ($p = 5/26$), nonvowel ($q = 21/26$)
(Here, vowel = {a, e, i, o, u}.)

e. Experiment: Guess on a five-part multiple-choice examination.
Outcomes: right ($p = .2$), wrong ($q = .8$).

f. Experiment: Carrier CF parents have a child.
Outcomes: no CF ($p = .75$), child develops CF ($q = .25$)

EXAMPLE 5.2.2 The following are examples of experiments that are not Bernoulli trials:

a. Roll a fair die and observe the number showing faceup. This is not a Bernoulli trial since the set of possible outcomes {1, 2, 3, 4, 5, 6} has more than two options.

b. Suppose we choose a letter at random from the alphabet without replacement (i.e., once chosen, the same letter can not be repeated). Consider a

FIGURE **5.2.1**
Tree diagram for a
Bernoulli trial.

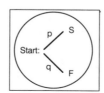

FIGURE **5.2.2**
(a) A fair coin; (b) a
loaded coin.

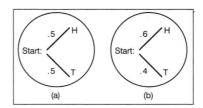

success to be a vowel {a,e,i,o,u}. On the first trial $p = 5/26$. If a vowel is chosen on the first trial, then on the second trial $p = 4/25$; if a consonant is chosen on the first trial, then on the second trial $p = 5/25$. Since the probability of success p is not constant under repeated trials, this is not a Bernoulli trial.

Binomial Experiment

A single **binomial experiment** may be thought of as either (1) a given Bernoulli trial repeated n times or (2) a duplicate set of n Bernoulli trials run simultaneously. For example, using the coin-flip model, consider the binomial experiment of flipping three coins (Figure 5.2.3). One may either (1) flip the same coin three separate times or (2) toss a handful of three coins all at once. Examples of binomial experiments include repeating the Bernoulli trials in Example 5.2.1: (a) flip three coins; (b) have three children; (c) draw five cards (with replacement) from a well-shuffled deck; (d) pick four letters at random with replacement from the alphabet; (e) guess on a ten-question multiple-choice examination where each question has four options and only one option is correct.

A binomial experiment with a small value for n (number of Bernoulli trials) is nicely visualized by a tree diagram. Figure 5.2.4 illustrates a binomial experiment where $n = 3$ and p (probability of success) $= .6$.

The advantage of such a tree diagram is that the probability for any possible outcome for the binomial experiment can be obtained quickly simply by multiplying the probabilities (multiplication rule of probability) along the path in the tree that yields the outcome. For example, the probability of the sequence success, failure, success is obtained by

$$P[SFS] = (.6)(.4)(.6) = 0.144$$

The probability for the sequence failure, failure, success is obtained by

$$P[FFS] = (.4)(.4)(.6) = 0.096$$

FIGURE **5.2.3**
Two coin-flip models for a binomial experiment. (a) Flip one coin three times; (b) flip three coins.

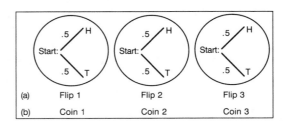

FIGURE **5.2.4**
A tree diagram for a
binomial experiment
with $n = 3$ and
$p = .6$.

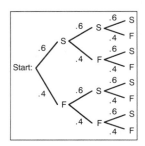

Also notice that there are eight branches in the tree diagram in Figure 5.2.4. This follows directly from the Fundamental Principle of Counting. At each stage of the tree, there are two options, success or failure. Since there are three stages in the tree, the total number of possible outcomes is obtained by

$$N = 2 \times 2 \times 2 = 8$$

In general, a **binomial experiment** is an experiment consisting of n independent and identical Bernoulli trials. The term **independent** means that the result from one trial does not affect the result from another trial. The term **identical** means that the probability of success is the same for all Bernoulli trials in the binomial experiment.

The total number of branches in a tree diagram for a binomial experiment consisting of n independent and identical Bernoulli trials is simply 2^n. Again, this follows directly from the Fundamental Principle of Counting since a binomial experiment has n stages, and each stage has two options (S or F).

Binomial Random Variable

Suppose we have a binomial experiment consisting of n independent Bernoulli trials each with probability of success p. The associated **binomial random variable** simply counts the number of successes in any run of the binomial experiment. A binomial RV is denoted by **Bino(n, p)**. The numbers n and p are called the parameters of the binomial RV.

Let $X = \text{Bino}(n, p)$. This means that X is the binomial RV associated with the binomial experiment consisting of n independent Bernoulli trials each with probability of success p. The binomial RV is a discrete RV whose possible values are $0, 1, 2, \ldots, n$; that is, in any run of the binomial experiment, the number of successes is a whole number between 0 and n inclusively. For example, the binomial RV X associated with flipping three fair coins is $X = \text{Bino}(3, .5)$. The possible number of heads (successes) that could show on any random toss of three fair coins is 0, 1, 2, or 3.

In Section 5.1 we illustrated how to compute the mean and standard deviation for a discrete random variable when provided with its probability density function. For a binomial random variable, that technique simplifies greatly. Suppose $X = \text{Bino}(n, p)$. Then to obtain the mean (expected value) and variance, simply apply the following formulas.

> ### Mean (expected value) and variance formulas for a binomial random variable $X = \text{Bino}(n, p)$
>
> Expected value (mean) $= E[X] = np$
> Variance of $X = V[X] = npq$

EXAMPLE 5.2.3 Consider a random family with six children. Let X count the number of girls in the family. Then $X = \text{Bino}(6, .5)$. So,

$$E[X] = np = (6)(.5) = 3$$
$$V[X] = npq = (6)(.5)(.5) = 1.5$$

and

$$\sigma_X = \sqrt{\text{variance}} = \sqrt{(1.5)} = 1.2$$

Hence, on average, a family with six children has three girls. A typical family with six children has 3 ± 1.2 girls.

Probability Density Function

In Section 5.1 we found that one needs a PDF in order to determine the probability of events of interest for a discrete RV. In order to specify a particular entry in the PDF for $X = \text{Bino}(n, p)$, we denote

$$f(x) = b(x; n, p).$$

Hence, $b(x; n, p)$ denotes the probability of exactly x successes in a binomial experiment with n Bernoulli trials each with probability of success p. For example, $b(2; 3, .6) = 0.432$ means that .432 is the probability of obtaining exactly two successes in a binomial experiment consisting of three Bernoulli trials where the probability of success in each trial is .6.

We present four methods for obtaining the PDF for a binomial RV.

Tree Diagram

If the number of Bernoulli trials is small, the binomial experiment is portrayed nicely by a **tree diagram**. For example, consider $X = \text{Bino}(3, .6)$. The tree diagram for the binomial experiment with probabilities for each outcome is displayed in Figure 5.2.5.

FIGURE 5.2.5
Probability tree diagram for $X = \text{Bino}(3, .6)$. The x column displays the number of successes in each branch of the tree.

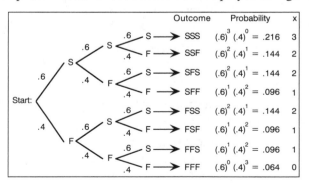

By reading the information in the tree diagram displayed in Figure 5.2.5, one can calculate the probabilities for the various possible values of the associated binomial RV.

$$P[X = 0] = P[\text{FFF}] = .064$$
$$P[X = 1] = P[\text{SFF or FSF or FFS}] = 3(.096) = .288$$
$$P[X = 2] = P[\text{SSF or SFS or FSS}] = 3(.144) = .432$$
$$P[X = 3] = P[\text{SSS}] = .216$$

The PDF for $X =$ Bino(3, .6) is displayed in Table 5.2.1.

TABLE **5.2.1**
A PDF for the binomial random variable $X =$ Bino(3, .6).

x	f(x)
0	.064
1	.288
2	.432
3	.216

Binomial Formula

One can compute the individual probability entries in the PDF for $X =$ Bino(n, p) by applying the following formula, called the **binomial formula**.

$$b(x; n, p) = C(n, x)p^x q^{n-x}$$

For convenience, a table of binomial coefficients (i.e., a table for C(n, x)) is provided in Table 1 of the Appendix.

EXAMPLE 5.2.4
$$\begin{aligned} b(3; 5, .4) &= C(5, 3)(.4)^3(.6)^2 \\ &= (10)(.064)(.36) \\ &= 0.2304 \end{aligned}$$

EXAMPLE 5.2.5 What is the probability that a family of five children has all girls? Here, $X =$ Bino(5,.5) where X counts the number of girls in the family. Thus,

$$\begin{aligned} b(5; 5, .5) &= C(5, 5)(.5)^5(.5)^0 \\ &= (1)(.03125)(1) \\ &= 0.03125 \end{aligned}$$

Hence, about 3 out of 100 families with five children have all girls.
The probability that the family has exactly three girls is computed by

$$\begin{aligned} b(3; 5, .5) &= C(5, 3)(.5)^3(.5)^2 \\ &= (10)(.125)(.25) \\ &= 0.31250 \end{aligned}$$

Hence, about 31 of 100 families with five children have exactly three girls.

Computers

Several computing packages have simple commands that can construct a PDF for any user-supplied binomial RV. We illustrate using Minitab.

To construct a PDF for $X = \text{Bino}(n, p)$, the general form is

MTB > PDF;
SUBC> BINO n p.

For example, the command with output for Bino(4, .5) is displayed in Figure 5.2.6. The general form of the command to obtain $b(x; n, p)$ is:

MTB > PDF x;
SUBC> BINO n p.

For example, the command with output to obtain $b(2; 4, .5)$ is displayed in Figure 5.2.7.

To construct a CDF for $X = \text{Bino}(n, p)$, the general form of the Minitab command is

MTB > CDF;
SUBC> BINO n p.

For example, the command with output to obtain a CDF for Bino(4, .5) is displayed in Figure 5.2.8.

Tables

One of the easier ways to solve problems involving a binomial RV is to make use of a handbook of statistical tables. Usually a binomial table in a handbook or a statistics text is a CDF. For reference, see Table 2 in the Appendix for a table of binomial probabilities.

EXAMPLE 5.2.6 An article by Olsson is followed by a Continuing Education Units (CEU) exam. The exam has ten questions. Each question has four options, of which exactly one option per question is correct. A passing score is seven correct answers. What is the probability of passing by guesswork alone?

Solution. Let X count the number of correct answers obtained by guessing alone. Then $X = \text{Bino}(10, 0.25)$. For passing,

$$P[X \geq 7]$$
$$= 1 - P[X \leq 6]$$
$$= 1 - .99649 \text{ (from Table 2, Appendix)}$$
$$= .00351$$

The probability that one will pass the exam by guesswork alone is .00351. Hence, only about 4 out of 1000 can be expected to pass by pure guesswork alone.

FIGURE **5.2.6**
Minitab output to display a PDF for $X = $ Bino(4,.5).

```
MTB > PDF;
SUBC> BINO 4 .5.

    BINOMIAL WITH N =    4   P = 0.500000
        K            P( X = K)
        0              0.0625
        1              0.2500
        2              0.3750
        3              0.2500
        4              0.0625
```

FIGURE 5.2.7
Minitab output to
obtain $b(2; 4, .5)$.

```
MTB > PDF 2;
SUBC> BINO 4 .5.

      K          P( X = K)
   2.00            0.3750
```

FIGURE 5.2.8
Minitab output to
obtain a CDF for
$X = \text{Bino}(4, .5)$.

```
MTB > CDF;
SUBC> BINO 4 .5.

   BINOMIAL WITH N =   4   P = 0.500000
      K  P( X LESS OR = K)
      0           0.0625
      1           0.3125
      2           0.6875
      3           0.9375
      4           1.0000
```

EXERCISES 5.2

Warm-ups 5.2

In Example 5.1.1 we considered the case of Jack and Jill, who wanted to plan a family. Each person was healthy; however, each was a carrier for cystic fibrosis (CF). Both Jack and Jill have a genetic makeup of Aa for CF. In Example 3.1.9 we determined that the probability a child will be healthy (not contract CF) is $3/4 = .75$; the probability a child will develop CF is $1/4 = .25$.

1. The physical health of the child with regard to CF is displayed in Figure 5.2.9.

FIGURE 5.2.9
Tree diagram for the physical makeup of a child whose parents both are healthy but carriers for cystic fibrosis (CF). OK means no CF.

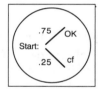

The graphic illustrates an example of

a. A categorical RV

b. A 2-trial

c. A Bernoulli trial

d. A tree diagram

e. All of the above

2. The parents are concerned about their original dream of having a family of three children. Their concern is displayed in Figure 5.2.10.
The diagram depicts

a. A 3-trial

b. A Bernoulli trial

c. A binomial experiment

d. Poor family planning

e. A tree diagram

FIGURE 5.2.10 A diagram of the concerns for two healthy CF carriers who are considering having a family of three children.

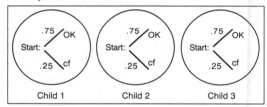

3. A binomial experiment is described by specifying the number n of independent Bernoulli trials each having probability of success p. Here, $n =$ ___ and $p =$ ___.

4. In general, the binomial RV

a. Counts the number of coin flips

b. Counts the number of Bernoulli trials

c. Counts the number of successes

d. Counts the number of failures

e. Determines the probability of success

5. In general, a binomial RV X counts the number of successes in a given binomial experiment with n Bernoulli trials each having probability of success p. The binomial RV X is denoted by $X = \text{Bino}(n, p)$. Here, $X = \text{Bino}($___, ___$)$.

6. Here, $X = \text{Bino}(3, .75)$ counts
   a. The number of children who get CF
   b. The number of children who are healthy (do not get CF)
   c. The number of children the parents have
   d. The probability of having a healthy child
   e. The probability of having a CF child

7. The mean (also called expected value) for $X = \text{Bino}(n, p)$ may be calculated by
   a. n **b.** $p + q = 1$ **c.** np **d.** npq **e.** $E[X]$

8. The mean for $X = \text{Bino}(3, .75)$ is
   a. 3   **b.** .75   **c.** .25   **d.** 2.25   **e.** μ

9. A genetics counselor tells the parents that the expected number of healthy (no CF) children in a family of 3 among carrier parents is 2.25. This means that
   a. The couple should have only 2.25 children.
   b. The couple will have 2.25 healthy children.
   c. The couple will have a CF child if they have 3 children.
   d. On average, a family with 3 children has about 2 healthy children.
   e. On average, a family of 3 children born to CF carrier parents has 2.25 healthy children.

10. The variance for a general binomial random variable $X = \text{Bino}(n, p)$ may be calculated by $V[X] = npq$. For $X = \text{Bino}(3, .75)$, $V[X] =$
   a. 3   **b.** .75   **c.** 2.25   **d.** .5625   **e.** σ_X

11. The general formula that the binomial RV $X = \text{Bino}(n, p)$ takes on the value x in a given experiment is given by $f(x) = C(n, x) p^x q^{n-x}$. The couple wants to know the chances that all three children will be healthy. This probability is computed by
   a. $C(3, 0)(.75)^3(.25)^0$
   b. $C(3, 3)(.75)^3(.25)^0$
   c. $C(3, 3)(.75)^0(.25)^3$
   d. $C(3, 0)(.75)^0(.25)^3$
   e. $3 \times .75$

12. The probability that all three children will be healthy is
   a. 1.266   **b.** .422   **c.** .048   **d.** .015   **e.** 2.25

13. The probability that at least one child will develop CF is
   a. .250
   b. .750
   c. .015
   d. .578
   e. Virtually 0; that is, with three children, there is no problem.

14. The probability table for $X = \text{Bino}(3, .75)$ displayed in Table 5.2.2 is called a

TABLE **5.2.2**
A probability table for the binomial random variable $X = \text{Bino}(3,.75)$.

x	$f(x)$
0	.015
1	.141
2	.422
3	.422
	1.000

   a. PDF
   b. CDF
   c. Frequency distribution table
   d. Binomial experiment
   e. Bernoulli trial

15. The event that at least one child is healthy (no CF) is specified by $X = 1, 2, 3$. Hence, the probability that at least one child is healthy is
   a. .015   **b.** .141   **c.** .422   **d.** 1.000   **e.** .985

Problems 5.2

1. A certain vaccine is reputed to be 90% effective in immunizing a person against the flu. Three people at random receive flu shots. Let X denote the number of these people who become immunized against flu. Hence, $X = \text{Bino}(3, 0.9)$.
   a. Construct a tree depicting the sample space of the experiment of giving flu shots to three random people. Use the tree to construct the PDF for X.
   b. Determine and interpret $E[X]$.
   c. Determine the variance of X.
   d. Determine the standard deviation of X.

e. What is the probability that
   i. Everyone is immunized?
   ii. No one is immunized?
   iii. Someone fails to become immunized?
   iv. Someone is immunized?

2. An article by Fritsch and Klein is followed by a multiple-choice exam consisting of ten questions. Each question has four options, of which only one option is correct. A passing score is seven correct answers. You can earn one CEU by mailing in your answer sheet with eight dollars and also passing the exam.

   a. Suppose you do not read the article and merely guess randomly on each question.
      i. What are your chances of getting exactly seven correct answers?
      ii. What is the probability that you will pass the exam?

   b. Suppose you read the article and are certain that five of your answers are correct; you are not sure about the other five questions, so you randomly guess on those. What are your chances of passing the exam?

3. The reported sensitivity of thallium scintigraphy for coronary artery disease is Sn = 0.78. Suppose four patients who actually have coronary artery disease undergo thallium scintigraphy. Let X denote the number of patients who receive positive scintigrams; that is, $X = \text{Bino}(4, 0.78)$.

   a. Construct a PDF for X.

   b. Determine and interpret E[X].

   c. Determine the variance and standard deviation of X.

   d. Among the four patients, what is the probability that
      i. All receive positive scintigrams?
      ii. Nobody receives a positive scintigram?
      iii. Somebody receives a positive scintigram?
      iv. Somebody receives a negative scintigram?
      v. The majority receives a positive scintigram?

4. One could earn two CEUs by officially passing the 16-question multiple-choice exam based on a journal article by Henneman and Henneman. Each question has five options, of which exactly one is the correct response. A passing score is 12 correct answers.

a. Suppose you do not read the article and merely guess randomly on each question.
   i. What are your chances of getting exactly 12 correct answers?
   ii. What is the probability that you will pass the exam?

b. Suppose you read the article and you are certain that 10 of your answers are correct. You are not sure about the other 6 questions, so you randomly guess on those questions. What are your chances of passing the exam?

5. Application: genetic counseling. A person's gender is determined by the makeup of the sex chromosome pairing: XX = female and XY = male. The genetic makeup for an offspring can be portrayed by a Punnett square as shown in Table 5.2.3.

TABLE **5.2.3** Punnett square for the genetic makeup that determines a person's gender.

↓ Mother \Father→	X	Y
X	XX	XY
X	XX	XY

By simple Mendelian genetics, the probability that the child is male is .5; female, also .5. The X chromosome carries much genetic information in addition to gender, such as color perception, A. Color blindness is caused by the recessive allele a occupying this gene. The Y chromosome has no effect on color blindness. We denote XA and Xa for the X chromosome with dominant allele A and recessive allele a, respectively. The resulting genetic possibilities are shown in Table 5.2.4.

TABLE **5.2.4** Genetic makeup for color blindness.

Female	Male
XAXA (normal)	XAY (normal)
XAXa (carrier)	XaY (color-blind)
XaXa (color-blind)	

Suppose that the parents are a carrier mother and a normal father.

a. Depict the genotypes of the child by means of a (i) Punnett square, and (ii) a tree.

b. What is the probability that a child (from these parents) is
   i. A color-perceptive girl?
   ii. A color-perceptive boy?

iii. A color-blind girl?

iv. A color-blind boy?

v. Color-perceptive?

vi. Color-blind?

c. Suppose the couple wants to plan for three children.

   i. What is the probability that all their children will have color perception?

   ii. What is the probability that at least one child will be color-blind?

   iii. What is the probability that all their children will be color-blind?

   iv. One of the parents asks: How many color-blind children can we expect? Provide both a technical and a humane response.

d. Same as (c) for a couple wanting to plan for five children.

6. (An experiment) Consider the experiment of taking five fair coins, shaking them, and rolling them. Then count the number of heads. We examine the RV X = number of heads in a toss of five coins. Note that X = Bino(5, .5). Table 5.2.5 displays a PDF for X = Bino(5, .5). Now take five coins, roll them, count and record the number of heads. Do this binomial experiment 100 times.

TABLE **5.2.5**
A PDF for X = Bino(5,.5).

x	f(x)
0	0.031
1	0.156
2	0.313
3	0.313
4	0.156
5	0.031

a. Complete Table 5.2.6 by recording your observed frequencies (i.e., how many times in your 100 tosses did you observe 0 heads? 1 head? 2 heads, etc.). What do you think—do the expected frequencies reasonably match the observed frequencies?

b. Explain how the expected frequencies in Table 5.2.6 were obtained from the PDF.

c. Determine E[X], the expected number of heads in a toss of five coins, by applying the binomial formula E[X] = $n \times p$.

d. In your 100 tosses of five coins, what was the average (mean, $\bar{x}$) number of heads? (See Example 5.1.12 for a computational demonstration.)

TABLE **5.2.6** Summary of 100 tosses of five coins.

Number of Heads	Observed Frequency	Expected Frequency
0		3.1
1		15.6
2		31.3
3		31.3
4		15.6
5		3.1
Total	100	100.0

e. How does the theoretical expected value obtained in (c) compare with your observed mean obtained in (d)?

f. Determine σ_X, the standard deviation for X = Bino(5, .5), by applying the binomial formula $\sigma_X = \sqrt{n \times p \times q}$.

g. Determine s, the observed standard deviation (see Example 5.1.12 for a computational demonstration).

h. How does the theoretical standard deviation obtained in (f) compare with your observed standard deviation obtained in (g)?

i. A general description of an observed "typical" toss is mean ± standard deviation ($\bar{x} \pm$ s).

   i. $\bar{x} - s = ?$

   ii. $\bar{x} + s = ?$

   iii. How many of your 100 tosses showed the number of heads between $\bar{x} - s$ and $\bar{x} + s$?

   iv. What proportion of your 100 tosses showed the number of heads between $x - s$ and $\bar{x} + s$?

7. Redelmeier presented the following scenario. Suppose that the hospital death rate for all patients with congestive heart failure (CHF) is p = .05 (i.e., the probability that a patient admitted with CHF dies while in the hospital is 5%). Suppose a hospital has 100 CHF patients admitted in a given time frame. Assume that deaths among CHF patients are independent.

a. What is the expected number of deaths in this group of 100 CHF patients?

b. What is the variance and standard deviation for the number of deaths?

c. What proportion of hospitals will experience
  i. No deaths?
  ii. Exactly five deaths?
  iii. Five or fewer deaths?
  iv. More than five deaths?

d. Suppose that an audit of the last 100 CHF admissions at Area Hospital showed six deaths during the time of hospitalization. General Hospital, however, only had two deaths for the last 100 CHF patients. A tabloid newspaper ran an "exposé" of the poor care given at Area Hospital, heralding a CHF death rate three times greater in Area Hospital than in General Hospital as evidence. What do you think: Is the tabloid justified in its expose?

8. Redelmeier also considered the following more complex scenario. Suppose that, upon admission, a patient can be easily classified into one of two groups.

Good prognosis group (Group a): probability of in-hospital death is low, $p_a = .01$.
Dismal prognosis group (Group b): probability of in-hospital death is high, $p_b = .80$.

Now suppose that there are n = 100 admissions for CHF, of which $n_a = 95$ and $n_b = 5$ (i.e., 95 patients fall in the good prognosis group, 5 patients fall in the dismal prognosis group).

a. What is the expected number of deaths in the good prognosis group?

b. What is the expected number of deaths in the dismal prognosis group?

c. The formula for determining the probability of death in the entire (combined) group is given by
$$p = \frac{n_a p_a + n_b p_b}{n}$$
Apply this formula to determine the probability that a randomly selected individual in the whole group will die. Compare this answer with your answers from (a) and (b).

d. Instead of applying the formula presented in (c), one can consider a probability tree diagram. Consider the two-stage experiment of a new CHF admission. The first stage is the placement of the patient into the good prognosis group or the dismal prognosis group. The second stage is whether the patient will live or die. Construct the probability tree diagram. Using the diagram, compute the probability that a new CHF admission will die in the hospital.

e. Determine the expected number of deaths in the entire group of $n = 100$ patients.

f. The variance V for the number of deaths is given by the formula
$$V = n_a p_a(1 - p_a) + n_b p_b(1 - p_b)$$
Note that this combined variance V is obtained by adding the individual group a and group b variances. Apply the formula to obtain the variance for the number of deaths in a random group of $n = 100$ new hospital admissions for CHF. How does this formulation of the variance compare with your answer in Problem 7b?

g. Repeat Problem 7d as a result of the information obtained in Problem 8a–f.

9. Suppose a diagnostic test has a sensitivity of 95% for a certain condition (Sn = .95; i.e., there is a 95% probability that a sick person receives a true-positive test result). Suppose 20 people who have this condition are tested. Let X count the number of these 20 people who test positive.

a. Then, $X = \text{Bino}(n, p)$ where $n = $ _____ and $p = $ _____.

b. Construct a PDF for X in Minitab as follows:

```
MTB > NAME C1 'X', C2 'F(X)', C3 'CF(X)'
MTB > SET C1
DATA> 0:20
MTB > PDF C1 INTO C2;
SUBC> BINO(20,.95).
MTB > CDF C1 INTO C3;
SUBC> BINO(20,.95).
MTB > PRINT C1-C3
```

c. What is the probability that all 20 people will be diagnosed correctly?

d. What is the probability that at least one person will be misdiagnosed?

e. What is the probability that at least 19 will be diagnosed correctly?

f. What is the probability that at least 18 will be diagnosed correctly?

g. What is the probability that at least 17 will be diagnosed correctly?

h. A tabloid reports that in its sponsored trial of the diagnostic test, 20 afflicted people were tested and one-quarter went undetected. How believable is this report?

Summary

A **quantitative** data set is a data set with numerical entries. An **interval** data set is a quantitative data set in which the numbers act like "real" numbers; that is, the numbers count or measure something rather than act as synonyms for names or ranks. An interval data set may be generated by either a discrete or a continuous random variable (RV).

A **discrete RV** counts something; a **continuous RV** measures. The key feature of a discrete RV is that its possible values may be listed. This feature enables one to construct a **probability density function table (PDF)** as a tool for working with the RV. Such a table consists of two columns. The first column lists all the possible values and the second column displays the accompanying probabilities. The key is that all possibilities may be listed. In contrast, a continuous RV may assume an interval of values. Given any two possible outcomes, all values "in-between" are also possible. This in-between property makes constructing a list of all values impossible.

The PDF is the basic tool for working with a discrete RV. In an applied problem, once one sees a discrete RV at work, obtain its PDF. Using the PDF, one may compute the **probability** for any event of concern. In addition to computing probabilities, one can apply the table to determine the **mean** and **standard deviation** for the discrete RV. The mean for an RV is also called its **expected value**.

We caution that when asked to compute a mean or standard deviation one should first determine the context of the request. One may compute the mean (or standard deviation) for a data set or for an RV. These computations are performed differently.

The **binomial RV** is the most common discrete RV. To understand the nature of this RV, one starts with the concept of a 2-trial. A **2-trial** is an experiment with exactly two outcomes, generically called **success** and **failure**. A **Bernoulli trial** is a 2-trial in which the probability of success does not change when the trial is repeated. A **binomial experiment** is an experiment consisting of n independent and identical Bernoulli trials. The Bernoulli trials are considered **independent** because the outcome of one trial does not effect the outcome of any other trial in the binomial experiment. The Bernoulli trials are considered **identical** because the probability of success is the same for all trials. The **binomial random variable** counts the number of successes obtained in a binomial experiment.

The notation $X = \textbf{Bino}(n,p)$ means that X counts the number of successes in a binomial experiment consisting of n independent Bernoulli trials, each with probability of success p. The key ingredients for computational purposes are identified in the notation: n (the number of Bernoulli trials) and p (the probability of success on any trial). With this information one can quickly determine the mean of X ($E[X] = np$) and the variance of X ($V[X] = npq$, where $q = 1 - p$).

The PDF (and CDF) is an important tool for working with any discrete random variable. There are four methods for constructing the PDF for a binomial random variable $X = \text{Bino}(n, p)$: (1) **tree diagram**, (2) the **binomial formula** $b(x; n, p) = C(n, x)p^x p^{n-x}$, (3) **computer**, (4) statistical **table**. In Minitab the PDF and CDF commands, used in conjunction with the BINOMIAL subcommand, are especially helpful.

Keywords

Bernoulli trial	interval random variable
cumulative density	mean
function (CDF)	model
coin flip	probability
binomial experiment	probability density
binomial formula	function (PDF)
binomial random variable	random variable
mean	binomial
standard deviation	continuous
variance	discrete
binomial table	raw data set
continuous random variable	standard deviation
discrete random variable	success
expected value	tree diagram
experiment	trial
failure	2-trial
frequency distribution table	Bernoulli trial
identical	variance
independent	variation

References

Alspach G: Critical care orientation programs: Reader survey report. *Crit Care Nurse* 10, no. 5 (May 1990): 22.

Botkin J and Alemagno S: Carrier screening for cystic fibrosis: A pilot study of the attitudes of pregnant women. *Am J Public Health* 82, no. 5 (May 1992): 723.

Constine L et al: Hypothalamic-pituitary dysfunction after radiation for brain tumors. *N Engl J Med* 328, no. 2 (14 January 1993): 87.

Fritsch D and Klein D: Ludwig's angina. *Heart Lung* 21, no. 1 (January 1992): 39.

Henneman E and Henneman P: Intricacies of blood pressure measurement: Reexamining the rituals. *Heart Lung* 18, no. 3 (May 1989): 263.

Redelmeier D: Explaining variations in hospital death rates. *JAMA* 265, no. 4 (23/30 January 1991): 458.

Normal Distributions

Chapter 6 is a natural extension of Chapter 5. In Chapter 5 we focused on the most common of the discrete random variables, the binomial random variable. In Chapter 6 we focus on the most common continuous random variables, the normal random variables. Section 6.1 deals with the details of describing, computing, and applying a normal distribution. In Section 6.2 we consider the problem of how to determine whether a given continuous random variable has a normal distribution.

SECTION 6.1

Normal Random Variables

OBJECTIVES   This section will

1 Describe the normal and standard normal distributions.

2 Compute probabilities relative to the standard normal distribution.

3 State the Standardization Theorem.

4 Determine the z-score of a value *x* of a given normal random variable *X* with specified mean and standard deviation.

5 Compute and describe probabilities relative to a normal random variable when given its mean and standard deviation.

The normal probability distribution is the most fundamental and common of the continuous random variables (RVs). The probability density function (PDF) is the basic tool in dealing with an interval (discrete or continuous) RV. For discrete RVs, the PDF takes the form of a *table*. For continuous RVs, the PDF takes the form of a *curve* (graph).

EXAMPLE 6.1.1 (Adapted from Chamberlin) Figure 6.1.1 displays a model for the distribution of birth weights of full-term babies in Great Britain born to nonsmoking, nondrinking mothers (right curve) and to mothers who are heavy drinkers (left curve).

FIGURE **6.1.1**
Birth weight (grams)
distribution among
(a) nonsmoking,
nondrinking mothers
and (b) heavy-drinking
mothers.

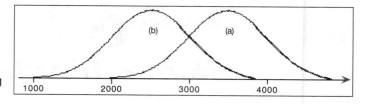

Among nonsmoking, nondrinking mothers, birth weight is (approximately) normally distributed with a mean of 3500 grams. Among heavy-drinking mothers, birth weight is (approximately) normally distributed with a mean of 2600 grams.

The graphic in Figure 6.1.1 clearly displays the effects on birth weight of babies born to mothers who drink heavily. The downward shift in the distribution of birth weights probably is due to the overall life-style of heavy drinkers, including cigarette smoking and maternal malnutrition.

The complete PDF for a continuous RV by necessity must be described by a curve rather than table. Since one cannot list all possibilities for a continuous RV, a comprehensive table is impossible. We begin our discussion of the normal distribution by displaying the properties of its PDF curve.

The Normal Distribution

Generally speaking, the normal distribution is described by the traditional "bell-shaped curve." This is the curve behind a student's question, Do you grade on the curve? A continuous RV has a **normal distribution** if the graph of its PDF has the following properties (see Figure 6.1.2):

1. The graph is continuous and positive. The graph is **continuous** if it is unbroken with no sudden jumps. The graph is **positive** if it lies completely above the horizontal axis.
2. The graph is **symmetrical about the mean**. The **mean** (μ) for a normal distribution is that point on the horizontal axis that cuts the curve into two mirror images. Locate the mean on the horizontal axis (Figure 6.1.2) and draw a vertical line

FIGURE **6.1.2** A normal distribution curve. The mean μ is that location on the horizontal that cuts the graph into two mirror images. The part of the graph from $\mu - \sigma$ to $\mu + \sigma$ is the dome of the bell-shaped curve. The parts of the curve to the left of $\mu - \sigma$ and the right of $\mu + \sigma$ bend upward (concave upward). The dome bends downward (concave downward). The total area under the curve (shaded region) is 1.

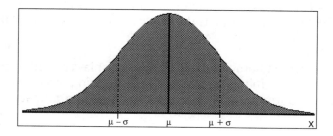

FIGURE **6.1.3**
The probability X is
between a (exclusively)
and b (inclusively)
corresponds to the
area under the curve
from a to b (shaded).

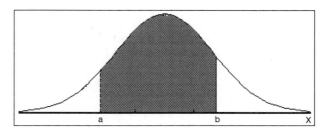

through it. The part of the graph to the left of the vertical line is a mirror image
of the part of the graph to the right of the mean. The mean centers the curve.
Tracing the curve from left to right, the curve ascends to the mean, peaks at the
mean, then descends after the mean.

3. The graph is **bell-shaped** with inflection points at one standard deviation unit
from either side of the mean. An **inflection point** is a point on the graph where
the direction of bending changes. Tracing the graph from the left, the graph
starts very close to the horizontal axis. From left to right one draws in a "curve
upward" (concave up) fashion, then draws a "curve downward" (concave down)
dome in the middle, finishing in a concave up fashion. The **standard deviation**
(σ) is the horizontal distance to either side of the mean that defines the dome of
the bell-shaped curve.

4. The total area underneath the curve is 1.

5. The area underneath the curve from $X = a$ to $X = b$ is the proportion of the
population whose value for X is somewhere between a and b (either inclusively
or exclusively). Figure 6.1.3 shows $P[a < X \le b]$. One uses the dotted line to
exclude a and the solid line to include b.

EXAMPLE 6.1.2 Among diabetics in the general U.S. population, the fasting blood glucose level
X is normally distributed (approximately) with mean 106 mg/dL and standard
deviation 8 mg/dL. The proportion of diabetics with fasting glucose levels between 90 and 120 mg/dL is depicted in the shaded portion of Figure 6.1.4.

6. The interval within one standard deviation of the mean accounts for 68% of the
distribution; two standard deviation units, 95%; 3 standard deviation units,
99.7% (see Figure 6.1.5).

Comment The Empirical Rule for data (Section 1.1.2) is based on the probabilities
for the normal distribution illustrated in Figure 6.1.5.

FIGURE **6.1.4**
The proportion of
diabetics with fasting
blood glucose level
between 90 and 120
mg/dL.

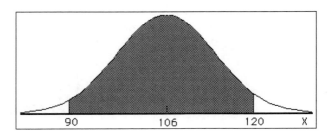

FIGURE **6.1.5**
The interval within one
standard deviation of
the mean accounts for
68% of a normal
distribution. The
interval within two
standard deviations of
the mean accounts for
95% of a normal
distribution. The
interval within three
standard deviations of
the mean accounts for
99.7% of a normal
distribution.

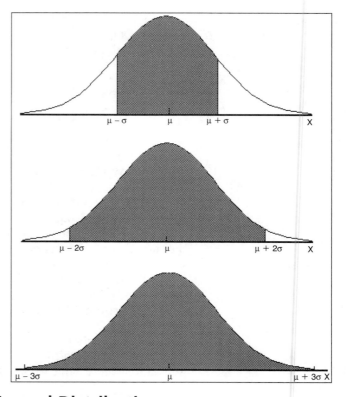

The Standard Normal Distribution

The **standard normal distribution** (Figure 6.1.6) is a normal distribution having a
mean of 0 and a standard deviation of 1. A continuous RV that has a standard normal
distribution is denoted by Z.

Computing Standard Normal Probabilities

One computes probabilities for a normal RV by converting to the standard normal.
We illustrate such computations by examples.

A key skill here is to be able to use standard normal tables. Table 3 in the
Appendix is a left-tail standard normal table from which one can read directly $P[Z <
z]$, where z is a given decimal number from -3.49 to 0.00. Table 4 is a right-tail

FIGURE **6.1.6**
The standard normal
distribution.

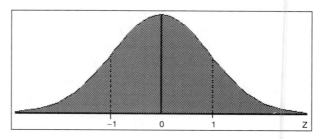

FIGURE *6.1.7*
(a) The shaded region
displays $P[Z < -1.27]$
$= .102$; (b) the
unshaded region
displays $P[Z \geq -1.27]$
$= .898$.

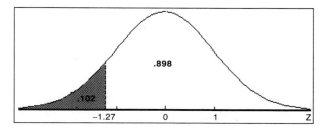

standard normal table from which one can read directly $P[Z > z]$, where z is a given decimal number from 0.00 to 3.49. Conceivably we need only one table (since a normal distribution is symmetrical); however, it is convenient for computational purposes to have them both. To guide the computations, we implore: *Draw a picture.*

EXAMPLE 6.1.3 Find $P[Z < -1.27]$. Here, we are asked to determine the probability that a standard normal value is under -1.27. First, draw a picture representing the problem (Figure 6.1.7).

Roughly locate -1.27 on the horizontal. It is positioned to the left of the mean (since -1.27 is negative), just to the left of the dome (the dome in the standard normal extends from -1 to $+1$ over the horizontal). Since we want the probability that $Z < -1.27$, shade in the area under the curve to the left of -1.27. Since a left-tail area is shaded, the picture suggests using Table 3 (Appendix). Use of Table 3 to find $P[Z < -1.27]$ is displayed in Figure 6.1.8.

To apply Table 3 to find $P[Z < -1.27]$, first locate -1.2 in the z column (leftmost column of the table). Second, locate the 0.07 column heading. Third, locate the intersection of the -1.2 row and the 0.07 column, obtaining the table entry of .102042. This entry is the probability that $Z < -1.27$; hence, $P[Z < -1.27] = .102$ (rounding to three places past the decimal point).

EXAMPLE 6.1.4
$$P[Z > -1.27]$$
$$= 1 - P[Z < -1.27]$$
$$= 1 - 0.102042$$
$$= 0.897958 \qquad \text{(see Figure 6.1.7, unshaded region)}$$

EXAMPLE 6.1.5 Find $P[Z > 0.73]$. The picture is displayed in Figure 6.1.9. From Table 4, $P[Z > 0.73] = .232695$. Hence, rounding, $P[Z > 0.73] = .233$.

FIGURE *6.1.8*
Determine
$P[Z < -1.27]$
using Table 3.

Table 3: CDF for the Standard Normal Distribution.				
z	0.00		0.07	
–3.4				
–1.2			.102042	

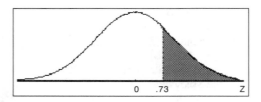

FIGURE **6.1.9**
Picture showing
$P[Z > .73]$.

EXAMPLE 6.1.6 Find $P[-1.72 \le Z \le 1.80]$. Refer to Figure 6.1.10. Note that we want the area of the shaded region. Our tables, however, provide us only with either left-tail (Table 3) or right-tail (Table 4) areas. We know that the total area under the curve is 1. Hence, to find the area of the shaded region, we find the combined area of the white tails, then subtract the area of the white region from 1 to obtain the area of the shaded region. First,

Unshaded (white) area	$P[-1.72 \le Z \le 1.80]$
$= P[Z < -1.72] + P[Z > 1.80]$	$=$ shaded area
$= .042716 + .035930$	$= 1 -$ white area
$= .078646.$	$= 1 - .078646$
	$= .921354$

Hence, $P[-1.72 \le Z \le 1.80] = .921$.

EXAMPLE 6.1.7 Find z such that $P[Z > z] = .085343$. Here, we want to determine the horizontal location z for which the area to the right is .085343 (Figure 6.1.11). A problem like this is similar to the game show "Jeopardy," in which the answer is given and the contestant is to provide the appropriate question. Hence, this problem may be phrased as, What number must I look up in Table 4 to get an answer of .085343? Scanning the body of Table 4, we observe that .085343 is the table entry for $z = 1.37$.

EXAMPLE 6.1.8 Find z such that $P[Z > z] = .748$. Although this is a right-tail problem, Table 4 cannot be used immediately. Table 4 extends only to the right half of the standard normal distribution and thus lists only right-tail areas for values of z from 0 to 3.49. The graph of this problem (Figure 6.1.12) suggests using the Complement Rule and finding the left-tail area using Table 3. The complement problem is to find z such that $P[Z < z] = .252$. Table 3 provides areas to five places past the decimal point. Find the table area entry closest to .252 (.251429). Then $z = -0.67$.

FIGURE **6.1.10**
$P[-1.72 \le Z \le 1.80]$.

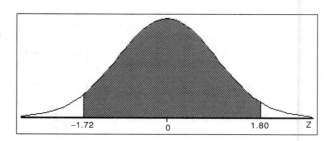

*FIGURE **6.1.11***
$P[Z > z] = .085343$.

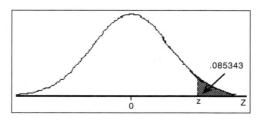

*FIGURE **6.1.12***
Display for
$P[Z > z] = .748$.

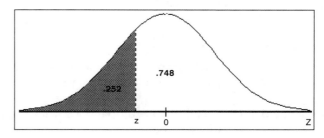

EXAMPLE 6.1.9 Find z so that $P[-z \le Z \le z] = .95$ (see Figure 6.1.13). Then $P[Z < -z] = .025$; so $z = -1.96$. Note that $P[Z < -1.96] = .025$ and $P[Z > 1.96] = .025$. Hence, $P[-1.96 \le Z \le 1.96] = .95$.

The Standardization Theorem

Do standard normal distributions really occur? The answer is an oxymoron: Hardly ever, and all the time! Nonstandard normal distributions occur frequently in the real world. However, *any* normal distribution can be easily converted to a standard normal distribution. Once it is converted, one can determine probabilities for interesting scenarios, as we did in computing standard normal probabilities. The process that allows one to convert a normal distribution into the standard normal distribution is formalized in the Standardization Theorem.

Let X be a normal random variable with mean μ and standard deviation σ. The **Standardization Theorem** states that the random variable Z given by

$$Z = \frac{X-\mu}{\sigma}$$

is *always standard normal* (mean of Z is 0 and standard deviation of Z is 1).

The Standardization Theorem is the key to computing probabilities involving a normal distribution. First, we note that

*FIGURE **6.1.13***
Diagram for
$P[-z < Z < z] = .95$.

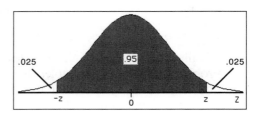

$$P[X < a]$$
$$= P\left[\frac{X-\mu}{\sigma} < \frac{a-\mu}{\sigma}\right]$$
$$= P\left[Z < \frac{a-\mu}{\sigma}\right]$$

Hence, to determine a probability for a normal distribution, merely standardize the problem and determine the corresponding probability using Table 3 or Table 4. We will shortly illustrate this idea with several examples. As a preliminary, we introduce the concept of a z-score.

The z-Score

The **z-score** is the number obtained by applying the Standardization Theorem to a particular value from a normal random variable.

EXAMPLE 6.1.10 Recall from Example 6.1.2 that the fasting blood glucose level for a diabetic is (approximately) normally distributed with a mean of 106 mg/dL and a standard deviation of 8 mg/dL. The z-score of a diabetic with a fasting blood glucose level of 120 mg/dL is:

$$z = \frac{120-106}{8} = 1.75$$

This means that a diabetic with a fasting blood glucose level of 120 mg/dL has a level that is 1.75 standard deviation units beyond the mean.

The z-score measures in standard deviation units how far a number is away from the mean. A number whose z-score is greater than 2 or less than -2 (more than two standard deviation units from the mean) is often considered to be an outlier (unusual).

Computing Normal Distribution Probabilities

Let X be an RV having a normal distribution with mean μ and standard deviation σ. Then from the Standardization Theorem:

a. $P[a < X] = P\left[\frac{a-\mu}{\sigma} < Z\right]$

b. $P[X < b] = P\left[Z < \frac{b-\mu}{\sigma}\right]$

c. $P[a < X < b] = P\left[\frac{a-\mu}{\sigma} < Z < \frac{b-\mu}{\sigma}\right]$

We illustrate how to apply these formulas to calculate probabilities for a normal distribution by using (1) the z-tables in the Appendix and (2) Minitab.

Using Tables

We illustrate the use of the z-tables (Appendix, Tables 3 and 4) to solve general problems with several examples. In each problem, note that a general normal distribution is solved by first standardizing it, then solving the corresponding standard normal problem by using the tables.

EXAMPLE 6.1.11 The height X of a U.S. male is (approximately) normally distributed with a mean of 69 inches and standard deviation of 2.5 inches. What proportion of the U.S. male population is under 6 feet tall? The solution is displayed in Figure 6.1.14.

$$P[X < 6 \text{ ft}]$$
$$= P[X < 72 \text{ inches}]$$
$$= P[Z < (72 - 69)/2.5]$$
$$= P[Z < 1.2]$$
$$= 1 - P[Z > 1.2]$$
$$= 1 - .115 \text{ (Table 4)}$$
$$= .885$$

About 88.5% of U.S. males are under 6 feet tall.

EXAMPLE 6.1.12 The systolic blood pressure (SBP) in a certain community is approximately normally distributed with a mean of 135.6 and standard deviation of 17.6. Hypertension is defined as a SBP of 140 or more. What proportion of the population is hypertensive? The solution is displayed in Figure 6.1.15.

$$P[SBP > 140]$$
$$= P[Z > (140 - 135.6)/17.6]$$
$$= P[Z > 0.25]$$
$$= .401 \text{ (Table 4)}$$

Thus, about 40% have hypertension in this community.

EXAMPLE 6.1.13 The weight W of a newborn baby is a normal (approximately) random variable with a mean of 7.1 pounds and a standard deviation of 1.1 pounds. What is the probability that a newborn will weigh between 6 and 8 pounds?

*FIGURE **6.1.14***
Diagram for $P[X < 6 \text{ ft}]$.

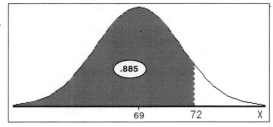

*FIGURE **6.1.15***
Diagram for $P[SBP > 140]$.

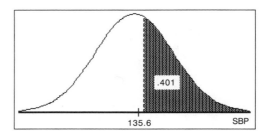

$$P[6 < W < 8]$$
$$= P[(6 - 7.1)/1.1 < Z < (8 - 7.1)/1.1]$$
$$= P[-1.00 < Z < 0.82]$$
$$= 1 - \text{white area}$$

See Figure 6.1.16 for the various shaded regions.

About 64% of newborns weigh 6 to 8 pounds.

white area
$$= P[Z \leq -1.00] + P[Z \geq .82]$$
$$= .158655 + .206108$$
$$= .364763$$

shaded area
$$= 1 - \text{white area}$$
$$= 1 - .364763$$
$$= .635237$$

EXAMPLE 6.1.14 What proportion of newborns will have low birth weight (under 5 pounds)? The solution is displayed in Figure 6.1.17.

$$P[W < 5]$$
$$= P[Z < (5 - 7.1)/1.1]$$
$$= P[Z < -1.91]$$
$$= .028067 \text{ (Table 3)}$$

Hence, about 3% of newborns have low birth weight (under 5 pounds).

EXAMPLE 6.1.15 A door manufacturer wants to manufacture doors of sufficient height that 95% of the male population can walk through the doorway without having to stoop. How high should the door be?

Let X be the RV of height of a U.S. male (see Example 6.1.11). Here, we want to find x so that $P[X < x] = .95$ (see Figure 6.1.18). We need to reformulate the problem into the equivalent complement problem since the table areas only go up to .5; that is, we cannot locate a left-tail area of .95 in Table 3. Note that $P[X < x] = .95$ is equivalent to the complement problem $P[X > x] = .05$. We examine the "answers" in Table 4 to obtain $z = 1.645$ (note that .05 is

FIGURE **6.1.16**
$P[6 < W < 8]$.

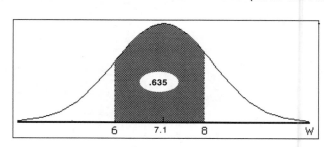

FIGURE **6.1.17**
$P[W < 5]$.

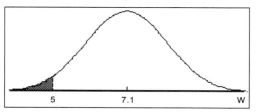

about halfway between .049471 and .050503). Now z is the standardization of x; that is,

$$1.645 = \frac{x - 69}{2.5}$$

Using algebra to solve for x, we find $x = 73.1$ inches. Hence, the doorway needs to be slightly over 73 inches to accommodate 95% of the male population.

Using Minitab

Minitab has built-in *left*-tail area capabilities but no corresponding right-tail capabilities. A left-tail table is a cumulative density function (CDF). Minitab's keyword to access a left-tail table is simply CDF. The area to the left of a given number x for a random variable X corresponds to $P[X \le x]$.

The general form of the Minitab command to find the area to the left of x for a normal distribution with mean M and standard deviation S is

```
MTB > CDF x;
SUBC> NORMAL M S.
```

In response, Minitab prints out x and the area to the left of x.

EXAMPLE 6.1.16 The height of a U.S. male is (approximately) normal with a mean of 69 inches and a standard deviation of 2.5 inches. What proportion of the U.S. male population is under 6 feet (72 inches)?

```
MTB > CDF 72;
SUBC> NORMAL 69 2.5.
    72.0000    0.8849
```

Hence, about 88.5% of the U.S. male population is under 72 inches.

One can direct Minitab to retain the probability value in a constant box K by

```
MTB > CDF X K;
SUBC> NORMAL M S.
```

The probability value retained in K can then be used in calculations.

EXAMPLE 6.1.17 The weight W of a newborn baby is (approximately) normal with a mean of 7.1 pounds and standard deviation of 1.1 pounds. What proportion of newborns weigh between 6 and 8 pounds? Using Minitab, we must set up the solution in terms of *left*-tail proportions only. Hence, $P[6 < W < 8] = P[W < 8] - P[W < 6]$:

FIGURE 6.1.18
Diagram for $P[X < x]$ = .95.

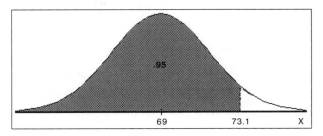

```
MTB > CDF 8 K1;
SUBC> NORMAL 7.1 1.1.
MTB > CDF 6 K2;
SUBC> NORMAL 7.1 1.1.
MTB > LET K3 = K1 - K2
MTB > PRINT K1 - K3
K1        0.793373
K2        0.158655
K3        0.634718
```

Hence, Minitab displays 79.3373% of newborns weigh 8 lbs or less, and 15.8655% weigh 6 lbs or less. Thus, 63.4718% weigh between 6 and 8 lbs. Such computational precision is beyond the precision of the given data. We report 63% of newborns weigh between 6 and 8 pounds.

EXAMPLE 6.1.18 Matthews et al studied serum progesterone levels as an aid in the diagnosis of ectopic pregnancy. On the basis of their study, suppose that serum progesterone is normally distributed in women with ectopic pregnancies with a mean of 5.63 ng/mL and standard deviation of 3.65 ng/mL. In women with normal pregnancies, serum progesterone is normally distributed with a mean of 30.85 ng/mL and standard deviation of 6.91 ng/mL. Suppose that one decides to use serum progesterone level as a diagnostic test for ectopic pregnancy. Consider a cutoff of 10 ng/mL; that is, a serum progesterone of 10 ng/mL or below is diagnostic for ectopic pregnancy.

a. What proportion of women with ectopic pregnancy will have a serum progesterone level of 10 ng/mL or less? What is the Sn for this diagnostic criterion? What is the F − R?

```
MTB > CDF 10;
SUBC> NORMAL 5.63 3.65.
    10.0000      0.8844
```

Hence, 88% of women with ectopic pregnancies will present a serum progesterone ≤ 10 ng/dl. Accordingly, Sn = 88% and F − R = 12%.

b. What proportion of women with a normal pregnancy will have a serum progesterone level greater than 10 ng/mL? What is the Sp for this diagnostic criterion? What is the F + R?

```
MTB > CDF 10 K1;
SUBC> NORMAL 30.85 6.91.
MTB > LET K2 = 1 - K1
MTB > PRINT K2
K2        0.998725
```

Hence, 99.9% of women with normal (nonectopic) pregnancies present a serum progesterone > 10 ng/dL. Accordingly, Sp = 99.9 and F + R = 0.1%.

Note that the clinician can manipulate the Sn and Sp of this test for ectopic pregnancy by manipulating the cutoff point.

Warm-ups
6.1

1. The standard normal distribution is a normal distribution with mean = ____ and standard deviation = ____.

2. The standard normal distribution is denoted by the letter ____.

3. The probability that a standard normal value is under -1.62 is denoted by

   a. $P[Z > 1.62]$

   b. $P[Z < 1.62]$

   c. $P[Z < -1.62]$

   d. $P[Z = -1.62]$

   e. $P[Z > -1.62]$

4. Directly from Table 3,
$P[Z \le -1.60] =$ ____ $P[Z \le -1.62] =$ ____
$P[Z \le -1.65] =$ ____ $P[Z \le -1.69] =$ ____

5. One can directly read Table 3 to obtain $P[Z \le a]$ for what values of a?

   a. -3.4 to -0.09

   b. -3.4 to 0

   c. Any negative value of a

   d. -3.49 to -0.09

   e. -3.49 to 0.00

6. The total area under the standard normal curve is ____.

7. A useful rule for computational purposes is: $P[Z > a] = 1 - P[Z \le a]$. This is an application of the

   a. Complement Rule

   b. Subset Rule

   c. Arrangement Rule

   d. Combinatorics

   e. Fundamental Principle of Counting

8. From Table 3, $P[Z \le -1.62] = .052616$. Hence,
$P[Z > -1.62]$
$= 1 - P[Z \le -1.62]$
$= 1 -$ ____
$=$ ____

9. $P[Z < a] = P[Z \le a]$. Hence, $P[Z < -1.62] =$ ____.

10. Table 4 provides $P[Z > a]$ for any number a between 0.00 and 3.49 inclusively. Reading directly from Table 4,
$P[Z > .7] =$ ____ $P[Z > .86] =$ ____
$P[Z > 2.40] =$ ____ $P[Z > 2.49] =$ ____

11. $P[Z \le 2.49] = 1 - P[Z > 2.49]$
$= 1 -$ ____
$=$ ____

12. Find the areas for regions 1 and 2 displayed in Figure 6.1.19.

FIGURE **6.1.19** Regions 1, 2, and 3 for Warm-ups 6.1.12 and 13.

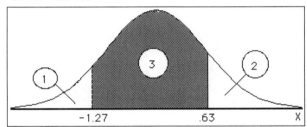

Region 1. From Table ____, $P[Z \le -1.27] =$ ____.
Region 2. From Table ____, $P[Z > .63] =$ ____.

13. The area of region 3 displayed in Figure 6.1.19 is denoted by

   a. $P[-1.27 < Z \le 0.63]$

   b. $P[-1.27 < Z] + P[Z \le .63]$

   c. $P[-1.27 < Z] + P[Z \ge .63]$

   d. $-1.27 < Z \le 0.63$

14. The area of region 3 can be calculated once we know the areas of regions 1 and 2. In particular,

Region 3 $= 1 - $ (region 1 + region 2)
         $= 1 -$ ____ $=$ ____

Hence, $P[-1.27 < Z \le 0.63] =$ ____.

15. Suppose X is a normal RV variable with mean 100 and standard deviation 10; that is, $X = \text{Normal}(\mu = 100, \sigma = 10)$. To standardize any x-value, one applies

$$z = \frac{x - \mu}{\sigma} = \frac{x - 100}{10}$$

A standardized x-value is called the z-score. What is the z-score for 115?

16. A probability problem involving a normal RV is solved by converting to the standard normal. Suppose $X = \text{Normal}(\mu = 100, \sigma = 10)$. Then,

$$P[X > 115] = P\left[Z > \frac{115 - 100}{10}\right]$$
$$= P[Z > \underline{}]$$
$$= \underline{}$$

17. For $X = \text{Normal}(\mu = 100, \sigma = 10)$,

$$P[X < 82] = P\left[Z < \frac{82 - 100}{10}\right]$$
$$= P[Z < \underline{}]$$
$$= \underline{}$$

18. $P[82 < X < 115] = P[\underline{} < Z < \underline{}]$
$$= 1 - (P[Z \leq \underline{}] + P[Z \geq \underline{}])$$
$$= 1 - (\underline{} + \underline{})$$
$$= 1 - \underline{}$$
$$= \underline{}$$

19. Suppose $X = \text{Normal}(\mu = 100, \sigma = 10)$. Suppose a subject's z-score is 1.13. What is the subject's x-value? This question involves the standardization procedure

$$\frac{x - 100}{10} = 1.13$$

First, multiply both sides by 10 to obtain: $x - 100 = \underline{}$.

Second, add 100 to both sides to obtain: $x = \underline{}$.

20. Suppose $X = \text{Normal}(\mu = 100, \sigma = 10)$. What x-value determines the top 25%? Here, we want to find x so that $P[X > x] = .25$. The corresponding z-problem is $P[Z > z] = .25$. From Table 4, $z = \underline{}$.

21. The z-score determining the top 25% in any normal distribution is 0.67. For $X = \text{Normal}(\mu = 100, \sigma = 10)$, the corresponding x-value is obtained from

$$\frac{x - 100}{10} = 0.67$$

Hence, $x = \underline{}$ is the cutoff score for the top 25%.

Problems 6.1

1. Determine each of the following using a standard normal table (Table 3 and/or 4). Include an appropriate diagram.
   a. $P[Z < -1.48]$ **b.** $P[Z \leq 2.57]$
   c. $P[Z > 0.64]$ **d.** $P[Z \leq -0.41]$
   e. $P[Z > 1.70]$ **f.** $P[-2.32 < Z \leq 0.83]$
   g. $P[0.72 \leq Z < 2.65]$ **h.** $P[-1.00 \leq Z \leq 1.00]$
   i. $P[-2.00 \leq Z \leq 2.00]$ **j.** $P[-3.00 \leq Z \leq 3.00]$
   k. $P[-1.59 \leq Z < 0.86]$ **l.** $P[-2.19 < Z \leq -0.43]$

2. Determine the value of z that yields the given probability. Include a diagram.
   a. $P[Z < z] = .085343$ **b.** $P[Z \leq z] = .091759$
   c. $P[Z \geq z] = .2709$ **d.** $P[Z > z] = .0038$
   e. $P[0 \leq Z < z] = .377$ **f.** $P[z \leq Z \leq 0] = .148$
   g. $P[-z < Z < z] = .95$ **h.** $P[-z < Z < z] = .90$
   i. $P[-z < Z < z] = .99$ **j.** $P[-z < Z < z] = .80$

3. Let X be a normal RV with a mean of 16 and a standard deviation of 3.
   a. Determine the z-score for
      i. 16 **ii.** 19 **iii.** 10 **iv.** 15 **v.** 13.2 **vi.** 11.7
   b. What value of x will produce the following z-score?
      i. 1.42 **ii.** 2 **iii.** -0.67 **iv.** -1.31 **v.** 0

4. Suppose X is a normal RV with mean 20 and standard deviation 4; that is, $X = \text{Normal}(\mu = 20, \sigma = 4)$. Determine
   a. $P[X < 20]$ **b.** $P[X > 20]$
   c. $P[X = 20]$ **d.** $P[X < 16]$
   e. $P[X > 24]$ **f.** $P[16 < X < 24]$
   g. $P[13 < X < 18]$ **h.** $P[22 < X < 27]$
   i. $P[14 < X < 23]$

5. Intelligence quotient (IQ) scores are based on a normal distribution with a mean of 100 and a standard deviation of 13.
   a. I. M. Smart has an IQ of 124. What proportion of the population has an IQ less than that of Ms. Smart? This proportion, converted to percent, is called a percentile. What percentile is Ms. Smart in?
   b. What IQ is needed to be in the top (i) half, (ii) third, (iii) quarter, (iv) 10%, (v) 5%, (vi) 1%?
   c. One organization advertises that its only requirement for membership is that one be in the

top 2% of the country in terms of IQ. What IQ level does one need to be qualified for membership in the organization?

d. Suppose we define a genius as "one in a million" in terms of top IQ. What IQ would one need to be considered a genius?

6. Suppose that as a result of the Bodai et al research on the oxygen insufflation suction catheter we assume that the change in PaO_2 during suctioning using the control technique is normally distributed with a mean change of 5.8 mm Hg and a standard deviation of 5.0 mm Hg. Here, change = start − end, where start means PaO_2 at the start of suctioning and end means PaO_2 at the end of suctioning. The raw data are given in Data Set 4, Group 3, Standard suction with valve adapter (control).

a. What proportion of these patients would show a drop in PaO_2 (i.e., change > 0)?

b. What proportion of these patients would show a gain in PaO_2 (i.e., change < 0)?

c. A drop of 20 mm Hg in PaO_2 is cause for clinical concern. What proportion show a drop ≥ 20 mm Hg? On this basis, would you consider the suctioning protocol safe?

7. Scholastic Aptitude Test (SAT) scores are scaled so that the resulting distribution is normal with a mean of 500 and a standard deviation of 100.

a. One state university system advertises a student must be in the top third in order to qualify for admission. What SAT score does the student need?

b. What SAT scores serve as boundaries for each of these categories?

Outstanding: top 5%
Superior: next 10%
Above average: next 15%
Average: middle 40%
Below average: lowest 30%

8. This simulation illustrates the interplay between sensitivity (Sn) and specificity (Sp) for diagnostic testing. Suppose researchers are studying the disease "Big D" and find that patients with the disease in general seem to have an elevated level of plasma Factor X. In the nondiseased population, plasma Factor X has a normal distribution with a mean of 80 and a standard deviation of 5. In Big D

patients, plasma Factor X has a normal distribution with a mean of 95 and a standard deviation of 4. Clinicians decide to use a Factor X level above 90 as a diagnostic indicator for Big D.

a. What proportion of Big D patients have a Factor X level above 90? What is the Sn of this Factor X test for Big D? What is the F − R for this diagnostic test?

b. What proportion of the nondiseased population has a Factor X level below 90? What is the Sp of this Factor X test for Big D? What is the F + R for this diagnostic test?

9. Matthews et al (Example 6.1.18) studied serum progesterone levels as an aid in the diagnosis of ectopic pregnancy. On the basis of their study, we supposed that serum progesterone is normally distributed in women with ectopic pregnancies with a mean of 5.63 ng/mL and a standard deviation of 3.65 ng/mL. In women with normal pregnancies, serum progesterone is normally distributed with a mean of 30.85 ng/mL and a standard deviation of 6.91 ng/mL. Suppose that one decides to use serum progesterone level as a diagnostic test for ectopic pregnancy. Consider a cutoff of 15 ng/mL; that is, a serum progesterone level of 15 ng/mL or below is diagnostic for ectopic pregnancy.

a. What proportion of women with ectopic pregnancy will have a serum progesterone level of 15 ng/mL or less? What is the Sn for this diagnostic criterion? What is the F − R?

b. What proportion of women with a normal pregnancy will have a serum progesterone level of 15 ng/mL or less? What is the Sp for this diagnostic criterion? What is the F + R?

10. Marik was interested in the 30-day survival rate of patients admitted to the coronary intensive care unit for acute myocardial infarction (AMI). Based on Marik's data, suppose that the prognostic score among survivors (SPS) is (approximately) normally distributed with a mean of 11.9 and a standard deviation of 4.0. The prognostic score among those who die within the first 30 days (DPS) is (approximately) normally distributed with a mean of 21.2 and a standard deviation of 5.9. The prognostic score (PS) is taken upon admission. Marik inquired about the utility of the PS as an indicator of short-term survival. Patients were classified as low-risk if their PS

at admission was < 12, as moderate-risk if PS was between 12 and 18, and as high-risk if PS > 18.

a. What proportion of survivors have a PS < 12?

b. What proportion of those who die within 30 days of admission for AMI have a low-risk classification?

c. What proportion of short-term survivors will be classified as having moderate risk?

d. What proportion of survivors have a moderate-risk classification?

e. What proportion of survivors will be classified high-risk?

f. What proportion of nonsurvivors will be classified high-risk?

g. (Challenge) Eighty-seven percent of the patients admitted for AMI survive over the short term. Suppose a newly admitted patient has a PS under 12 and is thus classified as low-risk. Low-risk patients are sent to the floor rather than being admitted to the intensive care unit.

  i. Construct a probability tree in which the first branch is survive or die, the second branch is PS < 12 or PS ≥ 12.

  ii. What is the probability that a newly admitted patient with a PS under 12 will survive?

  iii. What is the probability that a newly admitted patient with a high-risk PS will die?

11. Suppose that room temperature cardiac output among coronary care patients is (approximately) normally distributed with a mean of 4.50 liters/minute and standard deviation of 1.14 liters/minute (assumption based on the Daily and Mersch study).

a. What proportion of patients have a compromised cardiac output under 3.50 liters/minute?

b. What proportion of patients are under the low normal value of 4 liters/minute?

c. What proportion of patients are within the normal range of 4 to 8 liters/minute?

12. The National Cholesterol Education Program's (NCEP) cutoff for borderline high-risk total cholesterol is 200 ml/dL. Bachorik et al reported on screening total cholesterol levels for people enrolled in a heart disease prevention program.

a. Suppose that total cholesterol level in a certain population is (approximately) normally distributed with a mean of 223 mg/dL and standard deviation of 44 mg/dL. What proportion of people in the population have borderline high-risk total cholesterol?

b. Suppose that total cholesterol level in a certain population is (approximately) normally distributed with a mean of 208 mg/dL and standard deviation of 42 mg/dL. What proportion of people in the population have borderline high-risk total cholesterol?

13. (Continued from 12) The NCEP cutoff for borderline high-risk low-density lipoprotein (LDL) cholesterol concentration is 130 mg/dL. Suppose LDL cholesterol concentration in a group is (approximately) normally distributed with a mean of 139 mg/dL and standard deviation of 40 mg/dL. What proportion of people have borderline high LDL cholesterol?

Problems 14 and 15 are continuations of Example 6.1.1, which compares the distribution of birth weights of infants of heavy-drinking mothers with the birth weights of infants of nonsmoking, nondrinking mothers. Neonate low birth weight is defined as < 2500 grams.

14. Suppose that birth weight for infants of nonsmoking, nondrinking mothers is (approximately) normally distributed with a mean of 3500 grams and standard deviation of 450 grams. What proportion of babies of nonsmoking, nondrinking mothers are low birth weight?

15. Suppose that birth weight for infants of heavy-drinking mothers is (approximately) normally distributed with a mean of 2600 grams and standard deviation of 450 grams. What proportion of babies of heavy-drinking mothers are low birth weight?

16. Klag et al studied serum cholesterol as a risk factor for a midlife cardiovascular event in young males. They reported that young men with a serum cholesterol level ≥ 209 mg/dL were at increased risk for cardiovascular disease in midlife. In young men, serum cholesterol is (approximately) normally distributed with a mean of 190 mg/dL and a standard deviation of 30 mg/dL. What proportion of young men have a serum cholesterol ≥ 209 mg/dL (and hence are at increased risk for midlife cardiovascular disease)?

OBJECTIVE This section will

1 Determine if a given sample of a continuous random variable is consistent with normality by applying Minitab's nscores correlation test.

The normal distribution is the most common continuous distribution. Several statistical techniques for studying sample data are valid only for a sample drawn from a normal distribution. In practice, one often hypothesizes (assumes) that the distribution of a continuous RV of interest has a normal distribution, unless the data offer evidence to the contrary.

Since the normal distribution is the most common and easiest to use continuous RV, we take the position that "it is not unreasonable to assume normality," unless of course there is evidence to the contrary. An assumption made in this spirit is called a **null hypothesis**; that is, in the absence of evidence to the contrary (null evidence situation), we assume the null hypothesis (in this case, normality). When the sample offers evidence to the contrary, then we reject the null hypothesis. The main point here is that a researcher assumes normality unless the data offer sufficient evidence that such an assumption is unreasonable.

A protocol for deciding whether to retain or reject a null hypothesis is called a **Test of Hypothesis**. In this section we test the null hypothesis that the distribution is normal. A rejection of this assumption implies the alternative situation in which the distribution is nonnormal. A null hypothesis is symbolically denoted by H_0; the alternate hypothesis, H_a. Hence, we test

H_0: the distribution is normal

versus H_a: the distribution is nonnormal

The intent of this announcement is that, lacking evidence to the contrary, it is not unreasonable to proceed assuming a normal distribution. The key question now is: What is sufficient evidence for rejecting the null hypothesis of normality? We present a quick technique using Minitab.

Minitab's Nscores Correlation Test for Normality

The following algorithm uses Minitab to determine if a given sample contains sufficient evidence to reject the null hypothesis

H_0: the distribution is normal.

We refer to this algorithm simply as "Minitab's nscores correlation test for normality."

STEP 1. Enter the sample data and obtain the **sample nscores correlation** as follows:

```
MTB > SET C1
DATA> enter sample data
```

```
DATA> END OF DATA
MTB > PRINT C1    #check data entry
MTB > NSCORES C1 INTO C41
MTB > CORRELATION C1 AND C41
```

In response to the correlation command, Minitab displays the sample *nscores correlation*. The sample nscores correlation (always between 0 and 1) is a measure of the sample's consistency with normality.

Comment The use of column C41 for the sample nscores is arbitrary. One only needs to put the nscores into a column that is not being used.

STEP 2. Construct a **decision line** as displayed in Figure 6.2.1, where *r*, the **critical correlation**, is obtained from Table 6.2.1.

TABLE **6.2.1**
Critical correlation table for Minitab's nscores correlation test for normality.

Sample Size	Critical Correlation
5	.8320
10	.8804
15	.9110
20	.9290
25	.9408
30	.9490
40	.9597
50	.9664
60	.9710
75	.9757

Comment If the sample size lies between two table values, for a "quick" test use the *larger* corresponding critical value. For example, suppose the sample size is 34. The sample size 34 does not explicitly occur in Table 6.2.1. However, 34 is between 30 and 40. The corresponding critical correlations are .9490 (for sample size 30) and .9597 (for sample size 40). For a quick test, simply use the larger critical correlation (here, .9597).

The critical correlation is where we "draw the line" in order to decide if the sample contains sufficient evidence for rejecting the null hypothesis of normality. If the sample nscores correlation is greater than or equal to the critical correlation, then the sample is consistent with an assumption of normality. If the sample nscores correlation is less than the critical correlation, then the sample provides sufficient evidence to reject the null hypothesis of normality; that is, the data are inconsistent with normality.

STEP 3. Place the sample nscores correlation obtained in step 1 onto the decision line constructed in step 2. State the corresponding **conclusion**.

FIGURE **6.2.1**
Decision line for Minitab's nscores correlation test for normality.

Evidence for nonnormal	Consistent with normal

0   r   1

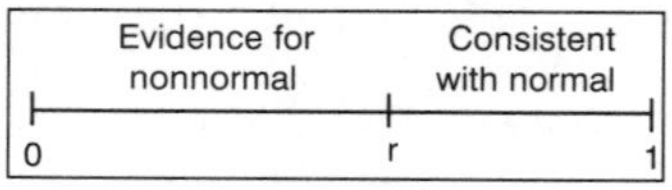

EXAMPLE 6.2.1 In Chapter 2 we studied the Daily and Mersch room temperature cardiac output data set. The histogram portraying this data set (see Figure 2.1.9) does not give the immediate impression of a supporting normal distribution. Minitab's nscores correlation procedure provides a method for testing

H_0: Room temperature cardiac outputs of cardiac intensive care patients are normally distributed.

versus H_a: Room temperature cardiac outputs of cardiac intensive care patients are not normally distributed.

STEP 1. Enter the room temperature cardiac outputs into column C1 and check for data entry accuracy. Then

```
MTB > NSCORES C1 INTO C41
MTB > CORRELATION C1 AND C41

Correlation of ROOMTEMP and C41 = 0.984
```

STEP 2. Here, since the sample size $n = 29$ lies between the table sample sizes of 25 and 30, we use the larger corresponding critical correlation of .9490. The decision line is displayed in Figure 6.2.2.

STEP 3. Since the sample nscores correlation of 0.984 is between the critical value of .9408 and 1, then the sample data set is consistent with normality. Hence, it is not unreasonable to assume that room temperature cardiac outputs follow a normal distribution (approximately) in the population of cardiac intensive care patients.

Comment In step 2 in Example 6.2.1, we were faced with the sample size $n = 29$. The sample size $n = 29$ is not included in the critical correlation table (Table 6.2.1). The sample size $n = 29$ falls between the two table sizes of $n = 25$ and $n = 30$ with critical correlations of .9408 and .9490, respectively. An alternative way to display the decision line is to represent the critical region from .9408 to .9490 as an ambiguous zone. If the sample nscores correlation is greater than .9490, then the sample nscores correlation is clearly in the *consistent with normal* region of the decision line; if less than .9408, then clearly in the *evidence for nonnormal* region. A decision line showing this feature is displayed in Figure 6.2.3.

The crosshatched region in the decision line in Figure 6.2.3 is an **ambiguous zone**. If the sample nscores correlation falls in the ambiguous zone, then the decision regarding a normal distribution is thus far inconclusive. In this event, apply the formula given at the bottom of Table 5 (Appendix, $\alpha = .01$). The formula calculates $cv(n)$, the critical value for a sample of size n. Usually, however, calculating this precise critical value is an unnecessary refinement for the purpose of reaching a decision about normality.

FIGURE **6.2.2**
Decision line for Minitab's nscores correlation test for normality for the Daily and Mersch room temperature cardiac output data set.

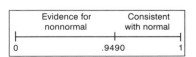

FIGURE **6.2.3**
Decision line for a sample size of 29. The
shaded region is the ambiguous zone.

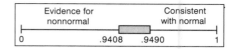

Comment When we test for normality, we are not concerned with whether the distribution is exactly normal. No real population is exactly normal. A normal distribution theoretically extends from minus to plus infinity. Cardiac outputs, for example, cannot be negative; hence, cardiac output cannot be a perfectly normal random variable. In real problems, we are interested if the distribution is approximately normal, that is, normal enough for practical purposes. Relatively small deviations from nonnormality are not going to hurt our ability to obtain correct conclusions. In this spirit, Minitab's nscores correlation test for normality serves us well.

EXERCISES 6.2

Warm-ups 6.2

Bridges et al measured blood hemoglobin (Hb) for each subject in a sample of 14 women. Figure 6.2.4 displays Minitab's output showing a print of the data and the information needed to test Hb for normality.

1. The sample size is ____.

2. Consult the critical correlation table (Table 6.2.1). Our sample of size 14 lies between what two sample sizes in column 1 of the table? ____ and ____.

3. The critical correlation for a sample of size

10 is ____
15 is ____

4. Fill in the empty boxes for the normality decision line shown in Figure 6.2.5.

5. What does the shaded region in the Figure 6.2.5 represent?

6. The sample nscores correlation is ____.

7. When the sample nscores correlation falls in the normal region, we are justified in stating that

FIGURE **6.2.4** Minitab output for the blood hemoglobin (Hb) data set.

```
MTB > PRINT C1

Hb
 15.5  13.6  13.5  13.0  13.3  12.4  11.1  13.1  16.1  16.4
 13.4  13.2  14.3  16.1

MTB > NSCORES C1 INTO C11
MTB > CORRELATION C1 AND C11

Correlation of Hb and NSHb = 0.959
```

FIGURE **6.2.5** Normality decision line for the Hb data set.

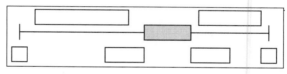

a. The sample is consistent with being drawn from a normal distribution.

b. It is not unreasonable to assume that the RV of interest is normally distributed in the population at large.

c. The sample contains insufficient evidence that the RV is nonnormal in the population.

d. We may proceed assuming a (approximately) normal distribution.

e. Any of the above.

Answer Warm-ups 8–11 true or false. If the sample nscores correlation falls in the normal zone, then

8. The sample is normally distributed.

9. We have proved that the RV of interest is normally distributed in the population as a whole.

10. The sample is typical of the kind of sample one would get if the RV of interest were normally distributed in the population.

11. The sample is consistent with the assumption that the RV is (approximately) normal in the population.

Problems 6.2

1. Consider the Daily and Mersch cardiac output data (Appendix, Data Set 1). Are the sample RTCO, ITCO, and Fick CO consistent with an assumption of normality?

2. Consider the Barcelona et al cardiac output data (Appendix, Data Set 2).

    a. Test the first iced injectate column and room temperature injectate (prefilled syringes) column for normality.

    b. Test the second iced injectate column and room temperature injectate (co-Set) column for normality.

3. Consider the Molyneaux et al coagulation study (Appendix, Data Set 3).

    a. Consider the 1.6-mL discard. Test the arterial, venous, and difference (arterial − venous) for normality.

    b. Consider the 3.2-mL-discard. Test the arterial, venous, and difference (arterial − venous) for normality.

    c. Consider the 4.8 mL-discard. Test the arterial, venous, and difference (arterial − venous) for normality.

4. Consider the Shively study about the effect of position change on mixed venous oxygen saturation (Appendix, Data Set 5). Check each of the following for normality.

    a. The baseline $S\bar{v}O_2$ for group 1.

    b. The baseline $S\bar{v}O_2$ for group 2.

    c. The baseline $S\bar{v}O_2$ for the combined groups (i.e., combine group 1 and group 2).

5. Consider the Clark and Hoffer data set (Appendix, Data Set 6). Test (a) age, (b) height, (c) weight, and (d) body mass index for normality.

6. Test the Sütsch et al data (Problem 2.1.12) for normality.

CHAPTER 6 OVERVIEW

Summary

The **normal distribution** is the most common continuous distribution. A normal distribution is specified by providing its **mean** and **standard deviation**. The mean centers the distribution. The standard deviation indicates the spread of the distribution. The graph of a normal distribution is the traditional **bell-shaped curve**. This curve is positive, continuous (unbroken), and symmetrical about the mean. The curve has three major components: a concave-up left tail, a concave-down dome centered over the mean, and a concave-up right tail. The total area under the curve is 1. The key aspect of the curve is that the **probability** that a value falls in some given interval corresponds to the area under the curve over the interval.

There are two common methods for computing probabilities for a normal distribution: computer and tables. Computations using Minitab are straightforward using the PDF and CDF commands. Computation by hand involves first converting a normal distribution to the **standard normal** distribution, then using standard normal tables.

Many statistical procedures are valid only for normal distributions. When a research study is conducted and a continuous data set is gathered, it is natural to inquire whether it is reasonable to assume that the data were obtained from a normal distribution. **Minitab** provides a computerized **nscores correlation test for normality**. The test measures a data set for consistency with normality. If a sample does not pass Minitab's nscores correlation test for normality, then it is improbable that the sample came from a normal distribution. Minitab's nscores correlation test allows us to decide whether a data set is consistent with an assumption of normality or whether the data set provides evidence for nonnormality.

Keywords

bell-shaped curve
continuous
critical nscores correlation
decision line
hypothesis
   alternate hypothesis
   null hypothesis
mean
normal distribution
normality

nscores correlation test for
   normality
positive curve
probability
standard deviation
standard normal distribution
Standardization Theorem
symmetrical
test of hypothesis
z-score

References

Bachorik P et al: Lipoprotein-cholesterol analysis during screening: Accuracy and reliability. *Ann Intern Med* 114, no. 9 (1 May 1991): 741.

Bridges N et al: Evaluation of a new system for hemoglobin measurement. *Am Clin Prod Rev* 22 (April 1987): 22.

Chamberlin G: Small for gestational age. *Br Med J* 302, no. 6792 (29 June 1991): 1592.

Klag M et al: Serum cholesterol in young men and subsequent cardiovascular disease. *N Engl J Med* 328, no. 5 (4 February 1993): 313.

Marik P: Myocardial infarction prognostic scoring system. *Heart Lung* 20, no. 1 (January 1991): 16.

Matthews C et al: Serum progesterone levels as an aid in the diagnosis of ectopic pregnancy. *Obstet Gynecol* 68 (1986): 390.

An Orientation to Descriptive Statistics
A REVIEW

We began our study of statistics for the health sciences by emphasizing the key role played by *variation*. In any serious study, the investigator begins by carefully specifying the population and random variable(s) of interest. Statistics is a tool that allows us to study a population as a whole, despite the fact that the individuals in that population differ. We began our practice of statistics by examining data sets from a variety of research studies. In order to get a handle on the data, we constructed a frequency distribution table and an accompanying graphic (bar graph, pie chart, dotplot, boxplot, stem-and-leaf diagram, or histogram). A frequency distribution table gives us a sense of how a random variable is distributed in a population. The distribution can be summarized succinctly by boiling down the data set to simply mean ± standard deviation.

An important feature of a frequency distribution table is the presentation of relative frequencies. These relative frequencies can be viewed in two important ways. The first is empirical in that a relative frequency describes the proportion of a study sample having a certain characteristic. The second is probabilistic in that a relative frequency estimates the probability that a randomly selected member of a population has the described characteristic. Hence, the concept of distribution has two important viewpoints: distribution of a random variable (RV) within a population, and a probability distribution for the RV applied to an RV in the population.

The important interpretations of probability in the health sciences are empirical and theoretical. Fundamental concepts supporting probability are experiment, sample space, and event. An experiment may be viewed as being simple or multistage. A multistage experiment may be portrayed by a tree diagram.

Computations involving probabilities usually involve combinatorics or the basic computational rules of probability. Combinatorics include the Fundamental Principal of Counting and the Subset Rule. Combinatorics allow one to count quickly the number of points in certain sample spaces and events of interest. The basic computational rules of probability are the Complement Rule and the Independence Rule. These allow one to compute the probability of a complex event made up of simpler events with known probabilities.

The important clinical role played by a basic understanding of probability is illustrated in diagnostic testing. Diagnostic testing utilizes several concepts based on simple notions from probability: sensitivity, specificity, false-positive and false-negative rates, predictive value, accuracy, and prevalence. Research data used to study diagnostics may be presented in the form of a two-factor frequency distribution table to facilitate making these computations.

Since serious study begins with a well-defined population and RV of interest, an understanding of the general concept of an RV is crucial. The two main types of RVs are categorical and quantitative. A categorical random variable classifies a member of a population into one of a list of exhaustive and mutually exclusive attributes. A quantitative RV assigns an appropriate number to any individual in the population.

A quantitative RV may be further classified as nominal, ordinal, or interval. A nominal number is used merely as a name for a subject in the study (i.e., an identification number). Ordinal numbers are used to rank an observation. An interval number is a number used to count or measure. Interval numbers have the key property of having an intrinsic notion of size so that a meaningful difference can be obtained between two different numbers. Interval numbers are numbers used as numbers, rather than merely as names or ranks.

There are two kinds of interval RVs: discrete and continuous. A discrete RV is one whose possible values can be enumerated (provided in a list). A continuous RV is accompanied by an interval of possibilities. A discrete RV counts; a continuous RV measures.

A discrete RV often is presented by means of a probability density function (PDF) table. Using the table, one can calculate the mean and standard deviation of the RV, as well as theoretical probabilities for events of interest. The most important of all the discrete RVs are the binomial RVs. The binomial RV $X = \text{Bino}(n,p)$ counts the number of successes in n independent Bernoulli trials, where each Bernoulli trial has a probability of success, p. A Bernoulli trial is an experiment that has exactly two outcomes, generically called success and failure, and having probabilities p and q, respectively.

When given the binomial RV $X = \text{Bino}(n,p)$, the mean and variance can be computed quickly using the expressions np and npq, respectively. The density function is given by

$$f(x) = C(n,x)p^x q^{n-x}$$

where $f(x)$ is the probability that $X = \text{Bino}(n, p)$ attains exactly x successes in any given binomial experiment. Skill using the binomial random variable is particularly useful in analyzing success and failure scenarios (e.g., genetics counseling).

A continuous RV often is presented with a graph of its PDF. One uses a continuous RV X by determining the probability that the value of X falls in some interval of interest. Such probabilities are often determined from tables. The most important continuous RVs are the normal RVs. A specific normal RV is given by supplying its mean and standard deviation. The Standardization Theorem allows one to calculate probabilities for any normal RV from a table of values for the standard normal random variable. The standard normal distribution is the normal distribution whose mean is 0 and standard deviation is 1.

A key research concern occurs when one wants to study a given continuous random variable within the context of a random sample. The researcher inquires whether the sample data are consistent with assuming that the RV has a normal distribution. Minitab's nscores and correlation provides a quick and easy method to test normality for a given interval data set.

PART I   Review Exercises

1. Varah et al obtained the following data set for the number of blood-clotting tests nurses performed at bedside in a study of 24 patients:

5 6 4 3 9 4 3 8 8 7 4 3
9 5 5 7 4 7 7 6 7 4 5 6

a. Determine n (sample size), Σx, and Σx^2.
b. Determine the sample mean, median, and range.

c. Apply the formula $s^2 = \dfrac{n(\Sigma x^2) - (\Sigma x)^2}{n(n-1)}$ to calculate the sample variance.
d. Determine the sample standard deviation.
e. Construct a frequency distribution table (ungrouped) that includes the frequency, relative frequency, and percent relative frequency. Construct a corresponding cumulative frequency distribution table.
f. Construct a bar graph and a pie chart that represent the data.

2. The data displayed in Table I-1 are adapted from LoBiondo-Wood and Haber.

TABLE **I-1**
Frequency distribution table adapted from LoBiondo-Wood and Haber.

Score	Frequency
50–59	2
60–69	10
70–79	23
80–89	15
90–99	1

a. The sample size is ____.
b. The unit of measurement is ____.
c. The class width is ____.
d. Construct a table that includes the class boundaries, relative frequencies, and cumulative relative frequencies.
e. Construct a relative frequency histogram for these data.
f. Construct a frequency polygon for these data.
g. Construct a relative frequency ogive for these data.

3. The PDF for a discrete random variable X is given in Table I-2.

TABLE **I-2** PDF for X.

x	0	1	2	3	4	5	6
$f(x)$	.12	.25	.27	.19	.10	.04	?

a. $f(2) =$ ____.
b. $f(6) =$ ____.
c. $\text{Prob}[2 < X \le 4] =$ ____.
d. Determine the mean of X.
e. Determine the variance and standard deviation of X.

4. Young et al reported on elevated fecal α_1-antitrypsin (αAT) as diagnostic for large-bowel cancer (LBC). Table I-3 is adapted from their report.

TABLE I-3 Data from Young et al.

		Large Bowel Cancer		
		Yes	No	
Elevated αAT	Yes	19	5	
	No	7	91	

a. Determine the Sn, F − R, Sp, F + R, PV+ , PV − , and accuracy of the test.
b. What is the prevalence of LBC in the research study?
c. Young et al noted that LBC prevalence is only .3% (3 out of 1000) in a target screening population. Assuming the Sn and Sp obtained in (a), determine PV + in the target screening population. (Hint: Construct a two-factor frequency distribution table for a large population of 100,000.)
d. Does αAT appear to be a useful test to diagnose LBC in a large screening population?
e. How might αAT be useful in diagnostics for LBC?

5. The sensitivity of a new diagnostic test for student's crud is 80%. Five sick students checked into the health center yesterday to obtain a medical release from their statistics examination (the students were really sick with student's crud, not test anxiety).

a. What is the probability that all five students will be correctly diagnosed?
b. What is the probability that at least one sick person will have to take the examination?
c. What is the expected number of this group of five students who will be correctly diagnosed by the test?

6. Matthews et al studied serum progesterone levels as an aid in the diagnosis of ectopic pregnancy. On the basis of their study, suppose that serum progesterone is normally distributed in women with ectopic pregnancies with a mean of 5.63 and standard deviation of 3.65 ng/mL. In women with normal pregnancies, serum progesterone is normally distributed with a mean of 30.85 and standard deviation of 6.91 ng/mL. Suppose that

one decides to use serum progesterone level as a diagnostic test for ectopic pregnancy.

a. Consider a cutoff of 20 ng/mL; that is, a serum progesterone level of 20 or below is diagnostic for ectopic pregnancy.
  i. What proportion of women with ectopic pregnancy will have a serum progesterone level of 20 or less? What is the Sn for this diagnostic criterion? What is the F − R?
  ii. What proportion of women with a normal pregnancy will have a serum progesterone level of 20 or less? What is the Sp for this diagnostic criterion? What is the F + R?

b. What cutoff criterion would make the sensitivity 99%?
c. What cutoff criterion would make the specificity 99%?

7. (Project) The following data are the exam scores of 51 students taken from LoBiondo-Wood and Haber.

54	58	62	64	64	64	64	66	66	68	68	68	70
72	72	72	72	72	72	72	72	72	74	74	74	74
74	74	74	76	78	78	78	78	78	80	80	80	80
80	82	82	84	84	84	84	84	84	86	88	90	

The professor is wondering how the students are doing and what grades to assign (A, B, C, D, F). Help the professor.

Remark This is an open-ended question that contains statistical and real-world implications. You are asked to "analyze the data." Part of your understanding of statistics includes knowing what to do with a data set. There is more to it than just finding the mean.

References

LoBiondo-Wood G and Haber J: *Nursing Research*, 2nd ed. C. V. Mosby, St. Louis, 1990, 295.
Matthews C et al: Serum progesterone levels as an aid in the diagnosis of ectopic pregnancy. *Obstet Gynecol* 68 (1986): 390.
Varah N et al: Heparin monitoring in the coronary care unit after percutaneous transluminal coronary angioplasty. *Heart Lung* 19, no. 3 (May 1990): 265.
Young G et al: α_1-Antitrypsin as a test for large bowel cancer. *Aust NZ J Med* 22, no. 1 (February 1992): 101.

An Orientation to Inferential Statistics

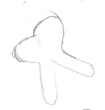

In general, the health sciences focus on behaviors and treatments. These correlate with the two major frameworks of the health sciences: holistic and intervention.

The holistic framework is oriented toward essentially well people. The goal is to assist growth in a healthy body, mind, and spirit by counseling appropriate behaviors. Colloquially, the approach in holistics is: Do this, it's good for you. More formally, the holistics health care professional counsels behaviors that are believed to sustain or improve the welfare of the patient.

The intervention framework is oriented toward people in need of an immediate treatment for a condition such as trauma, disease, or insanity. The hope of the health science professional is that as a result of an intervention the patient will be better off at discharge than at presentation. Colloquially, the intervention approach is: I'll make it better for you. More formally, the intervention health care professional counsels treatments that are believed (or at least hoped) to improve or sustain the presented condition of the patient.

In both frameworks of health care, the usual goal is an improvement in the condition of a patient or client. Fundamentally, one is to compare a present state with a desired better future state. The key for evaluation of the health care is a comparison of states.

As a scientist, the health science professional needs methods of assessment and comparison for the purpose of advancing policy or protocol. The basic tools of assessment and comparison in this regard are the confidence interval and test of hypothesis, which are the key topics in Part II: An Orientation to Inferential Statistics.

inference - reading between the lines.
holistic - whole person - keeping it, whole and good healthy
intervention - action to stop the bad, restore the good.

PART II
CONFIDENCE INTERVAL!

TEST OF HYPOTHESIS:

Confidence Intervals I

reading between the lines

In this chapter we begin inferential statistics—the process of drawing valid conclusions from data. In the previous chapters we focused on descriptive statistics and probability. In descriptive statistics we learned how to organize and present a sample data set. In probability we became acquainted with two standard models for describing variation: the binomial and normal distributions.

After one looks at the data, one wonders what it all means. Daily and Mersch were interested in patient care of cardiac patients in need of bedside hemodynamic monitoring. In particular, their research studied methods of determining cardiac output. They obtained data on 29 patients in whom cardiac outputs were obtained using three different methods. After examining the data, we ask: What does it all mean for patient care?

Daily and Mersch were interested in comparing whether there was any significant difference between cardiac output obtained using an ice-temperature injectate versus a room-temperature injectate. In this chapter we introduce how to construct confidence intervals for the mean. The confidence interval is a powerful tool for comparing the relative effectiveness of two methods, such as room-temperature versus ice-temperature cardiac output measurements. Using this tool, we can make confident inferences about the relative comparison of room- versus ice-temperature cardiac outputs among cardiac patients as a whole, not just in the study sample. This ability to generalize beyond the sample to the population at large makes statistics the useful tool that it is in the health sciences.

SECTION 7.1

Confidence Intervals for the Mean

OBJECTIVES   This section will

1   Describe the concept of estimate for the mean, distinguishing between a point estimate and an interval estimate.

2   Describe the term confidence interval for the mean.   *WIDE – 100%*
Narrow 90%.

3   Determine a c% confidence interval for the population mean of a continuous random variable X when provided with a random sample where either (a) the distribution is normal or (b) the sample size is large (> 30).

MARYANN   ↓thing of interest

A basic fact that every health science professional must cope with is that people differ. One way to get a handle on this variation is the following: *Instead of considering the individuals in the group, consider the group as an individual.* For a continuous random variable (RV), this usually is done by presenting the mean and the standard deviation. The mean is an idealized typical value that may be thought of as that value each person in the group would have if there were no variation. The standard deviation is a measure of the variation. Normally, a good majority of the population falls in the 1SD window, mean ± standard deviation. How does one obtain knowledge of the *population* mean? One begins with data.

EXAMPLE 7.1.1 Bridges et al studied new equipment for measuring blood hemoglobin (Hb). Hb is important in treating anemia. They obtained blood samples from 14 female and 15 male subjects. The sample data are presented in Table 7.1.1.

TABLE **7.1.1**
Hb data from Bridges et al (g/dL).

Female	Male
15.5	14.0
13.6	15.3
13.5	13.5
13.0	15.8
13.3	15.0
12.4	16.7
11.1	17.1
13.1	14.7
16.1	15.5
16.4	17.3
13.4	15.0
13.2	16.0
14.3	14.5
16.1	16.0
	16.9

Is Hb significantly different between men and women? Table 7.1.2 displays information about the sample and population means for females and males based on the Bridges et al data presented in Example 7.1.1.

TABLE **7.1.2**
Mean Hb (g/dL) for females and males based on data from Bridges et al.

	Sample	Population
Females	13.93	(13.02, 14.83)
Males	15.55	(14.92, 16.19)

Note that the *sample* of females uses only 14 women. The *population* of women, however, is much larger (millions). The sample mean is 13.93 mg/dL. This figure may be utilized as a crude estimate for the female population Hb mean. Of course, different samples will produce different sample means. Hence, a better way to provide an estimate for a population mean is to provide an interval, (13.02,14.83). Such an interval asserts that, based on the sample, the data provide evidence that the population mean Hb for women is somewhere between 13.02 and 14.83 g/dL.

Do men and women, in general, have the same Hb level? By looking at the individuals in the sample displayed in Example 7.1.1, one can see that some women have a higher Hb level than some men, and vice versa. In the *sample*, on average, men have a higher Hb reading. The key question now is, May one generalize from this sample to the population at large? Is it appropriate to assert that, in general, men have a higher Hb level than women? Sample means will differ, so just looking at the sample means does not provide the answer. A glance at the interval estimates in Table 7.1.2 provides the answer. The interval estimates do not overlap. Accordingly, we say that the mean Hb level for men is statistically significantly greater than the mean Hb level for women; that is, in general, men have a higher Hb level than women.

Generalizing, one considers a large background population of interest and a continuous random variable with population mean μ. The population mean μ is unknown to humans. To know μ one must census the entire population. However, a census usually is impractical due to lack of time and resources. Further, a census often is impossible due to a future outlook (e.g., the mean length of hospital stay for cardiac patients in the next 10 years). Hence, researchers must be content with an estimate of μ obtained from an unbiased sample. There are two kinds of estimates for μ that one can obtain from a sample: a point estimate and an interval estimate.

Point Estimate for the Mean μ

A sample produces a sample mean, $\bar{x}$. This sample mean is used as a **point estimate** for μ, that is, a single number used to estimate μ. For example, from Table 7.1.2, a point estimate for the mean Hb for females is 13.93 g/dL, and a point estimate for the mean Hb for males is 15.55 g/dL.

One denotes the use of $\bar{x}$ as a point estimate for μ by

$$\hat{\mu} = \bar{x} \qquad \text{estimating } \mu \text{ to equal sample mean}$$

The "hat" over the parameter μ indicates that we are estimating μ to be $\bar{x}$. For example, $\hat{\mu}_{\text{Female}} = 13.93$ g/dL, and $\hat{\mu}_{\text{Male}} = 15.55$ g/dL.

A sample is only a small part of the whole population. We would not expect the sample mean $\bar{x}$ to exactly equal the population mean μ; in fact, different samples have different sample means, but the population mean μ is fixed. Since a sample examines only a small part of the population, there is a risk that a random sample may be unrepresentative of the population, causing the sample mean $\bar{x}$ to differ significantly from μ. Hence, a researcher is concerned about the confidence that can be placed in a point estimate determined from a sample. Accordingly, the researcher expands the idea of a point estimate to an interval estimate.

Interval Estimate for the Mean

An **interval estimate** for μ is an interval (L, R) that claims that $L < \mu < R$. This claim, however, may or may not be true. An interval estimate simply admits that it does not know what μ is exactly, but rather offers a ballpark range in which μ is hoped to reside.

The numbers L and R are called the "left endpoint" and "right endpoint," respectively, of the interval. For example, from Table 7.1.2, an interval estimate for the mean Hb for females is (13.12,14.83) g/dL. The details of how we got this interval will be explained shortly.

We want a procedure that will regularly produce reliable interval estimates. Although sample data are different from sample to sample, a good procedure will produce an interval estimate that, from sample to sample, regularly contains μ. In addition, the interval must be sufficiently narrow to be useful. Although one can say with certainty that the mean age of a U.S. citizen is in the interval (1,200), such a "fact" is useless. Offering a very narrow interval, on the other hand, carries a great deal of risk that μ is in fact not in the interval. The trick is to balance utility with risk. The interval estimate must be narrow enough to be useful but wide enough to reliably contain μ.

0–100 meanmeaningless
1390–1395 too narrow

Confidence Interval for the Mean

A common statistical procedure producing an interval estimate is the confidence interval procedure. The interval estimate from this procedure is called a **confidence interval (CI)**. A key advantage of the CI procedure is that the user is free to select a **level of confidence**, c% (usually 90%, 95%, or 99%). The c% CI for μ procedure produces an interval estimate for μ from each random sample; of all these interval estimates, c% actually contain μ. Hence, constructing a 95% CI for μ from a random sample is like playing a 95% lottery. You randomly draw an interval from the CI barrel in which you know that 95% of the intervals actually contain μ; the other 5% do not contain μ. The 95% is a measure of the confidence you can put in a CI obtained from a random sample; the flip side, 5%, is the risk you take inherent with random sampling. Whether your CI is good (actually contains μ) or bad (does not contain μ) is merely the luck of the draw inherent with random sampling.

Summarizing, the c% CI for μ procedure has the following characteristics:

- For each random sample that can be drawn from the population, the procedure constructs an interval estimate for μ.
- c% of all these interval estimates actually contain μ.
- $(100 - c)$% of these interval estimates do not contain μ.

We will be able to construct a CI for μ within a statistical design that incorporates a continuous RV X, a large population, and a random sample of size n, where either:

1. X has a normal distribution; or
2. The sample size is large ($n > 30$).

Confidence Interval for the Mean Algorithm

The algorithm for constructing a c% confidence interval for the confidence interval for the mean is displayed in Figure 7.1.1. A CI for the mean is appropriate whenever (1) the RV of interest is (approximately) normal or (2) the sample size is large (> 30).

FIGURE *7.1.1* Method | STEPS
Algorithm for constructing a CI for the mean (n = sample size; $\bar{x}$ = sample mean; s = sample standard deviation).

STEP	NORMAL DISTRIBUTION NSCORES	LARGE SAMPLE SIZE ($n > 30$)
1. Sample Legend	n, $\bar{x}$, s standard deviation	n, $\bar{x}$, s
2. Critical Value	t (Appendix, Table 6) $df = n - 1$	z (Appendix, Table 7)
3. Endpoints	$L = \bar{x} - ts/\sqrt{n}$ $R = \bar{x} + ts/\sqrt{n}$	$L = \bar{x} - zs/\sqrt{n}$ $R = \bar{x} + zs/\sqrt{n}$
4. Conclusion	A c% CI for μ is (L, R).	An approximate c% CI for μ is (L, R).

$\bar{x}$ - sample mean

Comment Report the CI to the same level of precision as the given data. When rounding the answers in step 3 to report the CI in step 4, round down to obtain the left endpoint L and round up to obtain the right endpoint R. Such rounding will ensure that the stated level of confidence has been maintained.

In the four-step algorithm in Figure 7.1.1, step 1 displays the sample legend that contains the sample's contribution toward the construction of the CI. Step 2 contains a critical value that is obtained from a table. This critical value is a *stretch factor* that acts to control how wide the interval needs to be in order to ensure the degree of reliability specified by the level of confidence.

The algorithm in Figure 7.1.1 describes a procedure for transforming a sample into a CI for the mean. In particular, note that the *sample* mean is always at the center of the CI. When the RV of interest is normally distributed, the radius of the CI is $ts/\sqrt{n}$. Hence, to construct a CI for μ, start at the center $\bar{x}$ and then jump a distance $ts/\sqrt{n}$ to the left and right to obtain the left and right endpoints of the CI (Figure 7.1.2). Such a CI for μ interval is called a **t-interval**. When using the large sample size directions, the only change is that the critical value t is replaced by z. Accordingly, the resulting CI for μ is called a **z-interval**.

The t-interval algorithm is valid only for continuous RVs having a normal distribution. Hence, it is important to check the assumption of normality prior to applying this algorithm. If one has the raw data, apply Minitab's nscores correlation test for normality (Section 6.2). If one is supplied only with the sample legend and not the raw data, one should state explicitly that a normal distribution is assumed before invoking the t-interval algorithm.

The z-interval algorithm is valid for any continuous RV, normal or not. The only requirement is that the sample size is sufficiently large (>30).

FIGURE *7.1.2*
The general form for a t-CI for μ.

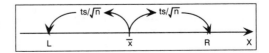

If one needs a CI based on a small sample that is inconsistent with an assumption of normality, then use Minitab to construct an s-interval (Section 8.1) for the population median. A flowchart for the general procedure to be followed in constructing a CI for an appropriate average value for a continuous RV is provided in Figure 7.1.3.

EXAMPLE 7.1.2 Henneman studied the effect of a music therapy program on patients with assumed myocardial infarction (MI). One RV of interest was a patient's peripheral temperature. Mean peripheral temperature of the 26 patients randomly assigned to the music therapy group was 87.80°F with a standard deviation of 5.79°F. Since the raw data were not provided, we assume that peripheral temperature is normally distributed in the population of interest. We now illustrate the four-step algorithm presented in Figure 7.1.1 by constructing 80%, 90%, and 95% CIs for the mean peripheral temperature of a patient with assumed MI upon the start of a music therapy program.

a. Construct an 80% CI for μ.
Step 1. $n = 26$, $\bar{x} = 87.80$, $s = 5.79$
Step 2. $t = 1.31636$ (Table 6, $df = n - 1 = 25$)
Step 3. $\bar{x} - ts/\sqrt{n} = 87.80 - (1.31636)(5.79)/\sqrt{26}$
$= 87.80 - 1.495 = 86.305$
$\bar{x} + ts/\sqrt{n} = 87.80 + (1.31636)(5.79)/\sqrt{26}$
$= 87.80 + 1.495 = 89.295$

FIGURE **7.1.3**
CI for an appropriate average value.

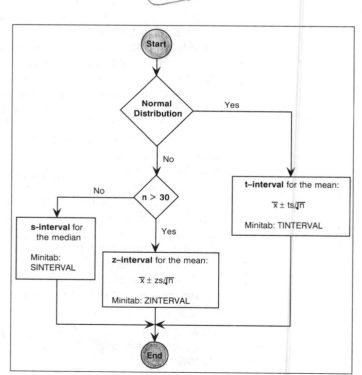

Step 4. Based on the given data, an 80% CI for the mean peripheral temperature of patients with presumed MI entering a music therapy program is (86.30, 89.30) degrees Fahrenheit.

b. Construct a 90% CI for μ.

Step 1. $n = 26, \bar{x} = 87.80, s = 5.79$

Step 2. $t = 1.70813$ (Table 6, $df = n - 1 = 25$)

Step 3. $\bar{x} \pm ts/\sqrt{n} = 87.80 \pm (1.70813)(5.79)/\sqrt{26}$
$$= 87.80 \pm 1.94$$
$$= 85.86, 89.74$$

Step 4. Based on the given data, a 90% CI for the mean peripheral temperature of patients with presumed MI entering a music therapy program is (85.86, 89.74) degrees Fahrenheit.

c. Construct a 95% CI for μ.

Step 1. $n = 26, \bar{x} = 87.80, s = 5.79$

Step 2. $t = 2.0595$ (Table 6, $df = n - 1 = 25$)

Step 3. $\bar{x} \pm ts/\sqrt{n} = 87.80 \pm (2.0595)(5.79)/\sqrt{26}$
$$= 87.80 \pm 2.339$$
$$= 85.461, 90.139$$

Step 4. Based on the given data, a 95% CI for the mean peripheral temperature of patients with presumed MI entering a music therapy program is (85.46, 90.14) degrees Fahrenheit.

These three CIs are displayed in Figure 7.1.4. Notice that the greater the confidence, the wider the CI, thus increasing the chance that a sample's CI may successfully capture the population mean.

Comment The quantity c% represents the "confidence" we can place in the CI generated by a random sample. Among all the random samples that could be drawn, c% of the associated CIs contain μ. While c% denotes our *confidence* in this procedure, the quantity $\alpha = 100 - c$ (percent) represents the *risk*; that is, α% of all the CIs generated by all possible random samples do not contain μ.

Comment When the RV of interest is normally distributed, step 2 of the CI algorithm directs one to obtain a t-value from a t-table for CIs (Appendix, Table 6). Alternatively, this t-value may be obtained by Minitab. Let c% be the level of confidence and *df* the degrees of freedom. Then, in general,

```
MTB > LET K1 = (1 + c/100)/2
MTB > INVCDF K1;
SUBC> T df.
```

FIGURE **7.1.4**
CIs for the Henneman data set, Example 7.1.2.

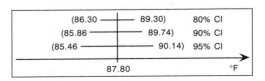

The t-values for the 80%, 90%, and 95% CIs we constructed for the Henneman example are obtained in Minitab as follows (recall, $df = 25$).

a. $c = 80\%$.
```
MTB > LET K1 = (1 + 80/100)/2
MTB > INVCDF K1;
SUBC> T 25.
    0.9000    1.3164
```
between 80% and 100%

b. $c = 90\%$.
```
MTB > LET K1 = (1 + 90/100)/2
MTB > INVCDF K1;
SUBC> T 25.
    0.9500    1.7081
```
Between 90% and 100%

c. $c = 95\%$.
```
MTB > LET K1 = (1 + 95/100)/2
MTB > INVCDF K1;
SUBC> T 25.
    0.9750    2.0595
```
Between 95% and 100%

EXAMPLE 7.1.3 We construct a 95% CI for the mean room-temperature cardiac output of critical care cardiac patients as reported in a study by Shellock and Riedinger. Shellock and Riedinger did not supply the raw data in their article. They reported that room-temperature cardiac output was 4.75 ± 2.35 (mean $\pm$ SD) liters/minute for their study of 45 critical care cardiac patients. Since the raw data are not given, we assume that room-temperature cardiac output is normally distributed in the population of critical care cardiac patients.

Step 1. $n = 45$, $\bar{x} = 4.75$, $s = 2.35$
Step 2. $t = 2.0211$ (Table 6, using $df = 40$)
Step 3. $\bar{x} \pm ts/\sqrt{n} = 4.75 \pm (2.0211)(2.35)/\sqrt{45}$
$\qquad\qquad\qquad = 4.75 \pm 0.71$
$\qquad\qquad\qquad = 4.04, 5.46$

Step 4. Based on the given study, an at least 95% CI for the mean room-temperature cardiac output of critically ill cardiac patients is (4.04, 5.46) liters/minute.

Comment Note that the sample size is $n = 45$. Table 6 does not have an entry for $df = 44$. Since $df = 44$ is between the adjacent Table 6 entries of $df = 40$ and $df = 60$, we take the *smaller df* and use $df = 40$. When we use a table t-value corresponding to a lower-level df than we are entitled to, the actual level of confidence has been slightly raised. Accordingly, we announce an *at least* 95% CI for the mean.

Comment A slightly sharper result may be obtained by using a more accurate t-value in step 2, rather than the crude method we applied and discussed in the previous comment. For the Shellock and Riedinger Example 7.1.3, we inquire, what is the t-value corresponding to $df = 44$? This t-value can be estimated by linear interpolation applied to Table 6, obtaining $t = 2.0157$. Using $t = 2.0157$ in step 3 yields the CI 4.75 ± 0.706. At the level of precision of the data, we still report the 95% CI as (4.04,5.46). Hence, in this example, no precision has been lost using our cruder approach.

The ultimate in precision can be achieved by obtaining the exact t-value from Minitab:

```
MTB > LET K1 = (1 + 95/100)/2
MTB > INVCDF K1;
SUBC> T 44.
    0.9750    2.0154
```

Minitab informs that t ($df = 44$) = 2.0154. Using t = 2.0154 in step 3 yields the CI 4.75 ± 0.706. Again, nothing has been lost at the level of precision of the given data with our cruder approach to the t-value in step 2.

In the event that a researcher did not want to invoke an assumption of normality for the distribution of room-temperature cardiac outputs, the above t-interval construction is not valid. However, when the sample size is large ($n > 30$), we may construct a z-interval.

EXAMPLE 7.1.4 We construct an approximate 95% CI for the mean room-temperature cardiac output of critically ill cardiac patients based on the Shellock and Riedinger data (Example 7.1.3) as follows:

Step 1. $n = 45, \bar{x} = 4.75, s = 2.35$
Step 2. $z = 1.960$ (Table 7)
Step 3. $\bar{x} \pm zs/\sqrt{n} = 4.75 \pm (1.960)(2.35)/\sqrt{45}$
$= 4.06, 5.44$
Step 4. Based on the given study, an approximate 95% CI for the mean room-temperature cardiac output of critically ill cardiac patients is (4.06,5.44) liters/minute.

Comment As with t-intervals, the z-value requested in step 2 may be obtained by Minitab. In general, suppose c% is the desired level of confidence. Then,

```
MTB > LET K1 = (1 + c/100)/2
MTB > INVCDF K1;
SUBC> NORMAL 0 1.
```

For example, the z-value for 95% confidence is obtained by

```
MTB > LET K1 = (1 + 95/100)/2
MTB > INVCDF K1;
SUBC> NORMAL  0  1.
    0.9750    1.9600
```

Confidence Intervals for the Mean with Minitab

When we have the sample raw data, we will have a much easier time with CIs since we will be able to leave the computing to Minitab. However, frequently one's source of data in the health sciences is the literature. Journal articles and texts seldom display the raw sample data but usually display some compact summary of the data. The most common presentation is "mean ± SD." When one does not have the raw data, one must either explicitly assume a normal distribution or, in the event of a large sample size, waive the assumption of a normal distribution and be satisfied with an approximate CI.

We now display how to proceed using Minitab when supplied with the raw sample data. First, SET the data into a column in Minitab's spreadsheet. Then, apply the nscores and correlation test for consistency with normality. If the sample data are consistent with normality, then use the TINTERVAL command to construct the t-CI. If the sample is inconsistent with normality and the sample size is large ($n > 30$), then use the ZINTERVAL command to construct the approximate z-CI. An example of each case follows.

EXAMPLE 7.1.5 We construct 80%, 90%, 95%, and 99% CIs for the mean room-temperature cardiac output data obtained by Daily and Mersch. The Minitab output is displayed in Figure 7.1.5. We have noted previously that the room-temperature cardiac output data are consistent with normality (Example 6.2.1). Hence we are justified in constructing CIs using the t-interval algorithm. The appropriate CIs are displayed in Table 7.1.3.

Notice again that increasing the level of confidence increases the width of the CI.

EXAMPLE 7.1.6 Barcelona et al studied cardiac output determination by the thermodilution method comparing ice-temperature injectate with room-temperature injectate

FIGURE **7.1.5**
Minitab output for CIs for the Daily and Mersch cardiac output data.

```
MTB > OW 65        # set output width to 65 characters
MTB > PRINT C1

RTCO
   2.60   5.16   6.18   3.22   4.99   3.62   3.31   4.11   5.24
   4.27   3.42   4.70   5.42   5.36   2.63   3.70   5.39   5.44
   3.86   6.68   5.35   3.26   4.06   2.64   5.40   5.93   5.90
   4.11   4.44

MTB > NOTE    Check for normal distribution:
MTB >
MTB > NAME C41 'NSRTCO'
MTB > NSCORES C1 INTO C41
MTB > CORRELATION C1 AND C41

Correlation of RTCO and NSRTCO = 0.984

MTB >
MTB > NOTE    The 80, 90, 95, and 99 percent CIs:
MTB >
MTB > TINTERVAL 80 C1

              N       MEAN    STDEV   SE MEAN    80.0 PERCENT C.I.
RTCO         29      4.496    1.139    0.212   (   4.219,    4.774)

MTB > TINTERVAL 90 C1

              N       MEAN    STDEV   SE MEAN    90.0 PERCENT C.I.
RTCO         29      4.496    1.139    0.212   (   4.136,    4.856)

MTB > TINTERVAL 95 C1

              N       MEAN    STDEV   SE MEAN    95.0 PERCENT C.I.
RTCO         29      4.496    1.139    0.212   (   4.063,    4.930)

MTB > TINTERVAL 99 C1

              N       MEAN    STDEV   SE MEAN    99.0 PERCENT C.I.
RTCO         29      4.496    1.139    0.212   (   3.912,    5.081)
```

CI = confidence intervals

	Level of Confidence		CI for mean room temp CO
	80		(4.21, 4.78)
	90		(4.13, 4.86)
	95		(4.06, 4.93)
	99		(3.91, 5.09)

TABLE **7.1.3**
Confidence intervals for the Daily and Mersch room-temperature cardiac output (CO) data set.

contained in prefilled syringes or a closed injectate delivery system (Appendix, Data Set 2). We determine a 95% CI for the mean cardiac output using iced injectates in the prefilled syringe portion of the study (first iced injectate column in the data set). Since we have the raw sample data, we carry out the needed computations in Minitab (Figure 7.1.6).

The preliminary check for normality shows that the data are inconsistent with an assumption of a normal distribution (Minitab nscores correlation 0.946, critical value 0.9597). Since the sample size is large ($n = 41 > 30$), we construct a z-interval that displays an approximate 95% CI for the mean cardiac output. Finally, we report that, based on the Barcelona et al study, an approximate 95% CI for the mean cardiac output of critically ill cardiac patients determined by using an ice-temperature injectate is (3.5, 4.3) liters/minute.

FIGURE **7.1.6**
Minitab output for CIs for the Barcelona et al ice-temperature injectates, prefilled syringes.

```
MTB > OW 65    # set output width to 65 characters
MTB > PRINT C1

Iced PFS
    3.8    3.8    3.2    3.5    4.0    3.8    4.0    3.9    3.1
    3.8    3.4    3.8    3.4    3.3    3.7    3.5    3.5    3.2
    3.4    3.5    4.5    4.6    4.2    5.0    5.3    4.7    4.8
    2.8    2.2    2.7    6.2    6.7    7.2    5.7    3.0    3.7
    3.4    2.4    2.9    2.7    3.8

MTB > NOTE      Check for Normal Distribution
MTB >
MTB > NAME C41 'NS Iced'
MTB > NSCORES C1 INTO C41
MTB > CORRELATION C1 AND C41

Correlation of Iced PFS and NS Iced = 0.946

MTB >
MTB > NOTE      Obtain and retain the standard deviation
MTB > LET K1 = STDEV (C1)
MTB >
MTB > NOTE      Obtain 95% and 90% z confidence intervals
MTB > ZINTERVAL 95 K1 C1

THE ASSUMED SIGMA = 1.09

                N    MEAN   STDEV  SE MEAN   95.0 PERCENT C.I.
Iced PFS       41   3.905   1.091   0.170  (   3.570,    4.239)

MTB > ZINTERVAL 90 K1 C1

THE ASSUMED SIGMA = 1.09

                N    MEAN   STDEV  SE MEAN   90.0 PERCENT C.I.
Iced PFS       41   3.905   1.091   0.170  (   3.624,    4.186)
```

(ICED + ROOM) *Below 40 readings on tables not normal

Background for Warm-ups 1–6. Stone et al studied the effect of lung hyperinflation and endotracheal suctioning on heart rate and rhythm in patients after coronary artery bypass graft (CABG) surgery. Baseline data for 26 patients 4 hours after CABG surgery were reported. Baseline heart rate (beats/minute) for these 26 patients was given as 93.0 ± 18.0 (mean ± SD). We determine a 95% confidence interval (CI) for the mean baseline heart rate of CABG surgery patients.

1. For samples of size $n \leq 30$, in order to construct a CI for the mean (μ), we need to assume that the distribution of the RV of interest is (approximately) normally distributed. In this illustration, the RV of interest is "heart rate 4 hours after CABG surgery." Hence, before proceeding to construct a CI for the mean baseline heart rate 4 hours after CABG surgery, we should explicitly state what assumption?

We now follow the four-step protocol for the construction of a 95% confidence t-interval for the mean (μ) baseline heart rate 4 hours after CABG surgery.

2. Step 1. The sample legend consists of the sample size (n), the sample mean ($\bar{x}$), and the sample standard deviation (s). Here,

$n =$ _____ $\bar{x} =$ _____ $s =$ _____

3. Step 2. Obtain t from Table 6: $df = n - 1 =$ _____
$t =$ _____

4. Step 3. Determine the left endpoint of the CI:

$L = \bar{x} - ts/\sqrt{n}$
$= (93.0) - (2.0595)(18.0)/\sqrt{26}$
$= 93.0 - 7.3$
$=$ _____

5. Step 3 continued. Determine the right endpoint of the CI:

$R = \bar{x} + ts/\sqrt{n}$
$=$ _____ $+ ($ ___ $)($ ___ $)/\sqrt{\text{___}}$
$=$ _____ $+$ _____
$=$ _____

6. Step 4. The conclusion should be stated as a full English sentence as follows. Based on the given data from Stone et al, a 95% CI for the mean baseline heart rate 4 hours after CABG surgery is 93.0 ± 7.3 beats per minute; that is, (85.7, ___) beats per minute.

7. The statement that "(85.7,100.3) is a 95% CI for μ (mean baseline heart rate)" means that
   a. Ninety-five percent of the time, μ is in the interval (85.7, 100.3).
   b. There is a 95% chance that μ is in (85.7, 100.3).
   c. The interval (85.7, 100.3) was constructed by a procedure that actually contains μ for 95% of all possible samples.
   d. Ninety-five percent of all the population means are in (85.7, 100.3).
   e. All of the above.

The following background applies to Warm-ups 8–14. Phibbs et al were interested in the study and treatment of hyaline membrane disease in neonates. In the reported rescue study, neonates were randomized into one of two groups, treated and control. The birth weight of 51 hyaline membrane disease neonates in the control group was 1332 ± 598 grams (mean ± SD).

First, we assume that birth weight in neonates presenting hyaline membrane disease is (approximately) normally distributed. Accordingly, we construct a 95% confidence t-interval for the mean birth weight based on the control data set. Warm-ups 8–11 present the details for constructing the t-interval.

8. Step 1. The sample legend is:

$n =$ _____ $\bar{x} =$ _____ $s =$ _____

9. Step 2. Obtain t from Table 6. $df = n - 1 =$ _____
$t =$ _____

10. Step 3. $L = \bar{x} - ts/\sqrt{n}$
$= 1332 - (2.0085)(598)/\sqrt{51}$
$=$ _____ $-$ _____
$=$ _____
$R = \bar{x} + ts/\sqrt{n}$
$=$ _____ $+ ($ ___ $)($ ___ $)/\sqrt{\text{___}}$
$=$ _____ $+$ _____
$=$ _____

11. Step 4. Based on the given control data set, a 95% CI for the mean birth weights of hyaline membrane neonates is (____, ____) grams.

Since the sample size is large ($n > 30$), we may construct an approximate 95% CI using the z-interval approach. In the z-interval construction, step 1 is the same as for the t-interval; that is, present the sample legend. In Warmups 12–14, we complete the construction of the z-interval.

12. Step 2. From Table 7, the z-value for 95% confidence is ____.

13. Step 3. $L = \bar{x} - zs/\sqrt{n}$
$$= \underline{\quad} - (\underline{\quad})(\underline{\quad})/\sqrt{\underline{\quad}}$$
$$= \underline{\quad} - \underline{\quad}$$
$$= \underline{\quad}$$
$R = \bar{x} + zs/\sqrt{n}$
$$= \underline{\quad} + (\underline{\quad})(\underline{\quad})/\sqrt{\underline{\quad}}$$
$$= \underline{\quad} + \underline{\quad}$$
$$= \underline{\quad}$$

14. Step 4. Hence, based on the control sample data set, an approximate 95% CI for the mean birth weight of hyaline membrane neonates is (____, ____).

Problems 7.1

1. Distinguish between a sample mean and a population mean.

2. Distinguish between a point estimate for μ and an interval estimate for μ.

3. Explain the phrase "95% CI for the mean."

4. Consider the Bridges et al data for Hb for females in Example 7.1.1, Table 7.1.1.

   a. Is the data set consistent with the assumption that Hb in females is (approximately) normally distributed?

   b. If valid, construct 90%, 95%, and 99% CIs for the mean Hb for females.

   c. What is the effect of increasing the level of confidence in (b)?

5. Consider the Bridges et al data for Hb for males in Example 7.1.1, Table 7.1.1.

   a. Is the data set consistent with the assumption that Hb in males is (approximately) normally distributed?

   b. If valid, construct 90%, 95%, and 99% CIs for the mean Hb for males.

   c. What is the effect of increasing the level of confidence in (b)?

6. The hematocrits of eight cardiac patients in a research study (see Problem 1.2.1) were:

   39.2 36.4 38.3 36.8 42.9 37.0 39.1 41.2

   Determine (a) 90%, (b) 95%, and (c) 99% CIs for the mean hematocrit of cardiac patients.

7. See Problem 1.2.6. The sample size is $n = 8$.

   a. Construct a 95% CI at each time for the V_T hyperinflation volume group.

   b. Construct a time series graph that portrays the 95% CIs for the mean, rather than mean ± SD intervals as displayed in Figure 1.2.7. Contrast and compare the two graphs.

   c. Repeat (a) and (b) for another hyperinflation volume.

8. Chulay reported the following data for a study of $n = 32$ patients (Table 7.1.4). All patients were male, aged 35–70, and scheduled for elective coronary artery bypass graft surgery.

TABLE **7.1.4** Data adapted from Chulay.

	Mean	SEM
PaO_2/PAO_2 ratio	0.48	0.03
Cardiac index	2.9	0.11
Ventilator settings		
Tidal volume (mL)	962	17.2
Rate (breaths/min)	10.6	0.17
FIO_2	0.52	0.01
PEEP (cm H_2O)	2.7	0.45

$SEM = SD/\sqrt{n}$.

   a. Determine a 90% CI for (i) the PaO_2/PAO_2 ratio, (ii) cardiac index, (iii) tidal volume, (iv) breathing rate, (v) FIO_2, and (vi) PEEP.

   b. What is the difference between a 90% CI for μ and the interval mean ± SD?

9. Chulay (see Problem 8) also presented the time series data on PaO_2 (mm Hg) for the 32 patients in the study (Table 7.1.5). Values are given as mean ± SEM (SEM = $SD/\sqrt{n}$). The suctioning episode began at time 0 and lasted for 2 minutes.

TABLE **7.1.5** Pao$_2$ data from Chulay.

Time (minutes)				
0	1	2	3	4
156 (9.01)	230 (2.3)	251 (13.7)	181 (9.7)	170 (9.0)

a. Determine a 95% CI for the mean Pao$_2$ at each time.

b. Construct a time series plot that displays the mean Pao$_2$ and the associated 95% CI at each time.

10. Consider the Bodai et al study of a clinical evaluation of an oxygen insufflation/suction catheter. The routine suctioning (control) data were examined in Section 1.2 (also see Appendix, Data Set 4, Group 2, routine suctioning [control]).

a. Determine a 95% CI for each of the given times: start, end, 1 minute, and 5 minutes.

b. Construct a plot of Pao$_2$ level versus time. At each of the four study times, plot the mean Pao$_2$ and the 95% CI rather than mean $\pm$ SD as done in Section 1.2. Describe the difference between these two graphs.

11. Mauro studied the effects of using the bell versus the diaphragm of the stethoscope on an indirect blood pressure measurement. Table 7.1.6 presents data adapted from her study of $n = 55$ patients.

TABLE **7.1.6** Data adapted from Mauro.

	Reading	Mean	SD
S1	Bell	113.82	11.16
	Diaphragm	112.29	11.75
D4	Bell	73.96	9.44
	Diaphragm	74.50	7.70
D5	Bell	64.82	9.43
	Diaphragm	66.43	8.05

S1 = systolic; D4 = fourth-phase diastolic; D5 = fifth-phase diastolic.

a. Determine a 95% CI for mean systolic (S1) blood pressure using (i) the bell and (ii) the diaphragm of the stethoscope.

b. Repeat (a) for the fourth-phase diastolic (D4).

c. Repeat (a) for the fifth-phase diastolic (D5).

12. Shellock and Riedinger reported that the ice-temperature cardiac output for the 45 patients in their study was 4.78 ± 2.11 (mean $\pm$ SD).

a. Assuming that the ice-temperature cardiac outputs are normally distributed, construct a 95% t-interval for the mean ice-temperature cardiac output of critically ill cardiac patients.

b. Construct a 95% z-interval for the mean ice-temperature cardiac output of critically ill cardiac patients.

c. Contrast and compare the two CIs.

13. Rice et al reported on the results of a patient education program. They evaluated the results of the education program by administering a mood adjective checklist (MACL). Their statistical design contained two groups: an experimental group and a control group. They reported the MACL scores for the two groups as shown in Table 7.1.7.

TABLE **7.1.7** Data adapted from Rice et al.

	Experimental Group	Control Group
Size	20	20
Mean	35.0	44.2
SD	15.0	14.4

Determine a 90% CI for the mean MACL score of both the experimental group and the control group. Do the intervals overlap? What do you think: Is there a significant difference in the MACL scores between the two groups?

14. Burek et al reported on the peak heart rate from an exercise thallium treadmill (ETT) test for two groups (Table 7.1.8): positive ETT group and negative ETT group. The positive group had a positive ETT for ischemia.

TABLE **7.1.8** Data adapted from Burek et al.

	Positive ETT Group	Negative ETT Group
Size	36	90
Mean	120.9	130.2
SD	21.4	14.4

Determine a 95% CI for the mean peak heart rate for both the positive ETT group and the negative ETT group. On the basis of your CIs, is the mean peak heart rate for one group different from the mean peak heart rate of the other group? Explain.

15. Consider the Bodai et al catheter study for group 3, standard suction with valve adapter (control) data set (Appendix, Data Set 4).

   a. Determine the sample legend displaying the sample size, mean, and standard deviation for start, end, 1 minute, and 5 minutes.

b. Construct a 95% CI for the mean Pa_{O_2} for each of the four times.

c. Construct a time series graph that displays the 95% CI for the mean Pa_{O_2} at each time.

16. Determine a 95% CI for mean aortic diameter among patients with type A dissection based on the data by Sütsch et al presented in Problem 2.1.12. Justify your choice of confidence interval (t- or z-interval).

SECTION 7.2	**OBJECTIVES** This section will
Paired Data	**1** Describe two classic paired-data situations in the health sciences.
	2 Determine a c% confidence interval for the mean of differences when given a random sample of paired data.

There are many ways that one can design a statistical study. One of the most common and most important designs in the health sciences is the paired-data design.

Classic Paired-Data Designs

There are two classic situations in the health sciences where one is interested in paired data:

1. Before and after, and
2. Method A versus method B.

The **before and after** case applies when one wants to study the effectiveness of an intervention therapy. One measures a given RV X at the start of an intervention, then again at the end of the intervention. A corresponding RV of interest is the change in X during the time of intervention. The change is measured by computing the **difference**, D:

$$D = \text{before} - \text{after}$$

Such a difference is of interest in a health program aimed at weight loss, lowering serum cholesterol, reduction of fever, or increasing physical endurance. Note that in an effectiveness study, each subject in the study yields a pair of measurements (before, after). The researcher then converts each pair into a difference. The data set of differences is analyzed as in Section 7.1.

   The **method A versus method B** situation applies when one wants to compare two different methods for obtaining the same measurement. For example:

1. Do the left and right arm yield the same blood pressure readings?

2. In taking a blood pressure with a sphygmomanometer and stethoscope, do the bell and diaphragm of the stethoscope yield the same results?
3. Are rectal and oral temperatures the same?
4. Is reduction of fever over a 1-hour period the same for aspirin as it is for Tylenol?
5. Do a room-temperature and an ice-temperature injectate yield the same cardiac outputs?

One compares two methods by determining whether there is any difference, D, between them. In a comparison study, each subject yields a pair of measurements (method A, method B). The researcher converts each pair into a difference. The data set of differences is analyzed as in Section 7.1.

In these paired-difference studies, it is important that one computes the difference for each patient individually. An appropriate CI is then calculated from these differences.

A before and after study is used to determine effectiveness, if any, of a therapeutic intervention. One starts with a random sample of patients and measures an RV X of interest. Then apply a treatment and measure X again. Thus each patient has a *before*-treatment and an *after*-treatment measurement of X; that is, each patient has a difference: D = before − after. Now the researcher determines an appropriate CI for the mean difference, μ_D. If zero belongs to the CI, then the data from the sample indicate that the treatment has no effect. If the CI lies to the right of zero (i.e., both endpoints are positive), then one has evidence to believe that the treatment is effective in lowering X. If the CI lies to the left of zero (i.e., both endpoints are negative), then one has evidence to believe that the treatment is effective in raising X.

A method A versus method B study is used to determine the difference, if any, between two competing methods. One starts with a continuous RV X of interest and a random sample. One measures the RV X on each subject in the sample by applying both method A and method B. If the two methods cannot be applied simultaneously, then a random procedure should be used to decide which method to apply first. For example, flip a coin. If it is heads, apply method A first; if tails, apply method B first. Thus each subject has a *method A* and a *method B* measurement of X; that is, each patient has a difference: D = method A − method B. Now the researcher determines an appropriate CI for the mean difference, μ_D. If zero belongs to the CI, then the data from the sample indicate that there is no difference between the two methods. If the CI lies to the right of zero (i.e., both endpoints are positive), then one has evidence that on average method A yields a higher reading. If the CI lies to the left of zero (i.e., both endpoints are negative), then one has evidence that on average method B yields a higher reading.

Paired-Data Confidence Intervals

A CI for the mean difference is computed using the techniques of Section 7.1. If the set of differences is consistent with normality, then a c% CI for the mean difference is computed by:

$$(\bar{d} - ts/\sqrt{n}, \bar{d} + ts/\sqrt{n})$$

Where $\bar{d}$ = sample mean difference,

s = sample standard deviation of the differences,

n = sample size (number of data pairs), and

t = confidence interval t-value obtained from Table 6 with $df = n - 1$.

If the set of differences is not consistent with normality, but the sample size is large ($n > 30$), then one replaces t by z (Table 7) in the preceding procedure to obtain an approximate c% CI for the mean difference.

EXAMPLE 7.2.1 The Daily and Mersch cardiac output study is a classic method A versus method B study. In particular, the research hypothesis is that cardiac output determined by using a room-temperature injectate is not significantly different than cardiac output determined by using an ice-temperature injectate. Cardiac output for each patient was determined using both methods. We first determine the difference for each patient. We then test for normality for the set of differences (the set of differences is consistent with normality). With these preliminaries completed, we determine a 95% CI for the mean of the differences. Here, D = room − ice. Since we have the raw data, we invoke Minitab for the computations (Figure 7.2.1).

A 95% CI for the mean of room − ice temperature cardiac output is (-0.18, 0.16). Based on the given sample, with 95% confidence the mean difference is not statistically significantly different from zero. Clinically, based on this study, on average there is no statistically significant difference in the cardiac outputs obtained by the two methods.

EXAMPLE 7.2.2 The Bodai et al evaluation of an oxygen insufflation suction catheter (see Appendix, Data Set 4) utilizes a typical before and after study. Let us define the difference D by D = before − after. The data for the six patients in group III control are shown in Table 7.2.1.

*TABLE **7.2.1***
Data adapted from Bodai et al.

− 1 Minute (Before)	0 Minute (After)	Difference
74	60	14
65	62	3
85	80	5
72	73	− 1
91	83	8
92	86	6

Since we have the raw data, we again invoke Minitab for the computations (Figure 7.2.2). Before constructing a 95% CI for D, we must check D for normality. Minitab's nscores correlation for D is 0.982 (critical value 0.8320); hence, the sample D is consistent with normality. Assuming now that D is normally distributed, we obtain a 95% t-CI for D.

A 95% CI for the mean difference in Pao_2 for the group III control is (0.5, 11.2). The study gives evidence of a statistically identifiable drop in Pao_2 as a result of

FIGURE *7.2.1*
Paired-difference CI for the Daily and Mersch cardiac output data set comparing room- with ice-temperature cardiac outputs. The room-temperature cardiac outputs are in column C1, ice-temperature cardiac outputs are in column C2.

```
MTB > NAME C3 'DIFF R-I'
MTB > LET C3 = C1 - C2
MTB > PRINT C1 - C3

 ROW   RTCO   ITCO   DIFF R-I

  1    2.60   3.02   -0.42000
  2    5.16   5.47   -0.31000
  3    6.18   5.72    0.46000
  4    3.22   4.22   -1.00000
  5    4.99   4.89    0.10000
  6    3.62   3.50    0.12000
  7    3.31   3.08    0.23000
  8    4.11   4.11    0.00000
  9    5.24   4.86    0.38000
 10    4.27   4.73   -0.46000
 11    3.42   3.78   -0.36000
 12    4.70   4.26    0.44000
 13    5.42   4.97    0.45000
 14    5.36   5.47   -0.11000
 15    2.63   2.62    0.01000
 16    3.70   3.87   -0.17000
 17    5.39   5.30    0.09000
 18    5.44   4.79    0.65000
 19    3.86   3.75    0.11000
 20    6.68   6.38    0.30000
 21    5.35   5.30    0.05000
 22    3.26   3.86   -0.60000
 23    4.06   4.28   -0.22000
 24    2.64   2.88   -0.24000
 25    5.40   5.63   -0.23000
 26    5.93   6.08   -0.15000
 27    5.90   6.15   -0.25000
 28    4.11   4.51   -0.40000
 29    4.44   3.26    1.18000

MTB > NOTE    Check for normality:
MTB > NAME C4 'NSDiff'
MTB > NSCORES C3 INTO C4
MTB > CORRELATION C3 AND C4

Correlation of DIFF R-I and NSDiff = 0.981

MTB > NOTE    Confidence Intervals:
MTB > TINTERVAL 95 C1 - C3
```

	N	MEAN	STDEV	SE MEAN	95.0 PERCENT C.I.
RTCO	29	4.496	1.139	0.212	(4.063, 4.930)
ITCO	29	4.508	1.043	0.194	(4.112, 4.905)
DIFF R-I	29	-0.0121	0.4298	0.0798	(-0.1756, 0.1514)

suction. The mean drop in PaO_2 during the suctioning period is at least 0.5 mm Hg, and may be as high as 11.2 mm Hg.

Comment The 95% CI for D in the previous example showed a *statistically significant* drop (on average) in PaO_2 from start to end of suctioning. This drop may or may not be *clinically* significant. Although a statistical analysis can detect a change in an RV, statistics do not determine whether the change is clinically important. In this particular study, a drop in PaO_2 of 20 mm Hg probably would be cause for clinical concern. The statistical problem of comparing the sample data against some clinically significant reference value is the major task of a Test of Hypothesis (introduced in Chapter 9).

FIGURE **7.2.2**
Minitab computations
for a 95% CI for the
mean difference in
Pao₂ for group III
control in the Bodai et
al study.

C 17
C 18

```
MTB > NOTE     Before = -1min (start of suctioning); column C1.
MTB > NOTE     After = 0min (end of suctioning); column C2
MTB >
MTB > NAME C3 'DIFF B-A'
MTB > LET C3 = C1 - C2
MTB > PRINT C1 - C3

 ROW  -1min   0min   DIV B-A

  1    74      60      14
  2    65      62       3
  3    85      80       5
  4    72      73      -1
  5    91      83       8
  6    92      86       6

MTB >
MTB > NOTE   Check differences for consistency with normal:
MTB >
MTB > NAME C4 'NSDiff'
MTB > NSCORES C3 INTO C4
MTB > CORRELATION C3 AND C4

Correlation of DIFF B-A and NSDiff = 0.982

MTB >
MTB > NOTE     95% Confidence Interval for the Difference:
MTB >
MTB > TINTERVAL 95 C1 - C3

              N     MEAN    STDEV   SE MEAN    95.0 PERCENT C.I.
-1min         6    79.83    11.09    4.53   (  68.19,   91.47)
0min          6    74.00    10.97    4.48   (  62.48,   85.52)
DIFF B-A      6     5.83     5.04    2.06   (   0.55,   11.12)
```

EXERCISES 7.2

Warm-ups
7.2

1. What are the two classic situations in the health
sciences that utilize a paired-data statistical design?

2. Paired-data statistical design means

   a. Each measurement is taken twice.

   b. Each measurement is done on two people.

   c. Two measurements are taken.

   d. Each member of the study group is measured
   twice.

3. Describe a before and after statistical design and
give an example.

4. Describe a method A versus method B statistical
design and give an example.

5. In a before and after study, one measures an RV at
two separate times: before and after an intervention. Let D = before − after. Match each inequality about D with the proper interpretation.

D		*Interpretation*
a. $D < 0$	***i.***	there is no change in the value of the RV.
b. $D = 0$	***ii.***	there is a drop in the value of the RV.
c. $D > 0$	***iii.***	there is a gain in the value of the RV.

6. In a method A versus method B study, one measures an RV using two different techniques. One
analyzes the data by computing the difference $D =$
method A − method B. Match the statement
about D with the appropriate interpretation.

D		*Interpretation*
a. $D < 0$	***i.***	Method A yields a higher measurement than method B.
b. $D = 0$	***ii.***	Method A yields a lower measurement than method B.
c. $D > 0$	***iii.***	The two methods yield the same measurement.

7. In a before and after paired-data study, the difference D = before − after was analyzed. A 95% CI for μ_D was (3.14, 9.62). On the basis of the CI, one may conclude with 95% confidence that, on average, there is

   a. A drop in the RV of interest

   b. An increase in the RV of interest

   c. No change in the RV of interest

8. For the CI in Warm-up 7, with 95% confidence

   a. $\mu_D = 0$

   b. $\mu_D > 0$

   c. $\mu_D < 0$

   d. $\mu_D = 6.38$

The following information applies to Warm-ups 9–12. Suppose a paired-data study on 20 subjects yields the sample data about the difference, D: the sample mean difference ($\bar{d}$) is 13.1, and the sample standard deviation of the differences (s) is 2.7.

9. What assumption must one state about D in order to construct a t-CI for μ_D?

10. Assuming that D is normally distributed, one may construct a t-interval for μ_D. For a 95% CI for μ_D, the appropriate value of t is ____.

11. The 95% CI for μ_D is computed by

$$\bar{d} \pm ts/\sqrt{n}$$

$$= \underline{13.1} \pm \underline{(2.903)}(\underline{2.7})/\sqrt{\underline{20}}$$

$$= \underline{13.1} \pm \underline{1.3}$$

12. The 95% CI obtained in Warm-up 11 is (____, ____).

Problems 7.2

1. See Problem 1.2.2. Construct (a) an 80%, (b) a 90%, (c) a 95%, and (d) a 99% CI for the mean temperature based on the given data.

2. See Problem 1.2.5. Construct a 95% CI for (a) first Pao_2, (b) second Pao_2, and (c) change.

3. Molyneaux et al studied the indwelling heparinized catheter (Appendix, Data Set 3). There are three tables of paired data.

   a. Are the paired data indicative of a before and after study or a method A versus method B study?

   b. Determine a 95% t-CI for the mean difference in each case where justified.

4. Consider the Daily and Mersch cardiac output (CO) study (Appendix, Data Set 1). The Fick CO was included in the statistical design as the "gold standard" for CO.

   a. Determine a 95% CI for RTCO − Fick.

   b. Determine a 95% CI for ITCO − Fick.

   c. What do you think: Does the mean RTCO or ITCO differ significantly from the mean Fick CO? What implications does this have for patient care?

5. Consider the Barcelona CO study (Appendix, Data Set 2).

   a. Determine a 95% t-CI (if justified) for the mean difference, D = iced − room, for
     i. The prefilled syringes group, and
     ii. The co-set group.

   b. Determine a 95% z-CI for the mean difference, D = iced − room, for
     i. The prefilled syringes group, and
     ii. The co-set group.

   c. Contrast and compare the t-CIs versus the z-CIs constructed in (a) and (b).

   d. What do you think; that is, what does it all mean for patient care?

6. Consider the Shively et al position change study (Appendix, Data Set 5).

   a. Determine a 95% CI for baseline for group 1.

   b. Determine a 95% CI for baseline for group 2.

   c. Based on the CIs obtained in parts (a) and (b), do the mean baseline $S\bar{v}o_2$ for the two groups appear to be significantly different (i.e., do the CIs overlap)?

   d. Determine a 95% CI for the difference RL0′ − RL1° for group 1. Is zero in the CI? Describe the significance of your answer.

   e. Repeat (d) for the difference RL0′ − RL2° for group 2.

Problems 7–11 are based on research reported in Bachorik et al. Subjects in the study were enrolled in a heart disease prevention program. Blood was drawn from each subject in the study. The blood sample was then split and analyzed for total cholesterol, triglycerides, and high- and low-density lipoprotein (HDL and LDL) cholesterol

using screening and standardized laboratory methods. All measurements were made in mmol/liter. The study utilized a set of 80 fasting and 74 nonfasting subjects. For each subject, the paired difference, D = screening − laboratory, value was determined. For Problems 7–11,

    a. Determine a 95% CI for the mean of the paired differences.

    b. Is this CI of the type $(+, +)$, $(−, −)$, or $(−, +)$? What conclusion can you draw about comparing the two methods (screening versus laboratory) in measuring the given RV?

7. Among the 80 fasting patients, the paired difference for total cholesterol was $−0.32 \pm 0.32$ (mean $\pm$ SD).

8. Among the 74 nonfasting subjects, the paired difference for total cholesterol was $−0.21 \pm 0.36$ (mean $\pm$ SD).

9. Among the 80 fasting subjects, the paired difference for serum triglycerides was reported as 0.14 ± 0.31.

10. Among the 80 fasting subjects, the paired difference for HDL cholesterol was $−0.18 \pm 0.26$.

11. Among 77 fasting subjects (3 samples were lost), the paired difference for LDL cholesterol was $−0.06 \pm 0.37$.

CHAPTER 7 OVERVIEW

Summary

This chapter is concerned with obtaining knowledge of the mean μ for a continuous RV of interest. One draws a random sample from the population, then utilizes the sample to provide information about the population mean μ. One uses the sample to calculate a **point estimate** and **interval estimate** for μ. The best point estimate for μ, based on the sample, is simply the sample mean. The best interval estimate is a **confidence interval (CI)**.

The most common level of confidence used in the health sciences is 95%. A 95% CI for μ is an interval estimate for μ. The interval actually contains μ for 95% of all possible samples. The other 5% of the samples do not contain μ. Whether a given sample yields a CI that contains μ or not merely depends on the luck of the draw. Any CI based on a sample is always at risk, but at least the risk is under the control of the investigator. However, there is a trade-off. The lower the risk, the wider the resulting CI for μ.

A CI for the population mean μ may be constructed whenever the RV of interest has a normal distribution or the sample size is large (greater than 30). When the RV has a normal distribution, one constructs a **t-interval** for μ. When the sample size is large, one may construct a **z-interval** for μ.

A CI always contains the sample mean. The sample mean is located in the middle of the CI. A CI is calculated by $\bar{x} \pm ts/\sqrt{n}$ for a t-interval and $\bar{x} \pm zs/\sqrt{n}$) for a z-interval. If one has the raw data set, one can easily check for **normality** by using Minitab's nscores correlation test. Minitab's

TINTERVAL and ZINTERVAL commands permit one to easily determine an appropriate CI for the mean.

A **paired-data** design is an important and common statistical design in the health sciences. The two classic situations calling for a paired-data design are (1) **before and after** and (2) **method A versus method B**. One applies a before and after design to study the effectiveness of an intervention. One commonly applies a method A versus method B design to compare two competing methods for performing a task.

In a paired-data study, one analyzes a sample by computing the **difference** for each pair of measurements. One can then obtain a CI for the mean of these differences. The CI is then compared with a reference of zero. If zero is in the CI, then the data do not show a statistically significant difference between the pairs. If the interval is positive or negative, then a statistically significant difference between the pairs has been detected.

Keywords

confidence
confidence interval
  t-interval
  z-interval
difference
endpoints
interval estimate
level of confidence
mean
normality

paired-data design
  before and after
  method A versus method B
point estimate
risk
sample legend
t-table
t-value
z-table
z-value

References

Bachorik P et al: Lipoprotein-cholesterol analysis during screening: Accuracy and reliability. *Ann Intern Med* 114, no. 9 (May 1991): 741.

Bridges N et al: Evaluation of a new system for hemoglobin measurement. *Am Clin Prod Rev* (April 1987): 22.

Burek K et al: Exercise capacity in patients 3 days after acute uncomplicated myocardial infarction. *Heart Lung* 18, no. 6 (November 1989): 575.

Chulay M: Arterial blood gas changes with a hyperinflation and hyperoxygenation suctioning intervention in critically ill patients. *Heart Lung* 17, no. 6 (November 1988): 654.

Henneman E: Effect of nursing contact on the stress response of patients being weaned from mechanical ventilation. *Heart Lung* 18, no. 5 (September 1989): 483.

Mauro A: Effects of bell versus diaphragm on indirect blood pressure measurement. *Heart Lung* 17, no. 5 (September 1988): 489.

Phibbs R et al: Initial clinical trial of EXOSURF. *Pediatrics* 88, no. 1 (July 1991): 1.

Rice V et al: Development and testing of an arteriography information intervention for stress reduction. *Heart Lung* 17, no. 1 (January 1988): 23.

Shellock F and Riedinger M: Reproducibility and accuracy of using room-temperature vs. ice-temperature injectate for thermodilution cardiac output determination. *Heart Lung* 12, no. 2 (March 1983): 175.

Stone K: Effect of lung hyperinflation and endotracheal suctioning on heart rate and rhythm in patients after coronary artery bypass graft surgery. *Heart Lung* 20, no. 5, pt. 1 (September 1991): 443.

Confidence Intervals II

In Chapter 7 we focused on finding a confidence interval (CI) for the mean. The mean is special in the health sciences because of the role of paired data. Determining the CI for the difference of paired data is especially useful in analyzing before and after studies and method A versus method B studies.

In this chapter we expand our concept of a CI to the median and the proportion. One needs the median to analyze a small ($n \leq 30$) nonnormal quantitative data set. One needs a proportion to analyze a categorical data set for a given attribute.

Accordingly, Section 8.1, focusing on the median, is a natural addition to Chapter 7. Section 8.2 focuses on the proportion. Analysis of the proportion is especially useful for some standard health sciences problems. A clinician wants to know whether a new intervention increases the proportion of those who are helped, or whether the proportion of those suffering certain side effects increases with the addition of steps to a given protocol. When one wants to deal with a fraction of the whole, an analysis of a proportion is called for. The proportion is also the vehicle applied in interpreting the results of opinion polls.

SECTION 8.1	**OBJECTIVE** This section will
Confidence Intervals for the Median	**1** Determine a c% confidence interval for the median by applying Minitab's SINTERVAL command to a given data set for a continuous random variable.

10/26/95

In Section 7.1 we determined a CI for the mean provided we were working with a continuous random variable (RV) where either (1) the distribution of the RV was normal or (2) the sample size was large ($n > 30$). When neither of these two conditions is met, we can still obtain a CI for an average value, provided we have the raw data. In this event, the appropriate average value is not the mean but the median.

In smaller data sets ($n \leq 30$) that are inconsistent with normality, one frequently is dealing with a nonsymmetrical distribution of data. Accordingly, the mean and median may differ substantially. The mean is heavily influenced by outliers. The median in such a case may be a preferred measure of central tendency.

The best point estimate for the population median is simply the sample median. In this section we concentrate on obtaining an interval estimate for the median.

S-Interval for the Median

An **s-interval** is a confidence interval for η, the population median. An s-interval can be constructed for any interval data set. There are no preliminary checks to conduct for an s-interval.

The theory behind the construction of an s-interval is the theory of coin flips. The main feature of the median for a continuous RV is that half the distribution lies below the median, half above. Suppose x is the measure of a randomly selected individual from the population. The probability that x is less than the median ($x < \eta$) is 50%. Note that $x < \eta$ is equivalent to $x - \eta < 0$. Hence,

$$P[X < \eta] = P[X - \eta < 0] = 0.5$$

When $x < \eta$ ($x - \eta < 0$), we say that the "sign of x" is negative with respect to the median. When $x > \eta$ ($x - \eta > 0$), the "sign of x" is positive with respect to the median. One constructs the CI for η on the basis of these "signs"; hence, the terminology of "sign interval," or s-interval for short.

This approach can be amazingly informative. Suppose one selects just three members at random from the population at large, then measures each member for some quantitative RV X. Then $\text{Prob}[X < \eta] = 1/2$. The probability that all three measurements are under the median is $(1/2)^3 = 1/8$. Similarly, the probability that all three measurements are above the median is also $1/8$. Hence, the probability that the three numbers are either all below or all above the median is $1/4$ ($1/8 + 1/8$). Hence, remarkably, there is a 75% probability that at least one of the numbers is below the median and at least one above. Accordingly, (minimum, maximum) is a 75% CI for the population median based on a random sample of just three people!

The "50-50" feature of coin flips is exploited by Minitab in constructing the sign CI (s-interval) for the median. In general, a sign CI for the median is obtained in Minitab by

1. SET data into column C
2. SINTERVAL conf C

where conf represents the desired level of confidence.

EXAMPLE 8.1.1 For illustration, we construct a 95% CI for the median for the Barcelona et al cardiac output data. In Example 7.1.6 we noted that the distribution of the sample data was inconsistent with normality, so we constructed a z-interval for μ, (3.5, 4.3). Our new analysis using Minitab is displayed in Figure 8.1.1. A 95% CI for the median is (3.4, 3.9) to the precision of the given data set. Since an exact 95% CI for the median η usually cannot be constructed, Minitab displays the next best interval above and below the requested 95% level. Here, a 94.04% CI for η is (3.4, 3.8) and a 97.25% CI for η is (3.4, 3.9). The 95% CI for the median,

(3.4, 3.9), is calculated from the 94.04% CI and 97.25% CI by a mathematical technique called "nonlinear interpolation" (NLI).

Comment Since the data set is inconsistent with normal, we do some exploratory data analysis (EDA) to see why (Figure 8.1.1). The DESCRIBE output indicates that the mean is a bit higher than the median. This indicates that the data may be skewed (trail off) toward the right. The DOTPLOT and BOXPLOT graphics clearly show this. The dotplot shows a somewhat bell-shaped distribution that trails off toward the higher end. The boxplot is enhanced using the NOTCH subcommand, which puts a set of parentheses in the box displaying the 95% s-interval for the median. Again, we see the outliers to the right. Hence, the Barcelona data are inconsistent with normal because of nonsymmetry due to the outliers.

Confidence Intervals for an Average Value

As a general rule for starting out, we recommend one proceed as follows in constructing a CI for an average value.

> CASE 1. Is the RV of interest normal? If so (either by Minitab's nscores correlation test for normality or by assumption), then construct a t-interval for the mean, μ. If not, proceed to case 2.
>
> CASE 2. Is the sample size sufficiently large (n > 30)? If so, then construct a z-interval for μ. If not, then proceed to case 3.
>
> CASE 3. Using Minitab, construct an s-interval for the median, η.
>
> This three-case protocol is only a suggestion for getting started in thinking about a CI. A deeper analysis might enhance case 2 as follows.
>
> Enhanced Case 2. Is the sample size sufficiently large ($n > 30$)? If not, go to case 3. If so, then some thought should be given to whether the mean or the median is a better guide to the average. One is justified in constructing both the z-interval for μ and the s-interval for η. Which is better depends on the nature of the problem one is studying.

Comment Many researchers interchange case 1 and case 2. Since real continuous RVs are only approximately normal (e.g., height, blood hemoglobin), in the case of a large-sample size the approximate large sample z-interval is about as good as can be expected anyway.

EXAMPLE 8.1.2 Consider the Barcelona et al cardiac output study, ice-temperature injectates, prefilled syringes. A 95% z-CI for μ is (3.57, 4.24). A 95% s-CI for η is (3.40, 3.82). Note that the s-CI is shorter (width .42) than the z-CI (width .67). The sample mean is 3.91; the sample median, 3.70. The sample mean is influenced by outliers, as seen in the boxplot in Figure 8.1.1.

Students interested in avoiding unnecessary work are initially overly tempted by the s-interval. Since an s-interval does not need preliminary checks for normality or

FIGURE **8.1.1**
Minitab output for
s-intervals for the
median for the
Barcelona et al
ice-temperature
injectates, prefilled
syringes.

```
MTB > PRINT C1

ITIPS
   3.8    3.8    3.2    3.5    4.0    3.8    4.0    3.9    3.1
   3.8    3.4    3.8    3.4    3.3    3.7    3.5    3.5    3.2
   3.4    3.5    4.5    4.6    4.2    5.0    5.3    4.7    4.8
   2.8    2.2    2.7    6.2    6.7    7.2    5.7    3.0    3.7
   3.4    2.4    2.9    2.7    3.8

MTB > NOTE    Exploratory Data Analysis:
MTB > DESCRIBE C1

                 N      MEAN    MEDIAN    TRMEAN     STDEV    SEMEAN
ITIPS           41     3.905     3.700     3.827     1.091     0.170

               MIN       MAX        Q1        Q3
ITIPS        2.200     7.200     3.250     4.350

MTB > DOTPLOT C1
                                     :
                             ::   :
                   . .  :.....:.:: ::.:  .  .... .   .     .    .
                 -+---------+---------+---------+---------+---------+-----ITIPS
                 2.0       3.0       4.0       5.0       6.0       7.0

MTB > BOXPLOT C1;
SUBC> NOTCH.

                    ----------
          ----------I ( + )  I-----------  *    *    *    o
         --+---------+---------+---------+---------+---------+----ITIPS
          2.0       3.0       4.0       5.0       6.0       7.0

MTB > SINTERVAL 95 C1

SIGN CONFIDENCE INTERVAL FOR MEDIAN

                            ACHIEVED
              N    MEDIAN   CONFIDENCE   CONFIDENCE INTERVAL   POSITION
ITIPS        41    3.700      0.9404     (  3.400,   3.800)        15
                              0.9500     (  3.400,   3.818)       NLI
                              0.9725     (  3.400,   3.900)        14

MTB > SINTERVAL 90 C1

SIGN CONFIDENCE INTERVAL FOR MEDIAN

                            ACHIEVED
              N    MEDIAN   CONFIDENCE   CONFIDENCE INTERVAL   POSITION
ITIPS        41    3.700      0.8827     (  3.500,   3.800)        16
                              0.9000     (  3.480,   3.800)       NLI
                              0.9404     (  3.400,   3.800)        15
```

sample size, why not bypass all the preliminary fuss and simply construct an s-interval? This is a good question. There are two reasons. First, the raw data may not be available. One *must* have the raw data to construct an s-interval, whereas one needs only the sample legend (size, mean, SD) to construct a t- or a z-interval. Second, for a normal distribution, the t-interval is shorter than the s-interval. Technically, statisticians say that the t-procedure is more powerful than the s-procedure for the mean (recall that in a normal distribution, the population mean and median are equal). In Example 7.1.5, we found using Minitab that a 95% t-interval for the mean RTCO is (4.06,4.93) liters/minute. We leave it for the student to verify that the corresponding 95% s-interval for the median RTCO is (3.83,5.36) liters/minute. Here, the s-interval is 76% wider than the t-interval!

Warm-ups
8.1

There are three types of CIs for an average value: t-interval for μ, z-interval for μ, and s-interval for η. Suppose one is presented with a data set for a continuous RV and asked to construct a CI.

1. The first necessary preliminary check to make is to
   a. Construct a histogram
   b. Construct the sample legend
   c. Test for a normal distribution
   d. Conduct EDA

2. In order to decide which type of CI to construct, one first checks for a normal distribution. If the data set is consistent with normal, then construct
   a. A t-interval for the mean
   b. A z-interval for the mean
   c. An s-interval for the mean
   d. An s-interval for the median

3. If one has a large sample size, then to obtain a confidence interval for μ, one may construct a (use the same options in Warm-up 2).

4. For the purposes of constructing a z-interval for μ, a large sample size is ____.

5. If one has a small quantitative data set that is inconsistent with normal, then to obtain a CI for an average value, one constructs
   a. A t-interval for μ
   b. A z-interval for μ
   c. A t-interval for η
   d. An s-interval for η
   e. An s-interval for μ

6. An s-interval is a confidence interval for the
   a. Sample size
   b. Sample mean
   c. Population mean
   d. Sample median
   e. Population median

7. The usual level of confidence in the health sciences is ____%.

8. In Figure 8.1.1, Minitab states that a 90% CI for the median cardiac output using an ice-temperature injectate in a prefilled syringe delivery system is (____, ____).

9. A CI should be reported using as many places past the decimal point as the raw data. Continuing from Warm-up 8, the CI stated by Minitab should be reported as (____, ____).

10. In Figure 7.1.6, Minitab states that a 90% z-CI for the mean cardiac output using an ice-temperature injectate in a prefilled syringe delivery system is (____, ____).

11. Continuing from Warm-up 10, the CI stated by Minitab should be reported as (____, ____).

12. Contrast and compare the two CIs in Warm-ups 9 and 11.

Problems 8.1

1. Consider the Clark and Hoffer metabolism data set (Appendix, Data Set 6). For each RV (age, height, weight, and body mass index), determine a 95% CI for an appropriate average value. If an RV is nonnormal, include an EDA analysis and verbally describe the nature of the distribution.

2. Consider the co-set group in the Barcelona et al cardiac output study (Appendix, Data Set 2). For each cardiac output method, iced and room, determine a 95% CI for an appropriate average value. If an RV is nonnormal, include an EDA analysis and verbally describe the nature of the distribution.

3. Consider the Molyneaux et al coagulation study (Appendix, Data Set 3), 1.6-mL discard. For the RVs arterial, venous, and D = arterial − venous, determine 95% CIs for an appropriate average value. If a sample is inconsistent with normal, include an EDA analysis and verbally describe the nature of the distribution.

4. Consider the Molyneaux et al coagulation study (Appendix, Data Set 3), 4.8-mL discard. For the RVs arterial, venous, and D = arterial − venous, determine 95% CIs for an appropriate average value. If a sample is inconsistent with normal, include an EDA analysis and verbally describe the nature of the distribution.

Meliones et al noted that pulmonary vascular resistance is an important determinant of cardiac output and is adversely affected by elevated mean arterial pressure. Part of the rationale for the study was to determine whether high-frequency jet ventilation (HFJV) could lower mean arterial pressure and result in an increase in cardiac output after a certain procedure (the Fontan procedure). Mean arterial pressure was measured in cm H_2O. Cardiac output was determined by cardiac index measured in liters/minute/m^2. The data are shown in Table 8.1.1. In Problems 5–12, analyze the specified data by determining an appropriate 95% CI. Justify your choice of CI.

5. Mean arterial pressure, Pre.

6. Mean arterial pressure, HFJV.

7. Mean arterial pressure, Post.

TABLE **8.1.1** Data adapted from Meliones et al.

	MEAN ARTERIAL PRESSURE			CARDIAC INDEX		
Patient	Pre	HFJV	Post	Pre	HFJV	Post
1	9.2	4.2	8.9	2.45	3.00	2.40
2	8.7	4.3	9.1	2.17	2.92	2.30
3	9.3	4.7	9.5	2.13	2.80	2.16
4	9.1	4.3	9.3	2.90	3.60	3.80
5	8.6	4.1	8.3	2.20	2.97	2.28
6	8.9	4.4	8.7	2.71	3.25	2.73
7	10.3	5.1	10.3	2.06	2.68	2.10
8	10.7	5.3	10.0	2.13	2.87	2.09
9	10.0	4.9	9.7	2.27	2.91	2.10
10	9.1	4.8	9.0	1.85	2.35	1.50
11	8.1	4.3	9.6	2.21	2.23	2.15
12	8.9	4.3	9.0	1.83	2.53	1.90
13	9.0	4.6	8.7	3.30	3.67	3.20

8. Mean arterial pressure, the difference Pre − Post. What does the CI tell you about the effect of HFJV on mean arterial pressure?

9. Cardiac index, Pre.

10. Cardiac index, HFJV.

11. Cardiac index, Post.

12. Cardiac index, the difference Pre − Post. What does the CI tell you about the effect of HFJV on cardiac index?

SECTION 8.2

Confidence Intervals for the Proportion

OBJECTIVES   This section will

1 Describe the term confidence interval for a proportion.

2 Determine an at least c% confidence interval for a population proportion of a given attribute when provided with a random sample.

3 Determine the sample size necessary to obtain an estimate of a proportion within a given degree of accuracy at c% confidence.

Many statistical studies in the health sciences eventually focus on the mean or the proportion for an RV of interest. One usually concentrates an analysis on the mean when dealing with a quantitative RV. When dealing with a categorical RV, the parameter of interest is the *proportion*.

The proportion describes what fraction of the population as a whole carries a characteristic of interest. Many problems in the health sciences have this feature:

- What proportion of Crohn's disease patients will be helped by cyclosporine therapy?
- What proportion of patients who have a heparin lock flushed with saline will develop phlebitis?
- What proportion of patients who develop atelectasis after abdominal surgery will present a fever $\geq 38°C$?
- What proportion of catheter-acquired bacteriuria cases in women will resolve following a single-dose therapy?
- What proportion of admissions to an adult trauma center transferred to intensive care test positive for alcohol or (nonprescription) drugs?

To obtain information about a proportion, one obtains a random sample for study. From the sample, one obtains a point estimate and an interval estimate for the proportion.

Estimating a Proportion

Consider a large background population and some well-defined attribute A of interest. Each member of the population either has attribute A or does not have attribute A. We focus on obtaining information about p, the proportion of the population that has attribute A.

Obtain a random sample of size n from the population. Examine each member of the sample to see whether it has attribute A. Let x be the number of sample members with attribute A. Then the **sample proportion** for attribute A is x/n. This results in a **point estimate** p: $\hat{p} = x/n$.

X (who has it)
π (everybody)

The real question is, What is p? The sample produces a point estimate $\hat{p} = x/n$ for the population proportion, but what good is it? That is where a CI for p comes in. A $c\%$ CI for the proportion p is an interval estimate for p constructed by a procedure which, of all possible random samples of size n, $c\%$ of these samples yields an interval estimate which actually contains p.

Confidence Interval for a Proportion

An at least $c\%$ CI for p is obtained by $(x/n) \pm z/(2\sqrt{n})$ where z is read from the z-table for confidence intervals (Appendix, Table 7). An *at least* $c\%$ CI means that of all random samples of size n that could be drawn, at least $c\%$ of the corresponding CIs will contain the population proportion p.

A four-step algorithm, similar to the algorithm used for constructing a CI for the mean, is applied for constructing a CI for a proportion.

Round right up
Leave L alone

Step 1. Determine the **sample legend**:
  n = sample size
  x = number in sample having the attribute of interest
Step 2. Determine **z** from the z-table for confidence intervals (Appendix, Table 7).
Step 3. Compute the **endpoints** of the CI:
  L (left endpoint) = $(x/n) - z/(2\sqrt{n})$ and
  R (right endpoint) = $(x/n) + z/(2\sqrt{n})$.
Step 4. An at least $c\%$ **CI for p** is (L,R).

Comment The CI for p sometimes is reported in the form $(x/n) \pm z/(2\sqrt{n})$. For example, $p = .59 \pm .14$. The example indicates that the sample point estimate for p is .59, while at the specified level of confidence, the population proportion p is in the interval $(.59 - .14, .59 + .14)$, which simplifies to $(.45, .63)$.

EXAMPLE 8.2.1 A newspaper article reported on an antirejection drug that appears to help some victims of Crohn's disease, a debilitating digestive tract disorder that afflicts as many as 1 million Americans. The article reported as follows: "In the new study, the first carefully designed test of the drug for these disorders, 71 patients with severe cases of Crohn's disease took either cyclosporine or a useless look-alike drug for four months. Twenty-two of the 37 patients taking cyclosporine experienced significant improvement in their condition."

We determine a point estimate and an at least 90% CI for the proportion p of Crohn's disease patients who took cyclosporine and experienced significant improvement in the 4-month period of the study.

The point estimate is given by: $\hat{p} = 22/37 = 0.59$; that is, 59% of the Crohn's disease patients in the study treated with cyclosporine showed improvement.

An at least 90% CI for p is constructed as follows.

Step 1. $n = 37, x = 22$
Step 2. $z = 1.645$ (Appendix, Table 7)
Step 3. $(x/n) - z/(2\sqrt{n}) = (22/37) - (1.645)/(2\sqrt{37})$
$= .459376428$ (calculator)   45
$(x/n) + z/(2\sqrt{n}) = (22/37) + (1.645)/(2\sqrt{37})$
$= .729812762$ (calculator)   73
Step 4. An at least 90% CI for the proportion of Crohn's disease patients who take cyclosporine and experience significant improvement in 4 months is $(.45, .73)$. Alternatively, $p = .59 \pm .14$.

Hence, based on the data contained in this study, with at least 90% confidence the proportion of all Crohn's disease patients who would be helped by cyclosporine therapy is at least 45%, and perhaps as high as 73%.

Comment How many decimal places should one use in reporting a proportion? We recommend the same guidelines as for reporting a relative frequency (see discussion after Example 1.1.8). In particular, use two places past the decimal point for a proportion if the sample size is ≤ 100. If the sample size is > 100, one may use three places past the decimal point to reflect the greater precision. More places past the decimal point should be used only to reflect the increased precision of a very large sample size.

EXAMPLE 8.2.2 Dunn and Lenihan compared a hospital policy of flushing heparin locks with a heparin solution to a protocol of flushing with a saline solution. Among several items in the research, the authors reported on data obtained in a study of 34 patients on a saline flush in which 5 developed phlebitis or infiltration. We determine a point estimate and a 95% CI for the proportion p of patients who develop phlebitis or infiltration while on a protocol of a saline flush for heparin locks.

The sample point estimate is given by: $\hat{p} = 5/34 = 0.15$.

An at least 95% CI for p is constructed as follows.

Step 1. $n = 34, x = 5$
Step 2. $z = 1.960$ (Table 7)
Step 3. $(x/n) - z/(2\sqrt{n}) = (5/34) - (1.960)/(2\sqrt{34})$
$$= -0.021009790 \text{ (calculator)}$$
$(x/n) + z/(2\sqrt{n}) = (5/34) + (1.960)/(2\sqrt{34})$
$$= 0.315127437 \text{ (calculator)}$$
Step 4. An at least 95% CI for the proportion p of patients with a heparin lock on a protocol of saline flushes who develop phlebitis or infiltration is (0.00,.32); that is, $p = .15 \pm .17$.

Comment Note that a proportion must be a number between 0 and 1. Hence, we take the interval [0, 1] to be the reality window for proportions; that is, any proportion must fall inside the [0, 1] window. A computed CI that has a portion falling outside the reality window, like $(-0.03, 0.32)$ in Example 8.2.2, has any unrealistic portion removed. Also note that 0 cannot be the population proportion since the sample proportion was 5/34. In this example an appropriate clinical conclusion is that with at least 95% confidence the proportion of patients on a heparin lock with a saline flush protocol who develop phlebitis or infiltration does not exceed 32%.

EXAMPLE 8.2.3 Roberts et al studied the use of fever (temperature greater than or equal to 38°C) as a diagnostic indicator for postoperative atelectasis as evidenced by X-ray observation. The data are given in the two-factor frequency distribution table displayed in Table 8.2.1.

TABLE **8.2.1**
Data adapted from
Roberts et al.

		X-ray film evidence for atelectasis		
		Yes	No	Total
Fever	Yes	72	37	109
$\geq 38°C$	No	82	79	161
	Total	154	116	270

In Example 4.1.1 we determined the sensitivity of fever as a diagnostic indicator of atelectasis: Sn = .468. We now expand this point estimate to an interval estimate by constructing a 95% CI for Sn (the proportion of patients with atelectasis who present fever).

Step 1. $n = 154, x = 72$
Step 2. $z = 1.960$ (Table 7)
Step 3. $(x/n) - z/(2\sqrt{n}) = (72/154) - (1.960)/(2\sqrt{154})$
$= 0.388561817$ (calculator)
$(x/n) + z/(2\sqrt{n}) = (72/154) + (1.960)/(2\sqrt{154})$
$= 0.546503118$ (calculator)
Step 4. Based on the given study, an at least 95% CI for the Sn of fever as a diagnostic test for atelectasis is (0.388, 0.547). Alternatively, Sn = .468 ± .079.

Comment Although the sample estimate of the Sn of fever as a diagnostic test for atelectasis is 46.8%, the true Sn (applied to the full population of all postoperative abdominal patients) is somewhere between 38.8% and 54.7%, with at least 95% confidence.

Sample Size

In order to obtain an at least c% CI for p in which the amount of *error* of the point estimate is at most d, one must use a sufficiently large sample size:

$$n = [z/(2d)]^2 \text{ rounded } up$$

The amount of error in an estimate is also called the **accuracy** of the estimate. For example, to estimate a proportion (p) within 5% accuracy (d) with at least 90% confidence, we need a sample size (n) of

$$n = [z/(2d)]^2 = [1.645/(2 \times .05)]^2 = [1.645/0.1]^2 = 270.6 + ;$$

hence, $n = 271$ (rounding *up* to the nearest whole number). We must take a random sample of at least 271 in order to assure we estimate the population proportion within 5% at the 90% level of confidence.

Table 8.2.2 illustrates the high cost of accuracy for obtaining the population proportion for a given attribute at an assured level of confidence.

TABLE **8.2.2**
Sample size needed to obtain a proportion at a given level of accuracy and confidence.

90% Confidence		95% Confidence		99% Confidence	
Accuracy	n	Accuracy	n	Accuracy	n
5%	271	5%	385	5%	664
4	423	4	601	4	1,037
3	752	3	1,068	3	1,842
2	1,692	2	2,401	2	4,148
1	6,766	1	9,604	1	16,577

EXAMPLE 8.2.4 A national newspaper carried a story about how we feel about "Baby M" (should a surrogate mother have the right to change her mind and keep the baby?). The inferences made in the article were based on a poll taken by International Communications Research. The footnote caption reads, "Results have a 3% margin of error." What sample size should be used to obtain this degree of accuracy at the

90%, 95%, and 99% levels of confidence? We can read the needed sample sizes from Table 8.2.2: 752, 1068, 1842, respectively. For illustration, we compute by formula the needed sample size for at least 90% confidence:

$$n = [z/(2d)]^2 = [1.645/(2 \times .03)]^2 = 752$$

The sample size used in the poll was 1020. By "playing jeopardy" in Table 8.2.2, this sample size corresponds almost to 95% confidence for results within 3% error. Hence, with high confidence the poll represents public opinion within 3% accuracy.

Summary

A condensed summary of the information needed to estimate a proportion is given.

Background. One is interested in the proportion p for some attribute of interest. Each member in the population either has or does not have the attribute.

Sample. A random sample of size n is drawn. One counts the number x in the sample who have the attribute of interest.

n = sample size

x = number in the sample with the attribute of interest

Point estimate. $\hat{p} = \frac{x}{n}$

Interval estimate. An "at least" CI for p is obtained by

$$\hat{p} \pm \frac{z}{2\sqrt{n}} \text{ (z is obtained from Appendix, Table 7)}$$

Sample size. To obtain a CI containing p within a degree of accuracy d, use a sample of size n where

$$n = \left[\frac{z}{2d}\right]^2 \text{ (round } up \text{ to the nearest whole number)}$$

EXERCISES 8.2

Warm-ups 8.2

Harding et al reported that single-dose therapy resolved infection in 30 of 37 asymptomatic women with catheter-acquired bacteriuria.

1. What is the population of interest?

2. What is the RV of interest?

3. Is the RV of interest categorical or quantitative?

The researchers are concerned with the proportion
p = **proportion of resolutions within 14 days among asymptomatic women with acquired bacteriuria treated with single-dose therapy**

4. The sample data "30 of 37" yields the point estimate for p:

$$\hat{p} = (\underline{\quad})/(\underline{\quad}) = \underline{\quad}$$

Report your answer to two places past the decimal point.

5. Stated as a percentage, the sample proportion is _____ %.

6. To get a handle on the population proportion p, we construct an at least 95% CI for p. From Table 7, z = ____.

7. An at least 95% CI for p is (L,R) where

$$L = \tfrac{30}{37} - \tfrac{1.960}{2\sqrt{37}} = .649699803 \text{ (calculator)}$$

What should one report for the left endpoint, L?

8. Determine the right endpoint R for the CI.

9. An at least 95% CI for p is 64% to 98%. This means that

   a. p is between 64% and 98%.

   b. p is in the interval (64%,98%) 95% of the time.

   c. There is a 95% chance p is between 64% and 98%.

   d. The interval (64%,98%) was constructed by a procedure for which, among all samples drawn from the population of interest, 95% of the resulting CIs for the proportion p will actually contain p.

10. An alternative way to report this CI is $81 \pm 17\%$. The number 17% is called the *degree of accuracy* for the CI. In order to obtain an at least 95% CI for p within 10% accuracy ($d = .10$), one applies the formula

$$n = \left\lceil \tfrac{z}{2d} \right\rceil^2 \text{ (rounded } up \text{ to the nearest whole number)}$$

Here, $n = \left\lceil \tfrac{z}{2d} \right\rceil^2 = \left[\dfrac{\boxed{}}{\boxed{}} \right]^2 = $ ____

Hence, $n = $ ____

11. In order to obtain an at least 95% CI for p within 5% accuracy, what sample size should be used?

Problems 8.2

1. See Exercise 1.1.2.

   a. Determine a point estimate for the proportion of CCU nurses who correctly diagnose VT.

   b. Determine 90%, 95%, and 99% CIs for the proportion in (a).

2. Kirby et al reported that during their study period, 496 patients were admitted by the adult trauma service, with 270 subsequently admitted to intensive care.

   a. Determine a point estimate for the proportion of patients transferred to intensive care from the adult trauma service.

   b. Determine 90%, 95%, and 99% CIs for the proportion in (a).

   c. Of the patients admitted to intensive care from the adult trauma service, 212 were screened for blood alcohol and drugs (the substance abuse kind, not prescription drugs). Fifty-eight percent of these 212 patients were positive for drugs and/or alcohol. Determine a 95% CI for the proportion of patients admitted to intensive care from the adult trauma service who screen positive for drugs and/or alcohol.

   d. Of the 212 screens given in (c), 75 were positive for marijuana. Determine a point estimate and 95% CI for the proportion of intensive care patients admitted from the adult trauma service who are positive for marijuana.

3. A newspaper article reported that the usual 5-year survival rate for lung cancer patients treated by the standard protocol (surgery) is only 33%. In a study with a new vaccine with 53 lung cancer patients, 33 survived 5 years after surgery.

   a. Determine a point estimate for the 5-year survival rate after surgery for lung cancer for patients who are given the new vaccine.

   b. Determine a 90% CI for the proportion specified in (a).

   c. Based on your CI obtained in (b), is the new vaccine effective in improving the 5-year survival rate for lung cancer patients after surgery?

4. A clinical study was made to determine the side effects of terazosin, a drug used to control hypertension. The study consisted of 859 patients on terazosin and 506 individuals on a placebo. Each person during a controlled time period was asked to keep track of general body ailments (headache, backache, asthenia). Of the 859 on terazosin therapy, 139 complained of general ailments; among the 506 on placebo, 80 such complaints were registered.

   a. Determine a point estimate for the proportion of patients on (i) terazosin and (ii) placebo who registered a complaint of general body ailment.

b. Determine a 95% CI for each of the proportions described in (a).

c. Based on your CIs, do you think a warning of general body ailment should be issued to patients on terazosin?

5. How large a sample is needed to ensure an estimate of a proportion within 2% with at least (a) 80%, (b) 90%, (c) 95%, (d) 98%, or (e) 99% confidence?

6. How large a sample is needed to ensure an estimate of a proportion within 10% with at least (a) 80%, (b) 90%, (c) 95%, (d) 98%, or (e) 99% confidence?

7. Jain et al studied 81,242 consecutive mother-infant pairs (deliveries) recorded by the Illinois regional perinatal network during 1982–86. Among these deliveries, there were 613 infants with a 1-minute zero Apgar score (apparently stillborn).

a. Determine a point estimate for the proportion of deliveries producing an infant with a 1-minute zero Apgar score.

b. Construct a 90%, 95%, and 99% CI for the proportion in (a).

8. (Continued from Problem 7) Of the 613 infants with a zero Apgar score at 1 minute, 520 were considered to be true stillborns (fetal deaths) since they showed no prebirth sign of life at the time of hospital admission for the delivery. The other 93 showed prebirth signs of life and were administered cardiopulmonary resuscitation (CPR). Of these 93 infants, 31 showed no response, while the other 62 were resuscitated and transferred to the neonatal intensive care unit (NICU). Determine a point estimate and 95% CI for each of the following:

a. The proportion of zero Apgar score deliveries who show no prebirth sign of life at the time of hospital admission for delivery.

b. The proportion of all deliveries who show no prebirth sign of life at the time of hospital admission for delivery.

c. The proportion of zero Apgar score deliveries showing prebirth life signs who are resuscitated by CPR and transferred to the NICU.

9. Harding et al in the study of catheter-acquired urinary tract infection in women (featured in the Warm-up exercises) also reported that bacteriuria resolved within 14 days without therapy in 15 of 42 subjects in the study.

a. Identify the proportion p of interest for the "15 of 42."

b. Determine a point estimate for p.

c. Construct an at least 95% CI for p.

10. (Continued from Problem 9) Harding et al also reported that in the group assigned to a 10-day therapy program, infection resolved in 26 of 33 patients.

a. Identify the proportion p of interest for the "26 of 33."

b. Determine a point estimate for p.

c. Construct an at least 95% CI for p.

11. (Continued from Problems 9 and 10) Harding et al also reported that infection more frequently was resolved within 14 days in women who were ≤ 65 years of age than in older women (62 of 70 versus 24 of 39).

a. Determine a point estimate and 95% CI for the proportion of women ≤ 65 years of age whose infection was resolved within 14 days.

b. Determine a point estimate and 95% CI for the proportion of women > 65 years of age whose infection was resolved within 14 days.

12. Venus et al reported that 71.6% of 1123 hospitals surveyed used the intermittent mandatory ventilation (IMV) protocol for weaning patients from a mechanical ventilator.

a. How many hospitals in the survey used the IMV protocol for weaning patients from a mechanical ventilator?

b. Determine a point estimate for the proportion of patients weaned from a mechanical ventilator by the IMV protocol.

c. Determine a 95% CI for the proportion of patients weaned from a mechanical ventilator by the IMV protocol.

13. The formula presented in this section for an "at least" c% CI for the proportion, p, is really an approximate CI. Although approximate, the formula has the nice feature that it can be used to estimate the sample size needed to obtain a CI for p within a prescribed desired degree of accuracy.

FIGURE **8.2.1** Minitab program for an exact CI for the proportion.

```
MTB > STORE 'CIP'
STOR> NOECHO
STOR> NOTE   This program constructs an exact confidence interval
STOR> NOTE        for the proportion.
STOR> NOTE
STOR> NOTE   Enter three numbers:
STOR> NOTE      x = number in sample with attribute of interest;
STOR> NOTE      n = sample size;
STOR> NOTE      c = desired percent level of confidence (usual, 95)
STOR> SET 'TERMINAL' C1;
STOR> NOBS 3.
STOR> LET K1 = C1(1)
STOR> LET K2 = C1(2)
STOR> LET K3 = C1(3)
STOR> LET K10 = K1/K2     # x/n
STOR> NOTE
STOR> NOTE The sample proportion is:
STOR> PRINT K10
STOR> NOTE
STOR> LET K4 = (100 - K3)/200     # alpha/2
STOR> LET K5 = K2 - K1 + 1        # n - x + 1
STOR> INVCDF  K4  K11;            # lower confidence limit
STOR> BETA  K1  K5.
STOR> LET K4 = 1 - K4             # 1 - alpha/2
STOR> LET K5 = K1 + 1             # x + 1
STOR> LET K6 = K2 - K1            # n - x
STOR> INVCDF  K4  K12;            # upper confidence limit
STOR> BETA  K5  K6.
STOR> NOTE The Level of Confidence (percent) is:
STOR> PRINT K3
STOR> NOTE The Confidence Interval for p is:
STOR> PRINT K11 K12
STOR> ECHO
STOR> END OF PROGRAM
```

To run the CIP program, simply execute 'CIP' and follow directions:

```
MTB > EXECUTE 'CIP'
MTB > #
   This program constructs an exact confidence interval
        for the proportion.

   Enter three numbers:
      x = number in sample with attribute of interest;
      n = sample size;
      c = desired percent level of confidence (usual, 95)
DATA> 20 100 95
The sample proportion is:
K10      0.200000

The Level of Confidence (percent) is:
K3       95.0000
The Confidence Interval for p is:
K11      0.126655
K12      0.291843
MTB > END OF PROGRAM
MTB >
```

The formula is also basically simple to apply from a computational viewpoint.

A somewhat sharper result (i.e., a narrower CI) can be obtained by applying the following (slightly more complex) formula to obtain an approximate CI for p.

$$\hat{p} \pm z\sqrt{\hat{p}\hat{q}/n} \quad \text{where } \hat{p} = x/n \text{ and } \hat{q} = 1 - \hat{p}$$

The formula gives good approximations for a CI for p when the sample size is sufficiently large and neither $\hat{p}$ nor $\hat{q}$ is too small. A good rule of thumb for "sufficiently large" is that both $n\hat{p} \geq 5$ and $n\hat{q} \geq 5$. For each of the following situations,

    i. Determine whether the approximate CI is appropriate.

   ii. If so, then construct an approximate 95% CI.

  iii. Compare with the corresponding "at least" 95% CI.

  a. The "30 out of 37" from the Harding et al study described in the Warm-up exercises

  b. The "15 of 42" from Exercise 8.2.9

  c. The "26 of 33" from Exercise 8.2.10

  d. The "62 of 70" from Exercise 8.2.11

  e. The "24 of 39" from Exercise 8.2.11

14. A Minitab project. This Minitab project will allow the user to construct an exact c% CI for the proportion p. The procedure is based on statistical procedures beyond the scope of this course. Nevertheless, the procedure can be exploited for our purpose of constructing an exact CI for the proportion, p.

First, enter the STOREd program called CIP presented in Figure 8.2.1. Once STOREd, one only needs to EXECUTE 'CIP' in Minitab.

Check your program out for $x = 20$ and $n = 100$. You should get lower and upper 95% confidence limits of 0.126655 and 0.291843, respectively. You would then report a 95% CI of (12.6,29.2) percent.

Use the 'CIP' program in Minitab to obtain exact 95% CIs for p for each of the five situations described in Exercise 8.2.13.

CHAPTER OVERVIEW

Summary

The most basic measures for an RV are an average value for an interval RV and a proportion for a categorical RV. Fundamental techniques of research include methods for estimating an average value or a proportion based on a sample. An estimate should offer both a **point estimate** and an **interval estimate**.

When an interval RV is (assumed) normal or the sample size is large, one may provide both point and interval estimates for the mean. If the distribution is nonnormal and the sample size is small, we cannot provide an interval estimate for the mean. However, using Minitab we can obtain an **s-interval** for the **median**. The s-interval may be helpful in describing the central tendency (average) for a nonnormal data set containing outliers.

When dealing with a categorical RV, one is concerned about the **proportion** of a particular attribute of interest. Based on a sample, one can obtain both a **point estimate** and an **interval estimate** for such a proportion. Exploiting the "at least" **confidence interval** for the proportion formula, one also can obtain the **sample size** needed in order to obtain an estimate of the proportion within a desired degree of **accuracy**.

Keywords

accuracy	sample
confidence interval	sample median
error	sample proportion
mean	sample size
median	s-interval (median)
normality	t-interval (mean)
point estimate	z-interval (mean)
proportion	

References

Dunn D and Lenihan S: The case for the saline flush. *Am J Nurs*, vol. 87, no. 6, (June 1987): 798.

Exact confidence limits for population proportions. *MUG Newsletter* 13 (March 1991): 6.

Harding G et al: How long should catheter-acquired urinary tract infection in women be treated? *Ann Intern Med* 114, no. 9 (1 May 1991): 713.

Jain L et al: Cardiopulmonary resuscitation of apparently stillborn infants: Survival and long-term outcome. *J Pediatr* 118, no. 5 (May 1991): 778.

Kirby J et al: Alcohol and drug use among trauma patients admitted to an intensive care unit. *Heart Lung* 18, no. 3 (May 1989): 297.

Meliones J et al: High-frequency jet ventilation improves cardiac function after the fontan procedure. *Circulation* 84, no. 3, suppl. III (November 1991): III-364.

New drug shows promise for those with Crohn's disease. *Eureka Times Standard*, 3 November 1989.

Poll: Give 'Baby M' to Father. *USA Today*, 12 March 1987, A3.

Roberts J et al: Diagnostic accuracy of fever as a measure of postoperative pulmonary complication. *Heart Lung* 17, no. 2 (March 1988): 166.

Vaccine raises survival rate of cancer patients. *Eureka Times Standard*, 23 March 1988.

Venus B et al: National survey of methods and criteria used for weaning from mechanical ventilation. *Crit Care Med* 15 (1987): 530.

9

An Orientation to Test of Hypothesis

The main topic in any introductory statistics course is test of hypothesis. Test of hypothesis is more than just a procedure for solving a specific problem; it is a general way of thinking in its own right.

This topic, once mastered, is beautiful in its simplicity. It is a model of KISS (Keep It Super Simple) problem solving. However, this topic is tough. Everybody catches on at his or her own rate. Chapter 9 is meant as an orientation to the subject. Take it as a general overview. It is not crucial that all the details be mastered here. Take what you get out of it and bring your unanswered questions into Chapter 10. The advice here is not to focus on what you don't understand but to be aware of and take heart in what you do pick up.

The rest of this text is devoted to various tests of hypothesis. The orientation usually produces some confusion. This confusion gets resolved as one progresses through the remaining chapters. Hang in there. Major clarification takes place when we perform these tests starting in Chapter 10. Most students realize a substantial level of mastery by Chapter 12.

SECTION 9.1	**OBJECTIVES** This section will
Test of Hypothesis	**1** Describe and distinguish between a problem of location and a problem of comparison.
	2 Determine the null and alternate hypothesis appropriate for a statistical test of hypothesis when provided with a health sciences problem that can be recast as a problem of comparison.
	3 Describe the concept of statistical test of hypothesis.
	4 Describe the errors that may result from a statistical test of hypothesis.
	5 Describe the general protocol for a statistical test of hypothesis.

Phase 1 of research is concerned with statistical design and descriptive statistics. The motivation is the collection and presentation of data so that a story of interest emerges. After basic knowledge is acquired, one inquires about how to manage or explain the situation. One then embarks on phase 2: inferential statistics, the process of drawing valid conclusions from the given data. The main feature of inferential statistics is that a conclusion is made about a population based on a sample.

The background props needed to set the stage for inferential statistics are (1) a population and (2) a random variable (RV). The population specifies *who* is of interest. An RV specifies *what* is of interest about a member from the population.

EXAMPLE 9.1.1 A public health worker is concerned with hypertension in a large community. As a working definition, she accepts hypertension as systolic blood pressure (SBP) exceeding 140 mm Hg. To orient herself to hypertension in her community of responsibility, she inquires,

■ What is the average SBP of adults ≥ 30 years of age?
■ What proportion of adults aged ≥ 30 years have hypertension?

Her public health guidelines direct that she commit resources to the development and implementation of a public education program if the proportion of hypertensives among adults ≥ 30 years of age exceeds 15%.

The population of interest is adults ≥ 30 years of age in the community. The public health worker specifies two RVs of interest: SBP, a continuous RV, and hypertension (yes or no), a categorical RV. The purpose of her orientation to hypertension in her community is to determine whether or not to commit resources to develop and implement a public education program about hypertension. Her problem is resolved by determining whether or not the proportion of hypertensives exceeds 15%.

Problems in inferential statistics are concerned with either (1) the distribution of an RV or (2) a population parameter. We already studied a distribution problem in section 6.2, testing for normality There we inquired whether a given continuous RV had a normal distribution. We resolved the problem by applying Minitab's nscores correlation test to a random sample drawn from the population. In the remainder of this text, we will be concerned with problems in the health sciences that can be formulated for resolution in terms of some parameter. For example, the public health worker in Example 9.1.1 determines whether to implement a public education program on hypertension by resolving whether $p \geq .15$, where p is the proportion of hypertensives in the community among adults ≥ 30 years of age.

In a first course in health sciences statistics, almost all parameter problems boil down to resolving a question that involves either a proportion or an average. When the RV of interest is categorical, the parameter of interest is a proportion. When the RV of interest is continuous, the parameter of interest usually is an average value. A challenging and creative part of inferential statistics in the health sciences is to take some loosely formulated problem of general concern (should I start a public education program about hypertension?) and recast it into a statement involving a population parameter (is $p \geq .15$?). We now concern ourselves with the awareness and phrasing of the two major types of parameter problems in inferential statistics.

Two Parameter Problems in Inferential Statistics

Statistics is a valuable tool to assist in addressing many concerns in the health sciences. This often occurs by recasting a specific health science problem into a statistics problem stated in terms of a population parameter. A **parameter** is a measure of a population, such as a proportion or an average. For example, the mean SBP in a community is 132 mm Hg. Here the parameter is the mean, and its value is 132. Also, the proportion of hypertensives in the community is 23%. Here the parameter is the proportion, and its value is 23%.

Comment We caution that the term *parameter* is used only in its technical statistical sense (a parameter is a measure of a population) in this section. It can be confusing because the word *parameter* has a technical meaning in several different areas, including mathematics and clinical health. In clinical health, a parameter is a number that specifies a limit or a boundary. For example, a physician may order a drug q4h but may hold the medication if blood pressure is too low (< 120 systolic or < 50 diastolic). In the physician's order, 120 and 50 are (clinical) parameters for the drug order. To assist in overcoming potential confusion wrought by multiple meanings, we will often use the term *population parameter*, even though the adjective *population* is an unnecessary redundancy in the technical statistical meaning of parameter.

In a single population, there are two key questions asked about a given parameter of interest namely,

Location: What is the value of the population parameter?
Comparison: How does the population parameter compare against a given reference value?

These two questions reflect the two key types of population parameter problems in inferential statistics: problems of location and problems of comparison. One is concerned about a **problem of location** when posing the question, What is the value of the parameter of interest? The two bulleted questions in Example 9.1.1 pose problems of location. A problem of location is resolved by displaying a confidence interval (Chapters 7 and 8). One is concerned about a **problem of comparison** when posing a question, Is the parameter equal to (less than, greater than) some reference value of interest? A problem of comparison is resolved by a test of hypothesis, a procedure introduced later in this section.

EXAMPLE 9.1.2 The public health worker described in Example 9.1.1 is concerned about the level of hypertension in her community, that is, the proportion of adults ≥ 30 years with SBP > 140. Her public health guidelines direct that if the proportion of hypertensives is greater than 15%, she should commit resources to the development and implementation of a public education program. The public health worker is faced with a problem of comparison. Her particular concern is whether p, the proportion of people with hypertension, is greater than .15 (15%). She does not want to act as a public health official without proper justification. Her "action hypothesis" (assumption under which she intervenes) is formally denoted by

$$H_a: p > .15$$

She gathers data specifically motivated by the determination of whether the proportion p of hypertensives is greater than .15, a reference value for when to commence action. The *action hypothesis* is prefaced by "H_a:." What follows "H_a:" is a statement of comparison of a parameter (p) to a specific reference value (.15).

A problem of comparison is presented by displaying appropriately framed hypotheses. A statistical **hypothesis** is a formal statement that can be tested on the basis of a random sample drawn from the population of interest. The specific skill of being able to formulate appropriate hypotheses to present a problem of comparison occupies most of the remainder of this section.

The Null Hypothesis and Alternate Hypothesis

A problem of comparison is formally launched by presenting a pair of competing hypotheses. These hypotheses are called the **null hypothesis** (denoted H_0) and the **alternate hypothesis** (denoted H_a). The hypotheses H_0 and H_a are competing in that one and only one of them is correct. Statistical etiquette requires that the null hypothesis, H_0, be presented first, followed by the alternate hypothesis, H_a.

The concepts of null and alternate hypotheses were introduced in Section 6.2, testing for normality. In this section we concentrate on those health science problems that can be recast as problems of comparison. As illustrated in Example 9.1.2, in such cases the original health science problem is reduced to a problem about a population parameter (a proportion or an average value).

We illustrate the presentation of hypothesis by several examples in which we describe a problem of comparison and state the appropriate null and alternate hypotheses. Each example is followed by a comment that highlights some special statistical facet in the example.

EXAMPLE 9.1.3 The public health worker in Example 9.1.2 is directed to develop and implement a public education program about hypertension if the proportion of adults aged ≥ 30 years with hypertension exceeds 15%. The set of hypotheses needed to formally launch her problem of comparison is displayed succinctly and informatively by

$$H_0: p \leq .15$$

$$H_a: p > .15$$

Comment Here, the term *null hypothesis* is very descriptive and appropriate. Without cause (i.e., null evidence situation), there is no justification for the public health official to expend public funds. The implication of the null hypothesis is that there is no reason to act on a health science problem unless there is evidence a problem exists. Lacking evidence to the contrary (null evidence situation), the appropriate stance of the official is that hypertension is under control ($p \leq .15$). In formal statistics, the alternate hypothesis is merely the opposite of the null hypothesis. However, in this example, it is the alternate hypothesis that motivates the health science problem. In such cases, the alternate hypothesis is also called an "action" or "intervention hypothesis" since it prescribes the condition for an action or intervention.

EXAMPLE 9.1.4 A new drug is being developed for use in the treatment of lung cancer. It is hoped that the drug will improve the current 5-year survival rate of .33 (33%) for patients who undergo treatment of lung cancer. Researchers wish to get evidence to support this hope. Here the population of interest is patients who have undergone surgery for treatment of lung cancer. The RV of interest is the categorical RV of whether the patient survives 5 years postoperatively (yes or no). The parameter of interest is p, the proportion of patients who survive at least 5 years after surgical treatment of lung cancer. The research motivation is to gather data to assess whether $p > .33$. Hence,

– only one is correct
– only one canbe

$H_0: p \leq .33$
$H_a: p > .33$

Comment When the health sciences concern is motivated by a research problem, the alternate hypothesis is usually called the **research hypothesis**. The research hypothesis is the "burden of proof" hypothesis. Note that with a lack of evidence (null evidence situation, hence, null hypothesis), there is no reason to believe that the drug will produce an improvement in survival rates. This general outlook applies to all tests of hypothesis involving an inequality; specifically, the alternate hypothesis is the "burden of proof" hypothesis. In this example, the number .33 is the **test reference value** in that the researchers specifically want to compare the 5-year survival rate of patients on the drug with the current survival rate of .33.

EXAMPLE 9.1.5 Nancy is considering randomizing patients into one of two groups, an experimental group and a control group, simply by flipping the coin she took from her pocket. She pauses to wonder if this coin-flipping procedure is really "fair." She plans on conducting a test by putting the coin in an empty coffee cup, shaking it, and tossing it on the table several times. She anticipates that if the coin is fair, it should show heads 50% of the time. Here, the (conceptual) population of interest is all the flips of the coin. The parameter of interest is p, the proportion of heads. The research motivation is to determine whether the results of the coin-tossing experiment are consistent with the "fair coin hypothesis"; that is, whether $p = .5$. The key here is that there is no reason to suspect that the coin is unfair unless it exhibits behavior to the contrary. Hence,

$H_0: p = .5$ (fair coin hypothesis)
$H_a: p \neq .5$

Comment This test of hypothesis concerns an "equals versus not equals" situation, rather than an inequality as in Examples 9.1.3 and 9.1.4. *In an "equals versus not equals" test, the equality is always placed in the null hypothesis*. Such a test is a **consistency test**. The data gathered in an experiment either will be consistent with the test reference value stated in the null hypothesis or will show that such an assumption is basically unreasonable.

EXAMPLE 9.1.6 The measurement of whole blood hemoglobin concentration (Hb) is one of the most common clinical laboratory tests and constitutes the first step in investigating anemia. Investigators evaluating a new system for Hb want to check whether the mean Hb determined by the new system is consistent with the accepted mean of 13.5 (g/dL) for women in the United States. Here the population of interest is U.S. women. The RV of interest is Hb, a continuous RV. The parameter of interest is μ, the mean Hb level. The research motivation is to check whether the mean Hb level of U.S. women for the new system is 13.5 g/dL. Hence,

$$H_0: \mu = 13.5 \text{ (g/dL)}$$
$$H_a: \mu \neq 13.5 \text{ (g/dL)}$$

Comment This basic test of hypothesis tests the situation of "equals versus not equals"; consequently, the equality is placed in the null hypothesis. The test reference value is 13.5.

EXAMPLE 9.1.7 A study is conducted to compare cardiac outputs taken using room-temperature and ice-temperature injectates. Room-temperature injectates are easier on both patient and clinician. The study is conducted to determine whether there is a discernible difference, on average, between cardiac outputs taken by both methods. A sample of patients is studied. For each patient in the study, the difference D (D = room − ice) is obtained. The population of interest is the set of cardiac patients who will undergo cardiac output determinations. The RV of interest is the difference D between room- and ice-temperature cardiac outputs. The RV D is continuous. The parameter of interest is μ_D, the mean value of D. The research motivation is to determine whether room-temperature cardiac outputs are consistent with ice-temperature outputs. Hence,

$$H_0: \mu_D = 0$$
$$H_a: \mu_D \neq 0$$

Note that the null hypothesis says that, on average, there is no difference between cardiac outputs taken with room- and ice-temperature injectates; that is, on average, D = room − ice = 0.

Comment In many paired-comparison studies (health or otherwise), the null hypothesis is that there is no discernible difference between two methods for performing a given task. One does not scientifically believe that there is a difference between two methods until one has evidence to support such a difference. Note that the test reference number is 0 for determining whether a difference exists or not.

EXAMPLE 9.1.8 Based on their experience, clinicians feel that endotracheal suctioning of respiratory care patients carries certain hazards. Researchers interested in measuring the effects of suctioning designed an experiment to see if 1 minute of controlled suctioning would decrease PaO_2 from the start of suctioning to the end of a 1-minute controlled suctioning session ($D = PaO_2$ before $- PaO_2$ after). The parameter of interest is μ_D, the mean value of D. The research motivation is the fear that, in general, suctioning reduces PaO_2. Hence,

$$H_0: \mu_D \leq 0$$
$$H_a: \mu_D > 0$$

Comment This problem of comparison is an example of a paired data intervention study. The research is motivated by a fear of the result of an intervention (does suctioning produce a potentially hazardous effect as shown by decreased PaO_2?). In this case the null hypothesis (no-evidence situation) may be described colloquially as the Alfred E. Newman (What! Me Worry?) hypothesis. The general sense of the null hypothesis is that without due reason there is no cause for alarm. The alternate hypothesis here is the research hypothesis, which carries the burden of proof. There is no need for worry unless evidence is produced showing that a real problem exists.

Once a health science problem has been converted to a statistical problem of comparison involving the two competing statements, the null and alternate hypotheses, we need to be able to decide which hypothesis to accept. The most common statistical procedure for making such a decision is test of hypothesis.

Test of Hypothesis

A statistical **test of hypothesis** (TOH) is a decision-making procedure that chooses between the null hypothesis H_0 and the alternate hypothesis H_a based on data obtained from a random sample and predicated on the assumption that H_0 is true unless the data warrant rejecting H_0 in favor of H_a.

In order for TOH to reject H_0 in favor of H_a, the sample must show itself to be highly improbable given that the null hypothesis H_0 is true. This explains why the formal TOH protocol always states H_0 first with H_a following. Initially, TOH operates from the assumption that H_0 is true. TOH will reject H_0 and accept H_a only when presented with a random sample that is highly improbable if H_0 is true. Hence, TOH sticks with H_0 until supplied with evidence that belief in H_0 is unreasonable.

The TOH procedure incorporates taking a random sample and making a decision based on information obtained from the sample. The nature of the decision is basically very simple: TOH either (1) retains H_0 or (2) rejects H_0 in favor of H_a. From this viewpoint, TOH merely acts as a judge who either sustains or overrules H_0. TOH gives "rights" to H_0 similar to the rights enjoyed by an accused person in American jurisprudence. An accused is assumed innocent until proven guilty. If the evidence is lacking or insufficient, the judge assumes

H_0: the accused is innocent

In order to convict, the prosecution must supply evidence to justify rejecting H_0; that is, the prosecution must present evidence sufficiently strong to infer that belief in H_0 is unreasonable. Consequently, the prosecutor's hypothesis

H_a: the accused is guilty

states the position that must assume the burden of proof.

Using American jurisprudence as a paradigm, the final decision announced by TOH is either (1) do not reject H_0 (retain H_0), or (2) reject H_0 and accept H_a. In order to reject H_0, one must display sufficient evidence to show that belief in H_0 is unreasonable. The decision "do not reject H_0" *does not mean that H_0 has been proven*. In American courts, some guilty people are not convicted due to lack of evidence. A judicial decision of "not guilty" does not mean that innocence has been proved but that innocence is presumed due to lack of evidence to convict. TOH holds a similar orientation about announcing a decision regarding H_0 versus H_a.

Is TOH always right in making its decision? Of course not! Anytime a decision is based on a random sample, one is always subject to the luck of the draw. However, TOH is right a surprising amount of the time! Since TOH is not infallible, however, it is very important that one understand and appreciate the type of errors that can be made by invoking the TOH procedure to resolve a statistical problem posing as a health sciences problem.

Acceptance and Rejection Errors

We discuss the nature of hypothesis testing in terms of H_0, the null hypothesis, from two viewpoints: *reality* and *decision*.

From the viewpoint of reality, H_0 must be either true or false. If one knows which of these options is correct, then there is no need for further study. The usual real-world situation is that we do not know which option is correct; we only know that H_0 must be either true or false. We need a decision-making procedure to assist in deciding which option, H_0 or H_a, to select. From the viewpoint of our decision, we either retain H_0 or reject H_0. In statistics, we make our decision by applying test of hypothesis (TOH).

TOH formally announces its statistical decision as either reject H_0 or do not reject H_0. On occasion, rather than using this formal language of statistics, we will adopt the corresponding language used in the clinical health sciences: Rule out H_0, or do not rule out H_0.

We now inquire how the two viewpoints about H_0, reality and decision, interact with each other when we apply TOH. The various pieces of the discussion fit together as displayed in Table 9.1.1. In reality, H_0 is either true or false, as displayed in the columns of Table 9.1.1. In order to uncover this reality, we obtain a random sample. Information from the sample is fed into a TOH procedure. A decision is produced. The decision about H_0 is either "do not rule out H_0" or "rule out H_0," as displayed in the rows of Table 9.1.1. To see how decision interfaces with reality, we first consider what can happen when H_0 is true; then second, what can happen when H_0 is false.

First, suppose that H_0 in reality is true. One of two outcomes can happen.

TABLE **9.1.1**
Reality and decision
can interact in four
different ways
about H_0.

		REALITY OF H_0	
		H_0 Is True	H_0 Is False
DECISION ABOUT H_0	*Do not rule out H_0*	Correct	Acceptance error (probability β)
	Rule out H_0	Rejection error (probability α)	Correct

TOH decides "do not rule out H_0." We obtain a correct decision. The decision is consistent with reality in that we retain H_0 and H_0 is true.

TOH decides "rule out H_0." An error is made. The sample directs TOH to rule out H_0 although in reality H_0 is true. This type of error is called a **rejection error** since an error is made by rejecting H_0. Formal statistical jargon refers to such an error as a type I error. Whenever a decision about a population is based on a sample, there is an inherent risk by the luck of the draw for the sample of making a rejection error. The probability that such an error will be made is called the **level of significance** (**LOS**) for the test of hypothesis. The LOS is usually denoted by α (Greek *a*). Alternatively, ($1 - \alpha$) measures the confidence we can have that TOH, based on a random sample, will correctly retain H_0 when H_0 in reality is true.

Second, suppose that in reality H_0 is false. One of two outcomes can happen.

TOH decides "do not rule out H_0." An error is made. The sample directs TOH to not rule out H_0, although in reality H_0 is false. This type of error is called an **acceptance error** (formally, type II error) since an error is made by accepting (i.e., not rejecting) H_0. The probability that such an error will be made is denoted by β (Greek *b*). Note that β is the probability of retaining H_0 when H_0 in reality is false. The corresponding probability $1 - \beta$ of correctly rejecting H_0 when H_0 is in reality false is called the **power** of the test.

TOH decides "rule out H_0." We obtain a correct decision.

A schematic of the general nature of hypothesis testing is shown in Figure 9.1.1. To initiate TOH, one inputs a set of hypotheses for testing (H_0 and H_a) and sets the α knob (LOS). A random sample from the population of interest is obtained and entered into TOH. In response, TOH then outputs the decision: Either do not reject H_0, or reject H_0 and accept H_a.

A major feature of TOH is that the user can preset the level of significance; that is, one can input the risk one is willing to take in making a decision based on a sample. The usual LOS setting in the health sciences is $\alpha = .05$. This means that *when the null hypothesis is true*, only 5% of all possible samples erroneously result in a "reject H_0" decision; 95% of all possible samples correctly result in a "do not reject H_0" decision. Hence, basing a decision on a sample is like playing a lottery, but the user gets to specify the level of risk one is willing to take.

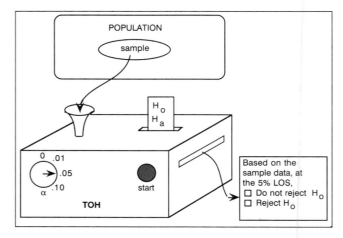

FIGURE **9.1.1**
TOH can be
conveniently thought
of as a decision-
making machine. One
inputs a hypothesis,
sets the α knob (LOS),
and enters the sample
data. TOH then
outputs the decision.

In general, there is no β knob on a TOH machine. Hypothesis testing for which both α and β must be controlled should be undertaken in consultation with an experienced statistician. The regulation of β usually is accomplished through adequacy of sample size. Hence, teamwork with a statistician must begin with the design phase of a study. Statistical consults after data are collected usually result in the sad news that the collected data are inadequate for analysis to resolve the health sciences problem of interest.

There are many parallels between statistical and diagnostic testing (see Figure 9.1.2). The two types of errors in a diagnostic test are the false negative and the false positive. Their probabilities, $F - R$ and $F + R$, respectively, correspond to α and β in TOH. The sensitivity and specificity of a diagnostic test correspond to $1 - \alpha$ and $1 - \beta$, the confidence and power of a statistical test. In a formal sense, a diagnostic test is a testing procedure for which, for a given condition of interest,

H_0: the patient does not have the condition
H_a: the patient has the condition

General Test of Hypothesis Protocol

A statistical test of hypothesis is carried out by applying the following seven-step protocol (procedure or algorithm). This general algorithm is presented only as a preview. In specific cases the user will be guided by an appropriate chart that provides the details.

Step 1. State the *null hypothesis* and the *alternate hypothesis*.
Step 2. State the *level of significance*.
Step 3. State the *test statistic*.
Step 4. Determine the *critical value* for the test.
Step 5. Construct a *decision line* that displays the "do not reject H_0" region and the "reject H_0" region.
Step 6. Determine the *sample value* when provided with a random sample drawn from the population.

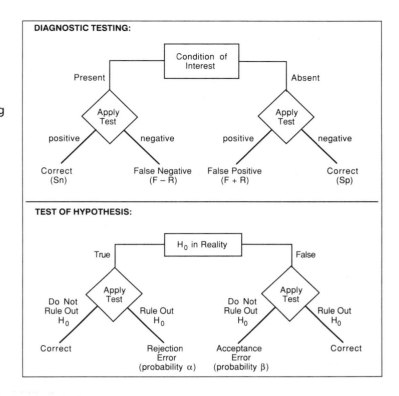

FIGURE **9.1.2**
The flowcharts display the decision-making process and consequences in diagnostic testing and a test of hypothesis.

Step 7. State the *conclusion*:

    a. Based on the given data, at the α LOS we do not reject (or rule out) the null hypothesis.

    b. Based on the given data, at the α LOS we reject (rule out) the null hypothesis and accept the alternate hypothesis.

Steps 1 and 2 are preliminary decisions that must be made by the user. In a good statistical design, these steps are done early in the research.

Steps 3 and 4 are read from provided charts or tables. These are automatic once steps 1 and 2 are completed.

Step 5 is also an automatic procedure that can be read from a provided chart. For each test it is essential that one construct a decision line utilizing the critical value obtained in step 4. The decision line becomes the automatic judge for retaining or rejecting the null hypothesis based on the given evidence (sample data).

Step 6 is a computational step that must be done by the user. In step 6 one runs the sample data through the test statistic, thereby boiling all the experimental (sample) work down to a single number. Do not perform these computations in step 3. The purpose of step 3 is to present an expression that tells the user what to do with data after they have been obtained. Ideally, steps 1 through 5 should be completed before data are collected.

Step 7 is the final step. One fits the sample value obtained in step 6 onto the decision line created in step 5. One then formally states the appropriate conclusion.

The conclusion should have three major components: the statistical conclusion, appropriate clinical implications, and the p-value for the test (Section 10.4). After all the computations, the bottom line is, what does it all mean for giving care?

This seven-step protocol will become clear after we have some practice and experience with performing statistical tests of hypothesis. Until then, note that statistical tests of hypothesis will be conducted according to this seven-step protocol. For each particular kind of problem presented in this text, there will be a prototype chart (see Appendix) to guide you through the steps.

EXERCISES 9.1

Warm-ups 9.1

1. Match each term in the first column to the appropriate description given in the second column.

Term	Description
a. Population	**i.** What is the value of a given population parameter?
b. Random variable	**ii.** The collection of all subjects of interest
c. Parameter	**iii.** An item of information appropriate for each member in the population
d. Problem of location	**iv.** A measure of the population at large
e. Problem of comparison	**v.** How does the population parameter match a given reference value?

2. A problem of location is resolved by presenting a
   a. Sample
   b. Parameter
   c. Confidence interval
   d. Test of hypothesis
   e. Null hypothesis

3. A problem of comparison is resolved by presenting a (same options as in Warm-up 2).

4. A problem of comparison that is concerned with the fraction of the population having a characteristic of interest is concerned with which population parameter?
   a. Mean

   b. Standard deviation
   c. Median
   d. Proportion
   e. A confidence interval

Background for Warm-ups 5–10. Dianne Lepley-Frey reported on dysrhythmias and blood pressure changes associated with thrombolysis. The population of interest was cardiac patients undergoing TPA therapy for treatment of an occluded artery. One of the four research questions posed in her article was, What is the frequency of dysrhythmias? In posing this question, the researcher was interested in determining the fraction of patients presenting one or more dysrhythmias.

5. This question is concerned with what population parameter? (Use the same options as in Warm-up 4).

6. This question states
   a. A problem of comparison
   b. A problem of location
   c. A problem of descriptive statistics
   d. A hypothesis to be tested
   e. A clinical problem, not a statistical problem

7. Suppose we were concerned with the statement "A majority of coronary patients administered TPA to alleviate an occluded artery will experience a dysrhythmia during the 3.5-hour TPA administration period." The statement identifies (use the same options as in Warm-up 6).

8. Let p be the proportion of patients who experience dysrhythmia. The concern that "the majority of patients experience dysrhythmia" translated in terms of p says that
    a. $p < .5$
    b. $p = .5$
    c. $p > .5$
    d. $p \le .5$
    e. $p \ge .5$

9. A problem of comparison is resolved by a test of hypothesis. The parameter of interest is p, the proportion of patients who experience a dysrhythmia. The research hypothesis for testing the given statement is
    a. $H_0: p > .5$
    b. $H_0: p \le .5$
    c. $H_a: p < .5$
    d. $H_a: p = .5$
    e. $H_a: p > .5$

10. The null hypothesis corresponding to the research hypothesis $H_a: p > .5$ is (use the same options from Warm-up 9).

Problems 9.1

A brief scenario is described in each problem. Complete (a)–(e) for each problem. If the scenario describes a problem of comparison, then also include (f)–(h).
a. What is the population of interest?
b. What is the random variable of interest?
c. Is the random variable of interest categorical or quantitative? If quantitative, is it nominal, ordinal, or interval? If interval, is it discrete or continuous?
d. What is the parameter of interest?
e. Is the scenario concerned with a problem of location or a problem of comparison?
f. Determine appropriate null and alternate hypotheses describing the Problem of Comparison.
g. Describe the practical effects of the consequences of a test of hypothesis if a rejection error is made.
h. Describe the practical effects of the consequences of a test of hypothesis if an acceptance error is made.

1. An obstetrics health manager is interested in knowing the average birth weight of neonates in a certain large community.

2. An obstetrics health manager is interested in knowing the proportion of very-low-birth-weight (<1500 grams) neonates in a certain large community.

3. An obstetrics health care manager is interested in her chances of getting a Health Department community education and services grant. Past experience has shown that the department funds well-prepared proposals where the documented proportion of low-birth-weight (<5 pounds) neonates in the community is greater than 10%.

Background for Problems 4–6 (see Section 1.2, An Application: Time Series Graphs). Researchers studied the potential hazard of airway suctioning on ventilator-dependent patients by measuring PaO_2 at the start of suctioning (baseline), at the end of a 1-minute suctioning protocol, 1-minute postsuction, and 5 minutes postsuction.

4. Researchers are interested in the average baseline PaO_2.

5. Researchers suspect that in general there is a discernible drop in PaO_2 as a result of suctioning.

6. Researchers are interested in whether PaO_2 returns at least to baseline after a recovery period of 5 minutes.

7. According to probability theory, if the chance of having a girl is .5, then the probability that a family with 6 children has a majority of girls (4, 5, or 6 girls) is .3438 [$X = \text{Bino}(6, .5)$, $\text{Prob}[X > 3] = .3438$]. A researcher decides to check this out by surveying a large number of families with 6 children and recording which families have a majority of girls. The researcher then wants to contrast the observed results with what one would expect based on theory.

Problems 8–11 are continued from Problem 4.1.2.

8. Researchers are interested in determining Sn and F − R of the diagnostic test "less than 25 microvolts in the last 40 milliseconds of the QRS waveform" as a positive indicator for the condition "prone to VT."

9. Researchers are interested in determining Sp and F + R of the diagnostic test "less than 25 micro-volts in the last 40 milliseconds of the QRS wave-form" as a positive indicator for the condition "prone to VT."

10. Researchers are interested in determining PV + of the diagnostic test "less than 25 microvolts in the last 40 milliseconds of the QRS waveform" as a positive indicator for the condition "prone to VT."

11. Researchers are interested in determining PV − of the diagnostic test "less than 25 microvolts in the last 40 milliseconds of the QRS waveform" as a positive indicator for the condition "prone to VT."

Background for Problems 12–15. Researchers are studying a new system for taking blood measurements. One measurement of importance is hemoglobin concentration (Hb); another, packed cell volume (PCV).

12. The Hb for a standard blood sample was determined to be 13.2 g/dL using standard calibration techniques. Researchers decided to assess the new system by taking several readings of the standard sample using the new system and contrasting the results with the value of 13.2 g/dL given by the standard calibration method.

13. Researchers wanted to know the average PCV for women determined by the new method. They decided to obtain the average by taking blood samples from women donors at the local blood bank.

14. Researchers wanted to contrast the average PCV for females as determined by the new system with the average value of 0.417 for women reported in the literature. The researchers used a random sample of female donors at the local blood bank.

15. Researchers wanted to contrast the average PCV for males as determined by the new system with the average value of 0.443 for men reported in the literature. The researchers used a random sample of male donors at the local blood bank.

16. Researchers were interested in comparing aPTT (a blood coagulation time) values using blood drawn from a patient with an arterial line against blood drawn by venipuncture. They were concerned with how much blood discard to use on the arterial line because of possible interference from heparin used to keep the arterial line patent. As part of the study, the researchers wanted to compare the aPTT from a set of patients who were on an arterial line. From each patient a blood sample was taken from the arterial line using a 1.6-mL discard, and by using a venipuncture. The researchers were interested in whether there was any discernible difference in aPTT using blood drawn by the two methods.

17. Woo et al studied comparison of thermodilution and transthoracic electrical bioimpedance cardiac outputs. The abstract for the paper began: "Current methods of measuring cardiac output require the invasive insertion of a thermodilution catheter with its concomitant risks and complications. We examined the noninvasive method of transthoracic electrical bioimpedance (TEB) in comparison with thermodilution cardiac outputs."

The goal of the research was stated as follows: "In this study, the following hypothesis was tested: ≥ 75% of the sample's TEB readings would be within 0.5 L/min of the simultaneous thermodilution cardiac outputs in a subpopulation of critically ill patients with heart failure."

CHAPTER **9** OVERVIEW

Summary

Inferential statistics is the process of making valid statements about a population based on data obtained from a random sample. Inferential statistics usually is concerned with the distribution of some random variable (RV) or some population parameter. Parameter problems are usually concerned with either a proportion or an average value. The two main types of problems concerning a parameter are a **problem of location** and a **problem of comparison**.

A **statistical hypothesis** is a formal statement that can be tested on the basis of a random sample drawn from the population. One launches a problem of comparison by presenting a set of competing hypotheses: the **null** hypothesis H_0 and the **alternate hypothesis H_a**. The null hypothesis is so named since it often reflects a "no evidence" situation; lacking evidence, one believes or proceeds as specified by H_0. When a problem of comparison is defined by statements reflecting "equal or not equal," then the equal statement must be placed in the null hypothesis H_0 and the not-equal statement in the alternate hypothesis H_a. In the health sciences, when a problem of comparison is defined by an inequality, H_a carries the research hypothesis or intervention hypothesis as suggested by a research or intervention motivation in the supporting health sciences problem.

The decision about which hypothesis to choose, H_0 or H_a, is made by a procedure called **test of hypothesis**. A statistical test of hypothesis is a decision-making procedure that chooses between H_0 and H_a based on data obtained from a sample and predicated on the assumption H_0 is true unless the data warrant rejecting H_0 in favor of H_a. Because of the pivotal role H_0 plays in test of hypothesis, when a statistical problem of comparison is presented, one presents H_0 first, with H_a following.

There is always a risk of error when one makes an inference about a population based on a sample. This error is merely the result of the chance luck of the draw in obtaining a random sample. There are two principal types of errors that can be made in conducting a test of hypothesis. If the null hypothesis is true, one might erroneously reject it. Such an error is called a **rejection error** (formally, type I error). The probability of making such an error is called the **level of significance** for the test of hypothesis. If the null hypothesis is false, one might erroneously retain it. Such an error is called an **acceptance error** (formally, type II error).

Diagnostic testing is a special application of test of hypothesis found in clinical and behavioral health sciences.

Keywords

acceptance error	problem of comparison
alternate hypothesis	problem of location
confidence interval	random variable
level of significance	rejection error
null hypothesis	research hypothesis
parameter	test of hypothesis
population	test reference value
power	

References

Lepley-Frey D: Dysrhythmias and blood pressure changes associated with thrombolysis. *Heart Lung* 20, no. 4 (July 1991): 335.

Woo M et al: Comparison of thermodilution and transthoracic electrical bioimpedance cardiac outputs. *Heart Lung* 20, no. 4 (July 1991): 357.

10

Tests of Hypothesis
for One Population

Does a new procedure for postoperative treatment of lung cancer really improve the current 5-year survival rate? Does a new, simpler method for measuring blood hemoglobin produce a result consistent with known reference values? In general, do ice-temperature and room-temperature injectates produce the same cardiac output?

Each of these questions suggests a problem of comparison in that each inquires how a given technique compares against some benchmark or reference value. Test of hypothesis is a procedure designed to resolve such problems.

The preceding questions are taken from the literature. We pose these questions in more detailed settings in the various sections in Chapter 10. Section 10.1 is concerned with the proportion. Section 10.2 is concerned with an average value. Section 10.3 extends Section 10.2 to deal with a common and very important statistical design in the health sciences: paired data.

The first three sections have two main objectives. The first objective is to master the general test of hypothesis procedure by analyzing problems of interest in the health sciences. Each problem solved adds clarity to the overall idea of test of hypothesis. There are several details to learn in test of hypothesis, and each problem has its own way of making some facet clear. The second objective is to add to our understanding of the general nature of proportion and average value; in particular, how to recast a problem in the health sciences into a statistical problem of comparison. It is amazing that so much in-depth analysis is geared to reducing a complicated health sciences situation into a mere statistical test of a proportion against a reference value. Usually, once a "word problem" can be reduced to a formal statement of hypothesis, one is well on the way toward resolving a problem at hand.

Section 10.4 introduces the concept of *p-value* into hypothesis testing. The *p*-value is a single-number summary of the entire test of hypothesis. Professionals writing in the literature usually report the *p*-value of a test. Professionals reading the literature know to look for the *p*-value of a test of hypothesis. In a "word," it tells them what they need to know as far as the statistics is concerned.

SECTION 10.1

Test of Hypothesis— Proportion

OBJECTIVES   This section will

1   Describe the design of one-population comparison studies in the health sciences.

2   Conduct a statistical test of hypothesis for the proportion when provided with an appropriate health sciences problem that contains a description of the population, a characteristic of interest, and a random sample with independent observations drawn from the population. The formal write-up should follow Chart 1 (Appendix).

Test of hypothesis is a procedure that makes a decision about a problem of comparison based on data. In this chapter we apply tests of hypothesis to resolve one-population problems of comparison.

EXAMPLE 10.1.1 (see Example 9.1.4) A new drug is being developed for use in the treatment of lung cancer. It is hoped that the drug will improve the current 5-year survival rate of .33 for patients who undergo surgery for treatment of lung cancer. Formally, we inquire whether

$$H_0: p \leq .33 \quad \text{null hypothesis}$$
$$H_a: p > .33 \quad \text{alternate hypothesis}$$

where p is the proportion of patients undergoing surgery for treatment of lung cancer who are also treated with the new drug. Researchers reported that in a study of 53 lung cancer patients who used the drug, 33 survived 5 years after surgery.

Although test of hypothesis is a procedure that makes a decision based on data, *not just any data will do*. Any test of hypothesis is based on assumptions about the design of the study that produced the data. These assumptions should be checked thoroughly before diving into calculations. This also explains why research articles usually pose the problem(s) of concern, then describe the design applied to obtain their data, then describe the analysis, and finally present the conclusions. Accordingly, we look further into the design of the study that produced the data in Example 10.1.1 (33 of 53 patients survived 5 years after surgery).

Design in a One-Population Problem of Comparison Study

Any study begins by specifying the populations (who) and the random variables (RVs) (what about them) of interest. A study that specifies just one population is called a **one-population** study. Example 10.1.1 displays a one-population study; the population of interest is patients undergoing surgery for treatment of lung cancer who are also treated with the new drug.

Statistics offers useful tools for providing insight into a health sciences concern that can be formulated into a problem of comparison. A problem of comparison is formally presented by displaying the null and alternate hypotheses. A problem of comparison posed in a one-population study is called simply a **one-population problem of comparison**. We note that Example 10.1.1 displays a one-population problem of comparison.

We will be able to resolve a one-population problem of comparison when given a *random sample with independent observations* taken from the population of interest.

Comment For convenience, the word *sample* is often used interchangeably to stand for either (1) the set of subjects who are studied, or (2) the data set obtained from those subjects. For example, in the Daily and Mersch cardiac output study (Appendix, Data Set 1), we say that the RTCO column is a sample of room-temperature cardiac outputs. Strictly speaking, the sample consists of the 29 patients in the study; the RTCO column is a data set of room-temperature cardiac outputs obtained from those 29 patients. Insisting on such strict language, however, makes for tedious communication. Context will imply which is meant: the person in the sample, or the reading associated with that person.

Random Samples

The reason for the requirement of a random sample is to allow one to assume that the sample is reasonably representative of the population at large. Ideally, the assumption of a random sample is met by utilizing a **simple random sample**, in which each member of the population has an equal chance of being chosen. This strict criterion, however, is not possible due to the common problems of time and money. For example, the question, Should a new drug be prescribed for patients undergoing surgery for treatment of lung cancer? applies not just to current patients but also to such patients in the near future (there is no way one can currently sample future patients!). Further, resource constraints usually prevent identifying and surveying everyone currently having a given condition, making a simple random sample of the population unfeasible. In the health sciences, one is usually content with a convenience sample rather than a simple random sample.

A **convenience sample** is a sample consisting of subjects who are currently available. Since the researcher takes from whoever happens to be there, the spirit of randomness usually is maintained. The intent of the word *convenience* is that the researcher conveniently takes from those currently available, rather than being inconvenienced with the burden of a simple random sample. For example, the researcher may take into a study the next 25 patients who give informed consent, or all patients admitted over the next 4 weeks. A study that samples from the next set of patients who happen to present is called a **prospective** study because of its future outlook. In contrast, a **retrospective** study has a past rather than a future orientation; it uses a sample of past patients. For example, a researcher may study the medical records of the past 25 patients or all patients over the past 4 weeks. In Example 10.1.1 the researchers at the onset used a convenience sample of 53 patients in a prospective study.

Convenience samples in the health sciences maintain the spirit of randomness when they avoid biasing the result with a confounding effect. A **confounding effect** is a characteristic that is not specified in the definition of a population in the study but is substantially present or absent in the sample. A classic example of confounding occurred during the Dewey versus Truman presidential election in 1944. Pollsters (using a random telephone sample) declared even on the eve of the election that Governor Dewey would win. The pollsters' result was confounded by restricting the polling to voters who had telephones (in 1944, telephone ownership was more common among wealthier people, who tended to be Republican and thus vote for Dewey). The biasing characteristic of "owning a telephone" was substantially present in the sample to an extent not found in the general electorate.

Whenever a convenience sample is used, one should give a full report of any exclusions in the study. An **exclusion** is a subject who is either screened from enrollment into a study or who is dropped from the sample during the course of the study. For example, a prospective study of coronary patients may enroll the next 50 admissions to a coronary care unit but exclude those with a pacemaker implant. Or a study of patients undergoing surgery for treatment of lung cancer may drop those who develop certain heart or liver conditions. Failure to report exclusions means failure to report conditions that may confound the results when applied to the general patient population.

Independent Observations

A sample contains **independent observations** if an observation made on one member of the sample does not affect or influence the observation made on any other member. This assumption is met by taking only one reading per member of the sample. For example, consider the Daily and Mersch cardiac output study (see Appendix, Data Set 1). The sample of room-temperature cardiac outputs is a sample of independent observations since there is one room-temperature cardiac output measurement recorded per patient. Similarly, the ITCO column displays another sample of independent observations, as does the Fick column.

A sample contains dependent observations if there are at least two observations recorded on the same individual. For example, the first row of cardiac outputs in the Daily and Mersch data table constitutes a sample with dependent observations since the room, ice, and Fick cardiac outputs were all taken on patient 1. Any research article that reports something like "47 observations on 32 patients" is not working with a sample with independent observations.

Independent observations are required so that the data set obtained from the sample maintains the random quality of the sample. If one were allowed to take several observations on a few individuals, then the resulting data set would be suspect of representing the population (much akin to "stuffing the ballot box"). We may assume that the observations in Example 10.1.1 are independent observations. In that study there was only one observation per patient (survived 5 years postsurgery, or died). Further, whether one particular patient survived or not did not influence whether any other patient in the study survived or not. Hence, it is reasonable to assume that the sample described in Example 10.1.1 (33 of 53 survived) is a random sample with independent observations.

For the methods presented in this text, the assumption of independent samples is crucial and cannot be violated. A sample containing dependent observations needs the services of a professional statistician for full analysis.

Once we have formally launched a one-population problem of comparison with an appropriate null hypothesis H_0 and alternate hypothesis H_a, we then want to decide between H_0 and H_a. We will be able to make that decision if we are provided with data from a random sample with independent observations. The decision is made by following the directions provided in a test of hypothesis chart.

Test of Hypothesis Charts

The purpose of test of hypothesis (TOH) is to decide between H_0 and H_a based on an appropriate data set. Toward this end, the Appendix contains several test of hypothesis charts to guide one through the details of the procedure. After selecting the appropriate chart (using H_0 and H_a as a key), carefully follow the directions to arrive at the appropriate decision based on the given data. The solution is written following the seven-step protocol outlined in Section 9.1. The charts in the Appendix contain the first five of these steps since details vary from test to test. The general nature of steps 6 and 7 are the same for all tests and therefore are not repeated in each chart.

Some tests have criteria. These preliminary criteria are assumptions on which a theoretical formulation and justification of the main TOH are based. One must first check any preliminary criteria to ensure that one's choice of test is valid. It is valid to apply the main test only if all preliminary criteria are satisfied. For example, Chart 1 carries a preliminary criterion to check for adequacy of sample size.

In the main TOH, we will need to know whether the test is one- or two-tailed. Review the form of the H_0 and H_a statements in Examples 9.1.3–8. Note that some hypotheses are presented as "equal versus not equal" statements, while the others involve inequalities ($<$ or $>$ in H_a). A TOH utilizing an "equal versus not equal" set of hypotheses (Examples 9.1.5–7) is called a **two-tailed test**. In a two-tailed test, the "equals" statement is *always* carried in the null hypothesis H_0; the "not equals" statement is *always* carried in the alternate hypothesis H_a. A TOH involving inequalities (Examples 9.1.3, 9.1.4, and 9.1.8) is called a **one-tailed test**. In a one-tailed test, the alternate hypothesis is *always* the "burden of proof" hypothesis, usually reflecting a research or intervention motivation from the associated health sciences problem. Each TOH chart is constructed so that alternate (a) is a two-tailed test, while alternates (b) and (c) are one-tailed tests.

Step 1 in the main TOH is to identify the nature of the hypothesis being tested. Each chart provides three alternates: (a), (b), and (c). Your write-up for step 1 should state three items: (1) the null hypothesis H_0 and alternate hypothesis H_a, (2) the test alternate (a, b, or c from the chart), and (3) whether the test is one- or two-tailed.

Step 2 states a level of significance (LOS). The usual standard in the health sciences is an LOS of .05; that is, the test will carry an inherent 5% risk of rejecting H_0 if H_0 is true.

Conducting a Test of Hypothesis for a Proportion

A one-population problem of comparison involving a proportion is resolved by applying the test of hypothesis detailed in Chart 1 (Appendix) to a given random sample with independent observations. Figure 10.1.1 displays the solution for the problem of comparison presented in Example 10.1.1 (the lung cancer problem). We now discuss the point-by-point details of writing up the test of hypothesis displayed in Figure 10.1.1.

The preliminary criteria specified in Chart 1 are criteria to determine whether the sample size is sufficiently large to justify applying the main test. The main test is valid only if both of the given sample size criteria are met. If the preliminary criteria are not met, halt the test (consult a statistician for further analysis). Here, the preliminary criteria are met, so we proceed to the seven-step main test.

Step 1 displays the null hypothesis ($H_0: p \leq .33$) and the alternate hypotheses ($H_a: p > .33$), and notes that they have the form of test alternate (c), a one-tailed test.

Step 2 informs that we will conduct the test at the 5% level of significance; that is, $\alpha = .05$.

Step 3 displays the test statistic. Note that the test reference number from the null hypothesis (here, $p_0 = .33$) is inserted into the test statistic in a specific problem. The test statistic tells the researcher what is to be done with data once the data have been obtained. Hence, the test statistic acts as a guide indicating to the researcher what data need to be collected. Here, we examine a sample of n patients (who use the drug after surgical treatment for lung cancer) and determine the sample proportion, p (the proportion of patients who survive ≥ 5 years). *Do not carry out the sample calculations yet*; that is, do not substitute the sample information into the test statistic (that comes in step 6).

FIGURE **10.1.1** The formal write-up for the lung cancer problem (Example 10.1.1) is given. The write-up presents a test of hypothesis for the proportion, single population, in the seven-step format following the protocol of Chart 1 (Appendix).

I. Preliminary Criteria. Note that n (sample size) = 53 and p_0 (test reference value from H_0) = .33. So,

  (a) $np_0 = (53)(.33) = 17.49 \geq 5$, and
  (b) $n(1 - p_0) = (53)(1 - .33) = (53)(.67) = 35.51 \geq 5$

Hence, a sample of size n = 53 is sufficiently large.

II. Main Test of Hypothesis.

1. Hypothesis. $H_0: p \leq .33$ Test alternate (c);
             $H_a: p > .33$ a one-tailed test.

2. LOS. $\alpha = 0.05$

3. Test Statistic. $\dfrac{\hat{p} - .33}{\sqrt{\dfrac{.33(1 - .33)}{n}}} = \dfrac{\hat{p} - .33}{\sqrt{\dfrac{.2211}{n}}}$

4. Critical Value. z = 1.645 (from Appendix Table 8, Z-Table for Test of Hypothesis, one-tailed test, LOS .05).

5. Decision Line. Use decision line alternate (c) since the test of hypothesis is of alternate (c).

      Do Not Reject H_0 | Reject H_0
      ———————————————————→ Z
                1.645

6. Sample Value.

  sample z $= \dfrac{\hat{p} - .33}{\sqrt{\dfrac{.2211}{n}}} = \dfrac{\frac{33}{53} - .33}{\sqrt{\dfrac{.2211}{53}}} = 4.531$

7. Conclusion. Based on the given data, at the 5% LOS we reject $H_0: p \leq 0.33$ and accept $H_a: p > 0.33$. The data strongly supports that the new drug is effective in increasing the 5-year survival rate for patients who undergo surgery for treatment of lung cancer.

Step 4 is to obtain the critical value for the test, a value needed in step 5. One obtains the critical value from a table as directed in the chart. Here, one is directed to the Z-Table for Test of Hypothesis (Appendix, Table 8). To use the Z-Table, one must know the LOS for the test (step 2) and whether one is applying a one- or two-tailed test (step 1). In our example we have a one-tailed test and LOS .05. The test critical value, $z = 1.645$, is read directly from the Z-Table.

Step 5 constructs the decision line. One uses decision line alternate (a), (b), or (c) in tandem with the test alternate identified in step 1. In this example, since the TOH is of alternate (c), then we also use a decision line of form (c). Draw the form (c) decision line as indicated in the chart. Using a ruler, draw a straight line segment, put an arrow on the right-hand end of the line, and label the decision line Z by the tip of the arrow. Put a tick mark on the decision line as indicated in the chart, and label the tick mark with the test critical value 1.645 obtained in step 4. The theory behind the 5% LOS decision line is that if the null hypothesis is true, then among all possible samples that can be drawn, only 5% of those samples, when run through the test statistic, will yield a sample value (step 6) that falls in the reject H_0 zone.

The key objective of these first five steps is to obtain the decision line. Ideally, these five steps should be done as part of the statistical design, before any fieldwork or data collection begins.

Step 6 carries out the calculations using the sample data. The sample data are substituted into the test statistic (displayed in step 3). The test statistic may be thought of as the test "trash compactor" since it compresses the sample data into a single number, the sample value (here, 4.531). As a rule of thumb, we recommend carrying out the computation of the sample value to as many decimal places as used in the critical value. Here, the critical value 1.645 (step 4) shows three places past the decimal point; hence, we also report the sample value to three places past the decimal point. The sample value is now sent to the decision line (displayed in step 5) for the verdict.

Step 7 announces the conclusion using at least two sentences. The first sentence states the simple statistical conclusion (reject H_0). Then, and most importantly, the practical implication is given. The bottom line is: What does it all mean for providing care? Here, we find that the data provide evidence that the drug does indeed statistically improve the 5-year survival rate for lung cancer patients. Clinicians should strongly consider incorporating this drug into the treatment protocol for patients undergoing surgery for treatment of lung cancer.

EXAMPLE 10.1.2 (see Example 9.1.5) To decide about the fairness of coin flips, Nancy posed the following problem of comparison:

$H_0: p = .5$ (fair coin hypothesis)
$H_a: p \neq .5$

where p is the proportion of heads showing in tossing a coin. To decide whether her coin is fair, Nancy flips her coin 100 times. She observes 54 heads and 46 tails. The TOH write-up for this example is given in Figure 10.1.2.

FIGURE **10.1.2**
The following displays the formal write-up for the coin flip (Example 10.1.2). The example illustrates a test of hypothesis for the proportion, single population, presented in the seven-step format following the protocol of Chart 1 (Appendix).

I. Preliminary. Note that $n = 100$ and $p_0 = 0.5$. Thus,

    (a) $np_0 = (100)(0.5) = 50 \geq 5$, and
    (b) $n(1 - p_0) = (100)(0.5) = (50) \geq 5$

Hence, the sample size is adequately large.

II. Main Test of Hypothesis.

    1. Hypothesis. $H_0: p = 0.5$ Alternate (a);
                      $H_a: p \neq 0.5$ two-tailed test.

    2. LOS. $\alpha = 0.05$

    3. Test Statistic. $\dfrac{\hat{p} - 0.5}{\sqrt{\dfrac{.5(1 - .5)}{n}}} = \dfrac{\hat{p} - 0.5}{\sqrt{\dfrac{.25}{n}}}$ *.5 two tailed test pg 443.*

    4. Critical Value. $z = 1.960$ (Appendix, Table 8)

    5. Decision Line. Alternate (a): *two tailed test*

        Reject H_0 Do Not Reject H_0 Reject H_0
               -1.960 1.960 z

    6. Sample Value.

$$\text{sample } z = \frac{\hat{p} - 0.5}{\sqrt{\dfrac{.25}{n}}} = \frac{\dfrac{54}{100} - 0.5}{\sqrt{\dfrac{.25}{100}}} = 0.800$$

    7. Conclusion. Based on the given data, at the 5% LOS we do not reject $H_0: p = 0.5$. The results of the coin toss are consistent with the toss of a fair coin.

Is the test of hypothesis in Example 10.1.2 justified? Note that Nancy's original concern is whether flipping her coin is "fair." She decides to resolve her concern by seeing if flipping the coin produces heads in a "50–50" fashion over 100 tosses. Her population of interest is a conceptual one: all possible flips of her coin. A simple random sample is impossible, so she decides on a convenience sample of the next 100 flips of the coin (a prospective study). At each flip, she makes one observation, heads (yes or no). She also takes steps in her study design to ensure that no one result affects any other result (place the coin in a cup, shake, and toss). Hence, we may assume that her sample of 100 tosses constitutes a random sample with independent observations. The resulting data are suitable to resolve the stated problem of comparison by applying the TOH detailed in Chart 1.

EXERCISES 10.1

Warm-ups 10.1

These Warm-ups are based on the research by Kirby et al (see Figure 1.1.10). Planners are concerned about the severity and causes of injuries of patients admitted to an adult trauma center (ATC). Clinicians felt that the severity of injury in the majority of cases necessitated transfer from the ATC to an intensive care unit (ICU). This feeling was incorporated as part of a larger study of ATC patients that took place at the University of Tennessee Medical Center beginning on 1 March 1988 and lasting for 5 months. During the course of the study, data were obtained on each new admission at a level 1 ATC. During the 5-month study period, there were 496 admissions to the ATC. Of these, 270 were transferred to an ICU.

1. The population of interest is
   a. Patients transferred to an ICU
   b. Patients admitted to an ATC
   c. Patients
   d. Trauma patients
   e. Admissions to the University of Tennessee Medical Center

2. The RV of interest is
   a. Transferred to an ICU (yes or no)
   b. Admitted to an ATC (yes or no)
   c. Trauma (yes or no)
   d. Admitted to the University of Tennessee (yes or no)

3. The parameter of interest is

   a. An ICU

   b. The ATC

   c. Trauma

   d. The proportion of ATC patients transferred to an ICU

   e. The majority

4. Clinicians felt that "the majority of admissions to an ATC are transferred to an ICU." Research is conducted to check this impression. Accordingly, the researchers formally state

$$H_0: p \leq .5$$
$$H_a: p > .5$$

Comparison

where p is the proportion of ATC patients transferred to an ICU. This formal statement of hypothesis presents

   a. A clinical problem of urgency

   b. A test of hypothesis

   c. A problem of location

   d. A problem of comparison

5. The study utilizes a sample of 496 admissions to a level 1 ATC. This sample constitutes

   a. A simple random sample

   b. The population of interest

   c. The data set

   d. A convenience sample

   e. A problem of comparison

6. Kirby et al reported that of these 496 admissions to the ATC, 270 were transferred to an ICU. Does this report describe a random sample with independent observations? (yes or no). YES

independent ADMISSION TO ICU each case was looked at.

7. A point estimate for p (proportion of ATC admissions transferred to an ICU) is calculated by

$$\hat{p} = \tfrac{270}{496} = .54 \ (54\%) \quad \text{NO.}$$

Does this verify that a majority of ATC admissions are transferred to the ICU? (yes or no).

We now conduct a test of hypothesis at the 5% level of significance following Chart 1 to resolve the problem H_0: $p \leq .5$ versus H_a: $p > .5$ based on the given data (270 of 496 ATC patients were transferred to an ICU).

8. What is the null hypothesis for this test? $p \leq .5$

9. What is the alternate hypothesis for this test? $p > .5$

10. What is the test reference value for this test? .5

11. According to Chart 1, we need to check preliminary criteria for adequacy of sample size. Here,

$$np_0 = 496 \times .5 = 248 \quad \text{and}$$
$$n(1 - p_0) = (496) \times (.5) = 248$$

Is the sample size adequate to conduct this TOH? yes

12. Is this a one- or two-tailed test? one

13. According to Chart 1, Step 1, which test alternate do we use: (a), (b), or (c)? c

14. From Table 8, at the 5% LOS, what is the test critical value?

15. Which form of the decision line do we use: (a), (b), or (c)?

16. Construct the decision line for this test.

17. To obtain the sample value (Chart 1, Step 6), the data are substituted into the test statistic:

$$\text{sample } z = \frac{\hat{p} - p_0}{\sqrt{\frac{p_0(1 - p_0)}{n}}} = \frac{\frac{270}{496} - .5}{\sqrt{\frac{.5(1 - .5)}{496}}} = \_\_\_$$

18. Does the sample z-value fall in the "do not reject H_0" zone or the "reject H_0" zone?

19. Does the result confirm or deny the research hypothesis?

20. What conclusion can you draw from this test of hypothesis?

Problems 10.1

Problems 10.1.1–3 are continuations of Warm-up 10.1 based on the research described by Kirby et al in Figure 1.1.10. Planners are concerned about the main causes for admission into an intensive care unit (ICU) among trauma patients. It is feared that a substantial proportion of such admissions are consequences of substance abuse by the patient. A study was made that screened patients for (nonprescription) drugs or alcohol at the time of admission into an adult trauma center (ATC).

1. During the study there were 496 patients admitted into the ATC. Of these, 270 were transferred to an ICU. Let p be the proportion of patients admitted to the ATC who are transferred to an ICU.

   a. Determine a 90% confidence interval for p. Is this result consistent with the TOH conducted in the warm-ups?

   b. At the 5% level of significance, test the research hypothesis that the proportion of patients admitted to the ATC who are transferred to an ICU is under 70%.

   c. At the 5% level of significance, are the study data consistent with the notion that 55% of admissions to the ATC are transferred to an ICU?

2. Drug and alcohol profiles were (randomly) obtained on 212 patients admitted to the ATC who were transferred to an ICU. Of these, 123 tested positive for drugs and/or alcohol. Let p be the proportion of those patients admitted to the ATC and transferred to an ICU who test positive for drugs and/or alcohol.

   a. Determine a point estimate for p.

   b. Determine a 90% confidence interval for p.

   c. At the 5% LOS, test the research hypothesis that the majority of patients admitted to the ATC and transferred to an ICU would test positive for drugs and/or alcohol.

   d. At the 5% LOS, test the research hypothesis that the proportion of patients admitted to the ATC and transferred to an ICU who would test positive for drugs and/or alcohol is under 75%.

   e. At the 5% LOS, are the study data consistent with the notion that 60% of patients admitted to the ATC and transferred to an ICU would test positive for drugs and/or alcohol?

3. The researchers stated that "over half of the patients who were positive for alcohol were also positive for drugs." Of the 81 patients who tested positive for alcohol, 51 tested positive for drugs. Let p be the proportion of patients who are admitted to an ATC, transferred to an ICU, testing positive for alcohol, who would also test positive for (nonprescription) drugs.

   a. Determine a point estimate for p.

   b. Determine a 90% confidence interval for p.

   c. At the 5% LOS, test the research hypothesis that over half of these patients would also test positive for drugs.

   d. At the 5% LOS, are the study data consistent with the notion that two-thirds of such patients would also test positive for drugs?

4. Rovner et al reported on a sample of 454 newly admitted nursing home patients who were enrolled in a study in 1987–88 in Maryland. In 1985 the National Nursing Home Survey (NNHS) announced that 20.5% of nursing home patients had cerebrovascular disease (CVD). In the Rovner et al study group, 121 of the 454 patients in the study were found to have CVD.

   a. Based on the study, determine a 95% confidence interval for p, the proportion of newly admitted nursing home patients who have CVD.

   b. Conduct an appropriate test of hypothesis at the 5% LOS to determine whether the proportion of patients with CVD in the study is statistically significantly different than the proportion announced by NNHS.

5. Klatsky et al reported on coffee drinking as a risk factor for heart attack. The researchers studied a population of patients who received health examinations at Oakland and San Francisco facilities of Kaiser Permanente Medical Care Program from January 1978 through December 1985. Of 1914 persons hospitalized for coronary disease, 740 were admitted to the hospital diagnosed with myocardial infarction (MI).

   a. Determine a 95% confidence interval for the proportion of coronary patients admitted to the hospital diagnosed with MI.

   b. Test the research hypothesis that the majority of coronary patients hospitalized for coronary disease have a diagnosis of MI.

   c. Are the data consistent with the hypothesis that 40% of coronary patients hospitalized for coronary disease have a diagnosis of MI?

6. (Continued from Problem 9.1.8) The research hypothesis of this study was that $\geq 75\%$ of the skin impedance results (transthoracic electrical bio-impedance, TEB) would have absolute differences

of ≤ 0.5 liters/minute from simultaneous thermodilution cardiac outputs in the subpopulation of critically ill patients with heart failure. In 80 cardiac output readings, 25 readings were within the 0.5-liters/minute range and 55 were outside it. Based on these data, should the research hypothesis be accepted?

7. Sorsensen et al studied the effects of a work-site nonsmoking policy as an incentive for employees to stop smoking. On 1 July 1985, the New England Telephone Company (NETCo) announced a companywide policy restricting smoking. This corporate policy was nontrivial since NETCo employed 27,374 people at about 600 sites. From 1 September 1985 smoking was banned in conference rooms and classrooms and was restricted in cafeterias and lounges. On 1 March 1986 smoking was banned in all work areas including individual offices.

   A random sample of employees was surveyed in November 1987. Of 375 survey respondents who were smokers when they first became aware of the policy, 79 said they had quit smoking altogether. Of the 79 respondents who were smokers when they first became aware of the policy but had since quit smoking, 32 reported that they quit smoking due to the policy.

   a. Determine a point estimate for the proportion of NETCo employees who were smokers when they first became aware of the policy but subsequently quit smoking.

   b. Determine a 95% confidence interval for the proportion specified in (a).

   c. The expected quit rate for this period was 5% (the reported quit rate in the general population is 2% to 5% per year). Based on the results of the survey, did the quit rate following NETCo's smoking policy exceed the expected normal quit rate of 5%?

   d. Determine a point estimate and a 95% confidence interval for the proportion of quitters who quit due to the policy.

   e. Determine a point estimate and a 95% confidence interval for the proportion of smokers who quit due to the policy.

   f. In (a) and (b), a "quitter" is defined as an employee who was smoking at the start of NETCo's smoking policy but was self-declared as not smoking at the time of the survey. A further look at the data showed that 13 of the quitters had quit smoking only within the past 3 months. Hence, 66 of the responders had quit for at least the past 3 months. Now use the definition of a quitter as an employee who was not smoking at the time of the survey and had stopped smoking for at least 3 months. Based on this definition, did the quit rate following NETCo's policy exceed the expected normal quit rate of 5%?

8. Harding et al studied catheter-acquired urinary tract infection in women. In their study, 112 asymptomatic female patients with catheter-acquired bacteriuremia were randomly assigned to various treatment groups. A group of 42 women was assigned to a control group and received no treatment. The other 70 women received treatment. The researchers recorded whether the infection was resolved within 14 days.

   a. The infection resolved in 15 of the 42 patients in the no-therapy group during the 14-day period. At the 10% level of significance, test the research hypothesis that the majority of infections were not resolved.

   b. Among the women who received treatment, 56 of 70 resolved. At the 10% level of significance, test the research hypothesis that most ($>60\%$) infections among women receiving treatment resolved.

9. Jonsbu et al claimed that over 10% of patients with a final diagnosis of myocardial infarction (MI) are incorrectly referred to the general ward (rather than the coronary care unit) on admission. Their data showed that of 503 MI patients in two major hospitals in Norway, 56 were incorrectly referred to the general ward. At the 5% LOS, do the given data support the stated claim?

10. Zwerling et al did a cost-benefit analysis of preemployment drug screening for the U.S. Postal Service in the Boston area. Their analysis focused on the economic costs and benefits to the Postal Service. The costs included the costs of drug screening and costs of hiring a new employee to replace the one screened out by a positive drug test. The benefits included savings resulting from lower absenteeism, injury, and accident rates. The

analysis showed that the cost-to-benefit result depended on the prevalence of drug use among applicants (this dependency is exactly the same as the role played by prevalence in diagnostic testing presented in Section 4.1). The break-even point is 3.2%; that is, if the prevalence of illegal drug use exceeds 3.2%, then a preemployment drug screening program would be cost-effective. In the study, 2533 applicants were screened for drugs by testing a urine sample. An applicant was considered drug-positive if the urine sample showed unprescribed marijuana, cocaine, phencyclidine, amphetamines, benzodiazepines, methaqualone, or propoxyphene. Among the 2533 applicants, 307 tested positive for drugs.

a. Determine a point estimate for the proportion of Postal Service applicants in Boston who test positive for drugs.

b. Determine a 95% confidence interval for the proportion of Postal Service applicants in Boston who test positive for drugs.

c. At the 5% LOS, does the prevalence of illegal drugs among Postal Service applicants in the Boston area exceed 3.2%? Answer by conducting an appropriate test of hypothesis.

d. What do you think—would you advocate a system of preemployment drug screening?

Problems 11–18 are based on research by Polednak, who studied data on all incident cancer cases diagnosed in people who were born in Puerto Rico but resided on Long Island during 1980–86. Polednak wanted to compare the incidence of cancer among the 9440 men and 10,500 women among these Puerto Rican–born residents of Long Island with (1) U.S. non–Puerto Ricans and (2) Puerto Rican residents. Polednak used data from the Surveillance, Epidemiology and End Results (SEER) Program of the National Cancer Institute to determine age- and sex-adjusted cancer rates for these comparison groups during the same 1980–86 time frame. Such studies of migrants can give insights into the role that the environment plays in cancer rates.

11. Polednak reported that there were 39 diagnosed cases of lung cancer among the 9440 Puerto Rican–born males living on Long Island during 1980–86. The corresponding lung cancer rate for the male U.S. non–Puerto Rican population was .004936.

a. Conduct a test of hypothesis to determine whether the observed proportion (39/9440) is consistent with the proportion (.004936) of cancer in the U.S. non–Puerto Rican population; that is, test $H_0: p = .004936$.

b. Assuming that the cancer rate for both groups is the same (.004936), how many lung cancer cases would you expect to see among the 9440 males? Is this expected number statistically significantly different from the observed number 39?

c. Do you feel that the incidence of lung cancer among Puerto Rican–born men living on Long Island during 1980–86 was less than, the same as, or greater than that for the U.S. non–Puerto Rican population. Explain.

12. (Continued from Problem 11) Using the SEER as a guide, Polednak determined that the corresponding lung cancer incidence rate for male Puerto Rican residents is .001367.

a. Conduct a TOH to determine if the observed proportion (39/9440) is consistent with the lung cancer rate for Puerto Rican residents.

b. Assuming that the cancer rate for both groups is the same (.001367), how many lung cancer cases would you expect to see among the 9440 males? Is this expected number statistically significantly different from the observed number 39?

c. Do you feel that the incidence of lung cancer among Puerto Rican–born men living on Long Island during 1980–86 was less than, the same as, or greater than that for Puerto Rican residents? Explain.

13. There were a total of 177 cancer cases among the 9440 Puerto Rican men living on Long Island during 1980–86. Using the SEER as a guide, Polednak determined that the corresponding incidence rate for all cancers for male U.S. non–Puerto Ricans is .02421.

a. Conduct a TOH to determine if the observed proportion (177/9440) is consistent with the total cancer rate for male Puerto Rican residents.

b. Assuming that the cancer rate for both groups is the same (.02421), how many cancer cases would you expect to see among the 9440 males? Is this expected number statistically significantly different from the observed number 177?

c. Do you feel that the incidence of cancer among Puerto Rican–born men living on Long Island during 1980–86 was less than, the same as, or greater than that for male Puerto Rican residents? Explain.

14. (Continued from Problem 13) The corresponding incidence rate for all cancers for the male residents of Puerto Rico was .01428. Is cancer incidence among Puerto Ricans on Long Island greater than in Puerto Rico?

15. There were 218 observed cancer cases among the 10,500 Puerto Rican women living on Long Island during 1980–86. The corresponding incidence rate for all cancers for the female non–Puerto Rican population is .02279.

a. Conduct a TOH to determine if the observed proportion (218/10500) is consistent with the total cancer rate for female U.S. non–Puerto Rican residents.

b. Assuming that the cancer rate for both groups is the same (.02279), how many cancer cases would you expect to see among the 10,500 women? Is this expected number statistically significantly different from the observed number 218?

c. Do you feel that the incidence of cancer among Puerto Rican–born women living on Long Island during 1980–86 was less than, the same as, or greater than that for U.S. non–Puerto Rican women? Explain.

16. (Continued from Problem 15) The corresponding incidence rate for all cancers for female Puerto Rican residents is .01295.

a. Conduct a TOH to determine if the observed proportion (218/10,500) is consistent with the total cancer rate for female Puerto Rican residents.

b. Assuming that the cancer rate for both groups is the same (.01295), how many cancer cases would you expect to see among the 10,500 women? Is this expected number statistically significantly different from the observed number 218?

c. Do you feel that the incidence of cancer among Puerto Rican–born women living on Long Island during 1980–86 was less than, the same

as, or greater than that for Puerto Rican women? Explain.

17. There were 62 observed breast cancer cases among the 10,500 Puerto Rican women living on Long Island during 1980–86 The corresponding incidence rate for breast cancers for the female non–Puerto Rican population is .00752.

a. Conduct a TOH to determine if the observed proportion (62/10,500) is consistent with the breast cancer rate for female U.S. non–Puerto Rican residents.

b. Assuming that the cancer rate for both groups is the same (.00752), how many cancer cases would you expect to see among the 10,500 women? Is this expected number statistically significantly different from the observed number 62?

c. Do you feel that the incidence of breast cancer among Puerto Rican–born women living on Long Island during 1980–86 was less than, the same as, or greater than that for U.S. non–Puerto Rican women? Explain.

18. (Continued from Problem 17) The corresponding incidence rate for breast cancers for the female Puerto Rican population is .0035. Is the incidence of breast cancer among Puerto Rican–born women living on Long Island greater than the incidence of breast cancer among the women of Puerto Rico?

19. Tiwary and Holguin studied obesity in dependent children of military personnel. They obtained a convenience sample of 1078 children ≥ 1 year of age admitted to the pediatric clinic at the Brooks Army Medical Center in San Antonio, Texas, from 1 October through 31 December 1986. They defined a child as very obese if the child was $> 140\%$ of ideal weight for age and sex. Of these 1078 children, 97 were very obese at the time of admission. Data from a large study in 1978 indicated that the proportion of very obese children was 5.5%. Based on the given data, is there evidence that the proportion of very obese children has statistically significantly increased from 1978 to 1986?

20. Berky et al reported on the incidence of allergy associated with the use of latex gloves. The researchers surveyed dentists in the U.S. Army. The researchers wanted to test several hypotheses based on their review of the literature. Their first hypothesis was that "the prevalence of latex glove-associated allergies will exeed 5%." Of 1043 dentists surveyed (all used gloves), 143 reported a latex glove allergy.

a. Determine a point estimate for the proportion of dentists who develop latex glove allergy.

b. Determine a 95% confidence interval for the proportion of dentists who develop latex glove allergy.

c. Conduct an appropriate TOH to determine whether or not the stated research hypothesis should be accepted. (Hint: recall the research hypothesis is H_a.)

Problems 21–24 are based on data from Chapman and Duff, who studied the frequency of glove perforations associated with selected obstetric surgery procedures. Obstetrics personnel at a Florida hospital double gloved for cesarean delivery, postpartum tubal sterilization, and vaginal deliveries. After surgery, each glove was carefully evaluated for a perforation.

21. Sixty-seven of 540 glove sets had at least one hole. Let p be the proportion of glove sets that have a postsurgery hole.

a. Determine a point estimate for p.

b. Determine a 95% confidence interval for p.

22. There were a total of 78 glove perforations. Of these, 52 occurred on a glove worn on the left hand, and 26 occurred on a glove worn on the right hand. Test the hypothesis that each hand is equally likely to get a perforation.

23. There were a total of 78 glove perforations. Of these, 52 occurred on a glove worn on the left hand, and 26 occurred on a glove worn on the right hand. Test the research hypothesis that the majority of perforations occur on a glove worn on the left hand.

24. The authors claimed that "more than half of the perforations (46/78, 59%) occurred on the thumb and the first two fingers of the left hand."

a. Are the authors justified in their claim?

b. Do these data support the research hypothesis that the majority of perforations occur on the thumb and the first two fingers of the left hand.

c. Explain why a test of hypothesis is needed to answer (*b*) but not (*a*).

SECTION 10.2

Test of Hypothesis— Average Value

OBJECTIVES This section will recast an appropriate health sciences problem into a problem of comparison about an average. To resolve the resulting problem of comparison, conduct an appropriate statistical test of hypothesis for an average when provided with a random sample with independent observations drawn from the population of interest:

1 t-test when the distribution is normal

2 z-test when the sample size is large

3 s-test otherwise when given the raw data

In Section 10.1 we introduced TOH for a proportion. In this section our focus is the average. At this point it is crucial that one is able to distinguish clearly between a problem concerned with a proportion and a problem concerned with an average. In a proportion problem, one is concerned with what fraction of the population has a certain characteristic. In an average value problem, one is concerned with a mean or median. We resolve an average value one-population problem of comparison by applying an appropriate test of hypothesis to a random sample with independent observations.

There are three tests of hypothesis about an average: t-test, z-test, and s-test. The preliminary analysis used to select the test of hypothesis option is analogous to that used for confidence intervals (see Section 7.1). The cascade of thinking to select an appropriate test option is as follows:

1. Check for normal. If normal, then t-test (Chart 2A).
2. Large sample size. If n (sample size) > 30, then z-test (Chart 2B).
3. Otherwise, STEST using Minitab on the raw data (Chart 2C).

The t-Test

When faced with a problem of comparison regarding the average, a t-test is appropriate *if the RV of interest has a normal distribution*. In that event, the t-test is a test of hypothesis about the *mean*.

When one is provided with the raw data set about a continuous RV, one can apply Minitab's nscores correlation procedure to test for normality (Section 6.2). When not provided with the raw data set, but only with the sample legend, one must assume that the distribution of interest is normal. This assumption of normality should be *explicitly stated* before proceeding with further analysis.

When one is dealing with a normal distribution, a problem of comparison concerning the average is best resolved by a t-test about the mean.

EXAMPLE 10.2.1 (See Example 9.1.6) Bridges et al wanted to check whether the mean blood hemoglobin (Hb) as determined by a new system was consistent with the reported mean of 13.5 mg/dL for U.S. women. The Hb using the new system on 14 random female blood bank donors was:

15.5   13.6   13.5   13.0   13.3   12.4   11.1
13.1   16.1   16.4   13.4   13.2   14.3   16.1

We are presented with a convenience sample of 14 Hb measurements. We assume that this data set is a random sample with independent observations. Thus, a TOH may be applied to resolve the problem of comparison:

$H_0: \mu = 13.5$
$H_a: \mu \neq 13.5$

Since the raw sample data are given, we can enlist Minitab to perform all the computational details. Minitab's output is displayed in Figure 10.2.1. The complete TOH write-up for this example is given in Figure 10.2.2.

Figure 10.2.1 shows Minitab's output for Example 10.2.1. A good output shows the commands that display (1) the raw data set, (2) the sample nscores correlation, and (3) the t-test. The general form of the command to conduct the t-test is

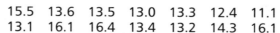

MTB > TTEST M C;
SUBC> ALTERNATE K.

FIGURE **10.2.1**
Minitab work-up and
output for the Hb
measurement study
(Example 10.2.1).

pg442 critical value
14 scores
.01 level of significance

Describe

Note: critical value .9110 - state
Normal or not normal

13.5 = reference value

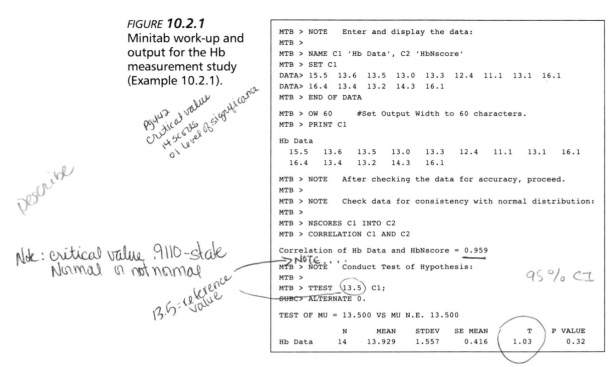

```
MTB > NOTE    Enter and display the data:
MTB >
MTB > NAME C1 'Hb Data', C2 'HbNscore'
MTB > SET C1
DATA> 15.5  13.6  13.5  13.0  13.3  12.4  11.1  13.1  16.1
DATA> 16.4  13.4  13.2  14.3  16.1
MTB > END OF DATA

MTB > OW 60      #Set Output Width to 60 characters.
MTB > PRINT C1

Hb Data
   15.5   13.6   13.5   13.0   13.3   12.4   11.1   13.1   16.1
   16.4   13.4   13.2   14.3   16.1

MTB > NOTE    After checking the data for accuracy, proceed.
MTB >
MTB > NOTE    Check data for consistency with normal distribution:
MTB >
MTB > NSCORES C1 INTO C2
MTB > CORRELATION C1 AND C2

Correlation of Hb Data and HbNscore = 0.959
> NOTE . . . .
MTB > NOTE    Conduct Test of Hypothesis:
MTB >
MTB > TTEST (13.5) C1;                              95% CI
SUBC> ALTERNATE 0.

TEST OF MU = 13.500 VS MU N.E. 13.500

              N      MEAN    STDEV   SE MEAN       T    P VALUE
Hb Data      14    13.929    1.557    0.416     1.03    0.32
```

where M is the test reference value used in the null hypothesis, C is the column that contains the raw data, and K is the test alternate. Minitab cannot use the test alternate designations (a), (b), and (c) in the charts but instead uses 0, −1, and 1, respectively. To conduct the needed t-test for Example 10.2.1 in Minitab,

```
MTB > TTEST 13.5 C1;
SUBC> ALTERNATE 0.
```

Note that 13.5 is the test reference value used in the null hypothesis and C1 is the column containing the Hb data. The TTEST command ends with a semicolon to indicate that we need to augment the main command by specifying the test alternate. Since we are applying a two-tailed test (test alternate (a) in Chart 2A), the test alternate in Minitab is 0.

In response to the TTEST command, Minitab prints the hypothesis being tested, followed by sample and test information. The number under T (here, 1.03) is the sample value (sample *t*). This number may simply be imported into step 6 of your TOH write-up. This refreshing step saves you from all sample calculations!

Check Minitab's statement of hypothesis (first line of output for the TTEST command) with your statement of hypothesis in step 1 to ensure Minitab is performing the test you want. If not, this usually means you failed to enter the test reference number correctly or failed to specify the test alternate in the ALTERNATE subcommand.

Figure 10.2.2 displays the write-up for the TOH following the guide of Chart 2A. First, the preliminary criterion for normality is checked. Since the sample is consistent with normality, the t-test is justified. The main test follows the usual seven-step protocol. Note in particular that step 1 states the hypotheses to be tested and identifies test alternate (a), a two-tailed test. The test is two-tailed since it is an "equal versus not equal" test. Steps 2–5 are routine, following Chart 2A. Note that step 5 displays a decision line using the same alternate (a) as identified in step 1.

Without Minitab, step 6 (sample value) in the TOH write-up (Figure 10.2.2) would have to be obtained "by hand." First, one would have to obtain the sample size (14), sample mean (13.93), and sample standard deviation (1.56). The "sample t" is then calculated by substituting these values into the test statistic specified in step 3:

$$\text{sample } t = \frac{\bar{x} - 13.5}{(s/\sqrt{n})} = \frac{13.93 - 13.5}{(1.56/\sqrt{14})} = 1.0314$$

It is simply much easier to let the computer do all these calculations.

EXAMPLE 10.2.2 Stone et al (see Problem 1.2.6) reported that the baseline (control) Pao_2 for the V_T group ($n = 8$) was 133 ± 27.7 mmHg (mean ± SD). Test the hypothesis that the mean Pao_2 is consistent with a mean value of 150. We first note that the raw data set is not given; only the sample legend is provided. We assume that the legend was obtained from a random sample with independent observations. We also assume that baseline Pao_2 values are (approximately) normally distributed in ventilation-dependent patients. This assumption of normality allows us to conduct a t-test about the mean.

We now test $H_0: \mu = 150$ versus $H_a: \mu \neq 150$ where μ is the mean baseline Pao_2 value among ventilated patients. A complete write-up for the TOH is given in Figure 10.2.3 following the protocol of Chart 2A.

(handwritten margin notes: t test 2A; Minitab does calculation you do write up.)

FIGURE 10.2.2
The figure displays a formal write-up for the blood hemoglobin example (Example 10.2.1). The presentation follows the protocol of Chart 2A: test of hypothesis for the mean, single population, normal random variable.

I. Preliminary Criterion. Since the raw sample data are given, we first check the sample Hb for consistency with a normal distribution. The sample size is n = 14. The critical nscores correlation is .8804 (n = 10), .9110 (n = 15). The shaded region in the following decision line is an "ambiguous zone."

Nonnormal |————————[░░░]————————| Normal
0   .8804   .9110   1

Since the sample nscores correlation is 0.959 (see Minitab output, Figure 10.2.1), we assume that Hb is (approximately) normally distributed in the female population.

II. Main Test of Hypothesis.
1. Hypothesis. $H_0: \mu = 13.5$ Test Alternate (a);
   $H_a: \mu \neq 13.5$ two-tailed test.
2. LOS. $\alpha = 0.05$
3. Test Statistic. $\frac{\bar{x} - 13.5}{(s/\sqrt{n})}$
4. Critical Value. t = 2.1604 (Table 9, df = n − 1 = 13)
5. Decision Line. Alternate (a):

Reject H_0 | Do Not Reject H_0 | Reject H_0
          −2.1604   2.1604 T_{13}

6. Sample Value. Sample t = 1.03 (Minitab)
7. Conclusion. Based on the given data, at the 5% LOS do not reject $H_0: \mu = 13.5$. The mean Hb level given by the new system is consistent with the reported mean of 13.5 mg/dL.

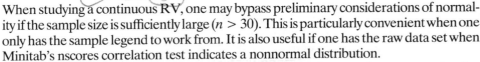

FIGURE **10.2.3**
This figure displays the formal write-up for the Pao_2 example from the research of Stone et al (Example 10.2.2). The presentation follows the protocol of Chart 2A: test of hypothesis for the mean, single population, normal random variable.

I. Preliminary Criterion. The raw data set is not given. We assume that baseline Pao_2 is (approximately) normally distributed in the population of ventilation dependent patients.

II. Main Test of Hypothesis.
1. Hypothesis. $H_0: \mu = 150$ Test alternate (a);
$H_a: \mu \neq 150$ two-tailed test.
2. LOS. $\alpha = .05$
3. Test Statistic. $\frac{\bar{x} - 150}{s/\sqrt{n}}$
4. Critical Value. 2.3646 (Table 9, df = 7)
5. Decision Line. Alternate (a):

Reject H_0	Do Not Reject H_0	Reject H_0
-2.3646		2.3646

6. Sample Value. Sample Legend: $n = 8$, $\bar{x} = 133$, $s = 27.7$

$$\text{sample } t = \frac{\bar{x} - 150}{s/\sqrt{n}} = \frac{133 - 150}{(27.7/\sqrt{8})} = -1.7359$$

7. Conclusion. Based on the given data, at the 5% level of significance, do not reject H_0: $\mu = 150$. The sample data are consistent with a mean Pao_2 value of 150 mmHg.

The z-Test

When studying a continuous RV, one may bypass preliminary considerations of normality if the sample size is sufficiently large ($n > 30$). This is particularly convenient when one only has the sample legend to work from. It is also useful if one has the raw data set when Minitab's nscores correlation test indicates a nonnormal distribution.

Like the t-test, the z-test also resolves a problem of comparison concerning the average of the RV by a test of hypothesis about the mean.

EXAMPLE 10.2.3 Tosata et al studied the effectiveness of conventional taping in stabilizing an endotracheal (ET) tube. A study of 50 patients showed ET tube displacement for patients using conventional taping was 1.26 ± 0.74 cm (mean $\pm$ SD). We inquire whether the mean displacement exceeds 1 cm, that is $H_a: \mu > 1$. We assume that the legend was obtained from a random sample with independent observations. Since we do not have the raw data, we cannot test for normality. However, since the sample size is large ($n = 50 > 30$), we can bypass this consideration and conduct a large-sample z-test for the mean. The analysis displayed in Figure 10.2.4 follows Chart 2B.

Note that step 1 states the hypothesis being tested and identifies this test as having the form of alternate (c), a one-tailed test. The designation "one-tailed" is utilized in step 4 in reading the critical z-value from Table 8. The designation "alternate (c)" is utilized in step 5 in choosing the correct form for the decision line.

The s-Test

When the t-test and z-test are inappropriate to resolve a problem of comparison about an average, one may have recourse to the s-test if one has the raw data. In the absence of the raw data set, one is stuck if neither the t-test nor z-test is appropriate—

FIGURE **10.2.4**

An analysis of the endotracheal displacement study for patients using conventional tape (Example 10.2.3) is presented. The analysis follows the protocol of Chart 2B. The test conducted is the large-sample z-test of hypothesis for the mean.

1. Hypothesis. $H_0: \mu \leq 1$ Test alternate (c);
$H_a: \mu > 1$ one-tailed test.
2. LOS. $\alpha = 0.05$
3. Test Statistic. $\dfrac{\bar{x} - \mu_0}{s/\sqrt{n}} = \dfrac{\bar{x} - 1}{s/\sqrt{n}}$
4. Critical Value. $z = 1.645$ (Table 8)
5. Decision Line. Alternate (c).

Do Not Reject H_0 | Reject H_0
1.645   Z

6. Sample Value. Sample Legend: $n = 50$, $\bar{x} = 1.26$, $s = 0.74$

sample $z = \dfrac{\bar{x} - 1}{s/\sqrt{n}} = \dfrac{1.26 - 1}{0.74/\sqrt{50}} = 2.484$

7. Conclusion. Based on the given data, at the 5% LOS reject $H_0: \mu \leq 1$ and accept $H_a: \mu > 1$. The data give strong evidence that the mean ET tube displacement for patients using conventional tape is greater than 1 cm.

one can only announce that one has insufficient information for further analysis about the average of the RV in the population as a whole.

Suppose now that the raw data set obtained from a random sample with independent observations is provided, and that neither the t-test nor the z-test is appropriate; that is, one has a small sample ($n \leq 30$) that is inconsistent with normality by Minitab's nscores correlation test. In that event, conduct an s-test to resolve a problem of comparison about the average of the RV of interest. The **s-test** is a test of hypothesis concerning the population median, η (not the mean, μ). To conduct the s-test, follow the protocol outlined in Chart 2C. The s-test is the only test in the charts that does not use the seven-step format. Instead, the s-test uses an abbreviated protocol that pivots on the so-called *p*-value of a test. The details of the *p*-value are presented in Section 10.4. For now, we concentrate on conducting the test and interpreting the conclusion.

EXAMPLE 10.2.4   Molyneaux et al studied activated partial thromboplastin time (aPTT) (Appendix, Data Set 3). They considered three different discard volumes to see whether, in general, aPTT measured from arterial blood taken from the indwelling catheter would match the aPTT measured from a venous sample (obtained by venipuncture). The arterial sample, if appropriate, would be much simpler from a nursing standpoint and would assist in patient comfort by saving the patient another needle stick. We consider the arterial blood sample with 1.6-mL discard. This convenience sample of 20 patients is a random sample with independent observations.

We pose two questions regarding the average aPTT value using blood obtained from an arterial line with a 1.6-mL discard. We inquire whether this average (1) is greater than 30 and (2) is consistent with a value of 35. Since we have the raw data, we enlist Minitab's help. The Minitab output is displayed in Figure 10.2.5.

Minitab's nscores correlation test indicates the sample is inconsistent with normality; hence, a t-test is not appropriate (critical nscores correlation for $n = 20$ is .9290). Since n (sample size) $= 20$, we are not justified in using the large sample size z-test. Hence, we formulate a test of hypothesis in terms of the median and conduct s-tests in Minitab. We have two problems of comparison to resolve: (1) H_0: $\eta \le 30$ versus H_a: $\eta > 30$, and (2) H_0: $\eta = 35$ versus H_a: $\eta \ne 35$.

Looking at Minitab's output, a statistician would say that the sample median ($\bar{x}$ = 33) is statistically significantly greater than 30 ($p = .0059$) and not statistically significantly different from 35 ($p = .1153$). This is a technical way of saying that, based on the given data, at the 5% level of significance, the population median is greater than 30, and further, the population median is consistent with a value of 35. A detailed write-up for the TOH for H_0: $\eta \le 30$ versus H_a: $\eta > 30$ is given in Figure 10.2.5 following the protocol of Chart 2C.

FIGURE **10.2.5** The formal write-up for an s-test of hypothesis for the Molyneaux et al aPTT example (Example 10.2.4) is displayed. The presentation follows the protocol of Chart 2C. Step 4a addresses the research inquiry whether the median aPTT is greater than 30. Step 4b addresses the research inquiry whether the median aPTT is 35.

```
1. Hypothesis.      H0: η ≤ 30       Test alternate (c);
                    Ha: η > 30       one-tailed test.
2. LOS. α = 0.05
3. Minitab
MTB > PRINT C2

Art 1.6
    33.1    30.2    34.6    32.2    26.0    41.8    30.5    41.2    29.3
    29.7    30.5    32.9    36.4    26.5    33.7    34.3    31.4   119.3
    50.8    48.7

MTB > NOTE      Test for normal distribution:
MTB > NSCORES C2 INTO C11
MTB > CORRELATION C2 AND C11

Correlation of Art 1.6 and NSArt1.6 = 0.697

MTB > NOTE     Test of Hypothesis:  H0:median <= 30 vs Ha:median > 30
MTB >
MTB > STEST 30 C2;
SUBC> ALTERNATE 1.

SIGN TEST OF MEDIAN = 30.00 VERSUS  G.T.   30.00

               N   BELOW  EQUAL  ABOVE   P-VALUE     MEDIAN
Art 1.6       20      4      0     16    0.0059      33.00
```

4a. Conclusion. Based on the given data, at the 5% level of significance we reject H_0: $\eta \le 30$ and accept H_a: $\eta > 30$. The sample provides evidence that the median aPTT is greater than 30 ($p = .0059$).

```
MTB > NOTE     Test of Hypothesis:  H0:median = 35 vs Ha:median N.E. 35
MTB >
MTB > STEST 35 C2;
SUBC> ALTERNATE 0.

SIGN TEST OF MEDIAN = 35.00 VERSUS  N.E.   35.00

               N   BELOW  EQUAL  ABOVE   P-VALUE     MEDIAN
Art 1.6       20     14      0      6    0.1153      33.0
```

4b. Conclusion. Based on the given data, at the 5% level of significance we do not reject H_0: $\eta = 35$. The sample data are consistent with a median aPTT value of 35 mm Hg ($p = .1153$).

Winklhofer-Roob et al studied vitamin E deficiency in children with cystic fibrosis. Vitamin E deficiency is a common problem for children with cystic fibrosis. The researchers measured erythrocyte cell vitamin E level (μmol/liter) in a convenience sample of ten children after an all-night fast and just before administration of an oral vitamin E dose. Cell vitamin E was then measured 9 hours later. The data are given in Table 10.2.1 (the full data set is given in the Appendix Data Set 7). Each column is a random sample with independent observations.

TABLE **10.2.1**
Cell vitamin E concentration in ten children with cystic fibrosis from the Winklhofer-Roob et al study.

Start	9 hours
1.5	5.4
4.1	7.8
1.0	3.3
3.5	5.9
1.9	3.1
2.1	5.6
2.3	8.1
1.5	6.7
3.1	3.9
1.7	6.0

A child is considered vitamin E deficient if cell vitamin E is under 4.5 μmol/liter. We test to determine whether the data indicate (1) a vitamin E deficiency at the start and (2) vitamin E recovery at 9 hours.

1. The population of interest in the study is
   a. Cystic fibrosis
   b. Vitamin E
   c. Cell vitamin E concentration
   d. Children with cystic fibrosis
   e. Erythrocytes

2. The RV of interest in the study is (use options of Warm-up 1).

3. We inquire whether the children in the study population present a vitamin E deficiency at the start. This inquiry poses
   a. A problem of location
   b. A problem of comparison
   c. A problem of descriptive statistics
   d. A nonstatistical problem

4. Cell vitamin E concentration (μmol/liter) is
   a. A categorical random variable
   b. A nominal random variable *for rank or name
   c. An ordinal random variable
   d. An interval random variable *counts or measures
   e. Not a random variable

5. To select the appropriate TOH about the average value, one first checks the data for
   a. Normality
   b. Large sample size
   c. Descriptive statistics
   d. Adequacy of sample size

6. Minitab's nscores correlation for the Start data is 0.969. Are the data consistent with an assumption of normality? *yes

7. When the RV of interest is (approximately) normal, what comparison test should one conduct?
   a. A t-test about the mean
   b. A z-test about the mean
   c. A z-test about the proportion
   d. An s-test about the mean
   e. An s-test about the median

8. To test whether the average cell vitamin E level at the start is under 4.5 μmol/liter, one conducts a TOH about
   a. A proportion
   b. The mean

c. The median

d. The standard deviation

e. Whether the child has cystic fibrosis

9. To resolve the problem of whether (on average) the children present a vitamin E deficiency (i.e., a vitamin E level under 4.5 μmol/liter), one should test

a. $H_0: \mu \leq 4.5$ versus $H_a: \mu > 4.5$

b. $H_0: p \leq 4.5$ versus $H_a: p > 4.5$

c. $H_0: \mu \geq 4.5$ versus $H_a: \mu < 4.5$

d. $H_0: p \geq 4.5$ versus $H_a: p < 4.5$

e. $H_0: \mu = 4.5$ versus $H_a: \mu \neq 4.5$

10. The researcher wants to confirm that the children actually present a vitamin E deficiency at Start. She tests $H_0: \mu \geq 4.5$ versus $H_a: \mu < 4.5$ where μ is the mean cell vitamin E concentration at Start. Based on Minitab's nscores correlation test, we assume cell vitamin E concentration is (approximately) normal. Accordingly, we conduct a t-test about the mean. To conduct the test based on the given data, we should follow the protocol specified in

a. Chart 1

b. Chart 2A

c. Chart 2B

d. Chart 2C

For Warm-ups 11–20, we consider the hypothesis $H_0: \mu \geq 4.5$ versus $H_a: \mu < 4.5$. The test of hypothesis is carried out following Chart 2A.

11. What alternate is this test of hypothesis—(a), (b), or (c)?

12. Is this a one- or a two-tailed test?

13. Chart 2A directs us to obtain the critical t-value from Table 9. Here,

n (sample size) = ____ $df = n - 1 =$ ____

14. At the 5% level of significance, the critical t-value is ____.

15. What decision line alternate should one use—(a), (b), or (c)?

16. Construct the decision line.

17. The sample t-value is obtained by evaluating the test statistic based on the sample. Here,

n (sample size) = 10
$\bar{x}$ (sample mean) = 2.270
s (sample standard deviation) = 0.991
μ_0 (test reference value) = 4.5

Hence,

$$\text{sample } t = \frac{\bar{x} - \mu_0}{(s/\sqrt{n})} = \frac{\boxed{} - \boxed{}}{(\boxed{} / \sqrt{\boxed{}})} = \underline{7.116}$$

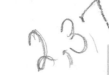

18. Using your decision line from Warm-up 16, what is your decision: reject H_0 or do not reject H_0?

19. What does the statistical decision in Warm-up 18 tell you about children with cystic fibrosis?

20. To determine whether children with cystic fibrosis in general present a fasting (overnight) cell vitamin E deficiency, researchers test

$H_0: \mu \geq 4.5$
$H_a: \mu < 4.5$

where μ is the mean cell vitamin E level at Start. The test is formally conducted using Chart 2, then Chart 2A. Following Chart 2A, write up the formal TOH in the seven-step format. Include the preliminary write-up for normality.

Problems 10.2

1. Bridges et al tested a new system for obtaining blood measurements. They were interested in whether the system gave results consistent with the published mean values for hemoglobin (Hb) and packed cell volume (PCV) for men and women. Random blood samples from 14 female and 15 male donors were obtained from a local blood bank. Hb and PCV were measured using the new system. The data are provided in Table 10.2.2.

a. Apply a TOH to determine whether the mean Hb as determined by the new system is consistent with the published mean of 15.25 g/dL for males.

b. Apply a TOH to determine whether the mean PCV as determined by the new system is consistent with the published mean of 0.397 for women.

TABLE **10.2.2** Hb data set from Bridges et al.

FEMALES		MALES	
Hb	PCV	Hb	PCV
15.5	.45	14.0	.41
13.6	.42	15.3	.45
13.5	.44	13.5	.43
13.0	.395	15.8	.46
13.3	.395	15.0	.43
12.4	.37	16.7	.47
11.1	.39	17.1	.475
13.1	.40	14.7	.45
16.1	.445	15.5	.45
16.4	.47	17.3	.44
13.4	.39	15.0	.43
13.2	.40	16.0	.455
14.3	.42	14.5	.44
16.1	.45	16.0	.44
		16.9	.47

c. Apply a test of hypothesis to determine whether the mean PCV as determined by the new system is consistent with the published mean of 0.443 for men.

d. Determine a 95% confidence interval for the mean Hb for women according to measurements using the new system.

e. Are the data consistent with the reported mean Hb for females of 13.45 ± 1.07 g/dL (mean ± SD)? Justify.

2. In the Bridges et al blood measurement study, in order to test the new system for consistency, 20 separate measurements from a single blood draw were taken. The new method gave a mean Hb of 13.275 g/dL with a standard deviation of 0.121 g/dL. The Hb of the same blood was determined to be 13.2 g/dL by using a standard reference method. Is the mean Hb measurement with the new system consistent with the reference value of 13.2 g/dL? Test at the 10% LOS.

3. Papadakis et al reported on eight patients with class 1 (a major finding at autopsy) abdominal abscesses, perforation, or infarction at the time of initiation of mechanical ventilation. The temperatures (°C) of the eight patients were reported as

36.9   35.9   36.5   36.4   38.2   36.8   37.0   39.1

a. Is the distribution of temperatures among the given patients consistent with normality?

b. Determine the sample size, mean, and standard deviation.

c. Determine a 95% confidence interval for the mean temperature of such patients.

d. Apply a test of hypothesis to determine whether the mean temperature of such patients is statistically significantly different from 37.0°C.

4. Tosata et al (Example 10.2.3) also studied a new tube holder designed to stabilize an endotracheal (ET) tube. There were 50 patients in the study. The amount of displacement of the ET tube was 0.43 ± 0.67 cm (mean $\pm$ SD). The amount of displacement using conventional tape usually was over 1 cm.

a. Assume that ET displacement is normally distributed. About what proportion of patients using the tube holder will have an ET tube displacement of over 1 cm?

b. At the 5% LOS, is the mean ET tube displacement for patients using the tube holder significantly less than
  i. 1 cm?
  ii. 0.75 cm?
  iii. 0.5 cm?
  iv. 0.4 cm?
  v. 0.3 cm?

5. The scores on an examination over TOHs for 23 students enrolled in a health sciences statistics course were:

37 67 70 81 81 83 85 86 86 87 91
92 92 92 93 95 95 96 97 97 98 99 100

The professor likes to gear the class so that the average exam score is 80 or better.

a. Conduct an appropriate test of hypothesis to determine whether the professor is meeting her goal.

b. Suppose the grading system is A, B, C, D, F. How would you assign grades to these test scores? (A histogram may help.)

Problems 6–23 are based on the Winklhofer-Roob et al study of vitamin E deficiency in children with cystic fibrosis (see Appendix, Data Set 7). In the Warm-ups we determined that initial cell vitamin E concentration is below the pediatric low normal level of 4.5 μmol/liter. In order to recover the cell vitamin E concentration, an oral dose was administered. Cell vitamin E concentration is considered recovered when it exceeds 4.5 μmol/liter.

6. Do the data support the research hypothesis that cell vitamin E concentration was still deficient after

   a. 1 hour?

   b. 3 hours?

   c. 6 hours?

7. Was cell vitamin E concentration recovered after 9 hours?

8. Do the data support the hypothesis that cell vitamin E concentration remains recovered after

   a. 12 hours?

   b. 24 hours?

The reference value used for cell vitamin E concentration (low normal pediatric level) was 4.5 μmol/liter. The reference value used for serum vitamin E concentration was 20.9 μmol/liter.

9. Test the hypothesis that mean serum vitamin E concentration is below 20.9 μmol/liter at

   a. Before (start; i.e., serum 0)

   b. 1 hour

   c. 3 hours

10. Test the research hypothesis that mean serum vitamin E concentration has recovered (exceeds 20.9 μmol/liter) at

    a. 6 hours

    b. 9 hours

    c. 12 hours

11. At 12 hours, we inquire whether the serum vitamin E concentration is consistent with the value of 20.9 μmol/liter. Accordingly, test H_0: $\mu = 20.9$ versus H_a: $\mu \neq 20.9$.

12. Make and test a conjecture for serum vitamin E concentration at 24 hours.

13. Conduct the tests stated in (a), (b), and (c) at 24 hours.

    a. H_0: $\mu \leq 20.9$ versus H_a: $\mu > 20.9$.

    b. H_0: $\mu = 20.9$ versus H_a: $\mu \neq 20.9$.

    c. H_0: $\mu \geq 20.9$ versus H_a: $\mu < 20.9$.

    d. Discuss the significance and differences between these three tests. Which test (a, b, or c) would you apply if you wanted to determine whether

    i. To administer another oral dose of vitamin E since serum vitamin E is below 20.9 μmol/L

    ii. Serum vitamin E still seemed to be above baseline

    iii. Serum vitamin E was about at the cutoff level, 20.9 μmol/L

Of the ten children in the study, five have cholestatic liver disease (CLD) and five do not. Problems 14–21 refer to the five children without CLD.

14. Test the research hypothesis that the baseline (Cell 0) cell vitamin E concentration is deficient (under 4.5) μmol/L.

15. Test the hypothesis that cell vitamin E level is deficient (under 4.5) at

    a. 1 hour

    b. 3 hours

    c. 6 hours

16. Test the hypothesis that cell vitamin E level is recovered (>4.5 μmol/L) at

    a. 9 hours

    b. 12 hours

    c. 24 hours

17. Test the research hypothesis that the baseline (serum 0) serum vitamin E concentration is deficient (below 20.9 μmol/L).

18. Test the hypothesis that serum vitamin E level is deficient (under 20.9 μmol/L) at

    a. 1 hour

    b. 3 hours

19. Test the hypothesis that serum vitamin E level is recovered (>20.9 μmol/L) at

    a. 6 hours

    b. 9 hours

20. Test the hypothesis that serum vitamin E level at 12 hours is consistent with the cutoff value of 20.9.

21. Make and test a conjecture for serum vitamin E level at 24 hours.

22. (Project) Analyze the serum vitamin E data for the five children with CLD.

23. (Project) Analyze the cell vitamin E data for the five children with CLD. What special difficulties do you find for these children?

OBJECTIVES   This section will

1   Recast an appropriate health sciences research problem utilizing a paired-data design into a paired-data difference problem of comparison.

2   Conduct a paired-data test of hypothesis when provided with an appropriate sample of paired data.

Paired-data tests are among the most common and important statistical tools needed in health sciences research. This section is a natural extension to Section 7.2, Confidence Intervals for the Mean (paired data), which introduced the notion of a statistical design that produces paired data which yields meaningful paired-data differences.

Paired-Data Difference

The key feature in a paired-data design is that each subject in the research study yields a pair of measurements, measurement A and measurement B, which are paired difference compatible (both A and B have the same units of measurement; e.g., both weight in kilograms or blood pressure in mm Hg). For analysis, each pair (A,B) is converted into a **difference**:

Difference = measurement A − measurement B

Briefly,

$$D = A - B$$

The data set of differences can now be tested. One performs tests of hypothesis about the average value of D using the methods presented in Section 10.2.

In a paired-data test, the test reference number is usually zero. This is a result of the usual type of study that calls for analysis by conducting paired data tests:

1. Before and after studies
2. Method A versus method B studies

EXAMPLE 10.3.1   The Bodai et al evaluation of an oxygen insufflation suction catheter (Section 1.2, An Application: Time Series Graphs) utilizes a typical before and after design. The research motivation is to determine whether a 1-minute suctioning protocol results in a significant drop in PaO_2. For each patient in the study, a PaO_2 measurement is taken at the start (before) and at the end (after) suctioning. For each patient, calculate the difference, D = before − after. If the before reading is greater than the after, then a drop in PaO_2 is observed and D > 0. To generalize, the research concern is whether on average D > 0. Hence, we test

H_0: $\mu_D \leq 0$
H_a: $\mu_D > 0$ (drop in PaO_2)

Comment Note how the general health sciences concern of the researchers (Is there a significant change in PaO_2?) is recast into a statement about μ_D, the average value of D = before − after. The possible clinical positions of interest regarding the effect of suctioning on PaO_2 are displayed in Table 10.3.1. Each clinical position is translated into a statement about the difference D = before − after. The statement is reformulated into a statistical statement involving the mean of D. The key utility of the final statistical statement is that it can be placed into an appropriate hypothesis that can be tested.

TABLE **10.3.1**
Association between the clinical concerns and statistical statements about the paired difference.

Clinical Position	D = Before − After	Statement
No change in PaO_2	On average, D = 0	$\mu_D = 0$
A drop in PaO_2	On average, D > 0	$\mu_D > 0$
A gain in PaO_2	On average, D < 0	$\mu_D < 0$

EXAMPLE 10.3.2 The Daily and Mersch cardiac output study utilizes a typical method A versus method B design. The research motivation is to determine whether cardiac output taken by using a room-temperature injectate (RTCO, method A) is consistent with those taken by using an ice-temperature injectate (ITCO, method B). For each patient in the study, cardiac output is taken using both methods. For each patient we calculate the difference, D = RTCO − ITCO. If the two readings are equivalent, then, in general, the room- and ice-temperature cardiac outputs are the same; that is, D = 0 on average. Accordingly, we test

H_0: $\mu_D = 0$ (methods equivalent)
H_a: $\mu_D \neq 0$

Comment Note how the general concern of the researchers is translated into a statement about μ_D, the average value of D = RTCO − ITCO. The possible clinical positions of interest regarding the comparison of RTCO and ITCO are shown in Table 10.3.2.

TABLE **10.3.2**
Clinical concerns of cardiac output in terms of the paired difference.

Clinical Position	D = RTCO − ITCO	Statement
They are the same	On average, D = 0	$\mu_D = 0$
RTCO > ITCO	On average, D > 0	$\mu_D > 0$
RTCO < ITCO	On average, D < 0	$\mu_D < 0$

Paired Data t-Test

Since the test reference number for a paired difference test frequently is 0, for convenience we include Chart 3 in the Appendix, which provides the protocol for this special paired-difference t-test, the test of choice when the set of differences D has a normal distribution. In general, one tests the RV D in the same way one would test for the average for a single population (Section 10.2).

EXAMPLE 10.3.3 Bodai et al presented the following set of paired data for their study (Table 10.3.3). We define the difference, D, as D = start − end. Since Bodai et al were concerned whether there is a statistically significant drop in PaO_2 as a result of applying the suction protocol, they tested

$H_0: \mu_D \leq 0$
$H_{a:} \mu_D > 0$ (drop in PaO_2)

TABLE **10.3.3**
The Bodai et al PaO_2 data.

Start	End	D
74	60	14
65	62	3
85	80	5
72	73	−1
91	83	8
92	86	6

As a necessary preliminary, we first test D for normality. Minitab's nscores correlation for D is 0.982 [critical value 0.8320 ($n = 5$), 0.8804 ($n = 10$)]. Hence, we assume that D is (approximately) normally distributed in the patient population of interest. An analysis using Minitab is presented in Figure 10.3.1. Figure 10.3.2 follows the protocol of Chart 3 to formally write up the TOH.

Comment Without Minitab, we would first need to assume normality. Then we would determine the sample legend "by hand": n (sample size) $= 6$, $\bar{d}$ (mean of sample differences) $= 5.8$, and s (standard deviation of sample differences) $= 5.0$. These values are then substituted into the test statistic to obtain the sample t:

$$\text{sample } t = \frac{\bar{D}}{(s_d/\sqrt{n})} = \frac{5.8}{(5.0/\sqrt{6})} = 2.84$$

FIGURE **10.3.1**
Paired-data t-test, Bodai et al PaO_2 suction study (Example 10.3.3). D = before − after. Enter 'Start' data into C1, 'End' data into C2.

```
MTB > NAME C1 'Start', C2 'End', C3 'D', C33 'Dnscores'
MTB > PRINT C1 - C3

ROW   Start   End     D

 1      74     60     14
 2      65     62      3
 3      85     80      5
 4      72     73     -1
 5      91     83      8
 6      92     86      6

MTB > NOTE      Test  D  for normal distribution:
MTB >
MTB > NSCORES C3 INTO C33
MTB > CORRELATION C3 AND C33

Correlation of D and Dnscores = 0.982

MTB > NOTE      Test of Hypothesis:
MTB >
MTB > TTEST 0 C3;
SUBC> ALTERNATE 1.

TEST OF MU = 0.00 VS MU G.T. 0.00

            N     MEAN    STDEV    SE MEAN     T    P VALUE
D           6     5.83     5.04      2.06    2.84    0.018
```

FIGURE **10.3.2**
Write-up for the Bodai et al PaO$_2$ suction study (Example 10.3.3), following Chart 3 for a paired-data t-test. D = before PaO$_2$ − after PaO$_2$.

I. Preliminary. Check D for normality. The shaded region in the decision line is an ambiguous zone. The sample nscores correlation is 0.982 (Figure 10.3.1).

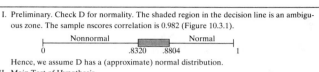

	Nonnormal			Normal	
0		.8320	.8804		1

Hence, we assume D has a (approximate) normal distribution.

II. Main Test of Hypothesis.

1. Hypothesis. H$_0$: $\mu_D \leq 0$ Alternate (c);
   H$_a$: $\mu_D > 0$ one-tailed test.

2. LOS. 0.05

3. Test Statistic. $\dfrac{\bar{D}}{(s_d/\sqrt{n})}$

4. Critical Value. t = 2.01505 (Table 9, df = 5)

5. Decision Line. Alternate (c):

   Do Not Reject H$_0$ | Reject H$_0$
   2.01505   T$_5$

6. Sample Value. sample t = 2.84 (Minitab)

7. Conclusion. Based on the given data, at the 5% LOS we reject H$_0$: $\mu_D \leq 0$ and accept H$_a$: $\mu_D > 0$. The data present evidence for a statistically significant drop in PaO$_2$ as a result of the one minute suctioning protocol with the oxygen insufflation catheter.

EXAMPLE 10.3.4 The Daily and Mersch cardiac output data are provided in Data Set 1 (Data Set Appendix). For each patient, calculate the difference D = RTCO − ITCO. We previously justified assuming that D is normally distributed in the patient population of interest (Example 7.2.1). Minitab's output is presented in Figure 10.3.3. We follow the protocol of Chart 3 to write up the paired-difference t-test of hypothesis (Figure 10.3.4).

FIGURE **10.3.3**
Minitab output for the paired-difference t-test for the Daily and Mersch cardiac output study (Example 10.3.4) is displayed.

```
MTB > NOTE     Enter RTCO into C1 and ITCO into C2.
MTB > NOTE     D = RTCO - ITCO
MTB > NAME C1 'RTCO', C2 'ITCO', C5 'D=R-I', C6 'NScoresD'
MTB > LET C5 = C1 - C2   #Calculate the column of Differences
MTB > NOTE     Check D for Normal Distribution:
MTB > NSCORES C5 INTO C6
MTB > CORRELATION C5 AND C6

Correlation of D=R-I and NScoresD = 0.981

MTB > TTEST 0 C5;     #conduct test of hypothesis
SUBC> ALTERNATE 0.

TEST OF MU = 0.0000 VS MU N.E. 0.0000

              N      MEAN     STDEV   SE MEAN       T   P VALUE
D=R-I        29   -0.0121    0.4298    0.0798   -0.15      0.88
```

FIGURE **10.3.4**
Write-up of the main test of hypothesis for the paired-data t-test for the Daily and Mersch cardiac output study (Example 10.3.4). The format follows the outline presented in Chart 3. D = RTCO − ITCO.

1. Hypothesis. H$_0$: $\mu_D = 0$ Alternate (a);
   H$_a$: $\mu_D \neq 0$ two-tailed test.

2. LOS. 0.10

3. Test Statistic. $\dfrac{\bar{D}}{(s_d/\sqrt{n})}$

4. Critical Value. t = 1.70112 (Table 9, df = 28)

5. Decision Line. Alternate (a):

   Reject H$_0$ | Do Not Reject H$_0$ | Reject H$_0$
   −1.70112   1.70112   T$_{28}$

6. Sample Value. sample t = −0.15 (Minitab)

7. Conclusion. Based on the given data, at the 10% LOS do not reject H$_0$: $\mu_D = 0$. There is no statistically significant difference on average between cardiac outputs obtained by the two methods.

Zillikens et al studied body composition of patients presenting cirrhosis of the liver. The patients were treated for ascites with paracentesis. The weight (kg) of each patient before and after treatment is given in Table 10.3.4.

TABLE **10.3.4**
Weight of patients before and after treatment.

Patient	Before	After
1	92.6	88.0
2	67.7	64.3
3	74.4	59.8
4	73.0	64.0
5	93.5	78.4
6	70.2	59.6
7	74.5	63.3
8	53.9	48.9
9	83.0	74.0
10	47.3	38.0
11	92.4	85.7
12	65.4	55.1

1. Does the Zillikens et al study present a paired-data design? (yes or no). Explain. *Yes ~ before and after*

2. What type of paired-data design is presented by the Zillikens et al study: before and after, or method A versus method B?

3. The population of interest is
   a. Patients with body composition
   b. Patients with a before and after weight
   c. Weight of patients
   d. Patients with cirrhosis of the liver
   e. Patients treated for ascites with paracentesis

4. In a paired-data design, the RV of interest is the difference, D, between the pairs. Here, D = ? *before - after*

5. Consider the difference D = weight before − weight after. A positive difference, D > 0, represents
   a. A weight gain
   b. No change in weight
   c. A weight loss
   d. Advanced cirrhosis

6. A negative difference, D < 0, represents (use same options in Warm-up 5).

7. D = 0 represents (use same options in Warm-up 5).

8. Zillikens et al tested the hypothesis that treatment of ascites with paracentesis results in a statistically significant loss in weight. Accordingly, they tested *want a loss*
   a. $H_0: \mu_D = 0$ versus $H_a: \mu_D \neq 0$
   b. $H_0: \mu_D \leq 0$ versus $H_a: \mu_D > 0$ *Ha*
   c. $H_0: \mu_D \geq 0$ versus $H_a: \mu_D < 0$
   d. $H_0: D \leq 0$ versus $H_a: D > 0$
   e. $H_0: D \leq 0$ versus $H_a: D > 0$

9. Minitab's sample nscores correlation for D is 0.982. What does this indicate? *Normality*

10. To test the research hypothesis that treatment of ascites with paracentesis in cirrhotic patients results in a statistically significant weight loss, conduct
    a. A paired-data s-test about the median weight loss
    b. A paired-data s-test about the mean weight loss
    c. A paired-data z-test about the mean weight loss
    d. A paired-data t-test about the mean weight loss

11. Following Chart 3, what is the critical t-value for the test at the 5% LOS?

12. The sample legend for D, the change in weight, is $n = 12, d = 9.07, s_d = 3.69$. Hence, the sample t-value is computed by

$$\text{sample } t = \frac{d}{(s_d/\sqrt{n})} = \frac{\boxed{}}{(\boxed{}/\sqrt{\boxed{}})} = \underline{}$$

13. At the 5% LOS, do you reject or retain $H_0: \mu_D \leq 0$?

14. What does this test tell you about cirrhotic patients undergoing treatment of ascites with paracentesis?

Problems 10.3

1. Consider the Daily and Mersch cardiac output study (Appendix, Data Set 1). At the 10% LOS, conduct a paired-data t-test to determine whether there is a statistically significant difference on average between

   a. RTCO and Fick cardiac output

   b. ITCO and Fick cardiac output

2. Consider the Barcelona et al cardiac output study (Appendix, Data Set 2). At the 10% LOS, is there a statistically significant difference on average between

   a. Iced injectate versus room-temperature injectate (prefilled syringes)?

   b. Iced injectate versus room-temperature injectate (Co-Set)?

3. Consider the Molyneaux et al aPTT study (Appendix, Data Set 3). At the 5% LOS, is there a statistically significant difference between arterial and venous aPTT

   a. Using 1.6-mL discard?

   b. Using 3.2-mL discard?

   c. Using 4.8-mL discard?

4. Brandstetter et al studied the concern that meal-induced hypoxemia may occur in asymptomatic patients with chronic obstructive pulmonary disease (COPD). The research group did a study on 11 patients in which arterial blood gas (ABG) samples were drawn on each patient just before and 30 minutes after the initiation of feeding through a nasogastric tube. In each ABG sample the oxygen partial pressure (Pa_{O_2}) was measured in mm Hg. The data are given in Table 10.3.5.

TABLE **10.3.5** Data from the Brandstetter et al study.

Patient	First Pa_{O_2}	Second Pa_{O_2}
1	60	62
2	83	85
3	87	85
4	52	50
5	86	84
6	95	93
7	59	58
8	101	99
9	80	77
10	91	88
11	89	82

On the basis of these data, at the 5% LOS, is there a decrease in Pa_{O_2} as a result of feeding; that is, is meal-induced hypoxemia in patients with COPD a problem?

5. Mauro conducted a study to determine the effects of using the bell versus the diaphragm of the stethoscope on indirect blood pressure measurement.

Based on theory and previous research, the following hypotheses were formulated and tested. As compared with the diaphragm of the stethoscope, use of the bell stethoscope for the indirect measure of blood pressure will result in (1) a higher systolic (S1) mean value, (2) a higher fourth phase diastolic (D4) mean value, and (3) a lower fifth phase diastolic (D5) mean value.

The study was done on 56 women (randomly selected nursing students registered for clinic courses at Rutgers University) in a randomized paired-data study. The author analyzed the data using the difference

$$D = \text{bell} - \text{diaphragm}$$

The results are summarized in Table 10.3.6. The t-column gives the sample value computed for a paired-data t-test.

TABLE **10.3.6** Summary results from the Mauro blood pressure measurement study.

Blood Pressure	t
S1	2.31
D4	0.60
D5	−1.91

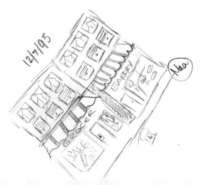

Utilizing the author's information, what conclusions can you reach about each of the three research hypotheses? Use a 5% LOS in your analysis.

6. Stäubli and Jakob studied anterior knee motion analysis. The study involved 16 patients, each of whom presented a chronic anterior cruciate ligament (ACL)–deficient knee on one leg with an ACL-intact knee on the other leg. The anterior knee motion (in millimeters) on each leg of each patient was measured just before surgery using two different methods: (1) the KT-1000 arthrometer and (2) simultaneous radiography. The data are given in Table 10.3.7.

TABLE **10.3.7** Data from Stäubli and Jakob.

| Patient | KT-1000 | | SIMULTANEOUS RADIOGRAPHY | |
	ACL Deficient	ACL Intact	ACL Deficient	ACL Intact
1	13.0	4.0	12.5	2.5
2	17.0	3.0	16.5	7.0
3	10.5	5.5	9.5	4.0
4	8.0	4.0	9.0	5.5
5	12.5	7.5	11.5	5.5
6	18.0	9.0	16.5	2.5
7	14.0	11.5	15.5	5.5
8	10.0	3.5	7.5	4.5
9	10.0	7.0	7.5	6.5
10	11.0	7.0	14.5	4.0
11	10.0	4.0	6.5	3.0
12	8.5	6.5	5.5	3.0
13	8.0	4.0	12.5	6.5
14	12.5	10.0	8.5	5.5
15	11.5	6.5	16.5	7.0
16	16.0	6.5	8.5	6.0

Conduct the following paired-data t-tests.

a. Is there a statistically significant difference in the anterior knee motion of the ACL-deficient knee as determined by the KT-1000 in comparison with simultaneous radiography?

b. Is there a statistically significant difference in the anterior knee motion of the ACL-intact knee as determined by the two methods?

c. Utilizing the K-1000, is the anterior knee motion of the ACL-deficient knee greater than the motion of the ACL-intact knee?

d. Utilizing simultaneous radiography, is the anterior knee motion of the ACL-intact knee less than that of the deficient knee?

e. A 3-mm difference in anterior tibial position between the two knees of a patient is considered diagnostic for ACL deficiency. Consequently, consider the difference (ACL deficient—ACL intact) for each patient as determined (i) by the KT-1000 and (ii) by simultaneous radiography. Is there a significant difference between these two differences? Answer in terms of both statistical and clinical significance.

7. Margolin et al reported baseline seated and standing diastolic blood pressures (DBPs) of 22 elderly (age ≥ 60) hypertensive subjects in a study group as shown in Table 10.3.8.

TABLE **10.3.8** Blood pressure data from Margolin et al.

Patient	Seated DBP	Standing DBP
1	93	98
2	85	85
3	98	108
4	96	96
5	98	102
6	97	96
7	88	90
8	86	90
9	100	98
10	95	96
11	93	89
12	95	94
13	102	101
14	99	110
15	91	89
16	91	101
17	98	100
18	95	98
19	94	100
20	100	100
21	99	102
22	93	102

a. Definite diastolic hypertension is defined as DBP > 90. Test the hypothesis

$H_0: \mu_{(DBP)} \leq 90$
$H_a: \mu_{(DBP)} > 90$

b. Repeat (a) for the standing DBP.

c. Test to determine whether there is evidence in this group for a difference between seated and standing DBP.

d. Determine 95% confidence intervals for the seated and standing DBP.

e. Determine the mean, standard deviation, and a 95% confidence interval for the difference between the seated and standing DBP. How do these results compare with your analysis in (c)?

8. Medley et al studied cardiac output in 21 critically ill adult patients. Cardiac output was obtained using an ice-temperature injectate. The researchers were interested in whether cardiac output obtained by putting the injectate into the proximal injectate lumen of the Swan-Ganz catheter gave comparable readings to cardiac output obtained by putting the injectate into the proximal infusion lumen. The infusion lumen is the manufacturer's recommended lumen to use for the injectate. However, on occasion that lumen may become occluded or be unavailable due to being used for infusion of medication. The reported data are given in Table 10.3.9. Is there a statistically significant difference on average between cardiac outputs taken by the two methods?

TABLE **10.3.9** Cardiac outputs obtained using ice-temperature injectate in the proximal injectate lumen and the proximal infusion lumen. Data from Medley et al.

Patient	Injectate Lumen	Infusion Lumen
1	9.85	9.21
2	5.15	5.20
3	10.39	11.36
4	4.58	4.78
5	4.21	4.39
6	6.79	6.04
7	11.98	11.72
8	4.35	4.58
9	10.76	11.76
10	5.69	5.52
11	7.82	6.54
12	9.37	10.37
13	6.93	7.32
14	15.95	13.43
15	7.93	8.82
16	6.18	5.72
17	6.35	5.85
18	2.41	3.10
19	4.40	4.07
20	5.84	5.52
21	8.67	9.24

9. Zillikens et al (see Warm-ups) also determined total body water (TBW) for the 12 patients in the study. TBW (in liters) was measured before and after treatment of ascites with paracentesis. The data are given in Table 10.3.10. Is there a statistically significant loss in TBW in cirrhotic patients treated for ascites with paracentesis?

TABLE **10.3.10** Data from Zillikens et al.

Patient	TOTAL BODY WATER Before	After	RESISTANCE Before	After	REACTANCE Before	After
1	37.3	35.1	562	601	52	58
2	34.3	32.6	537	568	39	50
3	38.5	28.3	450	637	42	75
4	40.4	36.2	508	574	56	69
5	47.4	42.5	417	470	29	32
6	38.4	34.6	508	570	51	62
7	35.6	32.3	565	630	44	53
8	29.6	26.9	682	761	35	43
9	44.4	36.5	448	556	40	53
10	34.3	30.3	456	524	30	36
11	36.0	31.6	572	662	54	72
12	38.7	31.3	475	602	42	51

10. Total body water (see Problem 9) is a quantity calculated from an equation. In order to use the equation, one must have measurements from bioelectrical impedance analysis, a noninvasive and safe procedure for measuring body composition. The procedure measures various facets of the body's ability to conduct an electrical current. Water and electrolyte portions of the body are good electrical conductors; bone and fat are poor conductors. Hence, a decrease in body water should correspond with an increase in the body's resistance to an electrical current.

a. To use a simplified form of the equation, one needs to know the body's resistance to an electrical current (measured in ohms). Based on the resistance data from Zillikens et al (Table 10.3.10), is there a statistically significant gain in resistance?

b. To use a more complex form of the equation for total body water, one also needs to know the body's reactance (an electrical property also measured in ohms). Based on the reactance data from Zillikens et al (Table 10.3.10), is there a statistically significant gain in reactance?

OBJECTIVES   This section will

1   Describe the concept of the *p*-value for a test of hypothesis.

2   Determine the *p*-value for a given test of hypothesis.

In the research literature, the most common number reported with any TOH is the test "*p*-value." Minitab, like most statistical software packages, automatically prints the *p*-value as part of the output for most tests of hypothesis. The *p*-value for a statistical TOH is intimately linked with the concept of level of significance.

Level of Significance

The **level of significance (LOS)** of a statistical TOH is the probability of rejecting the null hypothesis H_0 if in reality the null hypothesis is true. To illustrate this concept, suppose the null hypothesis is true and the LOS is 5%. Consider all random samples that can conceivably be drawn from the population at large. Compute the sample value for each sample. Then, only 5% of these sample values will fall in the "reject H_0" zone of the decision line; the other 95% will fall in the "do not reject H_0" zone. When drawing a single random sample, by the luck of the draw, one runs a 5% risk of making a rejection error (erroneously rejecting H_0 when H_0 in reality is true). The nature of the 5% LOS is depicted in Figure 10.4.1.

The standard LOS applied in most research in the health sciences is .05. Why 5%? Why not 1% or 10%? Why must we have an LOS at all? An answer to such questions has two components.

FIGURE **10.4.1**
Suppose the null hypothesis is true. The investigator wants to make a decision about the population based on a sample. The diagram traces the effect of a 5% level of significance in the decision-making process.

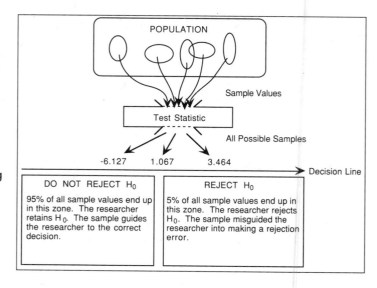

First, to conduct a test of hypothesis, one must "draw the line" somewhere to identify "do not reject H_0" and "reject H_0" regions in the decision line. Without an LOS, one has no test critical value to tell us where to "draw the line" to separate these regions (see Figure 10.4.2, for example). A TOH pits two competing statements, H_0 and H_a, against each other. The LOS merely states a criterion for retaining H_0 versus rejecting H_0. Without the LOS, we would be unable to resolve a statistical problem of comparison.

Second, in situations where we must "draw the line" somewhere, we must settle on where that "somewhere" is. Such situations are common in ordinary society. Lines may appear arbitrary, but they must be drawn. For example,

- The legal drinking and voting age in California is 21.
- The legal driving age for operating a motor vehicle on a public road in California is 16.
- A blood alcohol level $\geq .08$ is legal evidence for driving under the influence.
- A student with a cumulative grade point average under 2.00 is placed on academic probation.

The LOS most statisticians settle on for resolving a problem of comparison is .05. This usual level is sometimes raised or lowered depending on the seriousness of the consequences for making an acceptance or a rejection error. One can work around the apparent arbitrariness of .05 by inquiring: If the null hypothesis is true, how likely is it to get a sample value like the one obtained? Alternatively, how consistent is the sample with the null hypothesis? The answer to such an inquiry lies in the p-value.

The *p*-Value

The term p-value is short for "probability value." The **p-value** measures the probability, if the null hypothesis is true, of obtaining a random sample like the one being analyzed.

To illustrate the meaning of the p-value, consider the Bodai et al suctioning study (see Figure 10.3.2), which conducted a one-tailed t-test, alternate (c). The sample value was 2.84. In a TOH, this sample value is placed on a decision line for a verdict. The decision whether to reject or not reject the null hypothesis H_0 depends on where the sample value falls on the decision line. However, the demarcation of the rejection zone on the decision line can be manipulated by the LOS, as shown in Figure 10.4.2. At LOS .05 the critical value is 2.015; hence, reject H_0 (sample value 2.84 falls in the "reject H_0" zone). At LOS .025 the critical value is 2.571; again, reject H_0. But at LOS

FIGURE **10.4.2**
The decision line is portrayed for LOS .05, .025, and .01. The *p*-value is the LOS for which the sample value is equal to the critical value.

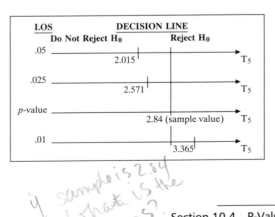

.01, the critical value is 3.365 and the sample value of 2.84 falls in the do "not reject H_0" zone! Somewhere between LOS .025 and .01 the decision switches. The LOS at which the decision switches is called the *p*-value for the test of hypothesis.

Once we know the sample value, we can actually manipulate the decision outcome by a judicious choice of the LOS! Continuing with the example shown in Figure 10.4.2, when LOS > .025, reject H_0, but when LOS < .01, do not reject H_0. The LOS at which the decision switches occurs precisely at that LOS whose associated critical value equals the sample value (here, 2.84). Since that particular LOS (called the *p*-value) occurs somewhere between .01 and .025, we simply report: .01 < *p*-value < .025.

The ***p*-value** of a statistical test is the LOS at which the sample value equals the critical value (see Figure 10.4.3). The *p*-value is the smallest LOS one can use and still retain the null hypothesis; alternatively, the *p*-value is the largest LOS one can use and still reject the null hypothesis. Honesty suggests that the *p*-value be reported with any test of hypothesis. Experienced people make a test decision merely by viewing the *p*-value:

1. **If *p*-value < LOS, reject the null hypothesis.**
2. **If *p*-value ≥ LOS, do not reject the null hypothesis.**

Since the *p*-value is a probability in decimal form, it is always a number between 0 and 1. A sample with a small *p*-value is unlikely to be obtained in a random draw if the null hypothesis is true. A sample with a small *p*-value does not "prove" the null hypothesis is incorrect but simply is an improbable sample if the null hypothesis is true. Hence, a sample with a small *p*-value is evidence against the null hypothesis. The level of significance defines how small is small enough.

DEFINITION **III** *p*-value

> The ***p*-value** of a test of hypothesis is the LOS at which the sample value equals the critical value.

If *p*-value < LOS, then reject the null hypothesis.
If *p*-value ≥ LOS, then do not reject the null hypothesis.

FIGURE **10.4.3**
When a single sample is drawn, the sample is run through the test statistic which compresses the sample data into a single number called the sample value. The sample value is then placed on the decision line for a verdict. The rejection zone(s) on the decision line are determined by the critical value, which in turn depends on the level of significance. The particular level of significance for which the critical value matches the sample value is called the *p*-value for the given test of hypothesis.

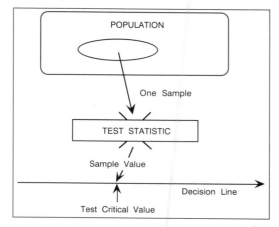

Obtaining the *p*-Value

Fortunately, computer statistical packages like Minitab usually print the *p*-value as part of the standard output for a statistical TOH (see Figures 10.2.1, 10.2.5, 10.3.1, 10.3.3). When one is working by hand, one must obtain the *p*-value by using the sample value in conjunction with the appropriate TOH table. This is a straightforward process for a two-tailed test.

EXAMPLE 10.4.1 We determine the *p*-value for a two-tailed z-test where the sample z-value is 3.147. Since a z-test was conducted, we start with Table 8 and locate 3.147 in the Z column. Note that 3.147 does not explicitly appear; however, 3.147 is located between Z column entries 3.090 and 3.291. The LOSs associated with these Z column entries for a two-tailed test are .002 and .001, respectively. Hence, we report that .001 < *p*-value < .002. This situation is summarized in Figure 10.4.4.

EXAMPLE 10.4.2 Consider the coin-flip example (Figure 10.1.2). A two-tailed z-test was performed on a sample that yielded a sample value of 0.800. Consult the Test of Hypothesis Z-Table (Table 8) and observe that the sample value 0.800 is smaller than any value in the Z column. Hence, one reports: *p*-value > .20.

EXAMPLE 10.4.3 Consider the Hb study (Figure 10.2.2). A two-tailed t-test was conducted on a sample that yielded a sample value of 1.03. Consult the Test of Hypothesis T-Table (Table 9), *df* = 13. The sample value of 1.03 is smaller than any table entry for *df* = 13. Hence, *p*-value > .20. This is consistent with the *p*-value of .32 reported by Minitab (Figure 10.2.1).

EXAMPLE 10.4.4 Consider the Daily and Mersch cardiac output study (Figure 10.3.4). A two-tailed t-test was conducted on a sample whose sample value was −0.15. Consult the Test of Hypothesis T-Table, *df* = 28. The magnitude of the sample value, 0.15, is much smaller than the smallest table entry of 1.31253 (LOS 0.20). Hence, *p*-value > .20. This is consistent with the *p*-value of .88 reported by Minitab (Figure 10.3.3).

 The situation is also straightforward for most one-tailed tests; specifically, when the sample value is either negative with test alternate (b) or positive with test alternate (c).

EXAMPLE 10.4.5 Consider the lung cancer drug example (Figure 10.1.1). A one-tailed z-test was conducted. The sample value was 4.531. To determine the *p*-value, consult the Test of Hypothesis Z-Table (Appendix, Table 8). Locate the sample value 4.531 in the Z column. Observe that the sample value 4.531 exceeds the largest table entry of 4.491; hence, the LOS associated with the sample value must be smaller than .000005. We report: *p*-value < .000005.

FIGURE **10.4.4**
Finding the *p*-value for a two-tailed z-test with sample z-value = 3.147.

LOS	Z	
.002	3.090	←
p-value	3.147	z-table entries
.001	3.291	←

Comment If the null hypothesis were true, obtaining a sample like the given sample by random chance is highly unlikely; specifically, less than 5 chances in 1 million. Rather than believing that the sample data set is most unusual, it seems evidently more prudent to reject the null hypothesis. In a TOH, "prudence" is defined by the level of significance.

EXAMPLE 10.4.6 Suppose a one-tailed z-test, test alternate (b), is conducted and the sample value is -2.413. In this case, with test alternate (b) and a negative sample value, one merely works with the *magnitude* (ignore the minus sign) of the sample value and the test of hypothesis table in order to obtain the p-value. In Table 8, we notice that 2.413 occurs between the Z column entries of 2.326 (LOS .01) and 2.567 (LOS .005). Hence, $.005 < $ p-value $< .01$.

The p-value situation is a bit tricky when the sample value is either positive with test alternate (b) or negative with test alternate (c). In that event, replace LOS with the quantity $1 - $ LOS.

EXAMPLE 10.4.7 Suppose a one-tailed test of alternate (c) is conducted and the sample value is -3.140. In Table 8, we note that 3.140 is between 3.090 (LOS .002) and 3.291 (LOS .001). Now replace each LOS by $1 - $ LOS:

LOS .002 $\Rightarrow$ LOS $1 - .002 = .998$
LOS .001 $\Rightarrow$ LOS $1 - .001 = .999$

Here, $.998 < $ p-value $< .999$.

Comment For a one-tailed test alternate (b), a positive sample value is overwhelming evidence to retain H_0. Similarly, for a one-tailed test alternate (c), a negative sample value is strong evidence to retain H_0. In most cases of a one-tailed test, the sign of the critical value and sample value are the same. When the sign of the critical value and sample value in a one-tailed test differ, one should go back and carefully check one's work. Often this signals either an arithmetic error or that one has stated the hypotheses "backward" (i.e., the inequalities in the null and alternate hypotheses are reversed).

Reporting the p-Value

Many research articles describe a TOH without specifying a level of significance, but report the p-value of the test. The practical purpose of the p-value is to provide a basis on which to decide whether the result of a TOH is statistically significant. A test result is **statistically significant** if the sample data provide sufficient evidence to reject the null hypothesis. A statistically significant result is indicated by a small p-value. How small should the p-value be for a test result to be proclaimed statistically significant? Although there is no definite answer to this question, the following guidelines are common in the health sciences:

If $.01 < $ p-value $< .05$, the result is significant.
If $.001 < $ p-value $< .01$, the result is highly significant.
If p-value $< .001$, the result is very highly significant.
If p-value $> .05$, the result is not significant (NS).

Comment When $.05 <$ p-value $< .10$, some articles report that "a trend toward significance is noted." We recommend against using this terminology; it would be far better simply to say "close call." Once the level of significance is set, one either retains or rejects the null hypothesis—there is no middle ground. This is akin to baseball, where a runner is either safe or out at first base (a trend toward being safe is a meaningless decision).

Comment Several articles make short shrift of the p-value by merely reporting "$p < .05$" or "NS." We strongly recommend against this practice. Report the exact value when relying on a computer output. Of course, the exact value should be appropriately rounded to one or two significant digits. When conducting a TOH by hand using the charts and tables, report the p-value to the extent allowable by the table.

For the remainder of the text, the conclusion to a TOH will *always* state the *p-value* for the test. A report on any statistical TOH should not be viewed as complete unless it contains the p-value for the test.

EXERCISES 10.4

Warm-ups 10.4

A large-sample z-test ($n > 30$) is carried out following the protocol in Chart 2B. A key purpose of Chart 2B is to provide direction for constructing the decision line (Chart 2B, steps 2–5). To construct the decision line, one obtains the test critical value from Table 8. For example, the critical value for a two-tailed z-test at the 2% LOS (.02 in decimal form) is 2.326. The decision line is shown in Figure 10.4.5.

FIGURE **10.4.5**
Decision line for a two-tailed z-test at LOS .02.

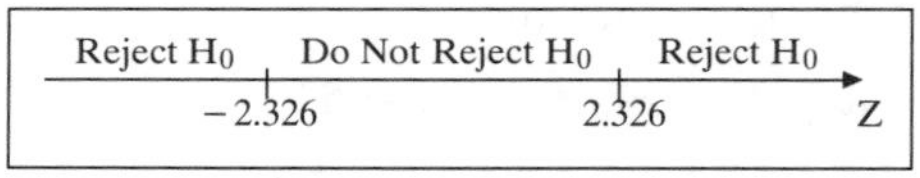

Reject H_0	Do Not Reject H_0	Reject H_0
-2.326	2.326	Z

1. Display the decision line for a two-tailed z-test at 1% LOS.

2. Display the decision line for a two-tailed z-test at 5% LOS.

3. Display the decision line for a two-tailed z-test at 10% LOS.

4. Display the decision line for a two-tailed z-test at 20% LOS.

5. As you increase the LOS, does the "do not reject H_0" region of the decision line
   a. Become shorter?
   b. Become longer?
   c. Stay the same?

6. As you increase the LOS, are you making it more or less likely of retaining H_0?

7. The p-value for a statistical test of hypothesis is
   a. The LOS at which the test critical z-value equals the sample z-value
   b. The largest LOS at which you can reject H_0
   c. The smallest LOS at which you can retain H_0
   d. All of the above

8. Suppose in a two-tailed z-test that the sample z-value is 2.137. This sample z-value falls between what two values in the Z column of Table 8?

9. What levels of significance are associated with the two Z column values in Warm-up 8?

10. Hence, ____ $<$ p-value $<$ ____.

11. The p-value for a two-tailed z-test with sample value 0.817 is reported by p-value $>$ _.20_.

12. The p-value for a two-tailed z-test with sample value 6.722 is reported by p-value $<$ ____.

13. The p-value for a one-tailed z-test with sample value 2.894 is reported by ____ $<$ p-value $<$ ____.

Problems 10.4

In Problems 1–25, determine the p-value for the specified test of hypothesis.

1. One-tailed z-test, alternate (c), sample $z = 2.411$

2. One-tailed z-test, alternate (b), sample $z = -3.164$

3. One-tailed z-test, alternate (c), sample $z = 1.037$

4. One-tailed z-test, alternate (c), sample $z = 6.487$

5. Two-tailed z-test, sample $z = 0.57$

6. Two-tailed z-test, sample $z = 1.893$

7. Two-tailed z-test, sample $z = 3.617$

8. Two-tailed z-test, sample $z = 4.82$

9. One-tailed z-test, alternate (b), sample $z = 2.5$

10. One-tailed z-test, alternate (c), sample $z = -2.2$

11. Two-tailed t-test, $df = 17$, sample $t = 2.3$

12. Two-tailed t-test, $df = 9$, sample $t = -3.1$

13. Two-tailed t-test, $df = 19$, sample $t = 0.97$

14. Two-tailed t-test, $df = 14$, sample $t = 5.3$

15. One-tailed t-test, alternate (c), $df = 20$, sample $t = 1.2$

16. One-tailed t-test, alternate (c), $df = 4$, sample $t = 9.3$

17. One-tailed t-test, alternate (c), $df = 24$, sample $t = 4.2$

18. One-tailed t-test, alternate (c), $df = 28$, sample $t = 2.3$

19. One-tailed t-test, alternate (b), $df = 23$, sample $t = -2.6$

20. One-tailed t-test, alternate (b), $df = 23$, sample t $= -4$

21. One-tailed t-test, alternate (b), $df = 23$, sample $t = -0.92$

22. One-tailed t-test, alternate (c), $df = 20$, sample $t = -2.2$

23. One-tailed t-test, alternate (c), $df = 20$, sample $t = -4.2$

24. One-tailed t-test, alternate (b), $df = 20$, sample $t = 0.79$

25. One-tailed t-test, alternate (b), $df = 20$, sample $t = 2.7$

26. Determine the p-value for the tests of hypothesis in Problems 10.1.

27. Determine the p-value for the tests of hypothesis in Problems 10.2.

28. Determine the p-value for the tests of hypothesis in Problems 10.3.

CHAPTER **10** OVERVIEW

Summary

A **test of hypothesis** (TOH) is a statistical procedure for resolving a problem of comparison. A **one-population problem of comparison** is resolved by applying a TOH to a **random sample with independent observations** drawn from the population of interest. In the health sciences, the assumption of a random sample usually is satisfied with a **convenience sample**, which maintains the spirit of randomness by taking precautions to avoid **confounding effects**.

One conducts a TOH by following the directions in an appropriate **chart** (Appendix) to guide one through the necessary computational details. The population parameter usually involved in a one-population test is a **pro-**portion or an **average**. A TOH about an average may be conducted about the median or the mean. An **s-test** tests the **median**. The **mean** may be tested by a **t-test** when the random variable of interest has a **normal distribution** or by a **z-test** when the sample size is large (>30).

In the health sciences, a TOH about the mean is often applied to analyze **paired data**. Paired data occur in **before and after** and in **method A versus method B** comparison studies. One analyzes paired data by computing the **difference** for each data pair. Since one can make a comparison between pairs by testing the mean of the differences against **zero**, zero is a common **test reference value** in a paired-data TOH.

A statistical TOH is summarized by presenting the **p-value** for the test. To decide between the null and alternate hypotheses, look at the p-value. If the p-value $\geq$ LOS, then retain H_0; otherwise, reject H_0 and accept H_a. In the health sciences literature, the p-value for a statistical test usually is reported.

Keywords

alternate hypothesis
before and after study
confounding effect
convenience sample
critical value
decision line
difference
hypothesis
independent observations
level of significance (LOS)
mean
median
method A versus method B
   study
normal distribution
null hypothesis
one-population study
one-tailed test
paired data
preliminary test
problem of comparison

problem of location
proportion
prospective study
p-value
random sample
random variable (RV)
retrospective study
sample legend
sample size
sample value
simple random sample
statistical significance
test alternate
test of hypothesis
   s-test
   t-test
   z-test
test reference value
test statistic
two-tailed test

References

Berky Z et al: Latex glove allergy. *JAMA* 268, no. 19 (18 November 1992): 2695.

Brandstetter R et al: Effect of nasogastric feedings on arterial oxygen tension in patients with symptomatic chronic obstructive pulmonary disease. *Heart Lung* 17, no. 2 (March 1988): 170.

Bridges N et al: Evaluation of a new system for hemoglobin measurement. *Am Clin Prod Rev* (April 1987): 22.

Chapman S and Duff P: Frequency of glove perforations and subsequent blood contact in association with selected obstetric surgical procedures. *Am J Obstet Gynecol* 168, no. 5 (May 1993): 1354.

Harding G et al: How long should catheter-acquired urinary tract infection in women be treated? *Ann Intern Med* 114, no. 9 (1 May 1991): 713.

Jonsbu J et al: Rapid and correct diagnosis of myocardial infarction: Standardized case history and clinical examination provide important information for correct referral to monitored beds. *J Intern Med* 229 (1991): 143.

Kirby J et al: Alcohol and drug use among trauma patients admitted to an intensive care unit. *Heart Lung* 18, no. 3 (May 1989): 297.

Klatsky A et al: Coffee use prior to myocardial infarction restudied: Heavier intake may increase the risk. *Am J Epidemiol* 132, no. 3(September 1990): 479.

Margolin G et al: Blood pressure lowering in elderly subjects: A double-blind crossover study of ω-3 and ω-6 fatty acids. *Am J Clin Nutr* 53, no. 3 (March 1991): 562.

Mauro A: Effects of bell versus diaphragm on indirect blood pressure measurement. *Heart Lung* 17, no. 5 (September 1988): 489.

Medley R et al: Comparability of the thermodilution cardiac output method: Proximal injectate versus proximal infusion lumens. *Heart Lung* 21, no. 1 (January 1992): 12.

Papadakis M et al: Treatable abdominal pathologic conditions and unsuspected malignant neoplasms at autopsy in veterans who received mechanical ventilation. *JAMA* 265, no. 7 (20 February 1991): 885.

Polednak A: Cancer incidence in the Puerto Rican–born population of Long Island, New York. *Am J Public Health* 81, no. 11 (November 1991): 1405.

Rovner B et al: Depression and mortality in nursing homes. *JAMA* 265, no. 8 (27 February 1991): 993.

Sorsensen G et al: Effects of a worksite nonsmoking policy: Evidence for increased cessation. *Am J Public Health* 81 (February 1991): 202.

Stäubli H and Jakob R: Anterior knee motion analysis: Measurement and simultaneous radiography. *Am J Sports Med* 19, no. 2 (March/April 1991): 172.

Tosata F et al: Evaluation of two methods used to stabilize oral endotracheal tubes. *Heart Lung* 16, no. 2 (March 1987): 140.

Winklhofer-Roob B et al: Short-term changes in erythrocyte α-tocopherol content of vitamin E–deficient patients with cystic fibrosis. *Am J Clin Nutr* 55, no. 1 (January 1992): 100.

Zillikens M et al: Whole-body and segmental bioelectrical-impedance analysis in patients with cirrhosis of the liver: Changes after treatment of ascites. *Am J Clin Nutr* 55, no. 3 (March 1992): 621.

Zwerling C et al: Costs and benefits of preemployment drug screening. *JAMA* 267, no. 1 (1 January 1992): 91.

11

Comparing Two Populations

One concept increasingly talked about in clinical circles is patient involvement in health care management. A single aspect of this large area is patient-controlled analgesia (PCA). A patient in the hospital can experience very uncomfortable pain for a few days, for example, after a large surgery. Should pain medication simply be administered as per a physician's order, or should the patient, who is the only one who can really feel the pain, essentially manage the pain control (analgesia)?

Important questions usually start in this nebulous "should" form. Such "should" questions are laden with psychological, sociological, cultural, legal, ethical, political, personal, and other considerations not appropriate for a scientific analysis. The important problem here is not to answer the given question but to pose one that can be answered. It can be agreed that with the rarest exception, postoperative patients need pain control during a short hospital recovery period. For discussion, suppose we decide that, in general, the less medication needed to be administered to control pain, the better. Consequently, one can reformulate the above "should" question into the following: Would patients in general receive less medication if (1) administered per standard physician's order or (2) self-administered for control of pain? Although this process of taking a general "should" problem and reformulating it into a specific question is summarized here in two paragraphs, this process is at the heart of statistical design and can take months. A statistical design can be no better than the question posed for study.

To answer the specific question, one can collect data using a sample of randomly presented patients. The sample of patients is then randomized into two groups of patients for pain control. One group, the *experimental group*, is a PCA group. Patients in the PCA group administered their own medication (Buprenex via Life Care PCA). The other group, the *control group*, received a traditional pain control protocol: intermittent injections of Buprenex 9.35 mg i.m. q3–6 hours prn pain. For each patient the amount of Buprenex administered was recorded. We can now compare to see which group in general undertook pain control with the least amount of Buprenex. In order to see how things turn out, we invite your attention to Problem 11.2.3.

This chapter is concerned with health science problems that want to contrast and compare either (1) a given effect in two different populations or (2) two different effects in the sample population. Such problems in the health sciences often can be recast into statistical problems of comparison. Section 11.1 focuses on those problems that may be resolved as statistical problems of comparison about proportions; Section 11.2, about averages.

OBJECTIVES   This section will

1   Describe the role and design of two-population comparison studies in the health sciences.

2   Resolve an appropriate health sciences problem by conducting a z-test of hypothesis for comparing the proportions of two populations when provided with data from independent random samples.

In Chapter 10 we introduced one-population comparison studies. In this chapter we extend to two-population comparison studies.

Two-Population Comparison Studies

The ability to assess the relative effectiveness of two different treatments is important in the health sciences. One needs this skill to assess whether, in general, a given intervention will improve the status of a patient (should congestive heart failure patients be treated with enalapril?) or whether a certain condition or behavior is detrimental to health (should a physician issue a warning for a side effect of headache when prescribing Cardizem to control hypertension?). Such assessment problems usually are resolved by research. Any statistical methods of resolution are dependent on the design strategies applied in the study to obtain the data used for analysis. The design strategies of choice in the health sciences are paired-data designs and those found in comparison studies.

A paired-data design is appropriate when *both* treatments can be applied to the *same* individual, such as

■   Room-temperature versus ice-temperature injectate to measure cardiac output
■   Sitting versus standing systolic blood pressure
■   Left or right arm for measuring blood pressure

In the preceding paired-data examples, each pair may be converted into a difference. The sample set of differences is then analyzed using a paired-difference test of hypothesis (Section 10.3). Whenever possible, such a paired-data design should be used to compare different treatments. Many treatments and conditions, however, are not candidates for a paired-data design. For example, to determine whether

■   Blood hemoglobin concentration is the same in men and women, a given patient cannot be both a male and female;
■   Cigarette smoking is correlated with lung cancer or heart disease, a study subject cannot be simultaneously a nonsmoker (never smoked) and a smoker;

■ Congestive heart failure patients are effectively recovered with enalapril, a study patient cannot be treated simultaneously with both enalapril therapy and placebo.

In such studies a given subject cannot be a representative member of both groups of interest simultaneously. Since a paired-data design is impossible, one must undertake a comparison study. A **comparison study** involves two different populations simultaneously. Independent and random samples with independent observations are obtained from each population. These samples are then compared against each other; hence the name, comparison study.

The assumptions of independent and random samples with independent observations are important requirements in a two-population comparison study. Samples are **independent** when an observation from one sample does not influence or affect an observation from another sample. In a multipopulation comparison study, the assumption of independent samples with independent observations is met with two design features: (1) *separate* random samples are taken from each population (ensuring independent samples), and (2) one measurement per subject per random variable (RV) (ensuring independent observations). For example, in the Bridges et al blood measurement study (see Table 10.2.2) male and female are independent since no one individual can belong to both samples. In contrast, the samples for hemoglobin (Hb) and packed cell volume (PCV) for females are not independent since both Hb and PCV were measured on the same women. For our needs in comparison studies, the assumption of independent samples with independent observations is crucial and may not be violated.

As with one-population studies, the strict sense of random samples may be relaxed as long as the spirit of randomness is maintained. In the health sciences, the assumption of random samples usually is met by taking carefully designed convenience samples. Since multipopulation studies encounter many new design problems regarding randomness, there are caveats to be issued and pitfalls to be avoided. Convenience samples that adhere to the following guidelines usually adequately maintain the spirit of randomness:

■ A research report should explicitly describe any exclusions in a study.
■ When a study is concerned with several different treatments (e.g., therapeutic drug versus placebo), if possible *randomly assign* subjects to the various treatment groups. A statistical design incorporating this feature is said to be **randomized**.
■ When comparing various treatments, if possible apply a double-blind design to the study. In a **double-blind** design, neither the patient nor the caregiver knows which treatment is being given or received. For example, in a double-blind study of enalapril versus placebo for treatment of congestive heart failure, neither the patient nor the person dispensing the medication to the patient knows whether enalapril or placebo is used.

The features of randomized and double-blind should be incorporated into the study design whenever appropriate. These features, however, are not always appropriate (or even possible). For an obvious example, to study the deleterious effects of fetal alcohol syndrome, it would be inappropriate to take a sample of nondrinking, nonpregnant women, randomly assign them to an alcoholics group and an abstainers group, induce pregnancy, and then gather data on their babies. In studying the effects of deleterious behavior like cigarette smoking or alcoholism, or traits that lead to a deleterious behavior like suicide, researchers use samples of people who have self-selected into the groups of interest rather than being randomly assigned to those groups. One must be particularly on guard for confounding effects when studying self-selected groups.

A health sciences professional must be versed in both paired-data studies (Section 10.3) and comparison studies. In this section we examine comparison problems concerned with proportions. A test of hypothesis to resolve such problems is called a comparison of proportions.

Comparison of Proportions

Comparison of proportions is a statistical test commonly applied in the health sciences to analyze data from a study evaluating the effectiveness of a treatment program. Subjects in the study are randomized into two groups. One group is the **experimental** group and receives the new treatment. The other group is the **control** group and does not receive the treatment (either no treatment or placebo). A standard for indicating improvement in the status of a subject is provided. One then carries out the study and determines the proportion of subjects helped in each group. The data are analyzed to determine whether the proportion of those helped in the experimental group is significantly greater than the proportion of those helped in the control group.

Our write-up for a test of hypothesis for the comparison of two proportions follows the instructions given in Chart 4 (Appendix). The test is valid assuming

- Independent and random samples from each population
- Independent observations within each sample
- Both sample sizes are adequately large

EXAMPLE 11.1.1 Galvao reported on the use of the drug enalapril in treating patients presenting congestive heart failure. The Enalapril Congestive Heart Failure study utilized a convenience sample of 256 patients in a randomized, double-blind, controlled design. Patients were randomly assigned to two groups: an enalapril group ($m = 126$) and a placebo group ($n = 130$). The investigators were interested in whether a patient showed an improvement in the New York Heart Association (NYHA) functional class after 4 weeks of therapy. In the enalapril group, 58 showed improvement; in the placebo group, 13 showed improvement. The study design and results are portrayed in Figure 11.1.1.

Let p_1 be the population proportion of congestive heart failure patients who show an improvement in NYHA functional class after 4 weeks of enalapril therapy. Similarly, let p_2 be the population proportion of heart patients who show an improvement in NYHA functional class after 4 weeks of placebo therapy. The motivation for the research is to test whether $p_1 > p_2$; accordingly,

$$H_0: p_1 \leq p_2$$
$$H_a: p_1 > p_2$$

FIGURE **11.1.1**
The Enalapril
Congestive Heart
Failure study.

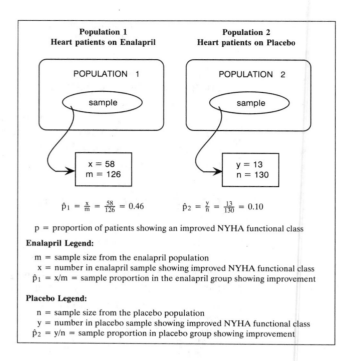

Since the study design used random and independent samples, and the sample sizes are large, we follow Chart 4 (Appendix) to conduct a z-test for comparison of proportions. The analysis is presented in Figure 11.1.2.

Our test of hypothesis for comparison of proportions (Chart 4) is a z-test since the test critical value (step 4) is obtained from a z-table. This z-test is permissible if the sample sizes are both adequately large. In a one-population study, a sample of size n for testing a hypothesized proportion p_0 is adequately large for a z-test if both $np_0 \geq 5$ and $n(1 - p_0) \geq 5$ (Chart 1). When comparing two populations, both samples must meet similar conditions for being adequately large (Chart 4, Preliminary Criteria). These conditions assure that both individuals with the attribute of interest and those without that attribute have a fair chance of being appropriately observed in the two samples. This fair chance is predicated on the assumption (null hypothesis) that both populations in the study have the same proportion of people with the attribute of interest.

EXAMPLE 11.1.2 Galvao also referred to the Consensus Trial, which examined the effect of enalapril on mortality in patients with severe congestive heart failure. The trial studied a convenience sample of 253 patients who were assigned to an enalapril group ($m = 127$) or a placebo group ($n = 126$) in a randomized, double-blind, controlled study. After 6 months the reported mortality rate was 26% for the enalapril group and 44% for the placebo group. We inquire whether mortality is statistically significantly lower in the enalapril group. Accordingly, we test

FIGURE **11.1.2**
The analysis of the Enalapril Congestive Heart Failure study (Example 11.1.1) is presented. The analysis follows Chart 4.

I. Preliminary criteria for adequacy of sample size.

$$\hat{p} = \frac{x+y}{m+n} = \frac{58+13}{126+10} = \frac{71}{256} \qquad \hat{q} = (1-\hat{p}) = 1 - \frac{71}{256} = \frac{256-71}{256} = \frac{185}{256}$$

$$m\hat{p} = 126\left(\frac{71}{256}\right) = 34.9 \geq 5 \qquad m\hat{q} = 126\left(\frac{185}{256}\right) = 91.0 \geq 5$$

$$n\hat{p} = 130\left(\frac{71}{256}\right) = 36.1 \geq 5 \qquad n\hat{q} = 130\left(\frac{185}{256}\right) = 93.9 \geq 5$$

II. Main Test of Hypothesis.

1. Hypothesis. $H_0: p_1 \leq p_2$ Alternate (c);

   $H_a: p_1 > p_2$ one-tailed test.

2. LOS. 0.05

3. Test Statistic. $\dfrac{\frac{x}{m} - \frac{y}{n}}{\sqrt{\hat{p}(1-\hat{p})\left(\frac{1}{m} + \frac{1}{n}\right)}}$ where $\hat{p} = \frac{x+y}{m+n}$

4. Critical Value. $z = 1.645$ (Table 8)

5. Decision Line.

   Do Not Reject H_0 | Reject H_0

   1.645   Z

6. Sample Value.

   $$\text{sample } z = \frac{\frac{x}{m} - \frac{y}{n}}{\sqrt{\hat{p}(1-\hat{p})\left(\frac{1}{m} + \frac{1}{n}\right)}} = \frac{\frac{58}{126} - \frac{13}{103}}{\sqrt{\left(\frac{71}{256}\right)\left(\frac{185}{256}\right)\left(\frac{1}{126} + \frac{1}{130}\right)}} = 6.438$$

7. Conclusion. Based on the given data, at the 5% LOS reject $H_0: p_1 \leq p_2$ and accept H_a: $p_1 > p_2$. The study provides very strong evidence that the proportion of patients on enalapril who show an improvement in NYHA functional class is statistically significantly greater than the proportion of patients on placebo. In this regard, enalapril therapy is effective (p-value $< .000005$).

$$H_0: p_1 \geq p_2$$
$$H_a: p_1 < p_2$$

where p is the proportion who die in a given group (1 = enalapril, 2 = placebo).

To conduct the test of hypothesis, we convert the given percentages to frequencies.

Enalapril Group:
    $m = 127$ (sample size)
    $x = 127(.26) = 33$ (number who died within 6 months)
    $\hat{p}_1 = 33/127$ (proportion of deaths in sample enalapril group)
Placebo Group:
    $n = 126$ (sample size)
    $y = 126(.44) = 55$ (number who died within 6 months)
    $\hat{p}_2 = 55/126$ (proportion of deaths in sample placebo group)

The test of hypothesis to compare the proportions of deaths between the two groups follows Chart 4 and is presented in Figure 11.1.3. Note that the preliminary criteria of independent random samples, independent observations, and large sample sizes are met.

Comment The Consensus Trial referred to in Example 11.1.2 began in April 1985. The study design was approved and monitored by an ethical review committee. In December 1986 the ethical review committee halted the trial on the basis of the analysis of the data collected up to that point. The committee concluded that enalapril statistically significantly reduced mortality in patients with congestive heart failure. The committee stated that it would be unethical to continue patients on placebo in the face of the accumulated evidence.

FIGURE **11.1.3**
A comparison of proportions analysis following Chart 4 for the Consensus Trial (Example 11.1.2) study is presented.

I. Preliminary criteria for adequacy of sample size.

$$\hat{p} = \frac{x+y}{m+n} = \frac{33+55}{127+126} = \frac{88}{263} \qquad \hat{q} = (1-\hat{p}) = 1 - \frac{88}{263} = \frac{263-88}{263} = \frac{175}{263}$$

$$m\hat{p} = 127\left(\frac{88}{263}\right) = 42.5 \geq 5 \qquad m\hat{q} = 127\left(\frac{175}{263}\right) = 84.5 \geq 5$$

$$n\hat{p} = 126\left(\frac{88}{263}\right) = 42.2 \geq 5 \qquad n\hat{q} = 126\left(\frac{175}{263}\right) = 83.8 \geq 5$$

II. Main Test of Hypothesis.

1. Hypothesis. $H_0: p_1 \geq p_2$ Alternate (b);
                 $H_a: p_1 < p_2$ one-tailed test.

2. LOS. 0.05

3. Test Statistic. $\dfrac{\frac{x}{m} - \frac{y}{n}}{\sqrt{\hat{p}(1-\hat{p})\left(\frac{1}{m}+\frac{1}{n}\right)}}$ where $\hat{p} = \frac{x+y}{m+n}$

4. Critical Value. $z = 1.645$ (Table 8)

5. Decision Line.

   Reject H_0 | Do Not Reject H_0
             -1.645 z

6. Sample Value.

$$\text{sample } z = \frac{\frac{33}{127} - \frac{55}{126}}{\sqrt{\left(\frac{88}{263}\right)\left(\frac{165}{263}\right)\left(\frac{1}{126}+\frac{1}{127}\right)}} = -2.950$$

7. Conclusion. Based on the given data, at the 5% level of significance we reject $H_0: p_1 \geq p_2$ and accept $H_a: p_1 < p_2$. Enalapril is effective in reducing the 6-month mortality rate in congestive heart failure patients ($.001 < p$-value $< .005$).

EXERCISES 11.1

Warm-Ups 11.1

A Dutch study group compared two doses of aspirin (30 mg versus 283 mg per day) for treating patients after a transient ischemic attack or minor ischemic stroke. In a double-blind, controlled clinical trial, 3131 patients were randomized into one of two groups. One group received a low dose (30 mg) of aspirin on a regular prescribed basis; the other group, 283 mg aspirin. The frequency of a vascular event (nonfatal stroke, nonfatal myocardial infarction, or death from a vascular cause—whichever came first) was 228 of 1555 for the 30-mg group, compared with 240 of 1576 in the 283-mg group during the 3-year study period. We inquire: Is the frequency of a vascular event significantly different between the two groups during the time frame of the study?

1. This study is double-blind means
   a. Blind people are used as study subjects in both groups.
   b. The researchers are blind to what is happening so that the results of the experiment will not be biased.
   c. The patients do not know what dose of aspirin they are getting.
   d. Neither the patient nor the administrator of the medication knows the treatment group of the subject.

2. The study is randomized means
   a. The patients are randomly assigned to receive a specific treatment during the course of the study.
   b. The aspirin dose is randomly determined at each administration.

   c. The patients are randomly assigned to a person giving the medication.
   d. The patients are randomly assigned to a mortality group.

3. Complete Table 11.1.1 for organizing the sample data.

TABLE **11.1.1**

	30-mg Group	283-mg Group
Sample size		
Number of events		

4. Let p be the proportion of subjects in a given group who have a vascular event during the study period. Then

$$\hat{p}_1 = 228/1555 = \underline{\quad} \text{ and } \hat{p}_2 = \underline{\quad}/\underline{\quad} = \underline{\quad}$$

where group 1 is the 30-mg group and group 2 is the 283-mg group.

5. The researchers wanted to test whether there was a statistically significant difference in vascular events between the two groups. State the null and alternate hypotheses for the comparison of proportions appropriate for the researchers' concern.

6. Our test of hypothesis for comparison of proportions (Chart 4) is valid only if both sample sizes are adequately large. To assess for adequacy of sample sizes, one needs the combined study proportion, $\hat{p} = (x + y)/(m + n)$ as defined in the preliminary criteria in Chart 4. What is $\hat{p}$ for this study?

7. To determine adequacy of sample sizes, one also needs the quantity $\hat{q} = (1 - \hat{p})$. What is $\hat{q}$ for this study?

8. Both sample sizes are adequately large if the four quantities $m\hat{p}$, $m\hat{q}$, $n\hat{p}$, and $n\hat{q}$ are all ≥ 5. Calculate these four quantities. Are both sample sizes adequately large?

9. At the 5% LOS, what is the critical z-value for a two-tailed test for a comparison of proportions?

10. Construct the decision line for testing $H_0: p_1 = p_2$ versus $H_a: p_1 \neq p_2$ at the 5% LOS.

11. What is the sample z-value?

12. At the 5% LOS, do we retain or reject $H_0: p_1 = p_2$?

13. Using Table 8, what is the p-value for the test?

14. How would you compare vascular events between the two groups?

Problems 11.1

1. The Enalapril Congestive Heart Failure Study made other inquiries of the patients beyond improvement in NYHA functional class. To determine patient perception, patients were interviewed to determine whether they "felt much better" as a result of the therapy program. Of the 126 patients in the enalapril group, 69 reported that they "felt much better," whereas 26 of the 130 in the placebo group "felt much better."

    a. Conduct a two-tailed test of hypothesis to determine whether there is a statistically significant difference in the proportion of patients who "felt much better" between the enalapril and placebo groups.

    b. Conduct a one-tailed test of hypothesis to determine whether the proportion of patients who "felt much better" is statistically significantly greater in the enalapril group.

2. The Consensus Trial examined the effect of enalapril on mortality in 253 patients with severe congestive heart failure. The 253 patients were randomly assigned to an enalapril group ($m = 127$) or a placebo group ($n = 126$). After 1 year, the reported mortality rate was 36% for the enalapril group and 52% for the placebo group. At the 5% LOS, is 1-year mortality for the enalapril group statistically significantly lower than 1-year mortality for the placebo group?

3. A clinical study was made to determine side effects of terazosin, a drug used to control hypertension. The randomized, double-blind, controlled study placed 859 patients on terazosin and 506 people on placebo. Each person during a controlled time period kept track of general body ailments (headache, backache, asthenia). Of the 859 on terazosin therapy, 139 complained of general body ailments; among the 506 persons on placebo, 80 such complaints were registered. Should a warning of general body ailments as a side effect be issued to patients on terazosin? Justify your answer with an appropriate test of hypothesis.

4. Burroughs Wellcome Co., a pharmaceutical firm, advertises its drug Retrovir in leading medical journals. They cite research describing a 1-year, randomized, double-blind, controlled study which reported that 33 of 453 HIV patients on placebo progressed to AIDS, whereas only 11 of 428 HIV patients on Retrovir progressed to AIDS. Is the proportion of HIV patients on Retrovir who progress to AIDS statistically significantly smaller than the proportion of HIV patients on placebo who progress to AIDS? Test at the 10% LOS.

5. Whitehall Laboratories, makers of Advil, published the following data in recent medical journals. The data were obtained in a single-dose, double-blind, randomized study. Patients were randomized into one of two groups: ibuprofen and placebo. Over the course of the study, patients indicated whether they experienced stomach upset (yes or no). The results are shown in Table 11.1.2. At the 5% LOS, is there a statistically significant difference in the proportion of patients who report upset stomach between ibuprofen and placebo?

TABLE **11.1.2** Data on ibuprofen.

	Yes	No	Total
Ibuprofen	8	664	672
Placebo	6	645	651
Total	14	1309	1323

6. Marion Merrell Dow, makers of Cardizem, a drug for control of hypertension, report the following results obtained in a randomized, double-blind, placebo-controlled hypertension study. Advertisements for Cardizem can be found in most recent medical journals. Of 315 patients on diltiazem (the active agent in Cardizem), 38 reported headache, while 17 of 211 placebo patients reported headache. Should an adverse reaction warning for headache be issued with a prescription of Cardizem?

7. Tatemichi et al studied 726 patients aged ≥ 60 with acute ischemic stroke. In particular, these patients were tested for the presence or absence of dementia.

   a. There were 392 female patients in the study; of these, 17.3% had dementia. There were 334 male patients in the study; of these, 14.4% had dementia. Is there a statistically significant difference in the proportion of those with dementia between the male and female populations of patients aged ≥ 60 with acute ischemic stroke?

   b. There were 709 patients in the study for whom a determination of previous myocardial infarction (MI) could be made. Of 128 patients with previous MI, 22.7% displayed dementia. Of the 581 patients with no history of MI, 14.1% displayed dementia. Is the presentation of dementia greater in patients with a previous MI than in those without MI?

   c. There were 702 patients in the study for whom a determination of previous stroke could be made. Of 168 with previous stroke, 30.4% were demented. Of 534 without previous stroke, 9.4% were demented. Is the occurrence of dementia lower among patients with no history of stroke?

   d. There were 718 patients for whom previous antiplatelet or anticoagulant drug use could be determined. Of the 93 patients with such drug history, 15.1% were demented. Of 625 with no history of such drug therapy, 16.0% were demented. Is dementia related to a history of antiplatelet or anticoagulant drug therapy?

8. Dening and Berrios studied the course of characteristic manifestations of patients with Wilson's disease. The study includes 195 cases of patients with unequivocal Wilson's disease. Index (baseline) measurements were taken for patients upon entry into the study. In this group, there were 84 neurological cases (patients with a certain neurological index). These neurological cases were further broken up into two groups: neuropsychiatric ($n = 58$) and neurological only ($n = 26$).

   a. What proportion of Wilson's disease patients are neurological cases? Determine both a point estimate and a 95% confidence interval.

   b. What proportion of the neurological cases are neuropsychiatric?

   c. Dysarthria was present in 51 of the 58 neuropsychiatric cases, and in 15 of the 58 neurological-only cases at entry into the study. Is the proportion of patients with dysarthria greater in the neurological-only group than in the neuropsychiatric group among neurological cases of patients with Wilson's disease?

   d. After an appropriate course of treatment, 35 of the 58 neuropsychiatric patients displayed dysarthria, while 7 of the 26 neurological-only patients displayed dysarthria. Is the proportion of patients after treatment with dysarthria greater in the neuropsychiatric group than in the neurological-only group?

9. Harding et al studied catheter-acquired urinary tract infection in hospitalized women. They randomized 112 asymptomatic female patients with catheter-acquired bacteriuria into treatment groups. They then observed whether infection resolved within 14 days. In each of the following, justify your answer with an appropriate test of hypothesis for comparison of proportions.

   a. Of the 112 patients in the study, 42 were randomized into a control group receiving no treatment for infection; the other 70 patients were randomized into treatment groups. In the control group, 15 women resolved infection within 14 days; in the treatment groups, 56 of 70 resolved. At the 5% LOS, is the resolution rate among treated women greater than among nontreated women?

b. There were two treatment groups. Group 1, the single-dose therapy group, received a single dose of antibiotic. Group 2, the 10-day therapy group, received a small dose of the antibiotic every day for 10 days. Of the 70 patients randomized to receive treatment, 37 were assigned to the single-dose group and 33 to the 10-day group. Infection from single-dose therapy was resolved in 30 of 37 patients; from 10-day therapy, in 26 of 33 patients. Are these results consistent with the hypothesis that the resolution rate is the same for both types of therapy?

10. (Continued from Problem 9) Support or refute the following claim made in the paper with an appropriate test of hypothesis for the comparison of proportions: Infection was resolved more often in women who were ≤ 65 years of age than in older women (62 of 70 versus 24 of 39).

Problems 11–14 are continued from the Warm-ups. Recall that the 30-mg aspirin group contained 1555 subjects, while the 283-mg aspirin group contained 1576 subjects.

11. There were 40 major bleeding complications in the 30-mg group and 53 major bleeding complications in the 283-mg group. Is there a significant difference in major bleeding complications between the two groups?

12. There were 49 minor bleeding episodes in the 30-mg group and 84 minor bleeding episodes in the 283-mg group. Is there a significant difference in minor bleeding episodes between the two groups?

13. There were 164 gastrointestinal symptoms reported in the 30-mg group and 179 gastrointestinal symptoms reported in the 283-mg group. Is there a significant difference in gastrointestinal symptoms between the two groups?

14. There were 73 other adverse effects in the 30-mg group and 90 in the 283-mg group. Is there a significant difference in other adverse effects between the two groups?

Problems 15–18 are based on a report by the First Seizure Trial Group, which conducted a 2-year study to investigate the effectiveness of antiepileptic drugs (AEDs) in preventing seizure recurrence in newly diagnosed patients with epilepsy. The study enrolled 397 patients who were randomized into either an immediate-treatment group or a no-treatment group.

15. Of the 204 patients in the treated group, 36 displayed a seizure recurrence during the study period. Of the 193 in the no-treatment group, 75 displayed a seizure recurrence. Is treatment with AEDs effective in reducing seizure recurrence?

16. Among the patients enrolled in the study, 270 were diagnosed as having generalized seizure and no previous uncertain seizures. Of these, 47 out of 138 patients randomized into the no-treatment group subsequently displayed a seizure recurrence, while 26 out of 132 randomized into the treated group subsequently displayed a seizure recurrence. Is AEDs treatment effective in reducing seizure recurrence among epileptics diagnosed as having generalized seizure with no previous uncertain seizures?

17. Among the 204 patients randomized into the immediate AEDs treatment group, 41 discontinued AEDs at some point during the study. Of these 41 patients, 11 displayed a seizure recurrence; 25 of 163 who complied with the AEDs treatment displayed a seizure recurrence. Is there statistically significantly less seizure recurrence among patients who complied with AEDs treatment?

18. In the study, 62 patients were diagnosed as having partial seizure and no previous uncertain seizures. Of these, 26 were in the no treatment group, and 12 subsequently displayed a seizure recurrence; 36 were in the treated group, and 3 subsequently displayed a seizure recurrence. Is AEDs treatment effective in reducing seizure recurrence among epileptics diagnosed as having generalized seizure with no previous uncertain seizures?

Problems 19–20 are based on results reported by Browman et al, who studied the effect of cigarette smoking on the effectiveness of therapy in treating head and neck cancer. The study enrolled a convenience sample of 115 consecutive patients who were diagnosed for head or neck cancer. The cancer was treated with surgery followed by radiation therapy. Of the 115 patients, 62 did not smoke during the course of postsurgery radiation therapy, while 53 smoked.

19. Browman et al reported that of the 53 patients who continued to smoke during the course of radiation therapy, 24 had a complete response to therapy. Of the 62 who did not smoke during the course of radiation therapy, 46 had a complete response to therapy. Is the proportion of patients presenting a complete response to radiation therapy following surgery for head or neck cancer significantly greater among nonsmokers than smokers?

20. Browman et al reported that the 2-year survival rate was 66% among the nonsmoking patients and 39% in the smoking group. Do the nonsmokers have a significantly greater 2-year survival rate than the smokers?

SECTION 11.2

Comparison of Average Values

OBJECTIVES   This section will

1 Describe the design of a comparison of averages study in the health sciences.

2 Determine which test of hypothesis to apply to resolve a comparison of averages problem.

3 Conduct an appropriate statistical test of hypothesis comparing the averages of two populations when provided with independent random samples with independent observations.

4 Construct a c% confidence interval for the difference in population means when provided with appropriate data.

In Section 11.1 we compared proportions between two populations. In this section we compare averages. In general, we will have two populations and a quantitative RV of interest. We inquire how the average of the RV in one population compares against the average of the RV in the other population; that is, is one average equal to, greater than, or less than the other average?

EXAMPLE 11.2.1 Vio et al were concerned that cigarette smoking compromises a nursing mother's ability to adequately support nutrition in her infant through breast-feeding. They conjectured that cigarette smoking induces decreased breast-milk production in nursing mothers. Accordingly, they investigated whether breast-milk production among smoking nursing mothers was less than breast-milk production among nonsmoking nursing mothers. Their study group consisted of 20 lactating mothers: 10 mothers never smoked, and 10 mothers smoked during pregnancy and continued to smoke during breast-feeding their infant. A smoker was defined as a person who smoked ≥ 4 cigarettes per day throughout both pregnancy and breast-feeding. Each mother-child pair also met the following criteria: infant age 1 to 3 months, normal birth weight, no morbidity, and exclusively breast-fed. The purpose of the selection process was that mother-infant pairs in the study were basically similar except for smoking habits.

Comparison of Averages

Vio et al (Example 11.2.1.) were concerned with a general health sciences problem: Does cigarette smoking compromise a nursing mother's ability to provide adequate nutritional support to her breast-fed infant? To gain insight into this health sciences problem, Vio et al formulated several problems of comparison; among them: "On average, is breast-milk production among smoking nursing mothers less than breast-milk production among nonsmoking nursing mothers?"

Vio et al pose a well-defined problem of comparison by specifying (1) the two populations of interest and (2) the RV of interest. The two populations of interest are nursing smoking mothers and nursing nonsmoking mothers. The random variable of interest is breast-milk production. A problem of comparison involving the average of an RV in two given populations is conveniently called a **comparison of averages** problem.

The advantage of recasting a general health sciences concern into a problem of comparison is that the problem of comparison can be resolved by statistical methods. These statistical methods all utilize some test of hypothesis. Our tests of hypothesis for resolving a comparison of averages problem require data from *independent random samples with independent observations*. Before starting the calculations in a test of hypothesis, one should check to verify this requirement is met.

EXAMPLE 11.2.2 The Vio et al breast-milk production study design (Example 11.2.1) incorporates a random sample of 20 lactating mothers (screened to meet enrollment criteria) taken from a larger convenience sample. Since the spirit of randomness is maintained, we may assume the data come from random samples. The samples are independent since the amount of breast-milk produced by a smoking mother does not influence the amount of milk produced by a nonsmoking mother. The study design called for independent observations within each sample (breast-milk production was to be measured and reported as a single number for each individual in the study).

Since the Vio et al study design utilizes independent random samples with independent observations, we resolve the comparison of averages problem with a test of hypothesis. We now need to select the appropriate test of hypothesis procedure.

Selecting a Test of Hypothesis for Comparing Averages

To analyze data obtained for comparing averages between two populations, we need to select the right test of hypothesis: t-test, z-test, or Mann-Whitney test. The selection process for which test of hypothesis to apply parallels the selection process for confidence intervals (Section 7.1). Our selection process starts by noting whether the raw data are available or we only have the data legend to work with.

Raw Data
When given the raw data, follow these checkpoints to determine which test of hypothesis for comparing averages to apply.

Checkpoint 1: Normal distributions. Perform an nscores correlation test for a normal distribution in Minitab on both samples. If both samples are consistent with normality, then apply a two-samples t-test for comparison of *means*; otherwise, go to checkpoint 2.

Checkpoint 2: Large sample sizes. If both sample sizes are large (> 30), then apply the large-samples z-test for comparison of *means* (Appendix, Chart 5C).

Checkpoint 3: Nonnormal, small sample size(s). If one or both samples are nonnormal and one or both samples are small (size ≤ 30), then compare the population *medians* by applying the Mann-Whitney test in Minitab.

Data Legend

Suppose that the raw data set is not available, but one has the data legend (sample size, sample mean, sample standard deviation). Selecting the right type of test of hypothesis to use is done simply by keying on the sample sizes.

Checkpoint 1: Large sample sizes. If both sample sizes are greater than 30, then apply the large-samples z-test for comparison of *means* (Appendix, Chart 5C).

Checkpoint 2: Small sample size(s). If one or both of the sample sizes is ≤ 30, then determine whether the RV of interest is continuous (Section 6.1).

a. If the RV of interest is continuous, make a statement assuming that the RV is normally distributed in each population. Then apply a two-samples t-test for comparison of means.

b. Otherwise, announce that you have insufficient information for analysis.

The basic tests of hypothesis for comparison of averages are the two-samples t-tests, large-samples z-test, and the Mann-Whitney test. Which one to apply depends on the nature of the data, as summarized in Figure 11.2.1. We now examine these three kinds of tests in more detail.

Two-Samples t-Tests

Suppose now that we have two populations, an RV of interest, and two independent random samples with independent observations drawn from the given populations. Suppose further that we are assuming that the RV is normally distributed in each population. Then, a **two-samples t-test for comparison of means** is appropriate.

EXAMPLE 11.2.3 The raw data set from Vio et al shown in Table 11.2.1 displays two independent random samples with independent observations: smoking mothers and

FIGURE **11.2.1**
Selecting a test to compare average values.

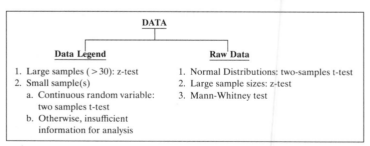

nonsmoking mothers. Since we have the raw data, we check both samples for normality. The critical nscores correlation at 1% LOS is .8804 (Table 5, Appendix). The respective sample nscores correlations are .981 and .947 (Figure 11.2.6). Hence, we assume that breast-milk production in nursing mothers is (approximately) normally distributed ($p > .10$).

TABLE **11.2.1**
Raw data set from Vio et al. The data present the average breast-milk production (g/day) over a 15-day period for each nursing mother in the study.

Smoking Mothers	Nonsmoking Mothers
621	947
793	945
593	1086
545	1202
753	973
655	981
895	930
767	745
714	903
598	899

The assumption that breast-milk production is normally distributed in both populations justifies applying a *t-test for comparison of means*. At the onset of our analysis of the Vio et al study, we noted only that we were going to compare the average breast-milk production of smoking mothers against the average breast-milk production of nonsmoking mothers. However, there are several ways to present an average, for example, the mean and the median. Establishing normality refines our task down to a two-samples *t-test* for comparison of *means*.

A normal distribution is controlled by two parameters: the mean and the standard deviation. The mean centers the distribution; the standard deviation controls the spread of the distribution. A t-test for comparison of means allows us to compare the means of the two groups, but what about the standard deviations (SDs)? For example, the SD for breast-milk production of smoking nursing mothers is 109.5 g/day; for nonsmoking nursing mothers, 120.0 g/day (see Figure 11.2.6). The two SDs are fairly close to each other. Hence, we may reasonably assume that variation in individual breast-milk production in the two groups is (approximately) the same. When the variation in the two groups is the same, then a powerful test for comparison of means called the "pooled t-test" should be applied. When an assumption of equal variation is not justified (or ignored), this is taken into account by applying a two-samples t-test (unpooled) for comparison of means.

Accordingly, there are two versions of a two-samples t-test for comparison of means: two-samples t-test (pooled) and two-samples t-test (not pooled). Figure 11.2.2 displays a rigorous (but simple) three-step protocol for deciding whether "pooling" is appropriate.

Comment Technically, the three-step procedure shown in Figure 11.2.2 describes a test of hypothesis for equality of population variances. If one wants to test

$$H_0: \sigma_1^2 = \sigma_2^2$$
$$H_a: \sigma_2^2 \neq \sigma_2^2$$

FIGURE *11.2.2*
Three-step procedure
to determine whether
to conduct a two-
samples t-test for
comparison of means
with or without
pooling. SD =
standard deviation.

Step 1. Calculate the quantity

$$\text{sample f-value} = \left(\frac{\text{larger sample SD}}{\text{smaller sample SD}}\right)^2$$

Record: L = sample size of sample with the larger SD,
S = sample size of sample with the smaller SD.

Step 2. From the LOS .01 F-Table (Table 10a, Appendix), determine the table entry in column L-1 and row S-1. This is the critical f-value for the decision line in Step 3 (f = critical f-value).

Step 3. Place the sample f-value obtained in Step 1 on the following decision line and then announce the verdict.

then apply the three-step procedure for the f-test given in Figure 11.2.2 with the decision line (step 3) adjusted as shown in Figure 11.2.3.

When the variances are equal, statisticians say the populations are **homoscedastic**; if not equal, **heteroscedastic**. Hence, the decision line may also be displayed as shown in Figure 11.2.4.

When the variances are equal (i.e., the populations are homoscedastic), statisticians have developed a powerful test for comparison of *means* called the two-samples t-test with pooling, or more simply, **pooled t-test**. *The pooled t-test should be used whenever justified*. The pooled t-test is more adept than any other test at recognizing when a null hypothesis for a comparison of means is false. The theory of the pooled t-test exploits the assumption of homoscedasticity; hence, the pooled t-test uses more information than a nonpooled version and accordingly may produce a stronger result.

The pooled t-test for the comparison of means is conducted by following Chart 5A, Appendix. The two-samples t-test without pooling is called the **Smith-Satterthwaite test** and follows Chart 5B. A glance at Chart 5B, step 4 (critical value) reveals a computational nightmare. Those who have not liked the computer up to this point often develop a sudden interest in Minitab.

The full summary of test selection options for comparison of averages follows.

Comparison of Averages

1. If normal distributions, then compare means by applying a two-samples t-test:
   a. If homoscedastic, then pooled t-test;
   b. If heteroscedastic, then Smith-Satterthwaite t-test.

2. If large sample sizes, then compare means by applying the large-samples z-test.

3. Compare medians by applying the Mann-Whitney test on Minitab.

FIGURE *11.2.3*
Decision line for equal
versus not equal variances.

FIGURE **11.2.4**
Decision line for homoscedastic
versus heteroscedastic populations.

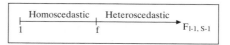

We illustrate the testing procedure by example, following the protocol outlined in Chart 5A for the pooled t-test and Chart 5B for the Smith-Satterthwaite test.

The Pooled Two-Samples t-Test for Comparison of Means

To justify conducting a pooled two-samples t-test for comparison of means, we need (1) independent random samples with independent observations, (2) normal distributions, and (3) homoscedasticity.

EXAMPLE 11.2.4   We continue with the Vio et al breast-milk study for smoking versus nonsmoking nursing mothers (Examples 11.2.1–3). We already noted independent random samples with independent observations (Examples 11.2.2 and 3) and normality (Example 11.2.3). We now consider homoscedasticity.

The sample standard deviation for the smoking mothers group is 109.5; for the nonsmoking mothers group, 120.0 (see Figure 11.2.6). The quotient of the larger to the smaller sample variance is given by $(120.0/109.5)^2 = 1.2$. The pool versus don't pool decision line is shown in Figure 11.2.5. The sample is consistent with homoscedasticity ($p > .05$). Hence, apply the pooled t-test.

We apply the pooled t-test for comparing mean breast-milk production in the two groups of nursing mothers. In particular, we test the formal statement of hypothesis

$H_0: \mu_1 \geq \mu_2$
$H_a: \mu_1 < \mu_2$ (smoking mothers produce less breast milk)

where μ_1 is the mean breast-milk production in smoking nursing mothers and μ_2 is the mean breast-milk production in nonsmoking nursing mothers.

Whenever we have the raw data, we conduct a two-samples t-test for comparison of means in Minitab. The general form of the two-sample pooled t-test in Minitab is

MTB > TWOSAMPLE C C;
SUBC> ALTERNATE K;
SUBC> POOLED.

To conduct the Smith-Satterthwaite test (the two-samples t-test without pooling), simply omit the POOLED subcommand.

FIGURE **11.2.5**
Decision line for pool versus
don't pool for the Vio et al study.

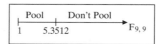

EXAMPLE 11.2.5 For the Vio et al study (Examples 11.2.3–4), we set the sample data into columns C1 (smoking mothers) and C2 (nonsmoking mothers). Minitab's work-up is displayed in Figure 11.2.6. For illustration, the detailed seven-step write-up for the pooled t-test comparison of mean breast-milk production for the two groups is given in Figure 11.2.7 and follows Chart 5A.

Note that virtually all the analysis can be done on the computer. In Minitab we can obtain the sample nscores correlation for each sample. One can then draw the normality decision line by hand to obtain that decision. To check for homoscedasticity, we need to know which standard deviation is larger. To get this quickly, issue the DESCRIBE command. Looking under the STDEV information, we see that the nonsmokers have the greater standard deviation. The LET K1 = . . . command following the DESCRIBE output produces the sample f-value for the homoscedasticity check. One can draw in the homoscedasticity decision line to obtain that verdict. We now know to issue the TWOSAMPLE command and attach the POOLED subcommand to conduct the pooled t-test.

FIGURE **11.2.6**
Minitab output for comparison of mean breast-milk production between smoking nursing mothers (data in C1) and nonsmoking nursing mothers (data in C2).

```
MTB > NOTE    Test for normal distributions:
MTB > NSCORES C1 INTO C11
MTB > CORRELATION C1 AND C11

Correlation of smokers and Nscores = 0.981

MTB > NSCORES C2 INTO C11
MTB > CORRELATION C2 AND C11

Correlation of no smoke and Nscores = 0.947

MTB > NOTE    Test for homoscedasticity:
MTB > DESCRIBE C1 C2

                N      MEAN    MEDIAN   TREMEAN    STDEV   SEMEAN
smokers        10     693.4     684.5     686.8    109.5     34.6
no smoke       10     961.1     946.0     958.0    120.0     37.9

               MIN       MAX        Q1        Q3
smokers      545.0     895.0     596.7     773.5
no smoke     745.0    1202.0     902.0    1007.3

MTB > LET K1 = (STDEV(C2)/STDEV(C1))**2
MTB > PRINT K1    #sample f-value
K1       1.20070
MTB >
MTB > NOTE    Conduct test of hypothesis (twosample pooled t-test):
MTB > TWOSAMPLE C1 C2;
SUBC> ALTERNATE -1;
SUBC> POOLED.

TWOSAMPLE T FOR smokers VS no smoke
                N      MEAN     STDEV    SE MEAN
smokers    10       693       109         35
no smoke   10       961       120         38

95 PCT CI FOR MU smokers - MU no smoke: (-376, -160)

TTEST MU smokers = MU no smoke (VS LT): T= -5.21  P=0.0000  DF= 18

POOLED STDEV =          115
```

FIGURE **11.2.7**

The write-up for the pooled t-test (main test) for the comparison of mean breast-milk production for smoking mothers versus nonsmoking mothers (Example 11.2.5) is displayed. The write-up follows Chart 5A. Population 1 = smoking mothers; population 2 = nonsmoking mothers.

1. Hypothesis. $H_0: \mu_1 \geq \mu_2$ Test alternate (b);
   $H_a: \mu_1 < \mu_2$ one-tailed test.
2. LOS. 0.05
3. Test Statistic. $\dfrac{\bar{x}_1 - \bar{x}_2}{\sqrt{s_p^2\left(\frac{1}{n_1} + \frac{1}{n_2}\right)}}$
   where $s_p^2 = [(n_1 - 1)s_1^2 + (n_2 - 1)s_2^2]/(n_1 + n_2 - 2)$
4. Critical Value. $df = n_1 + n_2 - 2 = 10 + - 2 = 18$
   $t = 1.73407$ (Table 9)
5. Decision Line.

   Reject H_0 No Not Reject H_0 $\rightarrow T_{18}$
   -1.73407
6. Sample Value. sample-t $= -5.21$ (Minitab, see Figure 11.2.6)
7. Conclusion. Based on the given data, at the 5% LOS reject $H_0: \mu_1 \geq \mu_2$ and accept $H_a: \mu_1 < \mu_2$. The data provide strong evidence that the mean breast-milk production in smoking nursing mothers is statistically significantly less than the mean breast-milk production in nonsmoking nursing mothers ($p < .00005$).

The real benefit of the computer output is that we can focus immediately on the *p*-value for the test (Minitab: p = 0.0000). We report $p < .00005$. Because of the very small *p*-value, without any further ado, we know to reject the null hypothesis! We can immediately report our conclusion: Smoking lactating mothers have less breast-milk production than nonsmoking lactating mothers ($t = -5.21, df = 18, p < .00005$).

Note the simple form of this verdict! The bottom-line conclusion is stated in plain English. The important test of hypothesis details follow, enclosed in parentheses: the sample value, the degrees of freedom if any, and the *p*-value. Professionals writing in the literature usually use this kind of brief summary format to report their results.

Comment With only the sample legend (without the raw data), you will need to go through the seven-step format following the directions given in a test of hypothesis chart. When working by hand using the sample legend, one must have the sample value in order to obtain the *p*-value. What makes a computer output so nice is that the *p*-value is issued and you have everything you need to make your decision. Recall that if *p*-value ≥ LOS, then do not reject the null hypothesis; if *p*-value < LOS, then reject the null hypothesis. It is precisely this facet of the *p*-value that was exploited to construct Chart 2C for the s-test. Any test of hypothesis can be reduced to this simplified form if one has the computer to issue the *p*-value. That is why, in a "word," the *p*-value tells an experienced professional what she or he needs to know about a test of hypothesis.

Comment As the Vio et al study shows, as does virtually any study having to do with smoking, don't smoke!

EXAMPLE 11.2.6 Schols et al studied 32 patients with chronic obstructive pulmonary disease (COPD). One of the characteristics measured for each patient in the study was body mass index (BMI). BMI for the 24 men in the study was 21.6 ± 2.5 (mean

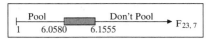

FIGURE 11.2.8
Decision line for pool versus don't pool for the Schols et al study.

± SD) kg/m². BMI for the 8 women in the study was 20.1 ± 2.1 kg/m². We inquire whether there is a statistically significant difference in BMI between male and female patients with COPD.

We will assume independent random samples with independent observations. Since we do not have the raw data, we cannot test for normality. Since we have the sample legend (but not the raw data), we will also assume that BMI is normally distributed in both the male and female populations of COPD patients. We now determine whether to apply the two-samples t-test for comparison of means with or without pooling (see Figure 11.2.2).

Step 1. Sample $f = \left(\frac{\text{larger SD}}{\text{smaller SD}}\right)^2 = \left(\frac{2.5}{2.1}\right)^2 = 1.4$

Step 2. The decision line is shown in Figure 11.2.8.

Step 3. Hence, apply the pooled t-test.

Comment The critical f-value displayed in step 2 can be obtained from Table 10a using a column heading of 23 and a row heading of 7. Note that although Table 10a does not have a column heading for 23, the value 23 falls between the table column headings of 20 and 25. Since the table f-value for $F_{25,7}$ is 6.0580 and for $F_{20,7}$ is 6.1555, we display an "ambiguous zone" in Figure 11.2.8. An exact critical f-value is obtained with Minitab by

```
MTB > INVCDF  .99;
SUBC> F  23  7.
0.9900    6.0921
```

This leads to the precise decision line shown in Figure 11.2.9.

The write-up for the pooled t-test for the Schols et al COPD study (Example 11.2.6) is given in Figure 11.2.10. The analysis follows the protocol provided in Chart 5A.

EXAMPLE 11.2.7 Arnold et al reported several characteristics of nonseptic versus septic subjects in their study. One of the characteristics was fat-free mass (FFM) measured in kilograms. The data are displayed in Table 11.2.2.

TABLE 11.2.2
Data from Arnold et al.

Nonseptic Patients	Septic Patients
36.4	47.0
58.8	38.7
45.9	44.7
53.7	41.8
34.3	42.2

FIGURE 11.2.9
Decision line for pool versus don't pool for the Schols et al study.

```
        Pool    Don't Pool
   |------|--------------→ F₂₃,₇
   1    6.0921
```

FIGURE 11.2.10
This figure illustrates the pooled t-test for comparison of means. The Schols et al study (Example 11.2.6) is analyzed to compare the mean BMI for male (population 1) against the mean BMI for female (population 2) COPD patients. The write-up follows the protocol outlined in Chart 5A.

1. Hypothesis. $H_0: \mu_1 = \mu_2$ Test alternate (a);
   $H_a: \mu_1 \neq \mu_2$ two-tailed test.

2. LOS. 0.05

3. Test Statistic. $\dfrac{\bar{X}_1 - \bar{X}_2}{\sqrt{s_p^2 \left(\frac{1}{n_1} + \frac{1}{n_2} \right)}}$

   where $s_p^2 = [(n_1 - 1)s_1^2 + (n_2 - 1)s_2^2]/(n_1 + n_2 - 2)$

4. Critical Value. $df = n_1 + n_2 - 2 = 24 + 8 - 2 = 30$
   $t = 2.0423$ (Table 9)

5. Decision Line.

   Reject H_0 | Do Not Reject H_0 | Reject H_0
   -2.0423 2.0423 T_{30}

6. Sample Value. $s_p^2 = \dfrac{23(2.5)^2 + 7(2.1)^2}{30} = 5.8207$

   sample $t = \dfrac{\bar{X}_1 - \bar{X}_2}{\sqrt{s_p^2 \left(\frac{1}{n_1} + \frac{1}{n_2} \right)}} = \dfrac{21.6 - 20.1}{\sqrt{5.8207 \left(\frac{1}{24} + \frac{1}{8} \right)}} = 1.523$

7. Conclusion. Based on the given data, at the 5% LOS we do not reject $H_0: \mu_1 = \mu_2$. There is no significant difference between the mean BMI for male and female COPD patients ($.10 < p\text{-value} < .20$).

We inquire whether the average FFM in the septic and nonseptic patients is the same. We assume independent random samples with independent observations. Since we have the raw data, we perform the analysis in Minitab. Minitab's output is exhibited in Figure 11.2.11. In examining the output, we first observe that both samples pass normality (critical nscores correlation 0.8320, $p > .10$). Hence, a two-samples t-test for comparison of means is appropriate.

We now check for homoscedasticity to determine whether to apply the pooled t-test or the Smith-Satterthwaite t-test for comparison of means (Figure 11.2.2). The sample f-value for this test is

(largest SD/smallest SD)^2 = 11.4763 (Minitab, Figure 11.2.11)

This sample f-value may be considered borderline in that it passes the test for homoscedasticity at the 1% LOS (critical value 15.9771) but not at 5% (critical value 6.3881). Hence, for the sake of illustration, we conduct both the pooled t-test (two-samples t-test with pooling) and the Smith-Satterthwaite t-test (two-samples t-test without pooling) in Minitab. With the raw data, these tests are easy to perform in Minitab.

From Minitab's output (Figure 11.2.11), we note that there is very little difference in the strength of these two two-samples t-tests. The p-value for the pooled t-test is .57; for the Smith-Satterthwaite t-test, .59. From these large p-values, we see that both tests yield the same result: retain $H_0: \mu_1 = \mu_2$. This contrast between the two versions of the two-samples t-test shows that it is not worth splitting hairs in close calls. The moral of the story is to use the pooled t-test, unless the sample *clearly* indicates heteroscedasticity.

Our formal conclusion is: There is no difference in fat-free mass between septic and nonseptic patients ($t = 0.59, df = 8, p = .57$).

FIGURE **11.2.11**
Minitab output for
comparison of means
for the Arnold et al
data of the lipid
infusion study
(Example 11.2.7).

```
MTB > PRINT C1 C2

  ROW   Septic   NoSeptic

   1     36.4      47.0
   2     58.8      38.7
   3     45.7      41.8
   5     34.3      42.2
MTB > NSCORES C1 INTO C11
MTB > CORRELATION C1 AND C11

Correlation of Septic and Nscores = 0.974

MTB > NSCORES C2 INTO C11
MTB > CORRELATION C2 AND C11

Correlation of NoSeptic and Nscores = 0.989

MTB > LET K1 = (STDEV(C1)/STDEV(C2))**2
MTB > PRINT K1
K1       11.4763
MTB >
MTB > TWOSAMPLE C1 C2;
SUBC> ALTERNATE 0;
SUBC> POOLED.

TWOSAMPLE T FOR Septic VS NoSeptic
             N      MEAN     STDEV   SE MEAN
Septic       5      45.8     10.6      4.8
NoSeptic     5      42.88    3.14      1.4

95 PCT CI FOR MU Septic - MU NoSeptic: (-8.5, 14.4)

TTEST MU Septic = MU NoSeptic (VS NE): T= 0.59  P=0.57  DF=  8

POOLED STDEV =        7.84

MTB > TWOSAMPLE C1 C2;
SUBC> ALTERNATE 0.

TWOSAMPLE T FOR Septic VS NoSeptic
             N      MEAN     STDEV   SE MEAN
Septic       5      45.8     10.6      4.8
NoSeptic     5      42.88    3.14      1.4

95 PCT CI FOR MU Septic - MU NoSeptic: (-10.8, 16.7)

TTEST MU Septic = MU NoSeptic (VS NE): T= 0.59  P=0.59  DF=  4
```

The sophisticated reader can see that a two-tailed test of hypothesis was performed to compare means. A t-test was conducted in which the sample t-value was .59. The p-value is .57, clearly much larger than the usual .05 level of significance. This sample result is very consistent with the null hypothesis. The only warning to be issued before embracing this result is that the sample sizes are very small (5 each). With such small samples, it is really quite difficult to determine differences.

Large-Samples z-Test for Comparison of Means

When the sample sizes are large (both > 30), we can compare averages in two populations by conducting a large-samples z-test for comparison of means.

EXAMPLE 11.2.8 George et al measured several variables among female small eaters and large eaters. Small eaters are women who eat by "grazing"; that is, although they may eat several times a day, they eat small amounts per eating session. Large eaters eat basically a full meal at each eating session. There were 40 women of each kind in the study. The body weight for the 40 small eaters was 50.6 ± 7.0 (mean ± SD) kg, whereas, the body weight for the 40 large eaters was 55.1 ± 9.5 kg. Is there a statistically significant difference in the average body weight between small eaters and large eaters?

We assume random and independent samples with independent observations. Since we do not have the raw data, we cannot check for normality. However, both sample sizes are large (> 30). Hence, we may apply the large-samples z-test for comparison of means. The write-up is displayed in Figure 11.2.12 and follows the protocol given in Chart 5C.

Mann-Whitney Test for Comparison of Medians

The **Mann-Whitney test** is a test for comparison of medians. The Mann-Whitney test is justified for any quantitative RV that is at least ordinal in nature (it doesn't make any sense to test nominal data). One needs the raw data set to carry out the Mann-Whitney test. If one has a raw data set that is inconsistent with normality and at least one of the sample sizes is small, then the Mann-Whitney test is the last recourse for being able to compare averages between the two populations.

EXAMPLE 11.2.9 We have been studying cardiac output from two studies: Barcelona et al, published in 1985, and Daily and Mersch, published in 1987. The data for the ice-temperature cardiac outputs indicate some significant differences between the two studies. For illustration, we inquire whether there is a significant difference between the average cardiac output, ice-temperature injectate, between the Barcelona et al study (prefilled syringes) and the Daily and Mersch study.

FIGURE 11.2.12
The large-samples z-test write-up comparing the mean body weight of small eaters (population 1) and large eaters (population 2) for women (Example 11.2.8) is displayed. The write-up follows Chart 5C.

1. Hypothesis. $H_0: \mu_1 \geq \mu_2$ Test alternate $H_a: \mu_1 < \mu_2$ one-tailed test.

2. LOS. 0.05

3. Test Statistic. $\dfrac{\bar{x}_1 - \bar{x}_2}{\sqrt{\dfrac{s_1^2}{n_1} + \dfrac{s_2^2}{n_2}}}$

4. Critical Value. 1.645 (Table 8)

5. Decision Line.

   Reject H_0 Do Not Reject H_0 z

   -1.645

6. Sample Value.

   sample $z = \dfrac{50.6 - 55.1}{\sqrt{\dfrac{(7.0)^2}{40} + \dfrac{(9.5)^2}{40}}} = -2.412$

7. Conclusion. Based on the given data, at the 5% LOS reject $H_0: \mu_1 \geq \mu_2$ and accept $H_a: \mu_1 < \mu_2$. The sample gives strong evidence that the mean body weight for female small eaters is signigicantly less than the mean body weight of large eaters ($.005 < p < .01$).

We may assume random and independent samples with independent observations. Since the Barcelona et al data set is inconsistent with normal, a t-test for comparison of means is inappropriate. Since the Daily and Mersch sample size is not large, the large-samples z-test for comparison of means is also inappropriate. Our final recourse, since we have the raw data, is to apply the Mann-Whitney test for comparison of medians on Minitab. The printout is exhibited in Figure 11.2.13.

The p-value for the test is contained in the last line of Minitab's output for the Mann-Whitney command about the "attained level of significance." Here, $p = .0107$, so we reject the null hypothesis that the medians are equal.

Since the confidence interval for the difference of the two medians is (-1.2297, -0.1703), we conclude that the Barcelona et al median is statistically significantly less than the Daily and Mersch median (note the ($-, -$) form of the confidence interval). This significance would lead us to reevaluate the two articles. In particular, we wonder whether Daily and Mersch perhaps excluded unstable or compromised patients from their study to an extent not done by Barcelona et al.

Confidence Interval for the Difference Between Averages

When we conduct a test of hypothesis for comparison of averages, we are able to tell whether or not one average is statistically significantly less than (or greater than) another average. When we detect that one average is significantly less than another, the next inquiry is: By how much? In order to estimate how much greater one average is than another, we will need to construct a confidence interval for the difference of the two averages.

One determines a confidence interval for the difference between two averages by using the same general approach used to conduct the test of hypothesis for

FIGURE *11.2.13*
Comparison of the median ice-temperature cardiac output between the Barcelona et al (prefilled syringes) and Daily and Mersch studies (Example 11.2.9). The Barcelona data are in C1; Daily and Mersch data, C2.

```
MTB > DESCRIBE C1 C2

                N      MEAN    MEDIAN    TRMEAN     STDEV    SEMEAN
ITCO B         41     3.905     3.700     3.827     1.091     0.170
ITCO DM        29     4.508     4.510     4.509     1.043     0.194

               MIN       MAX        Q1        Q3
ITCO B       2.200     7.200     3.250     4.350
ITCO DM      2.620     6.380     3.765     5.385

MTB > MANN WHITNEY C1 C2;
SUBC> ALTERNATE 0.

Mann-Whitney Confidence Interval and Test

ITCO B     N =  41     Median =       3.7000
ITCO DM    N =  29     Median =       4.5100
Point estimate for ETA1-ETA2 is      -0.7100
95.1 pct c.i. for ETA1-ETA2 is (-1.2297,-0.1703)
W = 1241.0
Test of ETA1 = ETA2  vs.  ETA1 n.e. ETA2 is significant at 0.0107
The test is significant at 0.0107 (adjusted for ties)
```

comparing those averages. Accordingly, one may construct a confidence interval for the difference between two means or the difference between two medians, depending on which average one is using.

To determine the confidence interval for the difference between two *medians*, one applies the Mann-Whitney command in Minitab. The confidence interval for the difference of the two medians is read directly from Minitab's output (e.g., Figure 11.2.13, confidence interval for ETA1 − ETA2).

To determine a confidence interval for the difference between two means, one determines a confidence t-interval or z-interval using the same guidelines used in choosing a t-test or z-test. If the sample sizes are large, one may construct a large-samples z-interval. If the distribution of the RV of interest is normal in both populations, then one determines either a pooled confidence t-interval or a Smith-Satterthwaite confidence t-interval.

Suppose the mean of population 1 is μ_1 and the mean for population 2 is μ_2. We determine a confidence interval for the difference of the two means (i.e., for $\mu_1 - \mu_2$). We illustrate by presenting the appropriate formula followed by an example.

Large-Samples Confidence z-Interval

A large-samples confidence z-interval is computed by

$$(\bar{x}_1 - \bar{x}_2) \pm z\sqrt{\frac{s_1^2}{n_1} + \frac{s_2^2}{n_2}}$$ where z is obtained from Table 7 (Appendix).

EXAMPLE 11.2.10 George et al compared body makeup of female small eaters and large eaters. The body weight for 40 small eaters was 50.6 ± 7.0 kg; for 40 large eaters, 55.1 ± 9.5 kg. In Example 11.2.8, a large-samples z-test determined that the mean body weight of female small eaters is significantly less than the mean body weight of female large eaters ($p < .01$). To determine the extent of the weight difference, we need a confidence interval. Since the sample sizes are large, we construct a 95% z-interval for the difference of the mean weights.

$$(\bar{x}_1 - \bar{x}_2) \pm z\sqrt{\frac{s_1^2}{n_1} + \frac{s_2^2}{n_2}}$$
$$= (50.6 - 55.1) \pm (1.960)\sqrt{\frac{7.0^2}{40} + \frac{9.5^2}{40}}$$
$$= -4.5 \pm 3.66$$
$$= (-8.2, -0.8)$$

Hence, the difference in weight on average is at least 0.8 kg, and may be as great as 8.2 kg. The unsatisfactory spread of this confidence interval indicates that a larger study needs to be made in order to obtain a more precise estimate of the difference in means.

Confidence t-Intervals

The key point here is that in order to construct a confidence interval for a normally distributed RV, one needs the appropriate t-value from Table 6 (Appendix). The *df* for the confidence interval for $\mu_1 - \mu_2$ is the same *df* that one uses in the two-samples t-test for comparing those same means. Accordingly, there is a pooled confidence t-interval and a Smith-Satterthwaite confidence t-interval for $\mu_1 - \mu_2$. The formulas for each follow.

The formula for the pooled confidence t-interval is

$$(\bar{x}_1 - \bar{x}_2) \pm t\sqrt{s_p^2\left(\frac{1}{n_1} + \frac{1}{n_2}\right)}$$

where t is obtained from Table 6 with $df = n_1 + n_2 - 2$
and $s_p^2 = [(n_1 - 1)s_1^2 + (n_2 - 1)s_2^2]/(n_1 + n_2 - 2)$

The formula for the Smith-Satterthwaite confidence t-interval is

$$(\bar{x}_1 - \bar{x}_2) \pm t\sqrt{\frac{s_1^2}{n_1} + \frac{s_2^2}{n_2}}$$

where t is obtained from Table 6 with

$$df = \frac{[s_1^2/n_1 + s_2^2/n_2]^2}{\left[\frac{(s_1^2/n_1)^2}{n_1 - 1} + \frac{(s_2^2/n_2)^2}{n_2 - 1}\right]} \quad \textbf{integer part only}$$

In taking the integer part only in the *df*, simply discard the decimal part of the answer; *do not round*.

EXAMPLE 11.2.11 We reconsider the Vio et al comparison study for breast-milk production between smoking and nonsmoking nursing mothers (Examples 11.2.1–5). The test of hypothesis is displayed in Figure 11.2.7. By testing we determined that the mean breast-milk production for smoking nursing mothers is significantly less than the mean breast-milk production for nonsmoking nursing mothers. We now consider the extent of the difference. Since the pooled t-test was justified to conduct the t-test for comparison of means, we determine a 95% pooled confidence t-interval for the difference between the means.

$$
\begin{aligned}
s_p^2 &= [(n_1 - 1)s_1^2 + (n_2 - 1)s_2^2]/(n_1 + n_2 - 2) \\
&= [9(109.5)^2 + 9(120.0)^2]/18 \\
&= 13195.125
\end{aligned}
$$

Then,

$$
\begin{aligned}
(\bar{x}_1 - \bar{x}_2) &\pm t\sqrt{s_p^2\left(\frac{1}{n_1} + \frac{1}{n_2}\right)} \\
&= (693.4 - 961.1) \pm (2.1009)\sqrt{\left(13195.125\left(\frac{1}{10} + \frac{1}{10}\right)\right)} \\
&= -267.7 \pm 107.93 \\
&= -376, -159 \quad \text{(round down for left endpoint, up for right endpoint)}
\end{aligned}
$$

Hence, a 95% confidence interval for $\mu_1 - \mu_2$ is $(-376, -159)$ g/day.

Notice that the general form of this confidence interval is (negative,negative). This form indicates that

$$\mu_1 - \mu_2 < 0;$$

that is, $\mu_1 < \mu_2$. This result is consistent with the result we obtained from the testing procedure that showed the mean breast-milk production for smoking nursing mothers was less than the mean breast-milk production for smoking nursing mothers. How much less? From the confidence interval, with 95% confidence, the mean breast-milk production for smoking nursing mothers is at least 159 g/day less than the mean breast-milk production for nonsmoking nursing mothers (and perhaps up to 376 less).

Now examine Figure 11.2.6, Minitab's output for the Vio et al breast-milk production comparison study. In particular, notice the output for the TWOSAMPLE command. As part of the output, Minitab displays a 95% confidence interval (95 PCT CI) for the difference between the means. This is another bonus for analyzing raw data in Minitab.

Comment Our calculated confidence interval in Example 11.2.11 is $(-376, -159)$. This differs slightly from Minitab's confidence interval of $(-376, -160)$ for the same study displayed in Figure 11.2.6. The difference, however, is due simply to rounding. We used approximations; Minitab carries out the computations with much greater precision. Also, Minitab simply rounds numbers and does not apply our confidence interval rule of rounding the left endpoint down and the right endpoint up.

EXERCISES 11.2

Warm-ups 11.2

Bridges et al studied new equipment for measuring blood hemoglobin (Hb). They obtained blood samples from 14 female and 15 male random blood donors. We inquire whether there is a statistically significant difference in the average Hb value between females and males. The data are presented in Table 11.2.3.

TABLE *11.2.3*
Hb data set.

Female	Male
15.5	14.0
13.6	15.3
13.5	13.5
13.0	15.8
13.3	15.0
12.4	16.7
11.1	17.1
13.1	14.7
16.1	15.5
16.4	17.3
13.4	15.0
13.2	16.0
14.3	14.5
16.1	16.0
	16.9

Minitab computer output for comparing Hb in the two groups is provided in Figure 11.2.14.

FIGURE *11.2.14*
Minitab output for analysis of the Hb data.

```
MTB > NOTE    Test for normal distributions:
MTB > NSCORES C1 INTO C11
MTB > CORRELATION C1 AND C11

Correlation of FemaleHb and Nscores = 0.959

MTB > NSCORES C2 INTO C11
MTB > CORRELATION C2 AND C11

Correlation of Male Hb and Nscores = 0.992

MTB > NOTE    Test for homoscedasticity:
MTB > DESCRIBE C1 C2

                N      MEAN    MEDIAN    TRMEAN     STDEV    SEMEAN
FemaleHb       14    13.929    13.450    13.958     1.557     0.416
Male Hb        15    15.553    15.500    15.577     1.139     0.294

               MIN       MAX        Q1        Q3
FemaleHb    11.100    16.400    13.075    15.650
Male Hb     13.500    17.300    14.700    16.700

MTB > LET K1 = (STDEV(C1)/STDEV(C2))**2
MTB > PRINT K1    #sample f-value
K1        1.86792
MTB >
MTB > NOTE    Conduct test of hypothesis:
MTB > TWOSAMPLE C1 C2;
SUBC> ALTERNATE 0.

TWOSAMPLE T FOR FemaleHb VS Male Hb
             N       MEAN     STDEV    SE MEAN
FemaleHb    14      13.93      1.56       0.42
Male Hb     15      15.55      1.14       0.29

95 PCT CI FOR MU FemaleHb - MU Male Hb: (-2.68, -0.57)

TTEST MU FemaleHb = MU Male Hb (VS NE): T=
-3.19  P=0.0041  DF=  23

MTB > TWOSAMPLE C1 C2;
SUBC> ALTERNATE 0;
SUBC> POOLED.

TWOSAMPLE T FOR FemaleHb VS Male Hb
             N       MEAN     STDEV    SE MEAN
FemaleHb    14      13.93      1.56       0.42
Male Hb     15      15.55      1.14       0.29

95 PCT CI FOR MU FemaleHb - MU Male Hb: (-2.66, -0.59)

TTEST MU FemaleHb = MU Male Hb (VS NE): T=
-3.22  P=0.0033  DF=  27

POOLED STDEV =       1.36
```

1. Do the given samples satisfy the assumptions for random and independent samples?

2. Is the Bridges et al data set presented as a raw data set or as a sample legend?

3. Construct a data legend for the Hb data shown in Table 11.2.3.

4. Is the sample Hb for females consistent with normality?

5. Is the sample Hb for males consistent with normality?

6. Since the sample Hb for both the female and male populations is consistent with a normal distribution, conduct a

   a. Two-samples t-test for comparison of medians

   b. Two-samples t-test for comparison of means

   c. Large-samples z-test for comparison of medians

   d. Large-samples z-test for comparison of means

   e. Mann-Whitney test

7. The two forms of the two-samples t-test for comparison of means are

   a. The Mann and the Whitney tests

   b. The mean and the median

   c. Pooled and Smith-Satterthwaite t-tests

   d. The Smith and Satterthwaite tests

   e. Homoscedastic and heteroscedastic

8. Since the Hb samples for females and males are consistent with normality, we conduct a two-samples t-test for comparison of means. We now need to decide whether to pool or not. The general decision line whether to pool or not is displayed in Figure 11.2.2. The sample f-value for this decision is calculated by (SD = standard deviation)

$$\text{sample f-value} = \left(\frac{\text{larger sample SD}}{\text{smaller sample SD}}\right)^2 = \left(\frac{\square}{\square}\right)^2 = \underline{\quad}$$

9. The larger SD is ____. The sample size of the sample with the larger SD is L = ____.

10. The smaller SD is ____. The sample size of the sample with the smaller SD is S = ____.

11. The critical f-value (f) for the pool versus don't pool decision is obtained from Table 10a (Appendix). Use the L-1 column (Warm-up 9) and S-1 row (Warm-up 10). Hence,
Column: L-1 = ____   Row: S-1 = ____
critical f-value: $f = $ ____

12. Fill in the boxes shown in Figure 11.2.15 for the pool versus don't pool decision line.

13. Should one conduct the two-samples t-test with or without pooling?

We conduct a two-sample pooled t-test for comparing the mean Hb in females (μ_1) against the mean Hb in males (μ_2). The test will follow the protocol of Chart 5A. In particular, at the 5% LOS we will test

$$H_0: \mu_1 = \mu_2$$
$$H_a: \mu_1 \neq \mu_2$$

14. The given test of hypothesis uses what test alternate: (a), (b), or (c)?

15. Is this a one- or two-tailed test of hypothesis?

FIGURE *11.2.15*   Pool versus don't pool decision line.

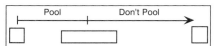

16. For a pooled t-test, the $df = n_1 + n_2 - 2$. Here, $df = $ ____?

17. Using the test of hypothesis t-table (Table 9, Appendix), what is the critical t-value?

18. Complete the comparison of means decision line shown in Figure 11.2.16.

19. What is the sample t-value for the two-sample pooled t-test?

20. At the 5% LOS, do you retain or reject the null hypothesis $H_0: \mu_1 = \mu_2$?

21. Provide a clinical interpretation for the statistical decision stated in Warm-up 20.

22. What is the *p*-value for the test of hypothesis?

23. Current clinical wisdom teaches that "Hb for females is less than Hb for males." To test this assertion using the Bridges et al study, one tests the hypothesis (group 1 = females, group 2 = males)

   a. $H_0: Hb_1 \geq Hb_2$ versus $H_a: Hb_1 < Hb_2$

   b. $H_0: \mu_1 \leq \mu_2$ versus $H_a: \mu_1 > \mu_2$

   c. $H_0: \mu_1 \geq \mu_2$ versus $H_a: \mu_1 < \mu_2$

   d. $H_0: p_1 \leq p_2$ versus $H_a: p_1 > p_2$

   e. $H_0: p_1 \geq p_2$ versus $H_a: p_1 < p_2$

Problems 11.2

1. Clapp studied delivery among two groups of women. The study enrolled 131 women who were either recreational runners (67) or aerobic dancers (64). All subjects had been exercising regularly for at least 6 months before conception. The women self-divided into two groups. Group A consisted of 87 women (46 runners and 41 aerobic dancers) who continued to exercise at or above 50% of their preconceptual level throughout pregnancy. Group B consisted of the other 44 women (21 runners and 23 aerobic dancers), who stopped their regular exercise routine by the end of the first trimester. Data on women birthing by vaginal delivery are shown in Table 11.2.4 (of the 87 women in group A, 82 delivered vaginally and 5 delivered by cesarean).

FIGURE *11.2.16*   Comparison of means decision line.

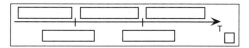

TABLE *11.2.4* Data from Clapp: women from Groups A and B giving birth by vaginal delivery.

Activity	Group A (n = 82)	Group B (n = 31)
Active labor (min) mean ± SD	264 ± 149	382 ± 275
Episiotomy done	38	25

a. Is there a difference in the time of active labor between the two groups?

b. Is there a difference in the episiotomy rate between the two groups?

2. Pierce et al studied the effects of two chest tube clearance protocols on drainage in patients after myocardial revascularization surgery. The two protocols are called (1) milking and (2) stripping. After a 30-minute admission period to the cardiac intensive care unit, the total chest drainage during the next 8 hours for the two chest tube clearance protocols are as shown in Table 11.2.5.

TABLE *11.2.5* Data from Pierce et al.

Protocol	n	Mean	SEM
Milking	100	541.6	38.0
Stripping	100	515.8	31.1

$SEM = SD/\sqrt{n}$.

a. What are the point estimates for the mean drainage for each protocol? Are they different? If so, which point estimate is larger?

b. Determine a 95% confidence interval for the mean drainage for each protocol. Do the intervals overlap? On the basis of these confidence intervals, is there evidence to suggest a difference in the mean drainages?

c. Determine a 95% confidence interval for the difference of the two means using the (i) pooled and (ii) Smith-Satterthwaite methods. Which interval is wider? Which method is justified? Which method is preferred? On the basis of this confidence interval, is there a perceptible difference between the two means?

d. Conduct an appropriate test of hypothesis to determine whether there is a statistically significant difference between the two means.

3. Lange et al studied patient-controlled analgesia (PCA) versus intermittent analgesia dosing. Actively involving patients in their own pain management by using PCA during the postoperative period is a relatively new concept. This method allows self-administration of small, frequent doses of an analgesic agent to maintain a state of constant pain control. Sixteen patients requiring posterolateral thoracotomy incisions were included in the study. The 16 patients were divided into two groups of 8 patients each. The control group of patients received intermittent injections of Buprenex 9.35 mg i.m. q 3–6 hrs prn pain. The other group, the PCA group, administered their own pain control medication (Buprenex via a Life Care PCA-preparation included preoperative teaching on the use of the device for PCA). The authors contended, "It is our hypothesis that by allowing patient participation in pain control using PCA, reduced sedation will occur."

For the control group, the mean amount of drug administered was 1.80 mg Buprenex with a standard deviation of 0.64 mg. For the PCA group, the mean amount of drug administered was 1.07 mg Buprenex with a standard deviation of 0.52 mg. Based on these data, what conclusion can you reach regarding the researcher's hypothesis?

4. Rice et al reported on a patient education program for relieving anxiety in patients about to undergo four-vessel arteriography. Forty patients agreed to participate in the study, of whom 20 were randomly assigned to an experimental program and the other 20 acted as controls and received only the normal hospital protocol. The experimental program consisted of the normal protocol plus a cassette tape education program regarding the angiography procedure. The Mood Adjective Checklist (MACL) was given to each patient to assess negative mood score (an indicator of stress) within 24 hours after the angiography procedure. A higher MACL score indicates greater stress. The data are given in Table 11.2.6.

TABLE *11.2.6* Data from Rice et al.

	Experimental Group	Control Group
Mean	35.0	44.2
SD	15.0	14.4
Size	20	20

The MACL for both groups upon admission was found to be statistically the same. Does this study give evidence that the patient education program is effective in reducing stress for patients undergoing arteriography?

5. Rakowski et al studied coagulation times on blood drawn from new (freshly installed) catheters versus blood drawn from old (7 days after installation) catheters. The data shown in Table 11.2.7 were presented on activated partial thromboplastin times (aPTT):

TABLE **11.2.7** Data from Rakowski et al.

	N	Mean	SD
Old	6	15.767	0.532
New	6	15.333	0.561

a. Construct a 95% confidence interval for
   i. The mean aPTT using the old catheters
   ii. The mean aPTT using the new catheters
   iii. The difference between the means

b. Based on your results in (a), is there evidence for a difference in aPTT from blood drawn from old and new catheters?

c. Conduct an appropriate test of hypothesis to compare the two means.

6. Shellock and Riedinger conducted thermodilution cardiac outputs on each of 45 acutely ill patients in the cardiac intensive care unit. These cardiac outputs were done by two methods. In method 1, an ice-temperature injectate was used; in method 2, a room-temperature injectate. The data shown in Table 11.2.8 were reported. Is the mean cardiac output of the two methods the same?

7. Shively studied effects of position change on mixed venous oxygen saturation ($S\bar{v}O_2$) in coronary artery bypass surgery patients. Her study incorporated 30 patients randomly divided into two groups. Group I consisted of 15 patients who were turned every hour; group II consisted of 15 patients who were

TABLE **11.2.8** Data from Shellock and Riedinger.

	Method 1	Method 2
Mean	4.78	4.75
SD	2.11	2.35

turned every 2 hours. Baseline $S\bar{v}O_2$ measurements were taken on each group. Other $S\bar{v}O_2$ measurements were also taken (Appendix, Data Set 5).

a. Is there sufficient evidence to indicate that the mean baseline $S\bar{v}O_2$ reading for the two groups is different?

b. Is there evidence to suggest that the mean $S\bar{v}O_2$ level in group II changed significantly in time while the patient was in a supine position?

8. Burek et al studied exercise capacity in patients 3 days after acute uncomplicated myocardial infarction (MI). The researchers studied 126 patients who were discharged from the hospital after acute MI. The discharge condition of these patients was classified as uncomplicated. The researchers studied the patients' postdischarge condition by giving them a low-level exercise thallium treadmill (ETT) test 3 days after discharge. Of these 126 patients, 36 had a positive test for ischemia (positive ETT). The peak heart rate for each patient was measured, with the results as shown in Table 11.2.9. Is the mean of the peak heart rate of the positive ETT group significantly lower than the mean peak heart rate of the negative ETT group?

TABLE **11.2.9** Data from Burek et al.

	Positive ETT	Negative ETT
n	36	90
Mean	120.9	130.2
SD	21.4	14.4

9. Kaplow compared two techniques for obtaining samples for coagulation studies: venipuncture and intra-arterial line. Kaplow stated, "It was hypothesized that no difference in mean clotting time would be found in coagulation specimens taken by venipuncture and by arterial line sampling." A venipuncture and arterial line blood sample was taken from each of 50 patients.

The mean clotting time for the venipuncture samples was 33.69 seconds with a standard deviation of 9.71 seconds. The mean clotting time for samples taken from the intraarterial catheter was 33.94 seconds with a standard deviation of 9.55 seconds. The range of differences was from -8.1 to 15.8 seconds with a mean difference of -0.26 seconds.

Results of the t-test analysis revealed no significant difference between the two methods ($t = -0.47, df = 49, p > 0.05$).

a. The second paragraph of the quote from the article refers to a t-test. What kind of t-test (pooled, Smith-Satterthwaite, paired-difference) is the author referring to? Justify. Conduct the appropriate test on the stated research hypothesis.

b. The author reported $p > .05$. Give a more precise p-value.

10. Schols et al, in their comparison study of men and women COPD patients, also reported measurements of inspiratory vital capacity (IVC) and forced expiratory volume in 1 second (FEV_1), as shown in Table 11.2.10.

TABLE **11.2.10** Data from Schols et al.

	Men (n = 24)	Women (n = 8)
IVC (liters)	2.8 ± 0.8	1.9 ± 0.5
FEV$_1$ (liters)	0.9 ± 0.5	0.8 ± 0.4

a. Is the mean IVC for men greater than the mean IVC for women? If so, by how much?

b. Is there a statistically significant difference between mean FEV_1 for men and women? If so, by how much?

11. George et al (Examples 11.2.8 and 10) also reported the energy and macronutrient intake data for female small eaters (SEs) and large eaters (LEs) shown in Table 11.2.11.

TABLE **11.2.11** Data from George et al.

	SEs (n = 40)	LEs (n = 40)
Energy intake (kcal)	1488 ± 312	2393 ± 509
Energy intake (kcal/kg)	27 ± 4	47 ± 4
Protein (%)	15 ± 2	14 ± 2
Fat (%)	35 ± 4	35 ± 4
Carbohydrate (%)	47 ± 6	49 ± 6

What energy and macronutrient RV are statistically significantly different between the two groups? By how much? Compare the nutritional results of the eating habits of the two groups.

12. In addition to the energy and macronutrient intake data, George et al also reported the body mass index (BMI), fat free mass (kg), and fat mass (kg) for the two groups.

a. For $n = 40$ SEs, BMI (kg/m^2) was 19.4 ± 2.2 (mean ± SD). For $n = 40$ LEs, BMI was 21.3 ± 3.2. Is there a statistically significant difference in mean BMI between the two groups? If so, by how much?

b. For fat free mass, data were collected on 33 SEs and 34 LEs. Fat free mass for SEs was 35.9 ± 5.3 kg; for LEs, 36.9 ± 4.7 kg. Is there a statistically significant difference between the two groups? If so, by how much?

c. For fat mass, data were collected on 33 SEs and 34 LEs. Fat mass for SEs was 14.5 ± 5.3 kg; for LEs, 18.7 ± 8.1 kg. Is there a statistically significant difference between the two groups? If so, by how much?

d. Based on your analysis in (a, b, c), verbally describe the differences between the two groups.

13. (Continued from Problem 11.1.8) Upon admission, the index neurological score for the 58 patients in the neuropsychiatric group was 6.4 ± 2.5 (mean ± SD); the neurological score was 4.6 ± 2.6 for the 26 patients in the neurological-only group. Assume that neurological score is normally distributed in the two study groups. Is the mean neurological score for the neuropsychiatric group statistically significantly greater than the mean neurological score for the neurological-only group?

14. (Continued from Problem 13) The general condition of the patients was measured by a Global Assessment Score (GAS). For the 58 patients in the neuropsychiatric group, the mean index GAS was 47.0 ± 16.0. For the 26 patients in the neurological-only group, the mean index GAS was 61.4 ± 16.0. Is the mean index GAS for the neuropsychiatric group significantly less than the mean index GAS for the neurological-only group?

15. (Continued from Problem 13) The mean hospital stay for the 58 patients in the neuropsychiatric group was 36.2 ± 56 days, whereas the mean hospital stay for the 26 patients in the neurological-only group was 17.1 ± 20 days. Is the mean hospital length for the neuropsychiatric patients significantly greater than for the neurological-only patients? If so, by how much?

16. Howenstine et al reported on an outbreak of pertussis in Indiana during 1984–85. They compared pulmonary functions of 22 infants with pertussis and 36 normal infants (controls). One of the pulmonary variates studied was functional residual capacity (FRC). FRC in the 22 pertussis infants was 176 ± 21 mL (mean $\pm$ SD). FRC in the 36 controls was 191 ± 33 mL. Is there a statistically significant difference in mean FRC between the two groups of infants?

17. Varsano et al compared efficacy of ceftriaxone and ampicillin for treatment of severe shigellosis in children. They studied 40 children infected with *Shigella* organisms. The children were randomly assigned to an ampicillin or ceftriaxone treatment group. The researchers reported the mean number of days $\pm$ SD until persistent negative stool culture as 11.7 ± 9.6 for the ampicillin group ($n = 20$) and 1.85 ± 0.6 for the ceftriaxone group ($n = 20$).

   a. You really don't need to be a statistician for this one. What is your intuitive conclusion?

   b. Assuming that the number of days to persistent negative stool culture is (approximately) normally distributed, conduct the statistical analysis; that is, is the mean number of days to recovery for the ceftriaxone group significantly less than for the ampicillin group?

18. Stähelin et al reported on the Basel study about β-carotene and cancer prevention. The report featured a 12-year cancer mortality study. The researchers were interested in a relationship between cancer mortality and plasma levels of β-carotene (μmol/liter), vitamin A (μmol/liter), and vitamin C (μmol/liter). The study group had 2421 survivors and 204 cancer deaths. The data shown in Table 11.2.12 were reported as mean $\pm$ SD. Determine whether or not there is a significant difference between survivors and cancer deaths in the mean plasma levels of

TABLE **11.2.12** Data from Stähelin et al.

	Survivors	Cancer
β-Carotene	0.436 ± 0.246	0.344 ± 0.229
Vitamin A	2.81 ± 0.49	2.81 ± 0.57
Vitamin C	52.76 ± 21.65	47.61 ± 25.42

   a. β-carotene   **b.** vitamin A   **c.** vitamin C

19. Knebel reported on several background studies in discussing current controversies about weaning patients from mechanical ventilation. The significance of these controversies is noted in the abstract introducing the article:

> As an acute episode of respiratory failure resolves for the patient who is receiving mechanical ventilation, the sometimes difficult task of resuming spontaneous ventilation begins. The resumption of spontaneous ventilation, commonly referred to as weaning, is often difficult for the patient with preexisting lung disease. The purpose of this article is to explore the current controversies related to weaning patients from mechanical ventilation.

One controversy concerned two weaning methods: intermittent mandatory ventilation (IMV) and T-piece. The random variable of concern is time ventilated in hours.

   a. In one study, Schachter et al reported 65 surgical patients weaned with IMV had a ventilation time of 145 ± 175 hours (mean $\pm$ SD). Another 65 nonsurgical patients with otherwise similar physical conditions weaned with a T-piece had a ventilation time of 142 ± 190 hours. Conduct a large-samples z-test to determine whether the mean duration of ventilation is significantly different between the two methods.

   b. In another study, Tomlinson et al reported 98 patients weaned with IMV had a ventilation time of 115.5 ± 479.1 hours (mean $\pm$ SD). Another 102 patients weaned with a T-piece had a mean ventilation time of 67.4 ± 100.0 hours. Conduct a large-samples z-test to determine whether the mean duration of ventilation is significantly different between the two methods.

   c. Construct a 95% z-confidence interval for the mean ventilation times for IMV and T-piece based on the Tomlinson et al data given in (b). Graph both intervals on the number line. What do you notice about the two confidence intervals?

   d. Conduct a test for homoscedasticity (i.e., equality of variances) between the ventilation times for the two methods based on the Tomlinson et al data. Do the variances appear to be different? If so, what significance might be attached to this difference?

e. Based on the results of the two studies presented in (a) and (b), what controversy, if any, do you feel exists?

20. Heather et al studied the effect of a bulk-forming cathartic on diarrhea in tube-fed patients. They gave the albumin level (g/dL) for experimental and control groups as shown in Table 11.2.13. Is there a statistically significant difference in the (a) standard deviations and (b) means between the two given groups?

TABLE **11.2.13** Data from Heather et al.

Group	Size	Mean	SD
Experimental	25	3.0	1.41
Control	24	2.8	0.023

21. Harding et al studied urinary tract infections in women. The infections were catheter acquired during a hospital stay.

a. In the study, 30 patients with symptoms of lower tract infection only were randomized into two groups. The number of days of catheter use for the single-dose therapy group was 3.7 ± 3.1 days (mean $\pm$ SD, $n = 14$); for the 10-day therapy group, 5.6 ± 6.8 days ($n = 16$). Is there a significant difference in the mean number of catheter days between the two groups?

b. There were 16 patients on a 10-day therapy program who had symptoms of lower tract infection only and 9 patients on a 10-day therapy program who had symptoms of upper tract infection. The mean number of days of catheter use for the two groups was 5.6 ± 6.8 for the lower tract infection only and 2.8 ± 1.9 for the upper tract infection group. Is there a significant difference between the means for the two groups?

22. Perez-Woods et al reported on pain control after cesarean birth, comparing the efficacy of patient-controlled analgesia (PCA) versus traditional morphine therapy. The article appeared as a state-of-the-art feature in the *Journal of Perinatology*. The 42 patients in the sample were randomly assigned to one of two groups. The PCA group had 25 patients, and the traditional therapy (control) group had 17 patients. No significant differences in demographic characteristics were identified between the two groups. The reported results are shown in Table 11.2.14.

The t-values in the right-hand column of Table 11.2.14 are the sample t-values calculated for the pooled t-test for comparison of means. Assume that the pooled t-test is valid for comparing the means for each variable between the two given groups.

a. Which variables are statistically significantly different between the two groups?

b. The purpose of the study was embodied in two proposed research hypotheses. The first research hypothesis was that "patient controlled administration of narcotics will be superior (i.e., increased satisfaction, reduced pain, decreased sedation, increased ambulation, and decreased length of stay)." Are the stated research hypotheses supported by the data?

c. The second research hypothesis was that "functional vital capacity will increase postoperatively with PCA." The researchers presented the data in Table 11.2.15. Is this research hypothesis supported by the data?

23. Tasota et al made a comparison between the amount of movement of an endotracheal (ET) tube held in place by (a) conventional tape and (b) a new tube holder. Both the conventional tape and

TABLE **11.2.14**
Data from Perez-Woods et al.

Variable	PCA GROUP (n = 25)		CONTROL GROUP (n = 17)		t
	Mean	SD	Mean	SD	
Time in recovery room	1.7	0.8	1.3	0.4	1.86
Satisfaction	3.9	1.1	4.7	1.1	−1.99
Ambulation	15.2	10.8	4.2	4.8	4.40
Amount of medication (mg)	96.6	43.3	49.1	17.6	4.92
Pain (nurse's assessment)	1.9	5.5	3.9	5.5	−1.44
Pain (patient's assessment)	4.1	5.1	6.4	9.6	−0.91
Sedation level	1.4	0.3	1.6	0.4	−2.06

TABLE **11.2.15**
Functional vital
capacity data from
Perez-Woods et al.

Variable	PCA GROUP (n = 25)		CONTROL GROUP (n = 17)		t
	Mean	SD	Mean	SD	
FVC presurgery	2.5	0.4	2.5	0.7	−0.03
FVC postsurgery	5.1	2.8	5.2	2.4	−0.10
FEV presurgery	2.2	0.4	2.1	0.5	0.53
FEV postsurgery	4.4	2.7	4.2	2.1	0.26
FVC/FEV presurgery	0.9	0.1	0.8	0.1	0.75
FVC/FEV postsurgery	1.9	1.2	1.8	0.9	0.30

FVC = forced vital capacity; FEV = forced expiratory volume.

new tube holder measurements were made on each of 50 patients with a reference point of movement placed at the lips. The research hypothesis was that the tube holder would allow less movement of the ET tube than conventional tape. The results from measurements taken from each of 50 patients are shown in Table 11.2.16.

TABLE **11.2.16** Data from Tasota et al.

	Tape	Tube Holder
Mean	1.26	0.43
SD	0.74	0.67

a. Describe why a comparison of means test is not appropriate to compare the amount of ET tube movement for both methods.

b. What test of hypothesis would be appropriate to compare the amount of ET movement with the ET tube stabilized by the two methods? Justify.

c. Can the test you specified in (b) be carried out with the given data? If so, carry out the test; if not, explain what further information you would need.

24. Crook et al investigated lipoprotein (a), Lp(a), as an indicator for cardiovascular disease. Serum Lp(a) levels were measured in two groups. The first group consisted of 26 premenopausal women with endometriosis. Lp(a) was measured at the start and at the end of a 6-month treatment program with danazol (a steroid). Start and 6-month Lp(a) levels were measured in 15 untreated women who served as controls. The data are presented in Table 11.2.17.

a. Is the mean baseline LP(a) of the control group significantly different from the mean baseline Lp(a) for the danazol treatment group?

b. Is there a significant change in the Lp(a) level after 6 months for the control group?

TABLE **11.2.17** Data from Crook et al.

CONTROL GROUP		
Patient	Start	6 Months
1	0.7	1.3
2	3.1	3.6
3	14.8	16.6
4	4.5	5.0
5	7.4	13.1
6	4.5	5.8
7	4.5	5.4
8	5.3	3.2
9	6.5	5.5
10	4.0	2.0
11	2.0	1.0
12	2.0	1.0
13	4.5	3.0
14	6.0	9.0
15	1.6	1.4

DANAZOL TREATMENT GROUP					
Patient	Start	6 Months	Patient	Start	6 Months
1	10.9	1.3	14	16.0	3.0
2	13.5	3.9	15	2.0	1.0
3	58.4	29.1	16	3.0	3.0
4	2.3	0	17	6.0	2.0
5	3.0	0	18	3.5	0
6	11.7	2.8	19	1.0	0
7	4.3	0	20	17.5	2.0
8	22.1	5.7	21	3.0	0
9	7.1	1.9	22	4.0	2.5
10	16.7	3.5	23	11.0	2.5
11	38.5	4.0	24	12.3	0
12	4.0	0	25	5.3	0
13	9.0	3.0	26	14.5	3.6

c. Is there a significant change in the Lp(a) level after 6 months of danazol therapy for the treatment group? If so, has Lp(a) increased or decreased? By how much?

d. Based on your analysis, is danazol an effective treatment for lowering Lp(a) in women with endometriosis?

25. Vio et al (see Examples 11.2.1–5) also monitored the weight of the infants during the 15-day study period. The data are presented in Table 11.2.18. Each infant was nurtured solely by breast-feeding. The ten mothers in the smoking group smoked an average of ≥ 4 cigarettes per day during pregnancy and continued to smoke while nursing their babies. The nonsmoking mothers never smoked.

TABLE **11.2.18** Neonate weight gain data from Vio et al. Weight in kg.

SMOKING MOTHERS			NONSMOKING MOTHERS		
Infant	Start	End	Infant	Start	End
1	3.83	4.10	1	5.95	6.45
2	4.05	4.20	2	4.50	4.85
3	4.70	5.05	3	4.90	5.41
4	4.80	4.95	4	4.12	4.68
5	3.97	4.41	5	4.90	5.30
6	3.90	4.30	6	4.47	5.25
7	4.39	4.95	7	4.59	5.16
8	3.73	4.35	8	3.69	4.23
9	4.94	5.27	9	4.40	5.10
10	4.39	4.50	10	3.90	4.48

a. Is there a significant difference in the weights of the two groups of babies at the start of the study?

b. Is there a significant difference in the weights of the two groups of babies at the end of the study?

c. Determine the weight gain for each baby. Is the change in weight significantly greater for infants with nonsmoking mothers? If so, by how much?

26. Falk et al studied treatment of progressive membranous glomerulopathy (a kidney disease). In particular, they wondered whether deterioration in kidney function could be halted by addition of a new drug to intravenous medication. A study randomized 26 patients into two treatment groups. Patients in the control group ($n = 13$) were treated with corticosteroids alone. Patients in the treatment group ($n = 13$) were treated with corticosteroids and intravenous cyclophosphamide. Blood pressure was closely monitored in these patients since the harmful effects of hypertension on the course of glomerulonephritis is well known. Mean blood pressure (MBP) for each patient for the protocol period was given as shown in Table 11.2.19.

TABLE **11.2.19** Mean blood pressure for kidney patients from Falk et al.

Control Group					Treatment Group				
94	95	100	104	106	69	88	94	96	97
109	109	112	117	120	105	106	108	108	109
122	127	130			111	112	118		

a. Determine a 95% confidence interval for MBP for the control group.

b. Determine a 95% confidence interval for MBP for the treatment group.

c. Compare the confidence intervals determined in (a) and (b). Do they overlap?

d. At the 5% LOS, is there a statistically significant difference in average MBP between the two groups?

e. Determine a 95% confidence interval for the difference in the mean MBP between the two groups.

CHAPTER *11* OVERVIEW

Summary

The ability to assess the relative effectiveness of two different treatments is an important skill in the health sciences. One needs this skill to determine whether a given intervention will, in general, improve the status of a patient, or whether a certain behavior or condition is detrimental to health. Such assessments often are made using studies that incorporate either a paired-data design or a comparison design. A **paired-data design** is appropriate if both treatments can be applied to each individual in the study. If not, a **comparison design** is utilized.

In a comparison design used to assess the relative effectiveness of two different treatments, there are two groups. One group, the **experimental** (treatment, therapy) group, receives a treatment of interest. The other, the **control** (placebo) group, does not. Ideally, both groups are alike except that one group receives the treatment while the other does not.

To assess the results of a study that utilizes a comparison design, one may apply a **comparison test of hypothesis**. There are two major types of comparison tests: tests of hypothesis for comparison of **proportions** and tests of hypothesis for comparison of **averages**. A comparison test of hypothesis is applied to **random** and **independent** samples with **independent observations**.

A **test of hypothesis for comparison of proportions** is a straightforward procedure. The only preliminary consideration is adequacy of sample size (both sizes exceed 30). A test of hypothesis for comparison of averages is more complex in that one must carefully consider which comparison test to apply (t-test, z-test, Mann-Whitney test). One may conduct a large-samples **z-test for comparison of means** to a data set of interval numbers if both sample sizes are large (>30). One may conduct a two-samples **t-test for comparison of means** if the random variable of interest is **normally distributed** in both populations. One may conduct a **Mann-Whitney test for comparison of medians** if one has a raw data set of numbers that are at least ordinal in nature.

When comparing averages, apply a two-samples t-test for comparison of means if the random variable of interest is normal in both populations. There are two t-tests for comparison of means. When the populations are **homoscedastic** (the variances are equal in the two populations), apply the powerful **pooled t-test** for comparison of means. Otherwise, apply the **Smith-Satterthwaite** t-test for comparison of means. Whenever justified, one should conduct the pooled t-test for comparison of means.

A test of hypothesis for comparison of averages may inform that one average is less than (or greater than) the other. To estimate the amount of the difference between the averages, construct a **confidence interval** for the difference of the averages. That confidence interval is obtained using the same procedure one used in selecting the test of hypothesis for comparing those averages.

Keywords

average
comparison test
   comparison of averages
   comparison of means
   comparison of medians
   comparison of proportions
confidence interval
confounding characteristic
degrees of freedom
double-blind
group
   control group
   experimental group
   placebo group
   treatment group
heteroscedastic
homoscedastic
large-samples z-test

legend
Mann-Whitney test
mean
median
normal distribution
pooled t-test
population
proportion
random samples
raw data set
sample
simple random sample
Smith-Satterthwaite test
t-test
test of hypothesis
two-samples t-test
z-test

References

Arnold J et al: Lipid infusion increases oxygen consumption similarly in septic and nonseptic patients. *Am J Clin Nutr* 53, no. 1 (January 1991): 143.

Browman G et al: Influence of cigarette smoking on the efficacy of radiation therapy in head and neck cancer. *N Engl J Med* 328, no. 3 (21 January 1993): 159.

Burek K et al: Exercise capacity in patients 3 days after acute, uncomplicated myocardial infarction. *Heart Lung* 18, no. 6 (November 1989): 575.

Clapp J: The course of labor after endurance exercise during pregnancy. *Am J Obstet Gynecol* 163, no. 6, part 1 (December 1990): 1799.

CONSENSUS Trial Study Group: Effects of enalapril on mortality in severe congestive heart failure. *N Engl J Med* 316, no. 23 (4 June 1987): 1429.

Crook D et al: Lipoprotein Lp(a) levels are reduced by danazol, an anabolic steroid. *Atherosclerosis* 92, no. 1 (January 1992): 41.

Dutch study group: A comparison of two doses of aspirin (30 mg vs 283 mg a day) in patients after a transient ischemic attack or minor ischemic stroke. *N Engl J Med* 325, no. 18 (31 October 1991): 1261.

D'Agostino R et al: Aspirin use and cardiovascular disease in women (letters). *JAMA* 267, no. 3 (15 January 1992): 364.

Dening T and Berrios G: Wilson's disease: A longitudinal study of psychiatric symptoms. *Biol Psychiatry* 28 (1990): 255.

Falk R et al: Treatment of progressive membranous glomerulophathy: A randomized trial comparing cyclophosphamide and corticosteroids with corticosteroids alone. *Ann Intern Med* 116, no. 6 (15 March 1992): 438.

First Seizure Trial Group: Randomized clinical trial on the efficacy of antiepileptic drugs in reducing the risk of relapse after a first unprovoked tonic-clonic seizure. *Neurology* 43, no. 3I (March 1993): 478.

Galvao M: The role of angiotensin converting enzyme inhibitors in congestive heart failure. *Heart Lung* 19, no. 5, pt. 1 (September 1990): 505.

George V et al: Further evidence for the presence of "small eaters" and "large eaters" among women. *Am J Clin Nutr* 53, no. 2 (February 1991): 425.

Harding G et al: How long should catheter-acquired urinary tract infection in women be treated? *Ann of Intern Med* 114, no. 9 (1 May 1991): 713.

Heather D et al: Effect of a bulk-forming cathartic on diarrhea in tube-fed patients. *Heart Lung* 20, no. 4 (July 1991): 409.

Howenstine M et al: Pulmonary function in infants after pertussis. *J Pediatr* 118, no. 4, Part 1 (April 1991): 568.

Kaplow R: Comparison of two techniques for obtaining samples for coagulation studies: Venipuncture and intraarterial line. *Heart Lung* 17, no. 6, pt. 1 (November 1988): 651.

Knebel A: Weaning from mechanical ventilation: Current controversies. *Heart Lung* 20, no. 4 (July 1991): 321.

Lange M: Patient controlled analgesia versus intermittent analgesia dosing. *Heart Lung* 17, no. 5 (September 1988): 495.

Perez-Woods R et al: Pain control after cesarean birth: Efficacy of patient-controlled analgesia vs traditional therapy (IM morphine). *J Perinatol* 11, no. 2 (1991): 174.

Pierce J: Effects of two chest tube clearance protocols on drainage in patients after myocardial revascularization surgery. *Heart Lung* 20, no. 2 (March 1991): 125.

Rakowski A et al: Minimum discard volume from arterial catheters to obtain coagulation studies free of heparin effect. *Heart Lung* 16, no. 6, pt. 1 (November 1987) 699.

Rice V et al: Development and testing of an arteriography information intervention for stress reduction. *Heart Lung* 17, no. 1 (January 1988): 23.

Schols A et al: Body composition by bioelectrical-impedance analysis compared with deuterium dilution and skinfold anthropometry in patients with COPD. *Am J Clin Nutr* 53, no. 2 (February 1991): 431.

Schachter E et al: Does intermittent mandatory ventilation accelerate weaning? *JAMA* 246, no. 11 (11 September 1981): 1210.

Shellock F and Riedinger M: Reproducibility and accuracy of using room-temperature vs ice temperature injectate for thermodilution cardiac output determination. *Heart Lung* 12, no. 2 (March 1983): 175.

Shively M: Effect of position change on mixed venous oxygen saturation in coronary artery bypass surgery patients. *Heart Lung* 17, no. 1 (January 1988): 51.

Stähelin H et al: The Basel study of β-carotene and cancer prevention. *Am J Clin Nutr* 53, no. 1 supplement, (January 1991): 265S.

Tasota F et al: Evaluation of two methods used to stabilize oral endotracheal tubes. *Heart Lung* 16, no. 2 (March 1987): 140.

Tatemichi T: Dementia in stroke survivors in the stroke data bank cohort. *Stroke* 21, no. 6 (June 1990): 858.

Tiwary C and Holguin A: Prevalence of obesity among children of military dependents at two major medical centers. *Am J Public Health* 82, no. 3 (March 1992): 354.

Tomlinson J et al: A prospective comparison of IMV and T-piece weaning from mechanical ventilation. *Chest* 96 (1989): 348.

Varsano T et al: Comparative efficacy of ceftriaxone and ampicillin for treatment of severe shigellosis in children. *J Pediatr* 118, no. 4, Part 1 (April 1991): 627.

Vio F et al: Smoking during pregnancy and lactation and its effects on breast-milk volume, *Am J Clin Nutr* 54, no. 6 (December 1991): 1011.

Wilson W: Ordering and administration of sedatives and analgesics during the withholding and withdrawal of life support from critically ill patients. *JAMA* 267, no. 7 (19 February 1992): 949.

An Orientation to Inferential Statistics
A REVIEW

Part II presents an orientation to the two major problems of concern in inferential statistics: problems of location and problems of comparison. Problems of location are solved by displaying an appropriate confidence interval (Chapters 7 and 8). Problems of comparison are resolved by tests of hypothesis (Chapters 9, 10, and 11).

A 95% confidence interval offers an interval that contains the parameter of interest for 95% of all possible samples. Common parameters of interest are proportions or averages (mean or median).

When concerned with an average, construct a t-interval, z-interval, or s-interval, depending on whether the underlying random variable is normal, the sample size is large (> 30), or neither, respectively. The t- and z-intervals are confidence intervals for the mean. An s-interval is a confidence interval for the median. A t- or z-interval for the mean can be constructed from the sample legend. To construct an s-interval, we need the raw data and apply Minitab.

A special application in the health sciences concerns paired-data that yield meaningful differences (paired differences). Paired-difference analysis is especially common in the health sciences due to the frequent application of before and after and method A versus method B studies. In such studies, one converts each data pair into a difference and then constructs the appropriate confidence interval for the difference. One can draw relevant conclusions by observing whether or not 0 is in the confidence interval.

Chapter 9 presents an orientation to test of hypothesis. Test of hypothesis is a useful tool for providing insight into those general health sciences problems that can be boiled down to a testable set of null and alternate hypotheses. Test of hypothesis then decides between these two rival hypotheses on the basis of data obtained from random samples.

The level of significance is a measure of the risk taken when applying a test of hypothesis. There are two fundamental kinds of possible errors inherent in hypothesis testing: rejection and acceptance errors. A rejection error is committed by rejecting the null hypothesis when

in reality the null hypothesis is true. An acceptance error is committed by retaining the null hypothesis when in reality the null hypothesis is false. The level of significance is the probability of making a rejection error.

Chapter 10 introduces one-population problems of comparison. Such problems are posed by a hypothesis that compares a parameter (proportion or an average) against a given reference value. Section 10.1 tested the proportion; Section 10.2, averages. Section 10.3 concentrated on paired-difference t-tests, one of the most common tests in the health sciences literature. Sections 10.1–3 detail the test of hypothesis protocol. In each situation, a test of hypothesis decides between the null and alternate hypothesis on the basis of a random sample with independent observations. In the health sciences, most random samples are convenience samples. A convenience sample usually maintains the spirit of randomness when precautions are taken to avoid confounding effects.

Section 10.4 presents the p-value, a way to compress all the computations in a test of hypothesis to a single number. The p-value is the most common test of hypothesis feature reported in the health sciences literature. The p-value measures the likelihood of obtaining a sample like the given sample if the null hypothesis is in reality true. Hence, a small p-value (usually $p < .05$) indicates that holding on to the null hypothesis is unreasonable. A larger p-value ($p > .05$) indicates that the sample drawn is consistent with the null hypothesis.

Chapter 11 deals with two-population problems of comparison. Section 11.1 compares two proportions; Section 11.2 compares averages. Comparison of proportions is a common test in studies where the effect of a treatment is compared with that of a placebo.

Comparison of averages parallels the construction of confidence intervals. Prior to testing one must ascertain whether the underlying random variable is normal in both populations, or one has large samples, or neither. If the random variable is normal in both populations, apply the pooled t-test or Smith-Satterthwaite t-test depending on whether the populations are homoscedastic (variances equal) or heteroscedastic.

The large-samples test is a z-test. The t-tests and z-test compare means. If neither normality nor large samples holds, one may conduct a Mann-Whitney test in Minitab. The Mann-Whitney test compares medians.

Understanding test of hypothesis is perhaps the raison d'être for health sciences statistics. From one perspective, test of hypothesis is the ultimate in KISS (Keep It Super Simple) methodology. The rather stunning simplicity is that a complex health science problem can be boiled down to a simple comparison statement embodied in a problem of comparison, which can then be resolved by a test of hypothesis on the basis of data from random samples (see Figure II-1).

The computational components of a test of hypothesis are basically straightforward. One can rely on well-formulated charts for guidance. For some, this imparts a "cookbook" flavor to health sciences statistics. However, for any test of hypothesis problem, the thought and care that go into problem formulation and design at the front end and interpretation toward providing care at the back end are anything but trivial.

PART II Review Problems

Problems 1–5 are based on the following study. Christensen et al studied neutrophils and opsonic capacity after intravenously administered immune globulin (IVGI) therapy. They enrolled 22 newborns with clinical signs of bacterial sepsis. The infants were randomized into two treatment groups: IVIG ($n = 11$) and placebo ($n = 11$). There were no differences in physiological measurements between the two groups at the start of treatment. Hemoglobin (g/dL) was one of the variates mea-sured to assess the effect of treatment. The data are shown in Table II-1.**

TABLE II-1 Data from Christensen et al given as mean ± SD.

Time	IVIG (n = 11)	Placebo (n = 11)
Start	15.0 ± 2.2	14.5 ± 1.6
24 Hour	15.4 ± 2.1	13.9 ± 0.09

1. Is there a significant difference between the two groups in mean hemoglobin at the start of therapy?
2. Test the 24-hour hemoglobin for homoscedasticity at the 1% LOS.
3. Conduct a Smith-Satterthwaite t-test for comparison of means for the 24-hour hemoglobin.
4. Conduct a pooled t-test for comparison of means for the 24-hour hemoglobin. Is the pooled t-test justified?
5. Explain why, based on the given information, one cannot test to determine whether or not there is a significant change in hemoglobin in the IVIG group from start to 24 hours.

Problems 6–9 are based on a study by Coates et al on the differences between black and white women with breast cancer. Coates et al observed several items in women who were newly diagnosed for breast cancer, including pain symptom and lump symptom. A woman had pain symptom if she recalled pain as a factor that led to medical consultation. A woman had lump symptom if she recalled feeling a lump in a breast as a factor that led to medical consultation. The data reported by Coates et al are shown in Table II-2.

FIGURE II-1
Interaction between test of hypothesis and health sciences problems.

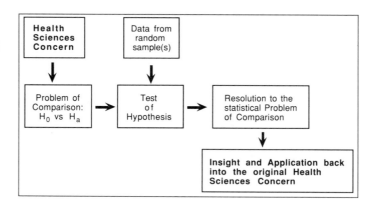

TABLE II-2 Data from Coates et al.

Symptom	Blacks (n = 410)	Whites (n = 325)
Pain	220	198
Lump	16	18

6. Determine a point estimate and 90% confidence interval for the proportion of blacks who report a pain symptom.
7. Determine a point estimate and 90% confidence interval for the proportion of whites who report a pain symptom.
8. Test the research (alternate) hypothesis that the proportion of blacks with pain symptom is significantly greater than the proportion of whites with pain symptom.
9. Is there a statistically significant difference between blacks and whites in the proportion with lump symptom?

Problems 10–14 are based on the following study. Margolin et al reported the baseline seated and standing systolic blood pressures (SBPs) of 22 elderly (aged ≥ 60) hypertensive subjects in a study group as shown in Table II-3.

TABLE II-3 Data adapted from Margolin et al.

Patient	Seated	Standing
1	183	180
2	169	167
3	146	145
4	173	158
5	178	184
6	193	181
7	177	178
8	173	163
9	175	173
10	142	137
11	157	149
12	135	130
13	170	167
14	131	127
15	151	137
16	155	148
17	179	172
18	186	180
19	177	176
20	155	148
21	151	152
22	161	168

10. Definite systolic hypertension is defined as > 150. Test the hypothesis that the mean seated SBP is > 150.
11. Repeat Problem 10 for standing SBP.
12. Test to determine whether there is evidence in this group for a difference between seated and standing SBP.
13. Determine 95% confidence intervals for (a) seated SBP and (b) standing SBP.
14. Determine the mean, standard deviation, and a 95% confidence interval for the difference between the seated and standing SBP. How do these results compare with your analysis in Problem 13?

Problems 15–27 are based on the following study. Paolisso et al studied the association between insulin resistance in nonobese elderly people with extracellular plasma and intracellular erythrocyte magnesium content. Paolisso et al utilized a convenience sample of 12 nonobese elderly patients. For contrast, Paolisso et al also studied a control group of 25 young healthy subjects. People in both groups led similar sedentary lives, eating weight-maintaining diets with similar daily protein intakes.

Among the 25 control subjects, erythrocyte magnesium ion (Mg^{++}) concentration was $2.18 \pm .20$ mmol/L and plasma magnesium was $.82 \pm .20$ mmol/liter (mean $\pm$ SD). The data for the 12 elderly patients in the study are given in Table II-4.

TABLE II-4 Data from Paolisso et al on elderly patients.

Patient	Gender	Erythrocyte	Plasma
1	M	1.78	.88
2	F	1.65	.71
3	F	1.99	.79
4	M	2.02	.81
5	M	1.78	.84
6	F	1.83	.64
7	F	1.88	.85
8	M	1.77	.82
9	F	2.03	.91
10	F	1.91	.84
11	M	1.89	.79
12	M	1.84	.69

15. Determine the mean and standard deviation of erythrocyte magnesium concentration for the 12 elderly patients.
16. Determine the mean and standard deviation of plasma magnesium concentration for the 12 elderly patients.

17. Determine a 95% confidence interval for the mean erythrocyte magnesium concentration for elderly patients.
18. Determine a 95% confidence interval for the mean plasma magnesium concentration for elderly patients.
19. Determine the mean and standard deviation of the difference between the erythrocyte and plasma magnesium concentrations.
20. Determine a 95% confidence interval for the mean difference between the erythrocyte and plasma magnesium concentrations.
21. Conduct a test of hypothesis to determine whether there is a statistically significant difference between the erythrocyte and plasma magnesium concentrations.
22. Conduct a test of hypothesis to determine whether the mean erythrocyte magnesium concentration is consistent with a value of 2.18 mmol/liter.
23. Is there a statistically significant difference in the average erythrocyte magnesium concentration between the elderly group and the control group?
24. Conduct a test of hypothesis to determine whether the mean plasma magnesium concentration is consistent with a value of 0.82 mmol/liter.
25. Is there a statistically significant difference in the average plasma magnesium concentration between the elderly group and the control group?
26. Is there a statistically significant difference in the mean erythrocyte magnesium concentration between elderly men and women?
27. Is there a statistically significant difference in the mean plasma magnesium concentration between elderly men and women?

References

Christensen R et al: Effects on neutrophil kinetics and serum opsonic capacity of intravenous administration of immune globin to neonates with clinical signs of early-onset sepsis. *J Pediatr* 118, no. 4, part 1 (April 1991): 606.

Coates R et al: Differences between black and white women with breast cancer in time from symptom recognition to medical consultation. *J Natl Cancer Inst* 84, no. 12 (17 June 1992): 938.

Margolin G et al: Blood pressure lowering in elderly subjects: A double-blind crossover study of ω-3 and ω-6 fatty acids. *Am J Clin Nutr* 53, no. 2 (February 1991): 562.

Paolisso G et al: Daily magnesium supplements improve glucose handling in elderly subjects. *Am J Clin Nutr* 55, no. 6 (June 1992): 1161.

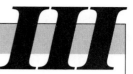

An Orientation to Multifaceted Statistics

Thus far we have been studying univariate statistics; i.e., we consider only one random variable at a time. In Chapter 10 we studied a single random variable in a *one*-population problem of comparison by comparing an appropriate parameter (proportion, mean, median) against a given reference value. In Chapter 11, we studied a single random variable in *two*-population problems of comparison by comparing an appropriate parameter in one population against the other population.

In problems of comparison involving a proportion, we considered only simple categorical random variables. A simple categorical random variable either observes or fails to observe a given attribute of interest, such as

■   In a mortality study, the patient either survives or dies.
■   In a treatment study, the patient either improves or does not improve.
■   In a headache study, the patient either reports a headache or doesn't.

The key point about these simple categorical variables is that they only have two attributes (usually, simply "yes" or "no" in response to some observation of interest).

In Part III of *Statistics: A Health Sciences Orientation* we extend our approach to tests of hypothesis by

■   Increasing the number of populations of interest (Chapter 12)
■   Increasing the number of options in the attribute list of a categorical random variable (Chapter 13)
■   Increasing the number of random variables on a given population (Chapter 13 and Chapter 14).

The emphasis in multifaceted statistics is on the *multi-*; that is, several populations, several attribute options, or several random variables of interest.

Aspects of multifaceted statistics are included in most advanced courses. Our presentation is strictly an orientation. We present three key topics: analysis of variance (ANOVA), chisquared tests, and linear regression. These topics are fundamental in a health sciences statistics course. Due to the complexity of the human condition, a health sciences study seldom is concerned with just one RV or a single group of subjects, and is often interested in categorical RVs with more than just one attribute. How do the many pieces fit together? What are the relationships between the multivariables? Such questions motivate Part III: An Orientation to Multifaceted Statistics.

Analysis of Variance

The usual treatment for gallstones used to be surgical removal. This procedure had all the discomforts associated with such an invasive technique, including risks associated with anesthesia, wound infection, discomforts of healing, and recovery time. Many cases of gallstones today can be treated by shock wave therapy, a noninvasive technique that bypasses risks from the invasive aspects of surgery. Shock wave therapy also eliminates the need for expensive care, like use of the recovery room, specifically associated with surgery.

Sackman et al were interested in researching the most effective method of shock wave therapy for treatment of gallstones. They considered three different general treatment methods:

1. Use of a model GM 1 lithotroper equipped with a water tank; patient partially submerged
2. Model MPL 9000 water cushion; low-energy shock wave
3. Model MPL 9000 water cushion; high-energy shock wave

In order to compare the three methods, Sackman et al utilized a convenience sample of patients who were then randomly assigned to the three groups. They then made assessments determining the effectiveness of the three treatment modalities. Which method performed best?

This question (Which method performed best?) poses a problem of comparison that is a natural extension of Chapters 10 and 11. In Chapter 10 we compared a single population parameter against a reference value of interest. In Chapter 11 we extended consideration to two populations; in particular, we compared two populations against each other. Here, we want to compare three different groups. And, of course, we may need to consider even more groups.

Analysis of variance (ANOVA) is a procedure for comparing the means of several populations against each other. Technically, it extends the two-tailed pooled t-test for equality of means from two to several populations. In Chapter 12 we study this procedure in two cases. Section 12.1 discusses the use of ANOVA when the raw data are provided. In Section 12.2 we consider the use of ANOVA when we are provided only with the sample legend (the raw data are unavailable).

In Problems 12.2.1–3 we invite you to apply the ANOVA technique to answer several concerns of Sackman et al regarding the three treatment modalities for gallstones.

SECTION 12.1

**Data Set
ANOVA**

OBJECTIVES   This section will

1 Determine whether one-way ANOVA is the appropriate procedure to test comparison of means when provided with a sample from each of several levels.

2 Apply ANOVA when presented with an appropriate health sciences problem for the comparison of means of several levels.

3 Apply an appropriate confidence interval procedure when ANOVA indicates a difference between level means.

4 Apply the Mood test for a comparison of medians.

ANOVA is a test of hypothesis procedure that extends a comparison of means for two populations to a comparison of means for several populations. In particular, ANOVA is an expansion of the two-tailed pooled t-test from two populations to several populations.

ANOVA is an acronym derived from *an*alysis *of* *va*riance. This sounds like a strange name for a test of hypothesis about means. It seems like a test comparing means should be called analysis of means. However, the theoretical basis on which the test is conducted is derived from considerations about the population variances. In particular, the formulas involved in computing the key sample value make heavy use of the homoscedastic assumption that the underlying variances in each of the given levels are all equal. Hence, the founding theoreticians called this statistical technique the analysis of variance. The name stuck, so the test is universally referred to as ANOVA.

The Background for ANOVA

ANOVA is used when one wants to determine whether or not the *means* for each population of interest are all equal. One common application for ANOVA in the health sciences involves comparing a variety of treatments (e.g., the Sackman et al gallstone study used to introduce this chapter). Another common application is to compare the effect of the same treatment on different groups.

EXAMPLE 12.1.1 A northern California health care team was engaged to conduct a general fitness program for a large corporation. The company believed that investing in the general health of its employees would be cost-effective by reducing the number of sick-leave days and increasing general productivity. A group of employees from each of the three plants operated by the company participated in a pilot study. Several baseline variables were measured for each subject, including weight, percent body fat, serum cholesterol, serum triglycerides, and high-density lipoproteins. These variables were measured again after 3 months. During the 3-month program, employees participated in a guided exercise program and attended classes in general health and nutrition conducted by the health care team. The health care team and the corporate sponsor of the program were interested in whether the program did any good.

Of course there are many ways to look at the general concern: Did the program do any good? One of the many concerns studied by the health care team was posed by the inquiry:

Was there a significant difference between the three plants in the way the 3-month program affected serum triglycerides?

This question was part of an evaluation to determine whether the same basic program worked equally well in all three plants, or whether the team would need to tailor a program to each plant.

In an ANOVA problem, a population of interest is called a **level**. In Example 12.1.1 the levels involved are the work forces at each of the three plants. We will simply refer to these three levels in Example 12.1.1 as plant A, plant B, and plant C.

The levels used in a design can be constructed with increasing layers of complexity. The simplest design is **one-way** ANOVA, where we make only one consideration at each level. In two-way ANOVA, one first constructs a primary set of levels, then on each level superimposes a secondary set of levels. For example, in the northern California health program (Example 12.1.1), for each primary group (plant A, B, or C), one could make a secondary inquiry about how the program affected men versus women. Such an extended study would call for a consideration of a two-way ANOVA since there are two levels of consideration: plant (A,B,C) and gender (female, male). In this section we will be concerned only with one-way ANOVA. Multiway ANOVA is a standard topic in many advanced statistics courses.

In a given problem, to determine whether ANOVA is justified for testing equality of means, we need to consider several preliminaries:

1. Type of design
2. Independent random samples with independent observations
3. Normality
4. Homoscedasticity

The first preliminary consideration (type of design) involves the way in which the levels are constructed and viewed. The two main designs for level formulation are the fixed treatments design and the random effects design.

Fixed Treatments versus Random Effects Design

The general setting for ANOVA displays several levels and a continuous random variable (RV) of interest. The levels involved are important choices in the design of the study. The levels can be set and defined by the researcher or they can be randomly selected from a large list of possible levels of interest. A **fixed treatment** level is well defined by the researcher; a *random effects* level is randomly selected from a collection of possible levels of interest.

EXAMPLE 12.1.2   Daily and Mersch (Appendix, Data Set 1) were interested in whether cardiac outputs taken by using a room-temperature injectate are statistically significantly different than cardiac outputs taken by using an ice-temperature injectate or the Fick method. The researchers applied a fixed treatments design. The cardiac output techniques are well defined by the three given methods (room-temperature injectate, ice-temperature injectate, Fick).

EXAMPLE 12.1.3   A clinician was interested in determining whether patients on certain prescription drugs had an affected heart rate. The clinician asked the pharmacist for a list of these prescribed drugs. The clinician was overwhelmed by the large number of drugs, so decided to randomly select four drugs, then from computer records randomly selected 15 patients receiving each of these four drugs. The clinician did not use a fixed treatment design but rather a random effects design. The drug protocols were not fixed but randomly selected. If the clinician was specifically interested in the four selected drugs at the outset, then we would have a fixed treatments design. In this random effects design, both the patients and the levels (here, drugs) are randomly selected.

EXAMPLE 12.1.4   The health care team conducting the northern California fitness program (Example 12.1.1) measured several variables at the start of the program and again at 3 months, including serum triglycerides. The health care team wondered whether the program's effect on serum triglycerides was the same in all three plants. This study uses a fixed treatments design since subjects are grouped according to the plant at which they work.

In most applications in the health sciences, a fixed treatments design is applied. If a random effects design is desired, one should consult a statistician regarding both the design and the analysis of the study. In this text we will conduct the analysis by ANOVA only on data obtained within a fixed treatments design.

Comment   The actual ANOVA comparison of means is the same for both the fixed treatments and random effects designs. However, if the level means are found to be significantly different, then the resulting course of action differs depending on the statistical design. In a fixed treatments design problem, if the level means are significantly different, then one wants to know how they differ. In a random effects design, however, which means are different is uninteresting. What is relevant is an explanation of the source of variation. We refer the interested reader to Sokol and Rohlf (especially Section 9.2) for further details.

Random and Independent Samples

The second preliminary consideration for ANOVA is that the samples obtained for each level must be independent random samples with independent observations.

The independent assumption is very important. If the samples are independent, the results obtained for one level do not influence (bias) the results for another level. In order to assure independent samples, one must have *a different random sample of subjects for each level*.

This assumption of independent samples is not met in many multilevel cases presented in the literature. If the independent samples assumption is not met, one should not carry out the ANOVA analysis presented in this section. Instead, one should consider an analysis of the problem by a **repeated measures** ANOVA (see Section 12.3). For example, the full Daily and Mersch cardiac output data set (Appendix, Data Set 1) should not be analyzed by one-way ANOVA. The Daily and Mersch data satisfy all the assumptions for one-way ANOVA except for independence of samples. In the Daily and Mersch study there are three cardiac output levels. However, all three methods were applied to each individual; hence, the assumption of independent samples is violated.

Normal Distributions

The third preliminary consideration for one-way ANOVA is that the RV of interest is normally distributed in each level. Accordingly, the sample for each level should be tested for normality.

EXAMPLE 12.1.5 One of the concerns in the northern California fitness program (Example 12.1.1 and 4) was whether the effect of the program on serum triglycerides was the same for all three plants. The changes in serum triglycerides from program initiation to 3 months are displayed in Table 12.1.1. Each measurement represents the quantity "start − end (3 months)" for serum triglycerides.

TABLE *12.1.1* Change in serum triglycerides.

Plant A			Plant B		Plant C	
25.78	34.82	28.87	66.17	− 0.96	2.27	38.85
6.41	4.76	68.89	33.69	82.03	10.08	16.95
− 52.25	64.90	25.01	0.65	34.52	81.96	38.84
− 135.28	85.54	42.69	-20.75	− 41.19	95.01	18.79
40.55	127.55	22.19	34.48	− 18.55	17.85	38.65
1.64	− 10.65	18.64	− 20.30	− 19.18	− 27.01	47.11
6.17	19.81	70.64	45.77	49.23	− 0.22	8.53
21.39					19.52	30.77
					147.54	

In Table 12.1.1, a positive number indicates a *drop* in serum triglycerides. For example, the first subject in plant A changed 25.78, a drop of 25.78 in serum triglycerides (start − end = 25.78). The third subject from plant A, however, displayed an *increase* of 52.25 (start − end = −52.25). Whether a person shows a positive or negative change in serum triglycerides is an artifact of the way change is defined: change = start − end.

To determine whether change in serum triglycerides is normally distributed in each of the plants, we apply Minitab's nscores correlation test (see Figure 12.1.3). The results for the triglycerides data (Example 12.1.5) are summarized in Table 12.1.2.

TABLE 12.1.2
Test for normality of triglycerides for the northern California fitness study.

Plant	Sample nscores Correlation	Sample Size	Critical Value (alpha = 0.01)
A	0.931	22	.9290–.9408
B	0.971	14	.8804–.9110
C	0.928	17	.9110–.9290

At the 1% level of significance (LOS), the sample from plant B is consistent with normality. However, the normality conclusion appears borderline for plants A and C since the sample nscores correlation falls in the ambiguous zone. Since there is insufficient evidence to reject outright a null hypothesis of normality, for the time being we will simply assume normality; that is, we assume that change in serum triglycerides is (approximately) normally distributed in each of the three plants.

Homoscedasticity

The final preliminary assumption to check to justify applying one-way ANOVA is homoscedasticity. This assumption is checked by the F_{max} **test**, outlined in Figure 12.1.1. The F_{max} test assumes that one is working with independent random samples with independent observations drawn from normal distributions. The F_{max} test is sensitive to normality; hence, if normality fails, do not conduct the F_{max} test.

EXAMPLE 12.1.6 We continue to consider the northern California fitness program's change in serum triglycerides study (Examples 12.1.1, 4, and 5). We noted there are three levels (plant A, plant B, plant C) in this study. The data legend is shown in Table 12.1.3.

TABLE 12.1.3
Data legend for the northern California corporate fitness study.

Plant	Sample Size	Mean	Standard Deviation
A	22	23.54	51.21
B	14	16.11	37.99
C	17	34.44	41.29

From Table 12.1.3 we observe that the largest sample standard deviation is 51.21 and the smallest sample standard deviation is 37.99. Hence, the sample value for the F_{max} test for homoscedasticity is calculated by

$$\text{sample } f_{max}\text{-value} = \left(\frac{\text{largest standard deviation}}{\text{smallest standard deviation}}\right)^2 = \left(\frac{51.21}{37.99}\right)^2 = 1.817$$

FIGURE **12.1.1**
Three-step F_{max} test
for homoscedasticity
for ANOVA.

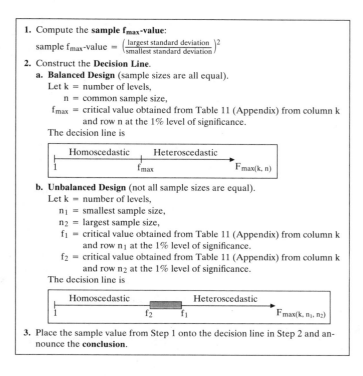

1. Compute the **sample f_{max}-value**:

   $$\text{sample } f_{max}\text{-value} = \left(\frac{\text{largest standard deviation}}{\text{smallest standard deviation}}\right)^2$$

2. Construct the **Decision Line**.

   a. Balanced Design (sample sizes are all equal).

   Let k = number of levels,

   n = common sample size,

   f_{max} = critical value obtained from Table 11 (Appendix) from column k and row n at the 1% level of significance.

   The decision line is

Homoscedastic	Heteroscedastic
1 f_{max}	$F_{max(k, n)}$

   b. Unbalanced Design (not all sample sizes are equal).

   Let k = number of levels,

   n_1 = smallest sample size,

   n_2 = largest sample size,

   f_1 = critical value obtained from Table 11 (Appendix) from column k and row n_1 at the 1% level of significance.

   f_2 = critical value obtained from Table 11 (Appendix) from column k and row n_2 at the 1% level of significance.

   The decision line is

Homoscedastic	Heteroscedastic
1 f_2 f_1	$F_{max(k, n_1, n_2)}$

3. Place the sample value from Step 1 onto the decision line in Step 2 and announce the **conclusion**.

The data legend (Table 12.1.3) reveals an unbalanced sampling design. The smallest sample size is 14 and the largest sample size is 22; that is, we have a sample size range from 14 to 22. These sample sizes do not specifically occur in Table 11 (Appendix). In order to cover our sample size range of 14 to 22, we use the Table 11 entries for $n = 13$ and $n = 31$. To obtain the ambiguous zone for the decision line at the 1% LOS, we read the Table 11 entries for three levels at $n = 13$ (6.1) and at $n = 31$ (3.0). The resulting decision line is shown in Figure 12.1.2

Our sample f_{max}-value of 1.817 clearly lies in the homoscedastic zone. Hence, on the basis of the F_{max} test, our samples are consistent with an assumption of homoscedasticity. Accordingly, we assume that the level variances are all equal.

We now summarize our results thus far for the northern California fitness program study so we can get a sense of the big picture of what is happening. The general *population* of interest is *employees of a large manufacturing company*. The *random variable* of interest is *change in serum triglycerides*. Our particular *problem* of interest is to determine *whether change in serum triglycerides is significantly different between plants*. Motivated by the problem of interest, each employee in the study is classified in one way: by plant. There are three fixed levels for plant: A, B, and C. Hence, we

FIGURE **12.1.2**
Homoscedasticity
decision line.

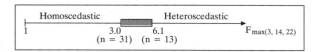

Homoscedastic	Heteroscedastic
1 3.0 6.1	$F_{max(3, 14, 22)}$
(n = 31) (n = 13)	

have a one-way fixed treatments design for change in serum triglycerides. An independent random sample is utilized from each plant. Based on Minitab's nscores and correlation test, we assume that the RV of interest, change in serum triglycerides, is (approximately) normally distributed in each level. Finally, we assume homoscedasticity based on the F_{max} test. The change in serum triglycerides data set (Table 12.1.1) is now a candidate for analysis by one-way ANOVA.

The design requirement of independent random samples with independent observations is crucial and may not be violated to justify ANOVA. Assumptions of normality and homoscedasticity are not so crucial and may be relaxed. A statistical test that yields a trustworthy conclusion despite violations in preliminary assumptions is called a **robust** test. ANOVA is a robust test. If all the assumptions of ANOVA are met, one may proceed with full justification in applying ANOVA. The p-value obtained will be exact. When assumptions of normality or homoscedasticity are even moderately violated, proceed with ANOVA with an appeal to robustness and report the p-value as approximate.

In the northern California fitness program's change in serum triglycerides study, the test for normality was borderline for two levels at the 1% LOS (Table 12.1.2). An appeal to robustness fully justifies the use of ANOVA to analyze the data since all other conditions for ANOVA are met. We proceed to the ANOVA analysis of the data.

Analysis of Variance Test

When applicable, ANOVA is the best test to determine whether the means of several levels are all the same or some means are different. The formal statement of hypotheses tested by ANOVA is

H_0: $\mu_1 = \mu_2 = \cdots = \mu_k$ (all level means are equal)
H_a: the means are otherwise

This null hypothesis is called the **omnibus hypothesis** (omnibus means dealing with several things at once). Note that the alternate hypothesis does not claim that all the means are different from each other but that at least two of the means are different.

After we fully consider the ANOVA assumptions, we are ready to analyze the data. The analysis should present two parts: (1) a boxplot diagram and (2) the ANOVA. The purpose of ANOVA is to test whether all the level means are equal. To get a good intuitive feel for this test, we present a **boxplot diagram**, which displays a boxplot for each level, all shown on the same scale. A boxplot diagram helps to give that important intuitive feel for comparing the distribution of the RV of interest between levels.

EXAMPLE 12.1.7 We analyze the northern California health program serum triglycerides data. In particular, we apply ANOVA to resolve the problem

H_o: $\mu_{plant\ A} = \mu_{plant\ B} = \mu_{plant\ C}$
H_a: the means are otherwise

Figure 12.1.3 displays a Minitab session for the ANOVA analysis.

FIGURE **12.1.3**
Minitab output for
ANOVA analysis of the
change in serum
triglycerides (Examples
12.1.1, 5, and 7).

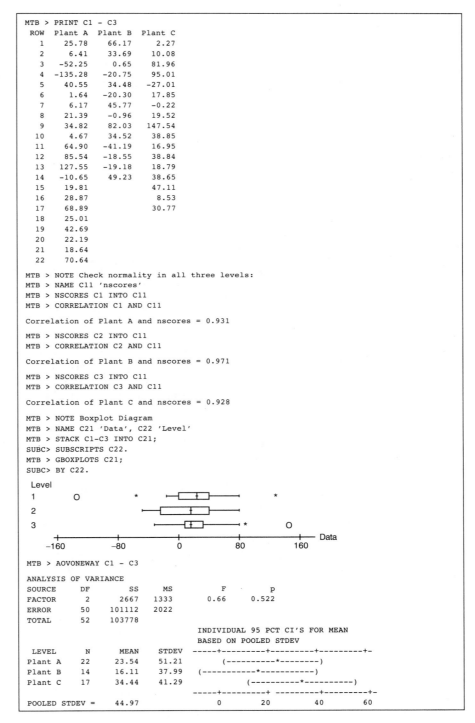

The raw sample data for the change in serum triglycerides are SET into columns C1–C3 in Minitab. The data for plant A employees are SET into column C1, plant B employees into column C2, and plant C employees into column C3. After data input, PRINT the data and inspect them for accuracy. Conduct an nscores and correlation for each column of data to obtain the information needed for the normality checks. Display a boxplot diagram. Conduct ANOVA by applying the Minitab command AOVONEWAY. The Minitab keyword AOVONEWAY stands for *analysis of variance one-way*.

There are three basic items that we need to obtain from Minitab's output to the AOVONEWAY command:

1. The **sample f-ratio**
2. The **degrees of freedom**
3. The **p-value**

The degrees of freedom are the first two entries in the DF column, the sample f-ratio is the number in the F column, and the *p*-value is the entry in the p column. Since the computer has given us the p-value for the test, we immediately announce the conclusion to the northern California fitness program change in serum triglycerides study:

> There is no significant difference between the three plants in change in serum triglycerides during the first 3 months of the northern California corporate fitness program $(f = .66, df = (2, 50), p \approx .5)$.

Minitab's output to the AOVONEWAY command (see Figure 12.1.3) has four components. The first component is the ANOVA table, which contains the sample information needed to carry out the ANOVA test of hypothesis. The items of interest from the ANOVA table are the degrees of freedom (DF column), sample f-ratio (F), and the *p*-value (p). The second component is the sample legend containing the sample size (N), mean (MEAN), and standard deviation (STDEV) for each level. The third component is a graphic, which displays a 95% confidence interval (CI) for each of the level means. The fourth component is the sample's estimate of the common standard deviation (recall that homoscedasticity is assumed). One obtains this estimate by reading "POOLED STDEV =." For example, in the northern California health program, the point estimate for the common standard deviation is 44.97.

A glance at either the boxplot diagram or the CI graphic in the AOVONEWAY output provides a rough general indication of how the level means relate to each other. In Figure 12.1.3, note that all three CIs clearly overlap, indicating no significant difference between level means. As a guideline, a common overlap by all the level CIs indicates that there is no statistically significant difference between level means.

When one rejects the null hypothesis in ANOVA, then the sample provides evidence that not all the level means are equal. We then want to proceed further with the analysis to determine which level means are significantly smaller or larger than other level means. One may use the CI picture as a rough guide to determine which levels have significantly different means.

EXAMPLE 12.1.8 Heini et al studied daily energy expenditure in pregnant Gambian women. A convenience sample consisted of 41 pregnant Gambian women who were then placed in one of three groups according to trimester of pregnancy. A convenience sample of 13 nonpregnant, nonlactating women served as controls. Figure 12.1.4

---

displays a Minitab session for analysis of daytime energy expenditure (measured as kilojoules per minute).

We leave it for the student to verify the preliminary assumptions for ANOVA. Based on Minitab's ANOVA output, we announce

There is a difference in daytime energy expenditure in pregnant Gambian women according to the trimester of pregnancy ($f = 8.11$, $df = (3, 50)$, $p < .0005$).

Since a statistically significant difference in mean daytime energy expenditure is detected by ANOVA, we naturally inquire further: How are these means different? The boxplot diagram and the CI graphic begin to tell the story. In particular, the CI graphic in Figure 12.1.4 clearly shows that daytime energy expenditure is greater for women in their third trimester than in the other three cases; further, there is no significant difference among the other three groups. In general, when ANOVA indicates that the level means are different, our next step is to look at appropriate CIs to determine which level means are significantly smaller or larger than the others.

ANOVA Confidence Intervals

There are a variety of powerful techniques for being able to discern which level means are significantly different from each other when ANOVA indicates that such differences occur. Minitab (release 8 or later) supports four subcommands (Tukey, Fisher, Dunnett, and MCB) to the ONEWAY command that provide these powerful techniques.

The Minitab command ONEWAY conducts an ANOVA analysis, just like the AOVONEWAY command but on a stacked data set rather than a data set presented level by level. In a stacked format the entire data set is presented in just two columns. The first column contains all the data from all the levels. The second column identifies the level of a given measurement. One then issues the ONEWAY command on the stacked data. The stacking is done in Minitab with the STACK command.

For the Heini et al study, recall that the original raw data were set in a level-by-level format in columns C1–C4 in Minitab's spreadsheet (see Figure 12.1.4). We stack this data set into new columns C21 and C22 (see Figure 12.1.5). Column C21 will contain the entire raw data set. Column C22 will contain 13 ones, 11 twos, 15 threes, and 15 fours, indicating that the first 13 items of data come from level 1, the next 11 items of data come from level 2, the next 15 items of data come from level 3, and the final 15 items of data come from level 4.

Note the form of the STACK command: STACK C1-C4 into C21. This command copies all the data into column C21 by copying the numbers first from C1, then C2, then C3, and finally C4. To keep track of what level a number belongs to, the SUBSCRIPTS subcommand accompanies the main STACK command. The subcommand SUBSCRIPTS C22 tells us that column C22 contains the level identifiers. We advise the student to PRINT C21 C22 to observe the form of the stacked data set. The ONEWAY command is then issued on the columns containing the stacked data and level identifiers; here, ONEWAY C21 C22.

Figure 12.1.5 displays a Minitab session that continues the analysis for the Heini et al data displayed in Figure 12.1.4. In Figure 12.1.5 observe that first the data are

FIGURE *12.1.4*
Minitab ANOVA
session for the Heini
et al data.

```
MTB > PRINT C1 - C4

ROW   Controls   First   Second   Third

  1     5.40     5.27     5.06     5.77
  2     4.64     5.52     5.31     6.03
  3     5.90     5.23     6.11     6.23
  4     4.69     5.10     5.31     6.32
  5     5.65     6.53     5.15     7.36
  6     5.27     5.94     6.32     5.48
  7     5.61     5.23     5.57     6.44
  8     5.44     4.94     5.23     6.61
  9     4.69     6.86     6.40     6.28
 10     4.90     5.73     5.65     6.74
 11     5.82     5.15     6.03     9.94
 12     6.49              5.57     7.87
 13     5.65              4.64     7.95
 14                       6.61     6.44
 15                       4.56     5.23

MTB > NSCORES C1 INTO C5
MTB > CORRELATION C1 AND C5

Correlation of Controls and Nscores = 0.974

MTB > NSCORES C2 INTO C5
MTB > CORRELATION C2 AND C5

Correlation of First and Nscores = 0.930

MTB > NSCORES C3 INTO C5
MTB > CORRELATION C3 AND C5

Correlation of Second and Nscores = 0.987

MTB > NSCORES C4 INTO C5
MTB > CORRELATION C4 AND C5

Correlation of Third and Nscores = 0.926

MTB > NOTE Boxplot Diagram
MTB > NAME C21 'Data', C22 'Level'
MTB > STACK C1 - C4 INTO C21;
SUBC> SUBSCRIPTS C22.
MTB > GBOXPLOTS C21;
SUBC> BY C22.
```

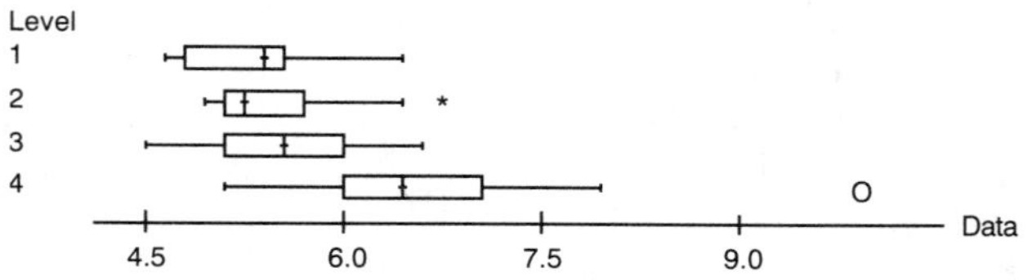

```
MTB > AOVONEWAY C1 - C4

ANALYSIS OF VARIANCE
SOURCE    DF       SS        MS        F         p
FACTOR     3    15.772    5.257     8.11     0.000
ERROR     50    32.426    0.649
TOTAL     53    48.198

                             INDIVIDUAL 95 PCT CI'S FOR MEAN
                             BASED ON POOLED STDEV
  LEVEL      N     MEAN    STDEV   --------+---------+---------+--------
Controls    13   5.3962   0.5506  (-------*-------)
First       11   5.5909   0.6214    (-------*-------)
Second      15   5.5680   0.6219    (------*------)
Third       15   6.7127   1.1806                       (------*------)
                                   --------+---------+---------+--------
POOLED STDEV =     0.8053              5.40      6.00      6.60
```

stacked, then the ONEWAY command is issued to conduct ANOVA. The ONE-WAY main command is augmented with a subcommand to display an appropriate confidence interval. In Figure 12.1.5 we issue all four subcommands (Tukey, Fisher, Dunnett, and MCB) only for the sake of illustration. Which subcommand to issue depends on the nature of the health science inquiry.

Comment Applying these subcommand ideas in a Macintosh or Windows environment is incredibly easy due to the point and click features in friendly dialog boxes.

A **Tukey confidence interval** is a CI for the difference between two level means. A **Tukey diagram** presents the Tukey CI for all possible pairs of level means. Since the Heini et al data involve four levels, there are $C(4, 2) = 6$ (Appendix, Table 1) level pairs. For example, a CI for the difference between the means for level 1 (controls) and level 2 (first trimester) is $(-955, 725)$. Since this CI has the form $(-, +)$, then 0 is in the interval and no statistically significant difference is detected between these two level means. Also, a CI for the difference between level 1 (control) and level 4 (third trimester) is $(-2247, -693)$. Since this CI has the form $(-, -)$, then $\mu_1 - \mu_4 < 0$, indicating that the level 1 mean is significantly smaller than the level 4 mean.

In a Tukey diagram, the level of confidence is a **simultaneous** level of confidence applying to all six intervals as a family. Specifically, with 95% confidence, *all* the six level mean differences are within the specified intervals. There is only a 5% risk (family error rate $= .0500$) that one or more of the intervals does not contain the difference of the level means. In simultaneous confidence, one is looking at the big picture, considering all applicable pairwise differences together, whereas with individual confidence one is looking at just one interval at a time. Individually, each of the Tukey CIs in Figure 12.1.5 is a 98.95% CI (individual error rate $= .0105$).

A **Fisher confidence interval** is an ordinary individual CI for the difference of the means between two levels. A **Fisher diagram** displays the Fisher CI for all possible pairs of level means. A Fisher diagram is exactly the same as the Tukey diagram with the single exception that the stated level of confidence applies to just one CI at a time rather than to the entire family of displayed intervals. For example, a 95% CI for $\mu_2 - \mu_3$ is $(-717, 513)$, indicating no detectable difference between the level means. In Figure 12.1.5 for the Fisher diagram, the "individual error rate" is .05, while the "family error rate" is .199. When you look at just one CI, the risk (error rate) that the interval does not contain the difference of the means is 5%—the confidence is 95%. When you look at the entire picture (family of intervals), the risk that at least one of the six displayed intervals does not contain the difference of the indicated means is 19.9%—family confidence is 80.1%.

A **Dunnett confidence interval** is a CI for the mean difference between a treatment level and the control. A **Dunnett diagram** displays a Dunnett CI for the difference between each noncontrol level and the control. For example, a simultaneous 95% CI for the difference between the means for level 2 (first trimester) and the control (level 1) is $(-649.4, 880.0)$. A simultaneous 95% CI for the difference between the means for level 4 and the control is $(763.0, 2177.6)$. Hence, there is no detectable difference between the level 2 mean and the control mean. There is a detectable difference between the level 4 mean and the control. Since the Heini et al study involves a control, the Dunnett subcommand is relevant. To apply the Dunnett

FIGURE **12.1.5**
Minitab ANOVA
session with
confidence intervals
for the Heini et al
data.

```
MTB > STACK C1 - C4 INTO C11;
SUBC> SUBSCRIPTS INTO C12.
MTB >
MTB > ONEWAY C11 C12;
SUBC> TUKEY .05;
SUBC> FISHER .05;
SUBC> DUNNETT .05 1;
SUBC> MCB .05 1.

ANALYSIS OF VARIANCE ON Data
SOURCE      DF       SS         MS        F        p
Level        3   20197308    6732436    11.32    0.000
ERROR       50   29747492     594950
TOTAL       53   49944800
                                     INDIVIDUAL 95 PCT CI'S FOR MEAN
                                     BASED ON POOLED STDEV
   LEVEL     N       MEAN      STDEV   -------+---------+---------+---------
      1     13      6971.2     613.0   (------*-----)
      2     11      7086.5     728.1      (-----*------)
      3     15      7188.3     744.7       (-----*----)
      4     15      8441.5     932.5                      (-----*----)
                                        -------+---------+---------+---------
POOLED STDEV =     771.3                  7000      7700      8400

Tukey's pairwise comparisons

    Family error rate = 0.0500
Individual error rate = 0.0105

Critical value = 3.76

Intervals for (column level mean) - (row level mean)

                 1          2          3

    2         -955
               725

    3         -994       -916
               560        712

    4        -2247      -2169      -2002
              -693       -541       -504

Fisher's pairwise comparisons

    Family error rate = 0.199
Individual error rate = 0.0500

Critical value = 2.009

Intervals for (column level mean) - (row level mean)

                 1          2          3

    2         -750
               520

    3         -804       -717
               370        513

    4        -2057      -1970      -1819
              -883       -740       -687

Dunnett's intervals for treatment mean minus control mean

    Family error rate = 0.0500
Individual error rate = 0.0192

Critical value = 2.42

Control = level 1 of Level
```

FIGURE **12.1.5** *(continued)*

```
    Level    Lower    Center    Upper ----------+---------+---------+---------+-
       2     -649.4    115.3    880.0  (----------*----------)
       3     -490.2    217.1    924.4   (---------*---------)
       4      763.0   1470.3   2177.6                         (---------*---------)
                                       ----------+---------+---------+---------+-
                                                 0       700      1400     2100


Hsu's MCB (Multiple Comparisons with the Best)

Family error rate = 0.0500

Critical value = 2.12

Intervals for level mean minus largest of other level means

    Level    Lower    Center    Upper -+---------+---------+---------+---------+
       1    -2089.9  -1470.3      0.0  (-----*-------------)
       2    -2004.1  -1355.0      0.0   (-----*------------)
       3    -1850.3  -1253.2      0.0    (-----*-----------)
       4       0.0    1253.2   1850.3                    (------------*-----)
                                       -+---------+---------+---------+---------+
                                     -2000     -1000       0       1000     2000
```

subcommand, one must specify which level is the control (hence, SUBC> DUNNETT .05 1, indicating that the family error [risk] rate is .05 and that level 1 is the control).

An **MCB confidence interval** is a CI for the mean difference between a treatment level and the "best" level (MCB stands for *m*ultiple *c*omparisons with the *b*est). An **MCB diagram** displays a CI for the difference between each level and the "best" level. One may choose the "best" level as the level with either the smallest level mean or the largest level mean. The choice is made in the MCB subcommand. Here we used SUBC> MCB .05 1, indicating a family error rate (risk) of 5% and the best level is the level with the largest level mean. To use the smallest level mean, simply replace 1 by −1 in the MCB subcommand. The MCB subcommand is useful for determining treatments intended to maximize or minimize something (e.g., what treatment will produce the *greatest* drop in serum cholesterol).

Summarizing, Minitab's ONEWAY command supports four subcommands: TUKEY, FISHER, DUNNETT, and MCB. Tukey and Fisher provide CIs for all pairwise differences between level means. Dunnett provides a CI for the difference between each treatment mean and a control mean. MCB provides a CI for the difference between each level mean and the best of the other level means. The general form for the Minitab subcommands for the ONEWAY main command are

```
SUBC> TUKEY [K].
SUBC> FISHER [K].
SUBC> DUNNETT [K] control is L.
SUBC> MCB [K] best is L.
```

In the DUNNETT subcommand, L specifies the control level. In the MCB command, L specifies the best level (use 1 for L when the best is the level with the largest mean; use −1 when the best is the level with the smallest mean). In each of the four subcommands, [K] represents an optional user-specified error rate (level of risk). If the risk is not specified, then a default error rate of 5% (95% confidence) is used. The error rate is the family error rate for TUKEY, DUNNETT, and MCB, and the individual error rate for FISHER. Error rates must be between .5 and .001. Values greater than 1.0 are interpreted as percentages. The *family* error rate is the maximum probability of obtaining one or more CIs that do not contain the true difference between level means. The *individual* error rate is the probability that a given CI will not contain the true difference in level means.

Comment In a highly technical situation, it is possible that ANOVA rejects the omnibus hypothesis, yet a Tukey diagram shows no significant difference between any pair of level means. This counterintuitive situation is indicative that ANOVA goes deeper than just the omnibus hypothesis that all the means are equal. The full theory of ANOVA is explained through the theory of linear contrasts, and problems are resolved with a Scheffé analysis. Such topics are meant for advanced courses and are beyond the scope of this text. The interested reader is invited to explore this subject in Zehna, a very readable reference for such an advanced topic.

When the assumptions for ANOVA are met, ANOVA is the best test for comparing averages between several levels. ANOVA specifically compares the means between the various levels. If ANOVA detects a difference in level means, one applies a CI technique to determine which level means are appropriately different. When normality badly fails, however, then to compare the various levels, one should consider the Mood test for comparison of medians.

The Mood Test for Comparison of Medians

The Mood test also assumes that the study being analyzed uses a fixed treatments model and independent random samples with independent observations. The omnibus hypothesis for the **Mood test** is that all the level *medians* are equal, in contrast to ANOVA, which tests whether all the level means are equal.

To apply the Mood test, first enter the data into Minitab's spreadsheet (just like in ANOVA). Before applying the MOOD command, one must represent the data in a stacked format. Stacking is done in Minitab with the STACK command. In a stacked format the entire data set is presented in two columns. The first column contains all the data from all the levels. The second column identifies the level of a given measurement. One then issues the MOOD command on the stacked data.

For the northern California fitness study, recall that the original raw data were set in columns C1–C3 in Minitab's spreadsheet (see Figure 12.1.3). We stack this data set into new columns C21 and C22 (see Figure 12.1.6). Column C21 will contain the entire raw data set. Column C22 will contain 22 ones, 14 twos, and 17 threes, indicating that the first 22 items of data come from level 1, the next 14 items of data come from level 2, and the final 17 items of data come from level 3.

EXAMPLE 12.1.9 For illustration, we apply the Mood test to the northern California fitness program's change in serum triglycerides data (Table 12.1.1). Minitab's output is displayed in Figure 12.1.6.

Looking at the output for the Mood test in Figure 12.1.6, we observe the *p*-value is very high (p = .980). Hence, we immediately conclude

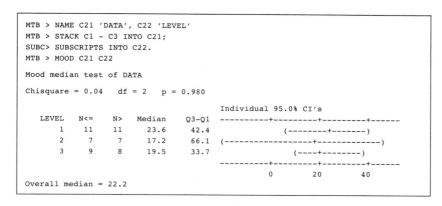

FIGURE **12.1.6**
The Mood test for comparison of medians applied to the change in serum triglycerides study (Examples 12.1.1, 5, and 7).

```
MTB > NAME C21 'DATA', C22 'LEVEL'
MTB > STACK C1 - C3 INTO C21;
SUBC> SUBSCRIPTS INTO C22.
MTB > MOOD C21 C22

Mood median test of DATA

Chisquare = 0.04    df = 2    p = 0.980

                                            Individual 95.0% CI's
    LEVEL    N<=    N>    Median    Q3-Q1   ----------+---------+---------+------
        1     11    11      23.6     42.4                  (--------+-------)
        2      7     7      17.2     66.1   (-----------------+-------------)
        3      9     8      19.5     33.7              (----+--------)
                                            ----------+---------+---------+------
                                                      0        20        40
Overall median = 22.2
```

There is no significant difference in the median change in serum triglycerides among the three plants ($\chi^2 = .04, df = 2, p = .98$).

Comment In the Mood test, the sample value is the number "Chisquare" (here, Chisquare $= .04$) and the degrees of freedom are denoted by df (here, df $= 2$). Chi is a Greek letter (see Appendix, Table 14). Hence, Chisquare is symbolically denoted by χ^2. We will see more about "chisquared tests" in Chapter 13. The key point here is that whenever we have a computer perform a test of hypothesis for us, if the computer provides the p-value we can immediately announce our conclusion in terms of the relevant health sciences problem. The technically important statistical numbers are provided in parentheses (sample value, degrees of freedom if applicable, p-value) following a relevant health sciences conclusion.

Minitab's output for the Mood test is similar to the output for ANOVA. In Figure 12.1.6 notice the diagram showing a 95% CI for the median for each of the three levels. Since these CIs so clearly overlap, the sample data detect no difference in the median change in serum triglycerides between the three plants. The CI diagram is especially useful for follow-up analysis when the omnibus null hypothesis is rejected.

EXAMPLE 12.1.10 For illustration, we apply the Mood test to the daytime energy expenditure data from Heini et al (Example 12.1.8). Minitab's output is shown in Figure 12.1.7. Since the p-value is small ($p = .003 < .05$), we reject the omnibus null hypothesis that all the medians are equal and announce our conclusion:

> There is a difference in daytime energy expenditure in pregnant Gambian women according to the trimester of pregnancy ($\chi^2 = 14.10, df = 3, p = .003$).

Because of the small p-value, we reject the omnibus null hypothesis that all the medians are equal. Hence, the Mood test indicates a difference among the level medians. We look at the CI graphic for guidance. The first three CIs clearly overlap, indicating no significant difference between the first three groups. The boundaries between the third and fourth intervals appear blurred (is there really an overlap?). However, because we know there is a difference in level medians, we infer from the graphic that women in their third trimester have a greater daytime energy expenditure than women in the other three groups.

FIGURE **12.1.7**
Minitab session
applying the Mood
test to the Heini et al
data.

```
MTB > NAME C11 'Data', C12 'Level'
MTB > STACK C1-C4 INTO C11;
SUBC> SUBSCRIPTS INTO C12.
MTB > MOOD C11 C12

Mood median test of Data

Chisquare = 14.10   df = 3   p = 0.003

                                     Individual 95.0% CI's
    Level   N<=   N>   Median   Q3-Q1  -+---------+---------+---------+-----
      1      10    3    5.44    0.94   (--------+--)
      2       7    4    5.27    0.79        (+----------)
      3      10    5    5.57    0.96        (-----+------)
      4       2   13    6.44    1.33                   (----+---------)
                                        -+---------+---------+---------+-----
                                        4.90      5.60      6.30      7.00

Overall median = 5.65
```

Comment Some students are tempted by the Mood test because one does not have to check out the normality and homoscedasticity assumptions needed for ANOVA. However, routinely using the Mood test rather than ANOVA is like examining the Andromeda galaxy in the night sky with binoculars when a telescope is available. Although a telescope is more trouble to use than binoculars, the telescope is much more powerful. There is a similar distinction in power between the Mood test (the binoculars) and ANOVA (the telescope). The CI graphics displayed in Figures 12.1.4 and 12.1.7 clearly show the greater power of ANOVA.

EXERCISES 12.1

Warm-ups 12.1

Examples 12.1.8 and 12.1.10 studied data from Heini et al about the daytime energy expenditure of pregnant Gambian women. Figure 12.1.8 displays a Minitab session for data from Heini et al about nighttime energy expenditure.

1. What are the four preliminary considerations for ANOVA?

2. Are nighttime energy expenditures in the four groups consistent with normality?

3. What is the largest sample standard deviation?

4. What is the smallest sample standard deviation?

5. The sample f_{max}-value is computed by
$$\text{sample } f_{max}\text{-value} = \left(\frac{\text{largest standard deviation}}{\text{smallest standard deviation}}\right)^2 = \left(\frac{\boxed{}}{\boxed{}}\right)^2 = \underline{}$$

6. Are the levels homoscedastic?

7. Is ANOVA justified?

8. What is the omnibus hypothesis for the ANOVA test?

9. Based on the boxplot diagram, give an intuitive description of the distribution of nighttime energy expenditure among the four groups of women.

10. What is the p-value for the ANOVA test?

11. Is the omnibus hypothesis retained or rejected?

12. What is the sample f-value for the ANOVA?

13. What are the degrees of freedom for the ANOVA?

14. An appropriate conclusion to be drawn from this ANOVA is:
There is a significant difference in (mean) nighttime energy expenditures between the four groups ($f = \underline{}$, $df = \underline{}$, $p < \underline{}$).

15. Based on the boxplot diagram and the CI graphic, describe the differences in mean nighttime energy expenditure among the four groups.

16. Does the Dunnett diagram confirm the CI and boxplot graphics?

17. In the Dunnett diagram, what does "family error rate = .0500" mean?

FIGURE **12.1.8**
Minitab session for the
Heini et al study of
nighttime energy
expenditures.

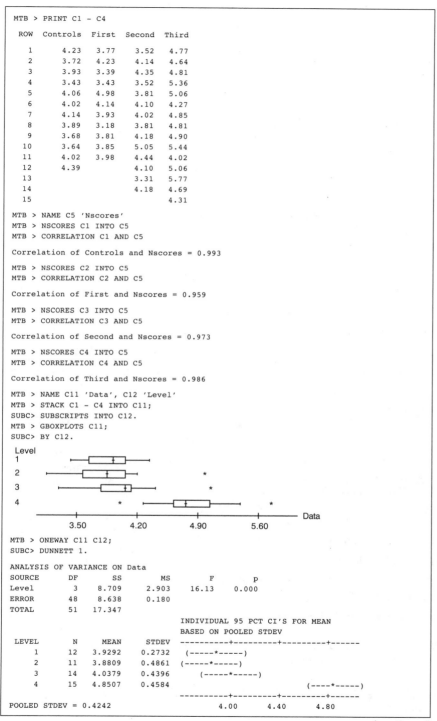

```
MTB > PRINT C1 - C4

ROW   Controls   First   Second   Third

 1      4.23      3.77    3.52     4.77
 2      3.72      4.23    4.14     4.64
 3      3.93      3.39    4.35     4.81
 4      3.43      3.43    3.52     5.36
 5      4.06      4.98    3.81     5.06
 6      4.02      4.14    4.10     4.27
 7      4.14      3.93    4.02     4.85
 8      3.89      3.18    3.81     4.81
 9      3.68      3.81    4.18     4.90
10      3.64      3.85    5.05     5.44
11      4.02      3.98    4.44     4.02
12      4.39              4.10     5.06
13                        3.31     5.77
14                        4.18     4.69
15                        4.31

MTB > NAME C5 'Nscores'
MTB > NSCORES C1 INTO C5
MTB > CORRELATION C1 AND C5

Correlation of Controls and Nscores = 0.993

MTB > NSCORES C2 INTO C5
MTB > CORRELATION C2 AND C5

Correlation of First and Nscores = 0.959

MTB > NSCORES C3 INTO C5
MTB > CORRELATION C3 AND C5

Correlation of Second and Nscores = 0.973

MTB > NSCORES C4 INTO C5
MTB > CORRELATION C4 AND C5

Correlation of Third and Nscores = 0.986

MTB > NAME C11 'Data', C12 'Level'
MTB > STACK C1 - C4 INTO C11;
SUBC> SUBSCRIPTS INTO C12.
MTB > GBOXPLOTS C11;
SUBC> BY C12.
```

```
 Level
 1                  +-----+-----+
                    |  +  |
 2              +----+--+--+----+         *
 3                 +------+-+-----+        *
 4                        *   +--+-+--+        *
        +---------+---------+---------+---------+----- Data
       3.50      4.20      4.90      5.60
```

```
MTB > ONEWAY C11 C12;
SUBC> DUNNETT 1.

ANALYSIS OF VARIANCE ON Data
SOURCE    DF      SS       MS       F       p
Level      3    8.709    2.903    16.13   0.000
ERROR     48    8.638    0.180
TOTAL     51   17.347
                             INDIVIDUAL 95 PCT CI'S FOR MEAN
                             BASED ON POOLED STDEV
 LEVEL     N     MEAN    STDEV  ---------+---------+---------+------
    1     12    3.9292   0.2732   (-----*-----)
    2     11    3.8809   0.4861 (-----*-----)
    3     14    4.0379   0.4396    (-----*-----)
    4     15    4.8507   0.4584                      (----*-----)
                                ---------+---------+---------+------
POOLED STDEV = 0.4242              4.00      4.40      4.80
```

(continued)

FIGURE **12.1.8** *(continued)*

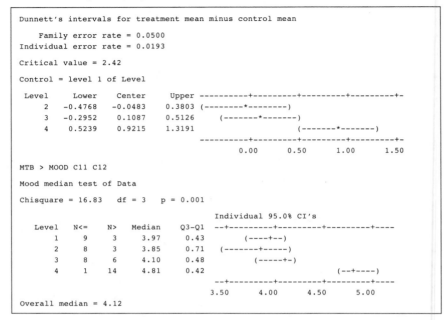

```
Dunnett's intervals for treatment mean minus control mean

     Family error rate = 0.0500
Individual error rate = 0.0193

Critical value = 2.42

Control = level 1 of Level

  Level    Lower    Center    Upper  ---------+---------+---------+---------+-
    2      -0.4768  -0.0483   0.3803  (--------*--------)
    3      -0.2952   0.1087   0.5126    (-------*-------)
    4       0.5239   0.9215   1.3191                  (-------*-------)
                                       ---------+---------+---------+---------+-
                                           0.00      0.50      1.00      1.50

MTB > MOOD C11 C12

Mood median test of Data

Chisquare = 16.83    df = 3    p = 0.001

                                      Individual 95.0% CI's
  Level   N<=   N>   Median   Q3-Q1  --+---------+---------+---------+----
    1      9     3    3.97     0.43        (----+--)
    2      8     3    3.85     0.71     (-------+-----)
    3      8     6    4.10     0.48         (-----+-)
    4      1    14    4.81     0.42                      (--+----)
                                      --+---------+---------+---------+----
                                      3.50      4.00      4.50      5.00

Overall median = 4.12
```

18. A CI for the difference between the mean for level 4 and the control is (____, ____).

19. What is the level of confidence for the CI in Warm-up 18?

20. What is the general form for the CI in Warm-up 18: $(-, -), (-, +), (+, +)$?

21. With ____ % confidence, the mean nighttime energy expenditure for pregnant Gambian women in their third trimester is greater than the mean for nonpregnant Gambian women (controls) by at least ____ and perhaps as much as ____.

22. What is the omnibus hypothesis for the Mood test?

23. What is the p-value for the Mood test?

24. Is the omnibus hypothesis for the Mood test retained or rejected?

25. An appropriate conclusion to be drawn from this Mood test is:
There is a significant difference in (median) nighttime energy expenditures between the four groups $(\chi^2 = \underline{\hphantom{xx}}, df = \underline{\hphantom{xx}}, p = \underline{\hphantom{xx}})$.

26. In this instance, which is preferable, ANOVA or the Mood test?

27. In terms of this example, explain what it means to say that ANOVA is more powerful than the Mood test.

Problems 12.1

1. Explain why one-way ANOVA is not appropriate for determining whether there is a statistically significant difference between the means for the four methods of cardiac output in the Barcelona et al cardiac output study (Appendix, Data Set 2).

2. Explain why the Mood test is not appropriate for comparison of averages for the Daily and Mersch cardiac output study.

3. Is either ANOVA or the Mood test an appropriate method to analyze the data in the Molyneaux coagulation study (Appendix, Data Set 3)?

4. For two populations, ANOVA is equivalent to the two-tailed pooled t-test. To illustrate, consider the Shively position change study (Appendix, Data Set 5).

    a. Conduct a two-tailed pooled t-test to determine whether there is a statistically significant difference in baseline $S\bar{v}O_2$ between the two groups.

b. Apply ANOVA to determine whether there is a statistically significant difference in baseline $S\bar{v}O_2$ between the two groups.

c. Contrast and compare the results from (a) and (b). How does the square of the sample t-value from the two-tailed pooled t-test compare to the sample f-ratio from ANOVA?

Problems 5–10 apply to the Bodai et al study (Appendix, Data Set 4). The Bodai et al study utilized a convenience sample of 16 patients randomized into three groups representing three different and well-defined treatment protocols. Each patient in the study was ventilatory-dependent. Care of such patients necessitates periodic suctioning. Each suctioning protocol was studied both without oxygenation (the control) and with oxygenation. Hence, each group of patients has two sets of measurements (a control set and an oxygenation set). Each set of measurements consists of PaO_2 readings at the start and end of a suctioning procedure, then again at 1 minute and 5 minutes postsuctioning to determine recovery.

5. For the control suctioning period, are the baseline (start) PaO_2 measurements significantly different between the three groups? Output from a Minitab session is displayed in Figure 12.1.9.

6. For the control suctioning period, is the change from suctioning (start − end) significantly different between the three groups?

7. For the control suctioning period, is the total change (start − 5 minutes) significantly different between the three groups?

8. For the oxygenated suctioning period, are the baseline (start) PaO_2 measurements significantly different between the three groups?

*FIGURE **12.1.9***
Minitab session for Problem 12.1.5

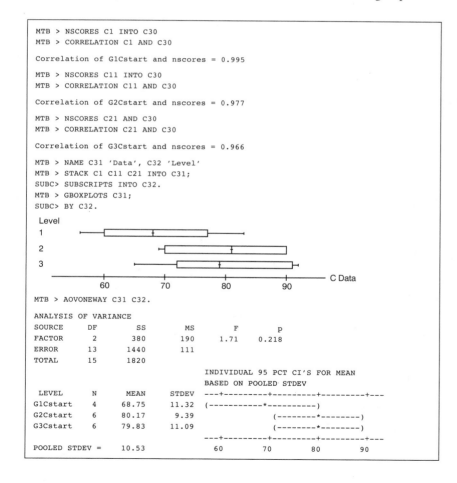

9. For the oxygenated suctioning period, is the change from suctioning (start − end) significantly different between the three groups?

10. For the oxygenated suctioning period, is the total change from suctioning (start − 5 minutes) significantly different between the three groups?

Problems 11–15 are based on research by Rolls et al, who studied aspects of the eating orders anorexia and bulimia. Rolls et al utilized a convenience sample of nine hospitalized patients with anorexia nervosa, nine hospitalized patients with bulimia nervosa, and nine controls (normal people recruited from the Johns Hopkins Hospital community). All subjects in the study were female. A sensitive research method for determining ability to adjust eating to match nutritional need is to provide a person with a fixed amount of food (preload) and then measure the subsequent food intake. The design of the study by Rolls et al measured the total energy intake during lunches that incorporated (1) a high-energy preload, (2) a low-energy preload, and (3) no preload.

11. Explain why a randomized study is inappropriate for the Rolls et al study.

12. Percent ideal body weight was measured for each person in the study (Table 12.1.4). Is there a statistically significant difference in percent ideal body weight between the three groups?

TABLE 12.1.4 Data from Rolls et al for percent ideal body weight.

Anorexics	Bulimics	Controls
65.7	104.4	90.2
71.8	85.7	86.5
66.4	96.0	103.2
50.0	87.8	93.4
73.4	86.4	95.6
67.8	83.9	90.7
80.0	91.9	87.1
78.4	107.0	103.6
64.3	115.0	99.2

13. The data for total energy intake (kJ) during lunch in a high-energy preload setting are shown in Table 12.1.5 (kJ = kilojoules, a metric measure of energy; 1 calorie = 4.1840 joules). Is there a statistically significant difference in the energy intake during a lunch with a high-energy preload for the three groups?

TABLE 12.1.5 Data from Rolls et al. Total energy intake during a lunch using a high-energy preload.

Anorexics	Bulimics	Controls
0.0	1705.8	2366.9
1158.5	1190.8	1037.6
1773.6	2729.2	1923.0
210.4	1204.6	730.1
184.9	5249.2	1420.9
919.2	1801.2	820.5
1369.0	3961.0	1213.8
4452.2	800.0	2733.0
0.0	4738.0	2674.8

14. The data for total energy intake (kJ) during lunch in a low-energy preload setting are shown in Table 12.1.6. Is there a statistically significant difference in the energy intake during a lunch with a low-energy preload for the three groups?

TABLE 12.1.6 Data from Rolls et al. Total energy intake (kJ) during a lunch using a low-energy preload.

Anorexics	Bulimics	Controls
707.5	1019.2	3454.7
2009.2	1822.1	2226.7
2081.5	1783.2	2281.5
1403.3	7129.1	1152.7
242.7	7933.7	2697.4
2392.4	2374.0	1181.6
2781.1	4973.9	3138.0
4502.0	234.7	3720.0
489.1	8094.8	2276.1

15. The data for total energy intake (kJ) during lunch in a no-preload setting are shown in Table 12.1.7. Is there a statistically significant difference in the energy intake during a lunch with no-preload for the three groups? Output from a Minitab session is displayed in Figure 12.1.10.

TABLE 12.1.7 Data from Rolls et al. Total energy intake (kJ) during a lunch with no preload.

Anorexics	Bulimics	Controls
943.5	1356.0	3423.3
1087.8	4254.7	2688.2
2351.8	3881.5	3156.0
1780.7	4263.1	1242.6
268.6	10493.0	3022.5
2778.6	2699.5	1592.0
3178.6	5571.8	3648.0
2809.1	1068.2	4238.4
930.1	9316.5	3484.8

FIGURE **12.1.10**
Minitab session for
Problem 12.1.15.

```
MTB > NSCORES C31 INTO C40
MTB > CORRELATION C31 AND C40

Correlation of Anorexic and Nscores = 0.970

MTB > NSCORES C32 C40
MTB > CORR C32 C40

Correlation of Bulimics and Nscores = 0.952

MTB > NSCORES C33 C40
MTB > CORR C33 C40

Correlation of Controls and Nscores = 0.958

MTB > NAME C41 'Data', C42 'Level'
MTB > STACK C31 - C33 INTO C41;
SUBC> SUBSCRIPTS INTO C42.
MTB > ONEWAY C41 C42;
SUBC> TUKEY.

ANALYSIS OF VARIANCE ON Data
SOURCE      DF        SS          MS         F        p
Level        2  40505220    20252610      4.81    0.018
ERROR       24 101079792     4211658
TOTAL       26 141585008

                                    INDIVIDUAL 95 PCT CI'S FOR MEAN
                                    BASED ON POOLED STDEV
  LEVEL       N      MEAN     STDEV  --------+---------+---------+--------
      1       9      1792      1032  (--------*-------)
      2       9      4767      3260                    (--------*--------)
      3       9      2944       970         (-------*--------)
                                    --------+---------+---------+--------
POOLED STDEV =       2052           1600      3200      4800

Tukey's pairwise comparisons

    Family error rate = 0.0500
Individual error rate = 0.0198

Critical value = 3.53

Intervals for (column level mean) - (row level mean)

               1          2

      2     -5390
             -560

      3     -3567       -592
             1263       4238

MTB > MOOD C21 C22

Mood median test of Data

Chisquare = 7.42   df = 2   p = 0.025

                                    Individual 95.0% CI's
   Level   N<=    N>  Median    Q3-Q1  -------+---------+---------+---------
       1     8     1    1781     1857  (--+---)
       2     3     6    4255     5416       (---------+----------------)
       3     3     6    3156     1426       (-----+)
                                    -------+---------+---------+---------
                                        2500      5000      7500

Overall median = 2809
```

Problems 16–21 are based on research by Heini et al, who studied daily energy expenditure in pregnant Gambian women. A convenience sample consisted of 41 pregnant Gambian women who were placed in three groups according to trimester of pregnancy (first trimester, second trimester, and third trimester). A convenience sample of 13 nonpregnant, nonlactating women served as controls. Measurements included weight (kg), body mass index (kg/m^2), fat-free mass (kg), total 24-hour energy expenditure (kJ/day), and weight-adjusted 24-hour energy expenditure (kJ $\cdot$ kg^{-1} $\cdot$ day^{-1}).

16. Is this a randomized study? Would a randomized study be appropriate?

17. The data for weight are provided in Table 12.1.8. Is there a statistically significant difference in weight between the four groups? If so, explain. Output from a Minitab session is provided in Figure 12.1.11.

TABLE *12.1.8* Data from Heini et al for weight (kg).

Controls	First Trimester	Second Trimester	Third Trimester
55.8	49.7	48.0	55.5
42.6	53.0	58.0	58.0
52.8	49.1	65.5	66.6
42.6	53.2	47.2	64.3
43.6	61.3	52.3	81.1
52.8	56.6	62.6	56.7
48.4	49.3	57.6	62.3
55.8	46.6	47.5	57.1
51.0	64.7	53.9	54.5
45.6	55.0	53.3	60.7
58.0	49.5	52.1	60.1
63.3		53.4	72.1
55.1		44.9	80.0
		71.4	66.0
		49.6	51.9

18. The data for body mass index (kg/m^2) are provided in Table 12.1.9. Is there a statistically significant difference in body mass index between the four groups? If so, explain.

19. The data for fat-free mass (kg) are provided in Table 12.1.10. Is there a statistically significant difference in fat-free mass between the four groups? If so, explain.

20. The data for 24-hour energy expenditure (kJ/day) are provided in Table 12.1.11. Is there a statistically significant difference in 24-hour energy expenditure between the four groups? If so, explain.

TABLE *12.1.9* Data from Heini et al for body mass index (kg/m^2).

Controls	First Trimester	Second Trimester	Third Trimester
23.8	20.7	19.7	20.4
17.5	21.9	22.7	24.1
20.0	19.7	22.1	24.8
18.9	21.0	16.7	24.2
16.4	22.2	19.8	25.3
21.9	20.2	24.6	23.4
18.7	18.0	22.4	23.2
20.0	20.0	20.0	23.6
21.6	23.8	20.3	21.7
19.2	22.7	21.1	23.6
20.5	19.1	20.2	22.6
24.9		21.5	25.2
21.5		19.6	30.7
		29.0	23.7
		20.4	21.2

TABLE *12.1.10* Data from Heini et al for fat-free mass (kg).

Controls	First Trimester	Second Trimester	Third Trimester
39.1	38.8	39.0	45.4
34.1	39.9	44.4	45.1
37.6	39.5	50.4	45.5
34.6	39.7	37.6	47.9
36.4	45.1	39.5	60.2
40.9	42.8	42.4	43.4
40.1	39.3	42.3	47.6
43.8	37.1	38.2	45.3
35.9	46.1	42.6	46.4
36.6	43.4	41.5	48.7
47.0	39.9	40.8	47.5
44.9		41.1	52.9
40.6		35.7	54.2
		49.8	51.6
		38.3	38.9

21. The data for weight-adjusted 24-hour energy expenditure (kJ/day) are provided in Table 12.1.12. Is there a statistically significant difference in weight-adjusted 24-hour energy expenditure between the four groups? If so, explain.

22. Jonsson et al studied the relationship between oxygen perfusion and collagen deposition in standardized, subcutaneous wounds in postoperative patients. The rate of collagen deposition is a major determinant in the adequacy of repair in closed wounds. A convenience sample of patients was

FIGURE *12.1.11*
Minitab session for
Problem 12.1.17.

```
MTB > NSCORES C1 INTO C10
MTB > CORRELATION C1 AND C10

Correlation of Controls and Nscores = 0.987

MTB > NSCORES C2 INTO C10
MTB > CORRELATION C2 AND C10

Correlation of First and Nscores = 0.954

MTB > NSCORES C3 INTO C10
MTB > CORRELATION C3 AND C10

Correlation of Second and Nscores = 0.961

MTB > NSCORES C4 INTO C10
MTB > CORRELATION C4 AND C10

Correlation of Third and Nscores = 0.953

MTB > NAME C11 'Data', C12 'Level'
MTB > GBOXPLOTS C11;
SUBC> BY C12.
```

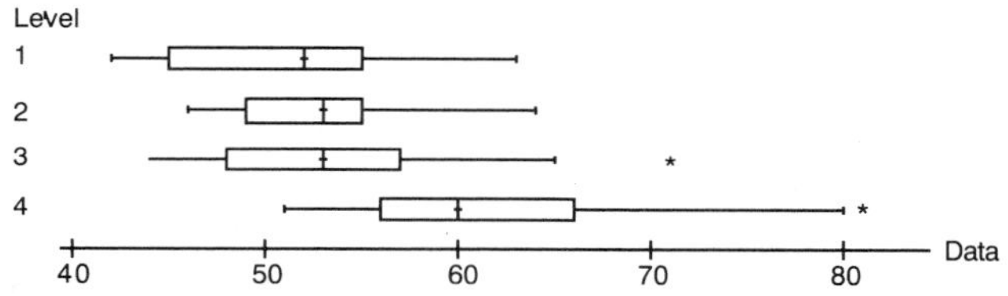

```
Level
  1        +------[   +   ]----------+
  2            +----[  +  ]------+
  3         +------[   +   ]--------+        *
  4                +-------[   +   ]----------+    *
        +-----+---------+---------+---------+---------+----- Data
       40        50        60        70        80
```

```
MTB > ONEWAY C11 C12;
SUBC> DUNNETT 1.

ANALYSIS OF VARIANCE ON Data
SOURCE     DF       SS       MS       F       p
Level       3    1149.6    383.2    7.18    0.000
ERROR      50    2670.1     53.4
TOTAL      53    3819.7

                              INDIVIDUAL 95 PCT CI'S FOR MEAN
                              BASED ON POOLED STDEV
LEVEL      N      MEAN    STDEV   --+---------+---------+---------+----
    1     13    51.338    6.455   (------*-----)
    2     11    53.455    5.599      (------*------)
    3     15    54.487    7.408       (------*-----)
    4     15    63.127    8.816                     (-----*------)
                                  --+---------+---------+---------+----
POOLED STDEV =   7.308           48.0      54.0      60.0      66.0

Dunnett's intervals for treatment mean minus control mean

     Family error rate = 0.0500
 Individual error rate = 0.0192

Critical value = 2.42

Control = level 1 of Level

Level  Lower   Center  Upper  ---------+---------+---------+---------+--
    2  -5.129   2.116   9.361  (------------*----------)
    3  -3.553   3.148   9.849  (----------*----------)
    4   5.087  11.788  18.489                  (-----------*----------)
                              ---------+---------+---------+---------+--
                                    0.0       6.0      12.0      18.0
```

TABLE **12.1.11** Data from Heini et al for 24-hour energy expenditure.

Controls	First Trimester	Second Trimester	Third Trimester
7138	6774	6469	7837
6163	7247	7000	7874
7393	6477	8063	8293
6067	6393	6573	8594
7343	8581	6636	9355
6996	7473	8088	7192
7268	6795	7092	8531
6979	6142	6674	8577
6192	8033	8590	8389
6389	7192	7314	9058
7263	6845	7786	7632
8197		7318	9828
7238		6029	10322
		7791	8279
		6402	6862

TABLE **12.1.12** Data from Heini et al for weight-adjusted 24-hour energy expenditure.

Controls	First Trimester	Second Trimester	Third Trimester
128.0	149.0	134.7	141.4
144.8	136.8	120.5	135.6
140.2	131.8	123.0	124.7
143.3	120.1	139.3	135.5
168.6	140.2	126.8	115.5
132.6	132.2	129.3	126.8
150.2	137.7	123.0	136.8
125.1	131.8	140.6	150.2
121.3	124.3	159.4	154.0
140.2	130.5	137.2	149.4
121.3	138.5	149.4	127.2
129.3		136.8	136.4
131.4		134.3	128.9
		109.2	125.5
		128.9	132.2

TABLE **12.1.14** Baseline serum triglycerides.

Plant A			Plant B			Plant C		
134.28	92.68	107.45	116.33	102.36	38.60	96.87	74.74	160.57
97.00	93.71	76.03	60.65	130.34	38.13	131.88	83.75	54.83
78.83	68.69	87.83	162.12	33.79	143.47	44.87	47.93	232.02
72.04	177.48	485.60	163.22	69.82	83.44	80.76	44.58	93.00
178.60	53.67	106.85	80.16	135.53		59.60	65.99	124.25
105.84	238.97	84.35				44.63	103.84	
144.27	61.99	53.72						
161.83								

divided into three groups according to level of oxygen perfusion—group 1, low perfusion; group 2, medium perfusion; and group 3, high perfusion. The 5-day collagen deposition (measured in μg/cm) was obtained for each patient (data in Table 12.1.13). Higher collagen deposition indicates greater wound healing.

TABLE **12.1.13** Data from Jonsson et al. The data represent 5-day collagen deposition (μg/cm) in postoperative patients.

Group 1	Group 2	Group 3		
0.40	2.47	2.55	2.78	3.00
0.70	2.36	3.16	1.94	3.55
0.46	2.90	3.09	3.23	3.61
2.09	1.04	4.11	6.51	4.53
2.26	2.88	4.74	4.67	3.21
3.17	3.42	6.33	5.11	5.42
	7.37			

a. Does this study use a randomized design? Explain.

b. Is there a statistically significant difference in collagen deposition between the three groups? Explain.

23. A measurement made at the start of a program is called a **baseline** measurement. In the northern California fitness program, we showed that the *changes* in serum triglycerides were not significantly different between the three plants involved in the study (Example 12.1.7). Table 12.1.14 gives the baseline serum triglycerides for this study. Is there a statistically significant difference in the average baseline serum triglyceride levels? Justify your answer by conducting and explaining both an ANOVA and a Mood test. Output from a Minitab session is provided in Figure 12.1.12.

FIGURE **12.1.12**
Minitab session for
Problem 12.1.23.

```
MTB > NAME C20 'Nscores', C21 'Data', C22 'Level'
MTB > NSCORES C11 INTO C20
MTB > CORRELATION C11 AND C20

Correlation of Base A and Nscores = 0.797

MTB > NSCORES C12 INTO C20
MTB > CORRELATION C12 AND C20

Correlation of Base B and Nscores = 0.976

MTB > NSCORES C13 AND C20
MTB > CORRELATION C13 AND C20

Correlation of Base C and Nscores = 0.916

MTB > DESCRIBE C11 - C13

                N       MEAN    MEDIAN    TRMEAN    STDEV    SEMEAN
Base A         22      125.5      95.4     111.1     93.1      19.8
Base B         14       97.0      92.9      96.7     45.7      12.2
Base C         17       90.8      80.8      84.5     49.6      12.0

               MIN        MAX        Q1        Q3
Base A        53.7      485.6      75.0     148.7
Base B        33.8      163.2      55.1     137.5
Base C        44.6      232.0      51.4     114.0

MTB > STACK C11 - C13 INTO C21;
SUBC> SUBSCRIPTS INTO C22.
MTB > GBOXPLOTS C21;
SUBC> BY C22.
```

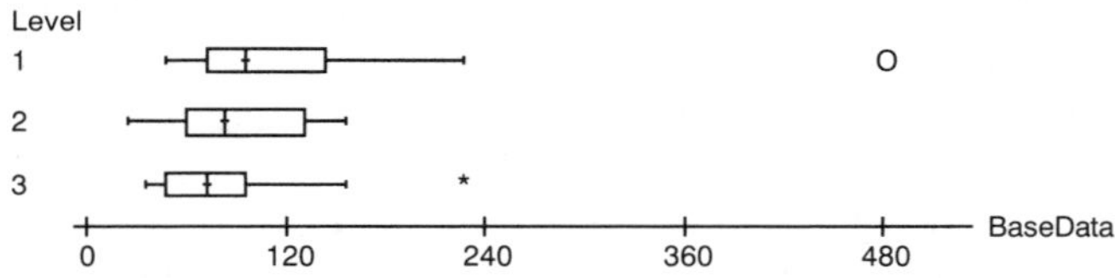

```
 Level
  1          ┌─┬─┐                              O

  2        ├─┤ ├─┤

  3        ├┬┐          *

         ─┼────────┼────────┼────────┼────────┼──── BaseData
          0       120      240      360      480
MTB > AOVONEWAY C11 - C13

ANALYSIS OF VARIANCE
SOURCE     DF        SS        MS       F       p
FACTOR      2     13400      6700    1.35    0.269
ERROR      50    248466      4969
TOTAL      52    261866
                                    INDIVIDUAL 95 PCT CI'S FOR MEAN
                                    BASED ON POOLED STDEV
 LEVEL      N      MEAN     STDEV    --+---------+---------+---------+----
Base A     22    125.53     93.08                    (---------*---------)
Base B     14     97.00     45.73       (-----------*------------)
Base C     17     90.83     49.58     (----------*-----------)
                                    --+---------+---------+---------+----
POOLED STDEV =    70.49              60        90       120       150

MTB > MOOD C21 C22

Mood median test of Data

Chisquare = 0.69   df = 2   p = 0.707

                                    Individual 95.0% CI's
 Level    N<=    N>    Median    Q3-Q1    ---------+---------+---------+-------
    1      10    12      95.4     73.6             (-----+--------------)
    2       7     7      92.9     82.4       (-----------+----------------)
    3      10     7      80.8     62.7     (---------+--------)
                                           ---------+---------+---------+-------
                                                   75       100       125

Overall median = 92.7
```

OBJECTIVE This section will

 Apply ANOVA when presented with an appropriate health sciences problem for the comparison of means and provided with a data legend.

In the health sciences literature, a raw data set is seldom provided. Journal articles that present an application of ANOVA usually present data in the form of a data legend: sample sizes, means, and standard deviations. The Minitab commands AOVONEWAY, MOOD, and ONEWAY can only work on the raw data set. This section presents techniques (Minitab and calculator) that work on a data legend.

Legend ANOVA

There are two main differences between conducting ANOVA with a raw data set and with a data legend. The first concerns the ANOVA preliminaries. One cannot test for normality without the raw data. When provided with only the sample legend, we issue a statement that we are assuming the RV of interest is normally distributed in each level in the study. We still need to check all the other preliminaries to ensure that the study uses a fixed treatments, one-way design, and independent random samples with independent observations. The test for homoscedasticity can also be conducted since the F_{max} test needs only the sample sizes and sample standard deviations.

The second difference concerns conducting the ANOVA test. The Minitab commands BOXPLOT and GBOXPLOT (for constructing a boxplot diagram), AOVONEWAY, ONEWAY, and MOOD must have the raw data set. We will resolve a multilevel problem of comparison of *means* by using the information in the sample legend to obtain the p-value for the ANOVA test. Once we know the p-value, we will be able to make the appropriate decision whether to retain or reject the omnibus null hypothesis of ANOVA that all of the level means are equal. With just the sample legend, it is impossible to conduct the Mood test for comparison of medians.

In order to use Minitab, we must first enter the STOREd program 'ANOVA-LEGEND' as presented in Figure 12.2.1.

Then, when a specific problem is presented:

```
MTB > READ C1–C3
DATA > enter the size, mean, and standard deviation for level 1
DATA > enter the size, mean, and standard deviation for level 2
DATA > continue
DATA > END OF DATA
MTB > EXECUTE 'ANOVALEGEND'
```

In response, Minitab will output the sample f_{max}-value for a preliminary test for homoscedasticity, the ANOVA information (sample f-value, degrees of freedom, and p-value), and a CI table giving the left and right endpoints of 95% CIs for each of the level means.

FIGURE **12.2.1**

Enter the following
two programs in
Minitab for analyzing
an ANOVA problem
with the data legend.

```
MTB > STORE 'ANOVACITABLE'
STOR> LET C22(K10) = C2(K10) - K6*SQRT(C13(2)/C1(K10))
STOR> LET C23(K10) = C2(K10) + K6*SQRT(C13(2)/C1(K10))
STOR> LET K10 = K10 + 1
STOR> END OF PROGRAM

MTB > STORE 'ANOVALEGEND'
STOR> NOECHO
STOR> NAME C1 'Size', C2 'Mean', C3 'SD'
STOR> ERASE C11 - C15, C21 - C23
STOR> NAME C11 'DF', C14 'F-ratio', C15 'p-value'
STOR> LET K1 = N(C1) - 1
STOR> LET K2 = SUM(C1) - N(C1)
STOR> LET C11(1) = K1
STOR> LET C11(2) = K2
STOR> LET C12(1) = SUM(C1*C2**2) - (SUM(C1*C2)**2)/SUM(C1)
STOR> LET C12(2) = SUM((C1-1)*C3**2)
STOR> LET C13(1) = C12(1)/C11(1)
STOR> LET C13(2) = C12(2)/C11(2)
STOR> LET C14(1) = C13(1)/C13(2)
STOR> LET K3 = C14(1)
STOR> CDF K3 K4;
STOR> F K1 K2.
STOR> LET C15(1) = 1 - K4
STOR> NOTE The sample legend is:
STOR> PRINT C1 - C3
STOR> NOTE The sample Fmax value is:
STOR> LET K5 = (MAXI(C3)/MINI(C3))**2
STOR> PRINT K5
STOR> NOTE
STOR> NOTE The ANOVA information is:
STOR> PRINT C11 C14 C15
STOR> NOTE 95% confidence intervals for each level:
STOR> INVCDF .975 K6;
STOR> T K2.
STOR> NAME C21 'Level', C22 'CI Left', C23 'CI Right'
STOR> LET K1 = K1 + 1
STOR> SET C21
STOR> 1:K1
STOR> LET K10 = 1
STOR> EXECUTE 'ANOVACITABLE' K1 TIMES
STOR> PRINT C21 - C23
STOR> NOTE END of ANOVA analysis.
STOR> ECHO
STOR> END OF PROGRAM
```

EXAMPLE 12.2.1 For illustration, we conduct an ANOVA analysis using the sample legend for the northern California corporate fitness program's change in serum triglycerides data (Table 12.1.3). We first enter the sample legend into Minitab as follows:

```
MTB > READ C1 - C3
DATA> 22   23.54   51.21
DATA> 14   16.11   37.99
DATA> 17   34.44   41.29
DATA> END OF DATA
MTB > PRINT C1 - C3
```

Note that the first row of DATA > entry contains the sample legend for plant A, the second row of DATA > entry contains the sample legend for plant B, and the third row of DATA > entry contains the sample legend for plant C. Once the sample legend is entered for each level in a study, PRINTed, and checked for accuracy, then

```
MTB > EXECUTE 'ANOVALEGEND'
```

Minitab's output is displayed in Figure 12.2.2. We obtain basically the same result as produced by applying ANOVA in Minitab to the raw data set (Figure 12.1.3). The differences are that ANOVALEGEND provides the sample f_{max}-value, gives the ANOVA sample f-value (F-ratio) and p-value to more decimal places, and displays a CI table instead of a graphic.

EXAMPLE 12.2.2 Rovner et al presented scores for the Mini-Mental State Examination (MMSE) and Activities of Daily Living (ADL) for three groups of nursing home patients classified by depression. A lower MMSE score is indicative of greater mental competence. A higher ADL score is indicative of greater activity and self-reliance. Rovner et al studied a convenience sample of 454 nursing home patients. After an examination, a patient was classified into one of three different depression levels. Each patient was given the MMSE and ADL tests. The results are summarized in Table 12.2.1.

TABLE **12.2.1**
Data from Rovner et al.

	Depression Disorders (n = 57)	Depression Symptoms (n = 82)	No Depression (n = 315)
MMSE	18.0 ± 8.8	20.0 ± 7.3	14.7 ± 10.0
ADL	14.1 ± 6.7	12.6 ± 7.3	15.0 ± 7.8

FIGURE **12.2.2**
Minitab session for the northern California corporate fitness program's change in serum triglycerides study using the data legend (Example 12.2.1).

```
MTB > EXECUTE 'ANOVALEGEND'
MTB > #
  The sample legend is:

ROW    Size    Mean      SD

  1      22    23.54    51.21
  2      14    16.11    37.99
  3      17    34.44    41.29

  The sample Fmax value is:
K5        1.81707

  The ANOVA information is:

ROW     DF    F-ratio     p-value

  1      2    0.659663    0.521467
  2     50

  95% confidence intervals for each level:

ROW   Level    CI Left   CI Right

  1      1     4.2830    42.7970
  2      2    -8.0300    40.2500
  3      3    12.5333    56.3467

  End of ANOVA analysis.
MTB > END
```

Comment Table 12.2.1 is a common way to display a data legend when several RVs are involved. Here we have the sample legends for three depression levels (depression disorder, depression symptoms, and no depression) and two RVs (MMSE and ADL). The n in each column heading refers to the level sample size. The numerical entry in each cell of the table is the sample's mean ± standard deviation.

We present an analysis of the MMSE data. The inquiry here is to determine whether, in general, MMSE score is indicative of the depression level of the patient. ANOVA specifically will test

H_0: $\mu_1 = \mu_2 = \mu_3$
H_a: the means are otherwise

We first note that the Rovner et al study is based on a fixed treatments, one-way design with respect to MMSE. Further, Rovner et al used independent random samples with independent observations.

Now note that the sample sizes are all large (all sample sizes are greater than 30). In particular, the sample sizes for depression symptoms ($n = 82$) and no depression ($n = 315$) are well beyond the scope of the F_{max} table (Appendix, Table 11) since the largest sample size in the F_{max} table is 61. In this event of large sample sizes, one may forgo considerations of normality and homoscedasticity. As long as one has data based on a fixed treatments, one-way design from random and independent samples, when presented with large sample sizes, simply conduct the ANOVA.

```
MTB > READ C1 - C3
DATA> 57   18   8.8
DATA> 82   20   7.3
DATA> 315  14.7  10
DATA> END OF DATA
MTB > PRINT C1 - C3
```

After checking the PRINT of the entered sample legend for accuracy, then

```
MTB > EXECUTE 'ANOVALEGEND'
```

Minitab's output is displayed in Figure 12.2.3. Based on Minitab's output (Figure 12.2.3), we announce our conclusion:

Mean MMSE scores are significantly different among depression levels in nursing home patients ($f = 11.7, df = (2, 451), p = .00001$).

Comment The ANOVALEGEND program may report the p-value simply as 0. This means p-value $< .0000000005$. One may simply report $p \approx 0$.

Once we know that a significant difference occurs, we want to dig a bit deeper. Which level or levels present a significantly higher mean MMSE score (implying compromised mental competence)? For this, we examine the CI table in Figure 12.2.3. We observe that the CIs for levels 2 and 3 are disjoint (they do not overlap). The intervals for levels 1 and 3 just barely overlap. At this point we can say that the mean MMSE score is significantly lower in nursing home patients with no depression than the mean MMSE score for nursing home patients with depression symptoms.

FIGURE *12.2.3*
Minitab session for the
Rovner et al MMSE
study using the data
legend (Example
12.1.2).

```
MTB > EXECUTE 'ANOVALEGEND'
MTB > #
  The sample legend is:

 ROW    Size    Mean      SD

   1      57    18.0     8.8
   2      82    20.0     7.3
   3     315    14.7    10.0

  The sample Fmax value is:
K5      1.87652

  The ANOVA information is:

 ROW     DF    F-ratio      p-value

   1      2    11.6543    0.0000116
   2     451

 95% confidence intervals for each level:

 ROW   Level    CI Left   CI Right

   1      1     15.5469    20.4531
   2      2     17.9548    22.0452
   3      3     13.6565    15.7435

 End of ANOVA analysis.
MTB > END
```

Although not surprising, the research is indicating that depression leads to decreased mental competence in nursing home patients. As is often the case, the use of statistical analysis serves to launch rather than completely resolve concerns in the health sciences. Here we would be interested in knowing exactly what effects depression has on mental competence. In the Rovner et al study, statistics in this context is acting as a check, verifying one's intuition or professional experience and pointing to an appropriate direction for further study.

The CIs for the mean MMSE score for nursing home patients with no depression and with depression disorder (levels 1 and 3) barely overlap. Hence, at this time we cannot assert that the mean MMSE scores for nursing home patients with no depression and depression disorders are significantly different. Although ANOVA is a powerful technique for indicating when all the level means are not the same, ANOVA does not inform which means are significantly different from each other. To identify which means are different, we have been relying on CIs. Our CI technique is acceptable as a rough guide, but it is not nearly as powerful as ANOVA itself. The means between the depression disorder level and the no-depression level may in fact be significantly different. It could be that our level CIs simply are not powerful enough to be able to pick up the significant difference. Like a previous analogy, ANOVA is a telescope for being able to indicate differences, but our CI technique is only a pair of binoculars for identifying precisely what those differences are.

Comment Section 12.1 presented a variety of powerful techniques for being able to discern which level means are significantly different from each other when ANOVA indicates such differences occur. However, the techniques needed for constructing these intervals by hand are beyond the scope of this text. Minitab has four subcommands (Tukey, Fisher, Dunnett, MCB) to the ONEWAY command that provide these powerful techniques, depending on the design of the study. However, one must have the raw data set to perform this analysis with Minitab.

Comment The sample sizes in the Rovner et al study (Example 12.2.2) are large (57, 82, and 315). Note that the maximum sample size in the F_{max} table (Appendix, Table 11) is only 61. Thus, the table is unsuitable for a test of homoscedasticity when the largest sample size exceeds 61. In that event, merely assume normality and homoscedasticity or rely on the robustness of ANOVA to provide a reliable resolution of the problem at hand. Any deeper analysis would necessitate having the raw data.

Calculator ANOVA

The industrious student may want to conduct an ANOVA on a sample legend by hand with the aid of a calculator. To do so, fill in the blank ANOVA table displayed in Table 12.2.2. The purpose of an ANOVA table is to guide one in computing the F-ratio, which is the sample f-value for the ANOVA test. The ANOVA test is carried out following the directions provided in Chart 6 (Appendix). The sample f-value (F-ratio) is placed on the decision line as shown in step 5 of Chart 6.

TABLE **12.2.2**
A blank ANOVA table.

	DF	SS	MS	F-ratio
FACTOR				
ERROR				

The blank ANOVA table (Table 12.2.2) is filled in using the following list of formulas, where

k = number of levels
N = grand sample size
n_i = sample size for level i
$\bar{x}_i$ = sample mean for level i
s_i = sample standard deviation for level i

$$DF\ FACTOR = k - 1$$
$$DF\ ERROR = N - k$$
$$SS\ FACTOR = \Sigma n_i \bar{x}_i^2 - \frac{\Sigma(n_i\bar{x}_i)^2}{N}$$
$$SS\ ERROR = \Sigma(n_i - 1)s_i^2$$
$$MS\ FACTOR = \frac{SS\ FACTOR}{DF\ FACTOR}$$
$$MS\ ERROR = \frac{SS\ ERROR}{DF\ ERROR}$$
$$F\text{-ratio} = \frac{MS\ FACTOR}{MS\ ERROR}$$

The sums in the expressions for SS FACTOR and SS ERROR are taken over all the levels in the given study.

As an aid in performing this list of computations, we recommend that the student first complete the worksheet shown in Table 12.2.3. The sum of the sample size (n)

column is the grand sample size (N). The sums of the n, $n\bar{x}^2$, and $(n\bar{x})^2$ columns are used in computing SS FACTOR. The sum of the $(n - 1)s^2$ column is SS ERROR.

TABLE **12.2.3**
Blank worksheet for ANOVA table computations.

Level	n	$\bar{x}$	s	$n\bar{x}$	$n\bar{x}^2$	$(n - 1)s^2$
1						
2						
...						
k						
SUM	N			$\Sigma n\bar{x}$	$\Sigma n\bar{x}^2$	$\Sigma(n - 1)s^2$

For illustration, we conduct an ANOVA analysis by hand using the sample legend for the northern California corporate fitness program's change in serum triglycerides data (Table 12.1.3). Table 12.2.4 displays the completed worksheet for the ANOVA computations.

TABLE **12.2.4** Worksheet for ANOVA computations for northern California fitness program's change in serum triglycerides.

Level	n	$\bar{x}$	s	$n\bar{x}$	$n\bar{x}^2$	$(n - 1)s^2$
1	22	23.54	51.21	517.88	12190.9	55071.7
2	14	16.11	37.99	225.54	3633.4	18762.1
3	17	34.44	41.29	585.48	20163.9	27277.8
SUM	53			1328.90	35988.2	101111.6

$$\text{DF FACTOR} = k - 1 = 3 - 1 = 2$$
$$\text{DF ERROR} = N - k = 53 - 3 = 50$$
$$\text{SS FACTOR} = \Sigma n_i \bar{x}_i^2 - \frac{(\Sigma n_i \bar{x}_i)^2}{N} = 35988.2 - \frac{(1328.90)^2}{53} = 2667.91$$
$$\text{SS ERROR} = \Sigma(n_i - 1)s_i^2 = 101111.6$$
$$\text{MS FACTOR} = \frac{\text{SS FACTOR}}{\text{DF FACTOR}} = \frac{2667.91}{2} = 1333.955$$
$$\text{MS ERROR} = \frac{\text{SS ERROR}}{\text{DF ERROR}} = \frac{101111.6}{50} = 2022.232$$
$$\text{F-ratio} = \frac{\text{MS FACTOR}}{\text{MS ERROR}} = \frac{1333.955}{2022.232} = .6596$$

The ANOVA table is the customary way of summarizing and reporting ANOVA computations leading to the F-ratio. Our ANOVA table is shown in Table 12.2.5.

TABLE **12.2.5**
ANOVA table for the northern California fitness program's change in serum triglycerides study.

	DF	SS	MS	F-ratio
FACTOR	2	2667.91	1333.955	.6596
ERROR	50	101112.6	2022.232	

From Table 10b (Appendix), at the 5% LOS the critical f-value with $df = (2, 50)$ is 3.1826. As directed by Chart 6 (Appendix), this leads to the decision line shown in Figure 12.2.4.

FIGURE **12.2.4**
ANOVA decision line.

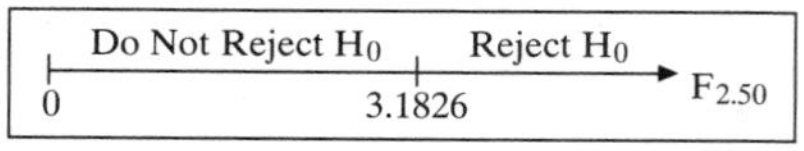

Do Not Reject H₀	Reject H₀	
0	3.1826	$F_{2.50}$

Hence, at the 5% LOS, do not reject the null hypothesis that all the level means are equal. Our final conclusion is the following:

There is no significant difference in the mean change in serum triglycerides between the three plants ($f = .659, df = (2, 50), p > .05$).

EXERCISES 12.2

Warm-ups 12.2

Figure 12.2.5 displays a Minitab session for the ANOVA analysis of the Rovner et al ADL data legend (see Example 12.2.2).

1. What preliminary test cannot be conducted when one is provided only with the data legend?

2. What can one do about normality?

3. What preliminary considerations of ANOVA can one forgo in the event of large sample sizes?

Warm-ups 4–13 apply to the ADL data from Rovner et al (see Example 12.2.2).

FIGURE **12.2.5** Minitab session for analyzing the data legend for the Rovner et al ADL study (Example 12.2.2).

```
MTB > EXECUTE 'ANOVALEGEND'
MTB > #
  The sample legend is:

 ROW   Size   Mean    SD

  1     57    14.1    6.7
  2     82    12.6    7.3
  3    315    15.0    7.8

  The sample Fmax value is:
K5      1.35531

  The ANOVA information is:

 ROW   DF    F-ratio    p-value

  1    2     3.32935    0.0366993
  2   451

  95% confidence intervals for each level:

 ROW  Level  CI Left  CI Right

  1    1     12.1261  16.0739
  2    2     10.9543  14.2457
  3    3     14.1603  15.8397

  End of ANOVA analysis.
MTB > END
```

4. Does the ADL data legend show large sample sizes?

5. What is the sample f-value for the ANOVA?

6. What are the degrees of freedom for the ANOVA?

7. What is the *p*-value for the ANOVA?

8. What set of hypotheses is being tested by the ANOVA?

9. Based on the p-value, at the 5% LOS, do we reject or not reject the omnibus null hypothesis?

10. State an appropriate conclusion in terms of the health science concern, indicating the key statistical numbers in parentheses at the end of the statement.

11. Do the 95% CIs for the level means overlap?

12. How can one reconcile the CI table with the ANOVA decision?

13. Based on the given output, at the 5% LOS, which level means would seem to be distinct?

Problems 12.2

In each of the following ANOVA problems, determine whether the preliminaries for ANOVA are met. If not, explain. If so, conduct the ANOVA. If the omnibus null hypothesis is rejected, explain the difference in level means and describe any insight this gives to the health sciences concern.

Problems 1–3 are based on research by Sackman et al, who studied the long-term results of three types of shock wave treatments for gallstones. A convenience sample of patients was randomly assigned to one of three groups:

A. Use of a model GM 1 lithotroper equipped with a water tank; patient partially submerged
B. Model MPL 9000 water cushion; low-energy shock wave
C. Model MPL 9000 water cushion; high-energy shock wave

Among the data collected on each patient, Sackman et al measured body mass index (BMI, kg/m^2) and the voltage (kV) applied during treatment. The data are summarized in Table 12.2.6.

TABLE **12.2.6** BMI and applied voltage data from Sackman et al.

	Group A (n = 184)	Group B (n = 242)	Group C (n = 285)
BMI	25 ± 4	26 ± 4	27 ± 5
Voltage	17.6 ± 0.9	18.2 ± 1.8	20.2 ± 2.2

1. Is there a significant difference between the three groups in BMI?

2. Is there a significant difference between the three groups in applied voltage?

3. Success of shock wave therapy on gallstones depends on the initial size and number of gallstones. Shock wave therapy "dissolves" a gallstone by breaking it into much smaller pieces. Sackman et al determined the diameter of the largest gallstone fragment resulting from shock wave therapy for each patient. Each patient was then assigned to a group as summarized in Table 12.2.7 (mean ± SD). The first group consisted of patients with a single gallstone whose diameter was ≤ 20 mm. The second group consisted of patients with a single gallstone whose diameter was > 20 mm. The third group consisted of patients with multiple stones. Is the diameter of the largest fragment significantly different between the three groups?

TABLE **12.2.7** Data from Sackman et al.

Single Stone ≤20 (n = 316)	Single Stone >20 (n = 257)	Multiple Stones (n = 138)
2.6 ± 1.8	4.0 ± 3.7	5.8 ± 3.8

Problems 4–7 are based on research by Foote and Erfurt, who studied the benefit-to-cost ratio of work-site blood pressure control programs. Foote and Erfurt conducted a 3-year blood pressure control program at three industrial sites. Each site received a different but well-defined blood pressure control program. A fourth site was selected to act as a control (there was no blood pressure control program at this site). After 3 years of the program, the researchers monitored the cost of subsequent health care claims for cardiovascular disease (CVD) and total health care claims for a period of 4 years. At each site, they selected a random sample of hypertensive employees and a random sample of normotensive employees. The data for hypertensive employees are summarized in Table 12.2.8. The data for normotensive employees are summarized in Table 12.2.9. In both tables the data are given as mean ± standard deviation.

4. Is there a significant difference in mean CVD claims for hypertensive employees between the four sites?

5. Is there a significant difference in mean total claims for hypertensive employees between the four sites?

6. Is there a significant difference in mean CVD claims for normotensive employees between the four sites?

7. Is there a significant difference in mean total claims for normotensive employees between the four sites?

Problems 8–11 are based on research by Stähelin et al, who reported on β-carotene and cancer prevention. In particular, Stähelin et al were interested in the relationship between plasma β-carotene concentration and mortality from cancer. The study period was 12 years. They also reported data for vitamins A and C. The data

TABLE **12.2.8**
Data from Foote and Erfurt on hypertensive employees.

Hypertensive Employees	Site 1 (n = 169)	Site 2 (n = 337)	Site 3 (n = 367)	Site 4 (n = 183)
CVD claims	1114 ± 4275	1174 ± 3584	987 ± 3568	475 ± 1753
Total claims	4326 ± 8722	4046 ± 7069	3407 ± 6581	2183 ± 3451

TABLE **12.2.9**
Data from Foote and Erfurt on normotensive employees.

Normotensive Employees	Site 1 (n = 179)	Site 2 (n = 321)	Site 3 (n = 343)	Site 4 (n = 184)
CVD claims	723 ± 3525	876 ± 3525	760 ± 5134	377 ± 2896
Total claims	2946 ± 6877	3196 ± 6998	2579 ± 6704	1875 ± 3915

provided in Table 12.2.10 are given as mean ± standard deviation.

8. Are the four groups significantly different in plasma concentration of β-carotene?

9. Are the four groups significantly different in plasma concentration of vitamin A?

10. Are the four groups significantly different in plasma concentration of vitamin C?

11. On the basis of these data, does there appear to be a relationship between cancer mortality and plasma level of β-carotene, vitamin A, or vitamin C?

Problems 12–21 are based on research by Caballero et al, who studied plasma amino acid concentrations in healthy elderly people. The study group consisted of 212 adults who were 20 to 90 years of age. The subjects were divided up into two groups: elderly (≥ 55 years, $n = 74$) and young (< 55 years, $n = 138$). Group characteristics measured were age (years), weight (kg), body mass index (BMI, kg/m^2), and obesity index (OI, expressed as weight/ideal body weight). These characteristics are displayed in Table 12.2.11. The measurements are shown as mean ± standard deviation.

12. Is there a significant difference between the four groups in age?

13. Is there a significant difference between the four groups in weight?

14. Is there a significant difference between the four groups in BMI?

15. Is there a significant difference between the four groups in OI?

16. Is there a significant difference between young and elderly males in weight?

17. Is there a significant difference between young and elderly males in BMI?

18. Is there a significant difference between young and elderly males in OI?

19. Is there a significant difference between young and elderly females in weight?

20. Is there a significant difference between young and elderly females in BMI?

21. Is there a significant difference between young and elderly females in OI?

22. Harding et al studied catheter-acquired urinary tract infection in women. The study is important since the urinary tract is the most common site of nosocomial (hospital-acquired) infections, accounting for 42% of such infections. Of these, about 80% develop after urinary catheterization. Further, 10% to 27% of hospitalized patients with an indwelling drainage catheter acquire catheter-associated urinary tract infection. Women have a higher incidence of such infections than men. Harding et al randomized a convenience sample of 119 female patients with catheter-acquired bacteriuria into three groups: group 1—no therapy; group

TABLE 12.2.10
Data from Stähelin et al.

	β-Carotene	Vitamin A	Vitamin C
Survivors (n = 2142)	.436 ± .246	2.81 ± .49	52.76 ± 21.65
Bronchus cancer (n = 68)	.295 ± .206	2.77 ± .58	52.38 ± 30.35
Stomach cancer (n = 20)	.281 ± .183	2.60 ± .36	42.86 ± 21.82
Gastrointestinal cancer (n = 37)	.365 ± .280	2.70 ± .55	45.90 ± 21.72

TABLE 12.2.11
Data from Caballero et al.

	YOUNG GROUP		ELDERLY GROUP	
Variate	Male (n = 68)	Female (n = 72)	Male (n = 32)	Female (n = 42)
Age	26 ± 4	25 ± 5	71 ± 7	72 ± 8
Weight	70.5 ± 10.3	61.4 ± 9.2	72.4 ± 9.3	62.4 ± 8.6
BMI	24.5 ± 2.5	26.1 ± 3.1	26.2 ± 2.1	28.1 ± 3.0
OI	1.06 ± .12	1.05 ± .14	1.12 ± .10	1.16 ± .14

2—single dose of therapy with trimethoprim-sulfamethoxazole; and group 3—10 days of drug therapy. Data for days of catheter use are shown in Table 12.2.12. Is there a significant difference in the mean length of catheterization between the three groups?

TABLE *12.2.12* Data from Harding et al.

Group	Size	Mean	SD
1	42	6.8	7.1
2	37	5.4	4.7
3	33	8.2	13.2

Problems 23–32 are based on research by Klatsky and Armstrong, who studied cardiovascular risk factors in Asian Americans. Subjects were classified into one of four ethnic groups: Chinese, Filipino, Japanese, and other. Variates measured included body mass index (kg/m^2), systolic blood pressure (mm Hg), diastolic blood pressure (mm Hg), total cholesterol (mmol/liter), and glucose (mmol/liter). Klatsky and Armstrong reported their data as mean $\pm$ SE (SE = $SD/\sqrt{n}$). The data for females are given in Table 12.2.13; for males, in Table 12.2.14. (ANOVA is justified due to the large sample sizes and robustness.)

23. Is there a significant difference between the four groups of female Asian Americans in BMI?

24. Is there a significant difference between the four groups of female Asian Americans in systolic blood pressure?

25. Is there a significant difference between the four groups of female Asian Americans in diastolic blood pressure?

26. Is there a significant difference between the four groups of female Asian Americans in cholesterol?

27. Is there a significant difference between the four groups of female Asian Americans in glucose?

28. Is there a significant difference between the four groups of male Asian Americans in BMI?

29. Is there a significant difference between the four groups of male Asian Americans in systolic blood pressure?

30. Is there a significant difference between the four groups of male Asian Americans in diastolic blood pressure?

31. Is there a significant difference between the four groups of male Asian Americans in cholesterol?

32. Is there a significant difference between the four groups of male Asian Americans in glucose?

33. Bajwa et al researched cholesterol levels in patients with panic disorder. They reported cholesterol level (mg/dL) as mean $\pm$ standard deviation in three groups. Cholesterol level in 30 patients with panic disorder was 224.7 $\pm$ 43.5; in 30 patients with major depression (but no panic disorder) was 189.8 $\pm$ 32.8; in 30 normal control subjects, 183.6 $\pm$ 37.7. Is there a significant difference in cholesterol level between the three given groups?

TABLE *12.2.13* Data from Klatsky and Armstrong on female Asian Americans.

Variate	Chinese (n = 3197)	Filipino (n = 2482)	Japanese (n = 1015)	Other (n = 623)
Body mass index	21.2 ± 0.1	22.6 ± 0.1	21.6 ± 0.1	22.2 ± 0.1
Systolic BP	116.3 ± 0.3	119.2 ± 0.3	115.7 ± 0.5	115.9 ± 0.6
Diastolic BP	71.7 ± 0.2	72.9 ± 0.2	70.3 ± 0.3	70.8 ± 0.4
Cholesterol	5.33 ± 0.02	5.35 ± 0.02	5.52 ± 0.03	5.26 ± 0.04
Glucose	5.22 ± 0.02	5.24 ± 0.02	5.26 ± 0.04	5.28 ± 0.05

TABLE *12.2.14* Data from Klatsky and Armstrong on male Asian Americans.

Variate	Chinese (n = 2754)	Filipino (n = 1729)	Japanese (n = 688)	Other (n = 543)
Body mass index	22.9 ± 0.1	23.9 ± 0.1	23.7 ± 0.1	23.6 ± 0.1
Systolic BP	122.2 ± 0.3	124.4 ± 0.4	121.3 ± 0.6	120.3 ± 0.7
Diastolic BP	75.5 ± 0.2	75.5 ± 0.2	73.9 ± 0.4	74.0 ± 0.4
Cholesterol	5.59 ± 0.02	5.67 ± 0.03	5.72 ± 0.04	5.52 ± 0.05
Glucose	5.45 ± 0.03	5.54 ± 0.03	5.54 ± 0.05	5.54 ± 0.06

OBJECTIVES   This section will

1   Apply one-way repeated measures ANOVA when presented with an appropriate health sciences problem for the comparison of means of several levels.

2   Apply two-way ANOVA when presented with an appropriate health sciences problem.

Graduate programs in the health sciences often contain a required specialized course dealing specifically with ANOVA, frequently in tandem with regression (Chapter 14). ANOVA is required when one wants to compare several groups or interventions with respect to several treatment variables. Accordingly, ANOVA can be an enormously complex subject. This section contains a very brief orientation to two advanced ANOVA techniques: one-way repeated measures ANOVA and two-way ANOVA.

One-Way Repeated Measures ANOVA

In Section 12.1 we noted that the Daily and Mersch cardiac output study satisfies all the assumptions of one-way ANOVA except for the requirement of independent samples. In the Daily and Mersch study, the population of interest is all cardiac patients needing cardiac output monitoring. The study recruited a convenience sample of 29 patients. Cardiac output was measured in three distinct ways: RTCO, ITCO, and Fick. RTCO and ITCO used a standard bedside thermodilution technique using either a room- or an ice-temperature injectate, respectively. The purpose of the study was to compare these simpler bedside techniques against the laboratory-intensive Fick method, the assumed gold standard for obtaining cardiac outputs. In particular, we inquire whether

$$H_0: \mu_{RTCO} = \mu_{ITCO} = \mu_{Fick}$$

Because each cardiac output method was applied to each patient, the one-way ANOVA requirement of random samples is not met. To meet the random samples requirement, we would need one sample of patients for the RTCO method, a second sample for the ITCO method, and yet a third sample for the Fick method.

Figure 12.3.1 displays Minitab's output for an inappropriate one-way ANOVA. Here the RTCO data are in column C1, the ITCO data in column C2, and the Fick data in column C3. The data are stacked into column C11 (named CO for cardiac output) with level identifiers in column C12 (named method). The ANOVA output in Figure 12.3.1 leads us to retain the null hypothesis that there is no significant difference in mean cardiac output taken by the three methods. But either a paired-data CI (Problem 7.2.4) or a paired-data t-test (Problem 10.3.1) shows a statistically significant difference in the mean cardiac output taken by RTCO versus Fick, or by ITCO versus Fick. As is usually the case, the wrong method applied to a statistical problem yields an incorrect result.

With a one-way comparison of means problem where the same sample of subjects is used for each level, the correct statistical methodology is one-way repeated measures ANOVA. Repeated measures ANOVA is more powerful than regular ANOVA when it is appropriate to apply the technique. In particular, the repeated measures feature eliminates the between-subjects variation that would occur from using different subjects for each level. Figure 12.3.2 displays a Minitab session for the one-way repeated measures analysis of the Daily and Mersch cardiac output study.

There are two features we need to clarify in the ANOVA output displayed in Figure 12.3.2: (1) the stacked form of the data and (2) the use of the ANOVA command.

For one-way repeated measures ANOVA, each item of data (cardiac output in column C11, named CO) must contain two identifiers. We must not only identify the method used to obtain the cardiac output (column C12, named method) but also must identify the patient on whom the measurement was taken. Hence, we set up column C13 (named patient). Column C13 contains three sets of the patient numbers from 1 to 29. Consequently, column C11 contains all 57 items of data. Column C12 contains either 1, 2, or 3, depending on whether the RTCO, ITCO, or Fick method was used. Column C13 contains the patient identifier.

The one-way repeated measures calculations are carried out by issuing the ANOVA command. Note the general form of the ANOVA command, a form unique in Minitab thus far to this command:

```
MTB > ANOVA CO = Method Patient;
SUBC> RANDOM Patient.
```

This command instructs Minitab to conduct an ANOVA where cardiac output (CO) is the RV of interest. Each data point is identified with two labels: method and patient. Further, the patients are randomly selected. Any data identifier that is a random effect rather than a fixed treatment is specified in the RANDOM subcommand. A data identifier not specified in the RANDOM subcommand (here method)

FIGURE *12.3.1*
Minitab session for inappropriate one-way ANOVA for the Daily and Mersch cardiac output study.

```
MTB > STACK C1 - C3 INTO C11;
SUBC> SUBSCRIPTS INTO C12.
MTB > ONEWAY C11 C12

ANALYSIS OF VARIANCE ON CO
SOURCE      DF       SS       MS       F       p
Method       2     2.18     1.09    0.86    0.426
ERROR       84   106.14     1.26
TOTAL       86   108.32
                                    INDIVIDUAL 95 PCT CI'S FOR MEAN
                                    BASED ON POOLED STDEV
LEVEL        N     MEAN    STDEV  ----+---------+---------+---------+--
    1       29    4.496    1.139  (----------*-----------)
    2       29    4.508    1.043  (-----------*-----------)
    3       29    4.838    1.186            (-----------*-----------)
                                    ----+---------+---------+---------+--
POOLED STDEV =     1.124            4.20     4.55     4.90     5.25
```

FIGURE **12.3.2**
Minitab session for
one-way repeated
measures ANOVA for
the Daily and Mersch
cardiac output study.

```
MTB > NAME C13 'Patient'
MTB > SET C13
DATA> 3(1:29)
DATA> END OF DATA
MTB > ANOVA CO = Method Patient;
SUBC> RANDOM Patient.

Factor      Type Levels Values
Method      fixed      3    1      2      3
Patient     random    29    1      2      3      4      5      6      7      8      9
                            10     11     12     13     14     15     16     17     18
                            19     20     21     22     23     24     25     26     27
                            28     29

Analysis of Variance for CO

Source      DF        SS        MS        F       P
Method       2    2.1807    1.0904     5.20   0.008
Patient     28   94.4091    3.3718    16.09   0.000
Error       56   11.7329    0.2095
Total       86  108.3227

MTB > NAME C21 = 'R - I', C22 'R - F', C23 'I - F'
MTB > LET C21 = C1 - C2
MTB > LET C22 = C1 - C3
MTB > LET C23 = C2 - C3
MTB > TINTERVAL 95 C21 - C23

            N     MEAN    STDEV  SE MEAN    95.0 PERCENT C.I.
R - I      29  -0.0121   0.4298   0.0798  ( -0.1756,  0.1514)
R - F      29   -0.342    0.654    0.121  (  -0.591,  -0.093)
I - F      29   -0.330    0.803    0.149  (  -0.635,  -0.024)
```

is assumed to be fixed. The Daily and Mersch CO data come from a study using a fixed treatments design (the CO methods RTCO, ITCO, and Fick are fixed treatments). Note especially that the column names CO, method, and patient are not put in single quotes when using the ANOVA command.

Comment An ordinary one-way ANOVA could be conducted by

```
MTB > ANOVA CO = METHOD
```

The output for this command is exactly the same as the ONEWAY command displayed in Figure 12.3.1.

Now let's interpret Minitab's output to the ANOVA command displayed in Figure 12.3.2. First, Minitab tells us that method represents a fixed treatment with 3 levels (labeled 1, 2, and 3). Then, patient represents a random effect with 29 levels (labeled from 1 to 29). Finally, we read the crucial sample f-value for method. Look in the "Analysis of Variance for CO" table, F column. The f-value corresponding to method, here 5.20, is our sample f-value. In order to use the sample f-value to come to some conclusion, we need a decision line.

The decision line for a one-way repeated measures ANOVA is an F-test decision line. In order to obtain a critical value for the F-test, we need both the column and row degrees of freedom. Our decision line will use two critical f-values, one liberal and one conservative. The use of two critical f-values will result in a decision line with three decision regions: do not reject H_0, an ambiguous zone, and reject H_0.

Comment For the technically minded, the liberal df is valid if a condition known as "sphericity" holds. If this condition does not hold, then the df for the F-test must be appropriately reduced. The reduction in df, however, never goes below the conservative df. If sphericity does not hold, then the accepted procedure is to multiply the liberal df by an adjustment factor, ϵ (epsilon). Depending on the circumstances, this adjustment factor is the Huynh and Feldt epsilon or the Greenhouse-Geisser epsilon. We refer the interested reader to Girden or Shott.

The smaller (liberal) critical value is the f-value with $(k - 1, (k - 1) \times (n - 1))$ degrees of freedom (df), where k is the number of fixed treatments and n is the number of patients in the study. In the Daily and Mersch CO study, $k = 3$ and $n = 29$. Hence, liberal $df = (2, 56)$. The larger (conservative) critical value is the f-value with $df = (1, n - 1)$; hence, conservative $df = (1, 28)$. These critical values are obtained in Minitab as follows:

```
MTB > INVCDF .95;
SUBC> F 2 56.
    0.9500    3.1619
MTB > INVCDF .95;
SUBC> F 1 28.    0.9500    4.1960
```

Hence, the critical values for the F-test are 3.1619 and 4.1960. The decision line to resolve H_0: $\mu_{RTCO} = \mu_{ITCO} = \mu_{Fick}$ for our one-way repeated measures ANOVA is displayed in Figure 12.3.3. The shaded region in Figure 12.3.3 is the ambiguous zone. If the sample f-value falls in this region, one needs further analysis (see Girden or Shott for further details).

Since the sample f-value 5.20 is larger than the liberal critical f-value, the sample f-value 5.20 falls in the reject H_0 zone; hence, we reject the omnibus null hypothesis that all the means are equal. To reinforce what was previously done for CIs and paired t-tests, Figure 12.3.2 displays a 95% CI for all three possible level differences. These CIs show that the means for RTCO and ITCO are statistically significantly smaller than the Fick mean.

One-way repeated measures ANOVA shows that mean cardiac outputs determined by the RTCO, ITCO, and Fick methods are significantly different. This difference would not be detected if one erroneously applied regular one-way ANOVA.

For convenience, Figure 12.3.4 presents a general summary for one-way repeated measures analysis of variance.

In the health sciences, one usually works with a convenience sample. As long as the spirit of randomness is maintained, such a sample is acceptable. Each treatment must be applied to each member in the sample in a manner that will obtain an independent measurement (within a given treatment, the result from one measurement should not influence or bias the result for the next measurement). When possible, the treatment should be randomized to avoid confounding from learning or carryover effects. There is no test for a multivariate normal distribution. However, if

FIGURE 12.3.3
Decision line for the Daily and Mersch study.

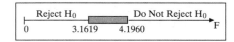

FIGURE 12.3.4
One-way repeated measures ANOVA.

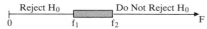

Assumptions. The basic assumptions for repeated measures ANOVA are:

1. random sample of subjects
2. fixed treatments applied to each subject in the sample (repeated measures)
3. independent observations within each fixed treatment
3. multivariate normal distribution

Decision Line. The decision in repeated measures ANOVA is based on an F-test using the following decision line.

f_1 = liberal critical f-value with $(k - 1, (k - 1) \times (n - 1))$ degrees of freedom
f_2 = conservative critical f-value with $(1, n - 1)$ degrees of freedom

The shaded region represents the ambiguous zone.

this assumption is met, then each level is normally distributed (however, the converse need not hold). Hence, the multivariate normality assumption can be partially checked by checking for normality for each of the fixed treatment samples. We will not test for homoscedasticity since it is involved with the multivariate assumption.

Comment Research using a repeated measures design should engage the services of a statistician from the inception of the study.

The statistical theory behind one-way ANOVA is rooted in mathematical models and a mathematical analysis of the various ways of looking at the variance. The main item of interest here is *variation*. Variation can be examined from several points of view:

- Within-subjects variation
- Within-treatments variation
- Total variation

One can look at each subject individually and then look at the variation within that subject produced by the different treatments. One can look at each treatment individually and look at the variation produced by the different subjects. Or one can forget about the treatments altogether and look at the variation, considering the entire data set as one big sample. Because the RV of interest can be studied from the viewpoints of two different factors (subjects and treatments), the actual theory of repeated measures ANOVA is founded on the theory for two-way ANOVA. Two-way ANOVA considers a population classified from two points of view (hence, the *two*-way).

Two-Way ANOVA

Two-way ANOVA is basically one-way ANOVA extended to two factors. In regular two-way ANOVA, one must have a random and independent sample for each level for each factor.

EXAMPLE 12.3.1 Fernicola and Roberts gave the data shown in Table 12.3.1 for the heart weight (grams) of a convenience sample of patients with previously normal mitral valves prior to infective endocarditis. The patients were classified by race (white, black) and gender (male, female).

TABLE **12.3.1**
Data from Fernicola and Roberts.

	White			Black		
Male	280	420	340	335	715	440
	370	390	440	620	520	600
	510	300	480	540	345	380
				270	485	500
				485	620	360
Female	205	280	195	210	390	360
	380	200		320	350	

In a two-way study, the raw data can be presented in a two-way data table. One factor defines the rows and the other factor defines the columns. In Table 12.3.1, since there are two row factors and two column factors, the table has four data cells. In general, if there are r rows and c columns, then there are $r \times c$ cells in the two-way table.

The basic assumptions for two-way ANOVA are

- Random and independent samples for each cell
- Independent observations within each cell
- Normal distributions within each cell
- Equal variances for the distribution for each cell

Two-way ANOVA allows us to test the following two hypotheses:

- The means between levels for the first factor are all equal
- The means between levels for the second factor are all equal

In addition, if there is more than one measurement for each cell, we can also test whether the two factors interact. In Example 12.3.1, there might be no difference in heart weight between black and white men but there might be between black and white women. If there is no interaction, we can make a general conclusion about the level factors (like heart weight for men is greater than for women). If there is interaction, conclusions will have to be made on a level-by-level basis.

For the Fernicola and Roberts study presented in Example 12.3.1, we thus have the following hypotheses to check:

Race hypothesis: Heart weight does not differ between races. Formally,

H_0: $\mu_{white} = \mu_{black}$

Gender hypothesis: Heart weight does not differ between genders. Formally,

H_0: $\mu_{male} = \mu_{female}$

Interaction hypothesis: Heart weight affects genders the same way among races.

H_0: there is no interaction between the race and gender

Since the calculations for two-way ANOVA are extensive, we proceed immediately to Minitab for the computational summary needed to test these hypotheses. To conduct two-way ANOVA in Minitab, the data must be presented in a two-way stacked format. First, the entire data set must be presented in a single column. The data column must be accompanied by two other columns acting as level identifiers for the two factors. Minitab then has a variety of commands that need to be considered.

There are two commands that can be used for *balanced* data sets. A balanced data set has the same number of entries in each cell of the two-way data table. Early versions of Minitab conducted balanced two-way analysis of variance with the TWO-WAY command. Later versions added the ANOVA command to allow statisticians to conduct an analysis based on mathematical models. For an unbalanced data set (unequal number of entries per cell), the GLM command must be used (GLM stands for general linear model). The format for the GLM command is the same as for ANOVA. The GLM command allows professional statisticians to obtain a great deal of technical and sophisticated information. We offer only a general orientation to these commands.

Figure 12.3.5 presents the Minitab analysis for the Fernicola and Roberts data (Example 12.3.1). We code the race factor with (1 = white, 2 = black) and the gender factor with (1 = male and 2 = female). Of course, these code numbers are completely arbitrary (any whole numbers could have been used). We recommend first entering the data in a cell-by-cell (unstacked) format, then stacking the data using the STACK command. For illustration, we present the data entry in Figure 12.3.5.

To interpret the output, we first need to determine whether there is any significant interaction between the factors of gender and race. In the "Analysis of Variance for HW" for the full GLM command, the p-value for gender * race is .851. This leads us to retain the interaction null hypothesis that there is no interaction between the two factors. The lack of interaction is portrayed clearly in Figure 12.3.6. Note that the *differences* in mean heart weight between males and females are the same for both races. It appears from the graph that blacks have a greater mean heart rate than whites, regardless of gender. In an interaction graph, no interaction is indicated when the line connecting the levels from one factor (here blacks) is parallel to the line connecting the levels from another factor (here whites). Interaction is usually indicated when these lines crisscross (i.e., interact).

We now apply appropriate factor tests of hypotheses to determine whether

- ■ Heart weight between races is significantly different
- ■ Heart weight between genders is significantly different

Before making this determination, we formally assume that race and gender do not interact ($p = .851$). In concordance with this assumption we rerun the GLM command without the interaction term:

```
MTB > GLM HW = Gender Race
```

After inspecting the "Analysis of Variance for HW" table output to the GLM command, we announce

FIGURE **12.3.5**
Minitab analysis of
the Fernicola and
Roberts data (Table
12.3.1).

```
MTB > NAME C1 'WM', C2 'WF', C3 'BM', C4 'BF'
MTB > SET C1
DATA> 280 420 340 370 390 440 510 300 480
MTB > SET C2
DATA> 205 280 195 380 200
MTB > SET C3
DATA> 335 715 440 620 520 600 540 345 380 270 485 500 485 620 360
MTB > SET C4
DATA> 210 390 360 320 350
DATA> END OF DATA
MTB > NAME C5 'HW', C6 'Cell'
MTB > STACK C1 - C4 INTO C5;
SUBC> SUBS INTO C6.

MTB > GBOXPLOTS C5;
SUBC> BY C6.
```

```
MTB > NAME C7 'Gender', C8 'Race'
MTB > SET C7        #enter Gender levels
DATA> 9(1) 5(2) 15(1) 5(2)
MTB > SET C8        #enter Race levels
DATA> 14(1) 20(2)
DATA> END OF DATA

MTB > GLM HW = Gender Race Gender*Race;
SUBC> MEANS Gender Race.

Factor    Levels Values
Gender       2     1     2
Race         2     1     2

Analysis of Variance for HW

Source       DF    Seq SS    Adj SS    Adj MS       F      P
Gender        1    177800    150847    150847   14.26  0.001
Race          1     57645     45860     45860    4.33  0.046
Gender*Race   1       378       378       378    0.04  0.851
Error        30    317416    317416     10581
Total        33    553239

Unusual Observations for HW

Obs.      HW        Fit  Stdev.Fit  Residual  St.Resid
 16   715.000  481.000     26.559   234.000      2.35R
 24   270.000  481.000     26.559  -211.000     -2.12R

R denotes an obs. with a large st. resid.

Means for HW

Gender      Mean     Stdev
    1      436.6     21.69
    2      289.0     32.53
Race
    1      322.1     28.69
    2      403.5     26.56

MTB > GLM HW = Gender Race
```

FIGURE **12.3.5** *(continued)*

```
Factor    Levels Values
Gender        2   1     2
Race          2   1     2

Analysis of Variance for HW

Source      DF      Seq SS      Adj SS      Adj MS       F       P
Gender       1      177800      152916      152916   14.92   0.001
Race         1       57645       57645       57645    5.62   0.024
Error       31      317794      317794       10251
Total       33      553239

Unusual Observations for HW

Obs.       HW       Fit Stdev.Fit  Residual   St.Resid
  16   715.000  479.295    24.588   235.705      2.40R
  24   270.000  479.295    24.588  -209.295     -2.13R

R denotes an obs. with a large st. resid.
```

FIGURE **12.3.6**
Interaction
graph for
gender and
race.

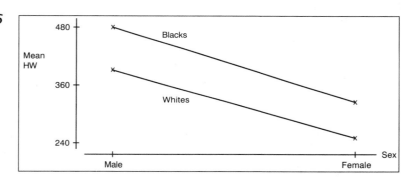

The mean heart weight for patients with previously normal mitral valves prior to active infective endocarditis differs significantly between males and females ($f = 14.92$, $df = (1, 31)$, $p = .001$).

The mean heart weight for patients with previously normal mitral valves prior to active infective endocarditis differs significantly between blacks and whites ($f = 5, 62$, $df = (1, 31)$, $p = .024$).

Hence, based on our two-way ANOVA analysis, we conclude that heart weight for patients with previously normal mitral valves prior to active infective endocarditis is related noninteractively to the race and gender of the patient.

Two-way ANOVA was developed by Sir Ronald Fisher in England to study the productivity of agricultural lands. A common design was to consider two soil types, say lowland valley and upper hillside. Suppose we wanted to test four fixed fertilizer treatments for growing crops. A plot of valley land is divided into four equal "blocks" and a fertilizer treatment is applied to each block. Similarly, a plot of hillside land is divided up into four equal "blocks" and a fertilizer treatment is applied to each block. The crop yield for each block is measured. Two-way ANOVA was designed to statistically compare yield for land type versus fertilizer treatment.

One-way repeated measures ANOVA can be considered as a special case of two-way ANOVA, where each patient in the study is considered a "block." The use of the same patients for each treatment, however, necessitates an adjustment in the straightforward two-way ANOVA decision procedure. The decision line in regular two-way ANOVA uses just the liberal critical f-value; hence, the decision line has only a do not reject H_0 and a reject H_0 region. Our adjustment for one-way repeated measures is simple. We use an adjusted decision line containing an ambiguous zone bounded by the conservative and liberal critical f-values. This adjusted decision line will serve our purposes well. In the rare case when the fixed treatments sample f-value from repeated measures ANOVA falls in the ambiguous zone, a complex refinement involving an adjustment epsilon will be needed, as mentioned in an earlier comment.

EXERCISES 12.3

Warm-ups 12.3

1. Repeated measures analysis is indicated when
   a. The same measurement is made repeatedly on a given subject.
   b. The study needs to be repeated several times.
   c. The statistical analysis needs to be repeated.
   d. The same sample of subjects is used for several treatments.
   e. The same number occurs repeatedly in a data set.

Warm-ups 2–14 are based on the Bodai et al suction study (Appendix, Data Set 4). We conduct a one-way repeated measures analysis on the data for group 2, oxygen insufflation alone. The data are reproduced in Table 12.3.2 for convenience. The numbers represent Pao_2 on each of four patients at the times start, end, 1 minute, and 5 minutes. A Minitab session is displayed in Figure 12.3.7.

TABLE **12.3.2** Pao_2 data from Bodai et al.

Patient	Start	End	1 Minute	5 Minutes
1	83	80	120	84
2	71	63	71	70
3	88	77	98	90
4	80	41	54	56
5	93	63	73	82
6	86	118	88	90

2. The factor time has four levels. What are they?

3. Is time a random effects factor or a fixed treatments factor?

4. The factor patient has six levels. What are they?

5. Is patient a random effects factor or a fixed treatments factor?

6. To construct the decision line to determine whether or not there is a significant difference in mean Pao_2 between the four given times, we need two critical f-values, a liberal critical f-value and a conservative critical f-value. The degrees of freedom for these critical f-values depend on k (number of levels in the fixed treatment factor) and n (number of subjects in the sample). For the Bodai et al data (Table 12.3.2), what are k and n?

7. The liberal df is $(k - 1, (k - 1) \times (n - 1))$. Here, liberal df = (____, ____).

8. The conservative df is simply $(1, n - 1)$. Here, conservative df = (____, ____).

9. At the 5% LOS, what is the liberal critical value?

10. At the 5% LOS, what is the conservative critical value?

11. What is the sample f-value to test the null hypothesis that there is no significant difference in mean Pao_2 between the four given times?

12. Should the time factor omnibus null hypothesis H_0: $\mu_{start} = \mu_{end} = \mu_{min1} = \mu_{min5}$ be rejected or not?

One-way repeated measures may be considered as a two-way ANOVA where the repeated levels, patients, are considered "blocks." Note that the common numbers in the analysis of variance tables from the ANOVA and the TWOWAY commands are the same. The decision line for

FIGURE **12.3.7**
Minitab session for
one-way repeated
measures for the
Bodai et al data.

```
MTB > NOTE   Enter raw data in a Time level by level format:
MTB > NAME C1 'Start', C2 'End', C3 'min1', C4 'min5'
MTB > READ C1 - C4
DATA> 83 80 120 84
DATA> 71 63 71 70
DATA> 88 77 98 90
DATA> 80 41 54 56
DATA> 93 63 73 82
DATA> 86 118 88 90
DATA> END
     6 ROWS READ

MTB > NOTE   Stack the data into a two-way format:
MTB > STACK C1 - C4 INTO C11;
SUBC> SUBSCRIPTS INTO C12.
MTB > SET C13
DATA> 4(1:6)
DATA> END OF DATA

MTB > NOTE   One-way repeated measures analysis of variance:
MTB > ANOVA PaO2 = Patient Time;
SUBC> RANDOM Patient.

Factor      Type Levels Values
Patient   random    6    1    2    3    4    5    6
Time      fixed     4    1    2    3    4

Analysis of Variance for PaO2

Source      DF       SS       MS      F      P
Patient      5   4292.2    858.4   4.46  0.011
Time         3    420.8    140.3   0.73  0.551
Error       15   2888.0    192.5
Total       23   7601.0

MTB > NOTE   Critical f-values:
MTB > INVCDF .95;
SUBC> F 3 15.
     0.9500 3.2874
MTB > INVCDF .95;
SUBC> F 1 5.
     0.9500   6.6079

MTB > NOTE   Two-way analysis of variance (consider patients as blocks):
MTB > TWOWAY C11 - C13;
SUBC> MEANS C12 C13.

ANALYSIS OF VARIANCE  PaO2

SOURCE      DF       SS       MS
Time         3      421      140
Patient      5     4292      858
ERROR       15     2888      193
TOTAL       23     7601

                        Individual 95% CI
    Time      Mean    --------+---------+---------+---------+--
       1      83.5            (------------*-----------)
       2      73.7    (-----------*-----------)
       3      84.0            (-----------*-----------)
       4      78.7        (-----------*-----------)
                        --------+---------+---------+---------+--
                           70.0     80.0      90.0     100.0

                        Individual 95% CI
  Patient     Mean    --------+---------+---------+---------+--
       1      91.7                     (-------*------)
       2      68.7          (------*-------)
       3      88.3                 (------*-------)
       4      57.7      (-------*------)
       5      77.7             (-------*------)
       6      95.5                    (-------*------)
                        --------+---------+---------+---------+--
                           60.0      80.0      100.0     120.0
```

both repeated measures and this two-way analysis is the same if the "sphericity" assumption holds. In that event, the liberal critical f-value is used to construct the decision line. Otherwise, our decision line showing the ambiguous zone should be used. Assuming "sphericity," we apply the TWOWAY command and augment it with a MEANS subcommand that displays individual 95% CIs for the specified levels. In Figure 12.3.7 we requested level means for both the time factor (in column C12) and the patient factor (in column C13).

13. Based on the CI graphics output from the TWO-WAY command, does there appear to be a significant difference in mean PaO_2 between times?

14. Based on the CI graphics output from the TWO-WAY command, does there appear to be a significant difference in mean PaO_2 between patients?

Problems 12.3

1. Conduct a one-way repeated measures analysis on the Barcelona et al data (Appendix, Data Set 2). For the sake of the exercise, assume multivariate normality.

2. Consider the Molyneaux et al data set (Appendix, Data Set 3). Determine the difference arterial − venous for each discard level. Conduct a one-factor repeated measures analysis to determine whether there is a significant difference between mean differences for the three discard levels. For the sake of the exercise, assume multivariate normality.

Problems 3–7 are based on the Bodai et al study (Appendix, Data Set 4). For each problem, for the sake of the exercise, assume multivariate normality. For each problem the fixed treatment factor is time with levels start, end, 1 minute, and 5 minutes. Conduct a one-way repeated measures analysis to determine whether there is a significant difference in mean PaO_2 between the four given times.

3. Group 1, routine suctioning.

4. Group 1, routine suctioning with insufflation catheter.

5. Group 2, routine suctioning.

6. Group 3, standard suction with valve adapter.

7. Group 3, oxygen insufflation with valve adapter.

Problems 8–13 are based on the Shively et al positioning study (Appendix, Data Set 5). For each problem, for the sake of the exercise, assume multivariate normality. For

each problem the fixed treatment factor is bed position. Conduct a one-way repeated measures analysis to determine whether there is a significant difference in mean SvO_2 between the given positions.

8. Group 1, all seven given positions.

9. Group 1, the three right lateral (RL) positions.

10. Group 1, the three supine (S) positions.

11. Group 2, all nine positions.

12. Group 2, the four RL positions.

13. Group 2, the four S positions.

14. Explain why one-way repeated measures analysis is not appropriate to analyze the Clark and Hoffer metabolism data (Appendix, Data Set 6).

Problems 15–20 are based on the Winklhofer-Roob cystic fibrosis study (Appendix, Data Set 7). For each problem, for the sake of the exercise, assume multivariate normality. For each problem the fixed treatment factor is time. Conduct a one-way repeated measures analysis to determine whether there is a significant difference in mean vitamin E between the given times.

15. Erythrocyte vitamin E, all ten children.

16. Erythrocyte vitamin E, the five children with cholestatic liver disease (CDL).

17. Erythrocyte vitamin E, the five children without CDL.

18. Serum vitamin E, all ten children.

19. Serum vitamin E, the five children with CDL.

20. Serum vitamin E, the five children without CDL.

21. Fernicola and Roberts (see Example 12.3.1) also gave the data shown in Table 12.3.3 for the heart weight of a convenience sample of patients with previously normal mitral valves prior to infective endocarditis. Conduct an appropriate two-way analysis of variance.

TABLE *12.3.3* Data from Fernicola and Roberts.

	White			Black	
Male	530	450	350	350	520
	650	500	530		
	530	535	505		
	540				
Female	600	480	275	400	360

22. Sütsch et al reported the data shown in Table 12.3.4 for aortic diameter (cm) in a convenience sample of patients presenting a dilated ascending aorta. Patients are classified according to gender (female, male) and aortic valve insufficiency (mild, moderate, severe). Conduct an appropriate analysis of variance.

TABLE *12.3.4* Data from Sütsch et al.

Gender	AORTIC VALVE INSUFFICIENCY								
	Mild			Moderate			Severe		
Female	4.4	4.1	5.7	4.5	9.0	5.9			
	5.5	6.0	6.0	7.0	5.5	7.1			
Male	6.5	4.9	5.3	5.4	6.3	3.7	6.3	6.2	6.7
	5.4	5.2	6.5	4.8	6.0	7.8	6.2	4.7	6.1
	5.0	5.5	5.5	6.9	7.1	5.8	6.2	5.9	
	4.7	6.4	6.2	6.6	7.6				
	5.1	4.0							

CHAPTER **12** OVERVIEW

Summary

ANOVA is statistical technique for resolving a multipopulation comparison of means problem. A population of interest in a multipopulation study is called a **level**. ANOVA extends the two-sided pooled t-test for comparison of means from two to several levels.

The set of hypotheses tested by ANOVA is

$H_0: \mu_1 = \mu_2 = \ldots \mu_k$
$H_a:$ the means are otherwise

where k is the number of levels in the study. The null hypothesis that all the means are equal is called the **omnibus hypothesis** for ANOVA.

The ANOVA alternate hypothesis merely says that at least two of the means are significantly different from each other. When ANOVA rejects the omnibus null hypothesis, then ANOVA is merely indicating a difference in means *without identifying which means are different*. To determine which means are different, one needs information about the level CIs.

Regular one-way ANOVA is valid assuming a **one-way, fixed treatments** design in a study utilizing independent random samples with independent observations. Further, the RV of interest must be normally distributed in each level and have the same standard deviation (or variance) in each level. Populations in which a given RV has the same variance are said to be **homoscedastic**. For normal distributions, homoscedasticity is checked by the F_{max} test. When the design does not utilize independent samples, but all fixed treatments are measured on the same sample, then a one-way **repeated measures** analysis should be used.

The computations for ANOVA are complex and should be done on a computer. When one has the raw data, using Minitab one may (1) display a **boxplot diagram** with the (G)BOXPLOT command and BY subcommand and (2) conduct an ANOVA analysis with the AOVONEWAY or ONEWAY commands. The command AOVONEWAY works only on an unstacked raw data set. The command ONEWAY works only on a stacked raw data set. A stacked data set is also needed to make a boxplot diagram. Section 12.2 provides a Minitab program ANOVALEGEND for conducting ANOVA when provided only with the data legend, as is the case with most journal articles in the health sciences. A one-way repeated measures analysis is conducted using the ANOVA command with the RANDOM subcommand.

The ANOVA decision whether to retain or reject the omnibus null hypothesis is made on the basis of the **p-value** provided by ANOVA. ANOVA is a robust test. A **robust** statistical test usually yields the correct decision even when preliminary assumptions are not all satisfied. ANOVA is robust even up to moderate violations of normality or homoscedasticity. When preliminaries are not technically met and one appeals to the robustness of the test, then the *p*-value offered by ANOVA is approximate.

When ANOVA rejects the omnibus hypothesis that all the level means are equal, then examine appropriate

CIs to determine which level means are different from each other. When one has the raw data, this may be accomplished in Minitab. The data are presented in a stacked form, and the ONEWAY command is applied. The ONEWAY command supports four subcommands: TUKEY, FISHER, DUNNETT, and MCB.

When the raw data set is provided and the assumption of normality badly fails, one may conduct the **Mood test** in Minitab. The Mood test's omnibus null hypothesis is that all the **medians** are equal. The Mood test, like ANOVA, assumes a one-way, fixed treatments design utilizing independent random samples with independent observations. But, unlike ANOVA, the Mood test does not need normality. ANOVA, however, is more powerful than the Mood test. ANOVA should be applied whenever valid.

Multiway ANOVA, like **two-way** ANOVA, can be carried out in Minitab for balanced designs with the ANOVA command. For unbalanced designs and studying underlying models, the GLM command is used.

Keywords

ANOVA	legend
one-way	level
repeated measures	level of significance
two-way	individual
balanced design	simultaneous
baseline	mean
boxplot diagram	median
comparison of means	Mood test
confidence interval (CI)	normal distribution
Dunnett	omnibus hypothesis
Fisher	one-way ANOVA
MCB	p-value
Tukey	random effects design
degrees of freedom	random samples
design	repeated measures
F_{max} test	robust
fixed treatment design	sample
general linear model	sample f_{max}-value
homoscedasticity	sample f-ratio
independent observation	test of hypothesis
independent samples	unbalanced design

References

Bajwa W et al: High cholesterol levels in patients with panic disorder. *Am J Psychiatry* 149, no. 3 (March 1992): 376.

Bodai B et al: A clinical evaluation of an oxygen insufflation/suction catheter. *Heart Lung* 16, no. 1 (January 1987): 39.

Caballero B et al: Plasma amino acid concentrations in healthy elderly men and women. *Am J Clin Nutr* 53, no. 5 (May 1991): 1249.

Foote A and Erfurt J: The benefit to cost ratio of work-site blood pressure control programs. *JAMA* 265, no. 10 (13 March 1991): 1283.

Girden E R: *ANOVA: Repeated Measures*. Sage University Paper Series on Quantitative Applications in the Social Sciences, no. 07–084. Newbury Park, Calif.: Sage, 1992.

Harding G et al: How long should catheter-acquired urinary tract infection in women be treated? *Ann Intern Med* 114, no. 9 (1 May 1991): 713.

Heini A et al: Twenty-four-hour energy expenditure in pregnant and nonpregnant Gambian women, measured in a whole-body indirect calorimeter. *Am J Clin Nutr* 55 (June 1992): 1078.

Jonsson K et al: Tissue oxygenation, anemia, and perfusion in relation to wound healing in surgical patients. *Ann Surg* 214, no. 5 (November 1991): 605.

Klatsky A and Armstrong M: Cardiovascular risk factors among Asian Americans living in northern California. *Am J Public Health* 81, no. 11 (November 1991): 1423.

Rolls B: Food intake, hunger, and satiety after preloads in women with eating disorders. *Am J Clin Nutr* 55 (June 1992): 1093.

Rovner B et al: Depression and mortality in nursing homes. *JAMA* 265, no. 8 (27 February 1991): 993.

Sackman M et al: The Munich Gallbladder Lithotripsy Study. *Ann Intern Med* 114, no. 4 (15 February 1991): 290.

Shott S: *Statistics for Health Professionals*. Philadelphia: W. B. Saunders, 1990.

Sokol R and Rohlf F J: *Biometry*. 2nd ed. New York: W. H. Freeman, 1981.

Stähelin H et al: β-Carotene and cancer prevention: The Basil Study. *Am J Clin Nutr* 53, no. 1 (January 1991): 265.

Sütsch G et al: Predictability of aortic dissection as a function of aortic diameter. *Eur Heart J* 12, no. 12 (December 1991): 1247.

Zehna P: *A Minitab Companion with Macros*. Reading, Mass.: Addison-Wesley, 1992.

13

Chisquared Tests

The favorite drink of adult Americans is coffee. But is drinking too much coffee bad for you? How much is too much? How could it be bad? Such concerns have reached the general public as a result of highly publicized research regarding coffee drinking as a possible coronary disease risk factor.

Klatsky et al undertook a massive study involving 101,774 adults in northern California over a 9-year period. Their concerns essentially boiled down to testable questions involving a proportion: What proportion of apparently healthy adults who drink coffee present a coronary event over a given time? What about the same concern for those who do not drink coffee? What about moderation? What about tea drinkers? Once one gets started, one opens a floodgate of "what abouts."

Chisquared tests are a collection of the most common testing techniques involving the proportion for multiattribute factors. We invite you to apply your chisquared skills in resolving concerns about coffee and tea drinking as a coronary disease risk factor in Problems 13.2.20–23.

SECTION 13.1	**OBJECTIVES** This section will
Goodness of Fit	**1** Describe the term *factor*.
	2 Determine the expected frequencies when provided with a factor of interest, the sample size, and a hypothesized set of proportions for the given factor.
	3 Conduct a chisquared goodness of fit test when provided with an appropriate problem from the health sciences.

The chisquared goodness of fit test presented in this section extends the case of one population with one attribute to one population with *multi*attributes. A viewpoint involving multiattributes is called a factor.

Factor

A **factor** is a general point of view specified by an exhaustive and mutually exclusive list of attributes. Many studies in the health sciences about a characteristic of interest are not presented in just a simple yes or no manner but can encompass a range of options. Examples include

Factor	Attributes
Eye color	Brown, blue, green, other
Gender	Male, female
Hospital ward	Medical-surgical, critical care, pediatrics, labor and delivery, postpartum, other
Hypertension	Normal, borderline, definite
Age of nursing home admission	≤ 64, 65–74, 75–84, ≥ 85

Each subject in a study is classified accordingly into a unique category from the viewpoint of any given factor. The attributes must be defined clearly so that each subject is unambiguously classified. For example, although the attributes for hypertension are given in general terms, they may be well defined by a systolic blood pressure reading as follows: normal (under 140), borderline (140–150), and definite (over 150).

A single attribute can be presented in the factor format by elevating the attribute to the rank of factor and noting whether it is present or absent in a given subject. For example,

Factor	Attributes
Gallstones	Present, absent
Fever	Yes, no
Hypertension	Present, absent
Pregnant	Yes, no

When given a population and a factor (with an accompanying list of attributes), one wants to know how these attributes are distributed in the population. Toward this end, one obtains a random sample and observes the factor attribute in each member of the sample. The results can be displayed by a simple frequency distribution table showing each attribute and corresponding frequency in the sample.

EXAMPLE 13.1.1 Rovner et al studied newly admitted patients to several nursing homes in 1987–88. The age distribution of these patients is shown in Table 13.1.1.

TABLE *13.1.1*
Frequency distribution for age at entry in the Rovner et al nursing home study.

Age at Entry	Observed Frequency
≤ 64	20
65–74	70
75–84	207
≥ 85	157
Total	454

Often in research, one has a model for the distribution of a factor in the population. A **model** specifies the proportion of each attribute in the factor. The model, which may be predicated on some theory or previous study, supplies a hypothesized set of proportions for the factor. The researcher then inquires whether the observed data in the sample are consistent with the given model. The researcher wonders whether the observed results fit the model; hence the term **goodness of fit**. In order to determine whether the sample results fit the model, the researcher determines what the sample should look like based on the model. The model provides the researcher with an idea of what to expect. Hence, the researcher wants to compare the *observed frequencies* (seen in the sample) to the *expected frequencies* (predicted by the model).

Expected Frequencies

The raw material needed for comparing a sample with a model is a table that presents the observed and expected frequencies for a given random sample. The expected frequencies are calculated on the basis of the proportions supplied by the model. These proportions are formalized into the null hypothesis for the goodness of fit test.

EXAMPLE 13.1.2 (Continued from Example 13.1.1) Rovner et al inquired whether the age distribution of the nursing home patients in their study was consistent with the age distribution of nursing home patients reported by the National Nursing Home Survey (NNHS). The NNHS reported the following age distribution: ≤ 64 (11.6%), 65–74 (14.2%), 75–84 (34.1%), and ≥ 85 (40.0%). The NNHS provides us with a model for the age distribution of nursing home patients at admission. Accordingly, the null hypothesis for testing whether the age distribution of nursing home patients in the sample is consistent with NNHS findings is

$$H_0: p_{\leq 64} = .116, p_{65-74} = .142, p_{75-84} = .341, p_{\geq 85} = .400$$

Comment Ideally, the sum of the proportions given in the null hypothesis should add up to 1.000. In Example 13.1.2 they add up to .999. This small deviation from the ideal is due to unavoidable round-off error in reporting results to three places past the decimal point. The sum of the NNHS percentages is 99.9% rather than the ideal 100.0%.

Expected frequencies are calculated on the assumption that the model (null hypothesis) is true. To calculate the sample expected frequencies, simply multiply the sample size by each attribute's hypothesized proportion. For example, in the Rovner nursing home study (Examples 13.1.1 and 2) the expected number of patients in each age category is computed as follows:

Sample Size	×	Hypothesized Proportion	=	Expected Frequency
454	×	.116	=	52.664
454	×	.142	=	64.468
454	×	.341	=	154.814
454	×	.400	=	181.600

In calculating an expected frequency, *do not round the answer*. Of course, one may round to a reasonable extent in reporting the expected frequency, but in further calculations extensive rounding leads to compounded round-off error in computing the sample value for the goodness of fit test.

Results are nicely summarized in a three-column table as follows:

Column 1: the attribute list of the factor of interest
Column 2: the sample observed frequencies for each attribute
Column 3: the sample expected frequencies for each attribute

For example, results for the Rovner et al study (Examples 13.1.1 and 2) are displayed in Table 13.1.2. We emphasize that observed and expected *frequencies* (not observed and expected proportions) are presented.

TABLE **13.1.2**
Observed versus expected frequencies for the Rovner et al age at entry nursing home study.

Age at Entry	Observed Frequency	Expected Frequency
≤ 64	20	52.664
65–74	70	64.468
75–84	207	154.814
≥ 85	157	181.600
Total	454	453.546

Comment Ideally, the sum of the expected frequency column should equal the sample size (here, 454). The close value of 453.546 for the total expected frequency is an artifact of round-off error. The expected proportions provided by the NNHS study added up to 99.9% rather than the ideal 100.0%. Hence, a small deviation from the ideal due to round-off error is to be expected here (99.9% of 454 is 453.546).

There are two key items to note about Table 13.1.2. First, the sample provides an **observed frequency** for each age at entry category. Second, the null hypothesis (NNHS model) produces a corresponding **expected frequency** for each age at entry category. The project now is to determine whether the observed frequencies are consistent with the expected frequencies; that is, do we have a good fit?

Chisquared Goodness of Fit Test

In order to determine whether the observed frequencies display a good fit with the expected frequencies, we need a measure for **goodness of fit**. This measure is supplied by an attribute's **chisquared** value, calculated by (observed − expected)^2/expected. For example, the chisquared value for each attribute in the Rovner et al nursing home study (Examples 13.1.1 and 2) is calculated as follows:

$$\text{Age} \le 64: (\text{observed} - \text{expected})^2/\text{expected} = (20 - 52.664)^2/52.664 = 20.259$$
$$65\text{--}74: (\text{observed} - \text{expected})^2/\text{expected} = (70 - 64.468)^2/64.468 = 0.475$$
$$75\text{--}84: (\text{observed} - \text{expected})^2/\text{expected} = (207 - 154.814)^2/154.814 = 17.591$$
$$\ge 85: (\text{observed} - \text{expected})^2/\text{expected} = (157 - 181.600)^2/181.600 = 3.332$$

Comment Note that each attribute's chisquared value is computed [from] the observed and expected *frequencies*, not the observed and expected [?]

The results are summarized in Table 13.1.3, which contains all the [?] we need in order to conduct a formal chisquared goodness of fit test. We c[onduct the] test at the 5% level of significance (LOS) in the usual format following the g[uidelines] presented in Chart 7 (Appendix). The total of the chisquared column is the [sample] **chisquared** value.

TABLE **13.1.3**
Chisquared goodness of fit table for the Rovner et al nursing home study.

Age at Entry	Observed Frequency	Expected Frequency	Chisquared
≤ 64	20	52.664	20.259
65–74	70	64.468	0.475
75–84	207	154.814	17.591
≥ 85	157	181.600	3.332
Total	454	453.546	41.657

The chisquared goodness of fit test has a preliminary consideration of sample size. In order for the chisquared test to be valid, the sample needs to be large enough so that each attribute has a fair chance of being adequately observed. The conventional conservative rule is that each expected frequency should be ≥ 5, in which case the sample is large enough to invoke the chisquared goodness of fit test. Experience has shown that as long as each expected frequency is ≥ 1, with no more than 20% of the attributes having an expected frequency under 5, then the chisquared test gives satisfactory results for testing goodness of fit. In the Rovner et al nursing home study, a glance at Table 13.1.3 shows that all expected frequencies are ≥ 5; hence, the chisquared goodness of fit test is valid. The formal write-up is displayed in Figure 13.1.1.

The alternate hypothesis accompanying the given null hypothesis for a chisquared goodness of fit test is simply H_a: the proportions are otherwise. This alternate hypothesis does not mean that all the proportions are different than what the

FIGURE **13.1.1**
Formal write-up for the chisquared goodness of fit test for the Rovner et al nursing home study (Examples 13.1.1 and 2).

> I. Preliminary. All the expected frequencies are greater than five. Hence, the sample size is adequately large to apply the chisquared goodness of fit test.
> II. Chisquared Goodness of Fit Test.
>   1. Hypothesis.
> H_0: $p_{\leq 64} = .116$, $p_{65-74} = .142$, $p_{75-84} = .341$, $p_{\geq 85} = .400$
> H_a: the proportions are otherwise
>   2. Level of Significance. 0.05
>   3. Test Statistic. $\Sigma(\text{Observed} - \text{Expected})^2/\text{Expected}$
>   4. Critical Value.   df $= 4 - 1 = 3$
> $\chi^2 = 7.8147$ (Table 12, Appendix)
>   5. Decision Line. 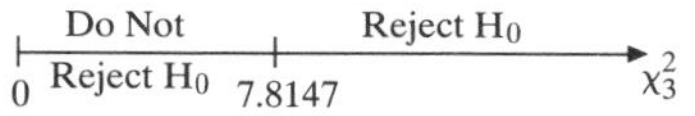
>
>   Do Not | Reject H_0
>   0 Reject H_0 7.8147 ————→ χ_3^2
>
>   6. Sample Value. The sample chisquared value is 41.657 (Table 13.1.3).
>   7. Conclusion. Based on the given data, at the 5% level of significance we reject H_0. The sample gives very strong evidence that the age distribution in the sample is not as specified in the National Nursing Home Survey ($\chi^2 = 41.7$, df $= 3$, p < 0.005).

'l hypothesis specifies, but that at least two of the proportions are different than 't is stated in the null hypothesis.

'ince the null hypothesis is rejected (Figure 13.1.1), we inquire where the aber-
from the hypothesized proportions occur; that is, which specific age categories
'rrepresented or overrepresented? We reexamine the expected versus ob-
'quency distribution table for those attributes that resulted in the greatest
'values. Note that the test critical value was 7.81. Both the ≤ 64 and 75–84
'ies produced a chisquared value in excess of the test critical value. In
'ular, the 20 patients observed in the ≤ 64 age category is statistically significantly less than the expected 52.664 patients, as indicated by the high (20.259) chisquared value for this category. Also, the 207 patients observed in the 75–84 age
group is statistically significantly more than the 154.814 expected, as indicated by the
high (17.591) chisquared value for this group.

An attribute's sample chisquared value is a measure of "goodness of fit." The
chisquared value measures a statistical distance between an observed frequency and
its corresponding expected frequency. The closer an observed frequency is to the
expected frequency, the smaller the chisquared value. Hence, a small overall sample
chisquared value indicates good agreement between the set of observed frequencies
and the corresponding set of expected frequencies; that is, we have a good fit. A large
chisquared value indicates poor agreement between what is observed and what is
expected. Accordingly, a large chisquared value provides evidence for rejecting the
set of proportions specified in the null hypothesis.

Often the hypothesized proportions (model) for a goodness of fit test come from
theory, such as some intrinsic notion of "fairness" or equiprobability.

EXAMPLE 13.1.3 A die was rolled 120 times, and the number showing on top was observed. The
resulting observed frequencies were

Face value	1	2	3	4	5	6
Frequency	27	15	17	25	15	21

Are the observed frequencies consistent with the results expected from a fair
die? That is, are the observed frequencies consistent with the results projected by
a fair die that each face value should show one-sixth of the time? The formal test
of hypothesis write-up is displayed in Figure 13.1.2.

The result of this die-rolling experiment is not unusual. Upon rolling a fair die 120
times, one can expect to obtain a sample chisquared value of 6.70 or larger over 25%
of the time (that's the message from the p-value).

Comment We strongly recommend displaying the chisquared table (Table 13.1.4)
as shown in step 6 of Figure 13.1.2 to organize and show your computations. A good
chisquare goodness of fit table has four columns:

Column 1 displays the factor attributes.
Column 2 displays the observed frequencies.
Column 3 displays the expected frequencies.
Column 4 displays the attribute chisquared values.

FIGURE **13.1.2**
Chisquared test of
hypothesis write-up
for the die-rolling
experiment (Example
13.1.3).

I. Preliminary. In 120 rolls of a fair die, each face value's fair share is 20 observations. Since each expected frequency of 20 is greater than 5, then the sample size is sufficiently large to apply the chisquared goodness of fit test.
II. Chisquared Goodness of Fit Test.
  1. Hypothesis.
    H_0: $p_1 = p_2 = p_3 = p_4 = p_5 = p_6 = 1/6$ (fair die hypothesis)
    H_a: the proportions are otherwise
  2. LOS. 0.05
  3. Test Statistic. Σ(Observed − Expected)^2/Expected
  4. Critical Value. df = 6 − 1 = 5
            $\chi^2 = 11.0705$ (Table 12, Appendix)
  5. Decision Line.

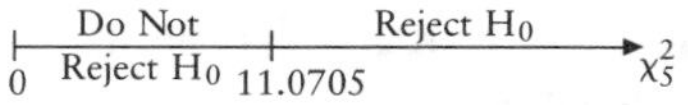

Do Not	Reject H_0	
Reject H_0		

0   11.0705 χ^2_5

  6. Sample Value. The sample chisquared value is 6.70 (Table 13.1.4).

TABLE **13.1.4**
Chisquared good-
ness of fit table
for the die-
tossing data.

Face Value	Observed	Expected	Chisquared
1	27	20	2.45
2	15	20	1.25
3	17	20	0.45
4	25	20	1.25
5	15	20	1.25
6	21	20	0.05
Total	120	120	6.70

  7. Conclusion. Based on the given data, at the 5% level of significance, we do not reject the null hypothesis. The observed frequencies are consistent with those expected from tosses of a fair die ($\chi^2 = 6.7$, df = 5, .10 < p < .25).

The sums for columns 2, 3, and 4 should also be displayed. Column 2 adds up to the sample size. Column 3 also adds up to the sample size (within round-off error). The sum of column 4 is the sample chisquared value.

EXERCISES 13.1

Warm-ups 13.1

1. What are the two main types of chisquared tests?
    Goodness of fit, independence of attributes

2. Chisquared tests focus on what parameter?
  a. Mean
  b. Median
  c. Proportion
  d. Standard deviation

3. A general point of view specified by an exhaustive and mutually exclusive list of attributes is called a
  a. Proportion
  b. Factor

  c. Goodness of fit
  d. Chisquared test

4. Suppose a model for the distribution of a factor is given. The model
  a. Specifies the proportion for each attribute in the factor
  b. Is used to formulate the null hypothesis for a chisquared goodness of fit test
  c. Is used to calculate expected frequencies in a sample
  d. All of the above

Background for Warm-ups 5–12. Chisquared goodness of fit tests are applied in genetics to verify that a given trait is inherited by some genetic model, like the simple dominant-recessive Mendelian model. Several inherited conditions are of this type, including Klinefelter's syndrome, Huntington's chorea, cystic fibrosis, sickle-cell anemia, Tay-Sachs disease, and the gender of the child. To illustrate the use of the chisquared test in genetics, we consider a simple botanical experiment using flower colors of pea plants (just like Mendel did). The student probably was introduced to a similar experiment in an introductory course in biology.

Flower color is determined by a single gene, which may be dominant (R) or recessive (r). Flower color is genetically determined by RR (red), Rr (pink), and rr (white). From basic Mendelian theory, if pink flowers are crossed, flower color in the progeny plants should appear red:pink:white::1:2:1. This means that for every four plants, there should be one red flower, two pink flowers, and one white flower. Hence, the predicted proportions of flower colors are red .25, pink .50, and white .25. You can verify these theoretical proportions by constructing a Punnett square or a probability tree diagram.

5. An experiment was conducted by crossing pink-flowered plants. Suppose 200 progeny are produced in which 54 plants have red flowers, 99 plants have pink flowers, and 47 plants have white flowers. The numbers 54, 99, and 47 are called the

   a. Hypothesized proportions

   b. Observed frequencies

   c. Expected frequencies

   d. Attribute chisquared values

   e. Test reference values

6. The null hypothesis in a goodness of fit test for flower color is

   $H_0: p_{red} = .25, p_{pink} = .50, p_{white} = .25$

7. The expected frequency for each attribute is calculated by multiplying the total sample size (200) by the attribute's hypothesized proportion (Warm-up 6). Here,

   expected frequency of red-flowered plants = 200 × .25 = 50

   expected frequency of pink-flowered plants = 200 × .50 = 100

   expected frequency of white-flowered plants = 200 × .25 = 50

8. Each attribute's chisquared value is obtained by calculating

   $\frac{(observed - expected)^2}{expected}$. So,

   $chisquared(red) = \frac{(54-50)^2}{50} = .32$

   $chisquared(pink) = \left(\frac{99-100}{100}\right)^2 = .01$

   $chisquared(white) = \left(\frac{47-50}{50}\right)^2 = .18$

9. Complete the chisquared goodness of fit Table 13.1.5.

TABLE **13.1.5** Chisquared goodness of fit table for flower color.

Flower Color	Observed Frequency	Expected Frequency	Chisquared
Red	54	50	.32
PINK	99	100	.01
WHITE	47	50	.18
Sum	200	200	.51

10. The preliminary check for the chisquared goodness of fit test is to determine whether

    a. The proportions in the null hypothesis add up to 1.

    b. The expected frequencies add up to the sample size.

    c. The sample size is adequately large.

    d. The observed frequencies add up to the sample size.

11. A sample size is adequately large if all expected frequencies are at least 1, and at most 20% of the attributes have an expected frequency less than 5. Is the sample size for the flower experiment adequately large? yes

12. State the null and alternate hypotheses to test the conjecture that the proportions of red, pink, and white flower colors follow simple Mendelian genetics.

13. What are the degrees of freedom for this test?

14. From Table 12 (Appendix), what is the critical chisquared value for this test at the 5% LOS?

15. Construct the decision line for this test.

16. What is the sample chisquared value?

17. Is the null hypothesis retained or rejected?

18. What is the p-value? *.25*

19. The statistical summary is: ($\chi^2 = $ *.5*, $df = $ *2*, p *.26*).

20. What does this experiment tell you about flower color in these plants?

Problems 13.1

1. In the nursing home study by Rovner et al, 77.3% of 454 new admissions to nursing homes were female. Is this figure (77.3% female) consistent with the notion that men and women are equally admitted to nursing homes, that is, that the ratio of women to men admitted to nursing homes is "fifty-fifty"?

   a. Test this notion by performing the z-test for the proportion $H_0: p = .5$, where p is the proportion of females admitted to nursing homes.

   b. Test this notion by conducting a chisquared test for goodness of fit for the hypothesis

   $$H_0: p_{\text{female}} = .5, p_{\text{male}} = .5$$

   where p is the proportion of each specified gender admitted to a nursing home.

   c. The chisquared test for a factor with two attributes is an extension of the two-tailed z-test for a proportion for one population, one attribute. In theory, $\chi^2 = z^2$. Is your sample chisquared value from (b) equal to the square of the sample z-value from (a)?

2. (Continued from Problem 1) The 1985 NNHS study reported that 71.5% of individuals admitted to nursing homes were female. Is the sample proportion of 77.3% female consistent with that reported by the NNHS?

   a. Test by performing an appropriate z-test for the proportion.

   b. Test by conducting a chisquared goodness of fit test.

3. The distribution of ABO blood types among U.S. whites is reported (Keeton) to be type A (41%), B (10%), AB (4%), and O (45%). A sample of 200 U.S. whites yielded 79 type A, 25 type B, 5 type AB, and 91 type O. At the 5% LOS, is the sample ABO blood type distribution consistent with that reported for whites by Keeton?

4. The distribution of ABO blood types among U.S. blacks is reported (Keeton) to be type A (28%), B (20%), AB (5%), and O (47%). A sample of 200 U.S. blacks yielded 64 type A, 35 type B, 10 type AB, and 91 type O. At the 5% LOS, is the sample ABO blood type distribution consistent with that reported for blacks?

5. A coin was tossed 100 times and yielded 54 heads and 46 tails. Is this result consistent with a result obtained from a fair coin? Determine your answer using a suitable chisquared goodness of fit test.

6. Tatemichi et al studied dementia in patients aged ≥ 60 with acute ischemic stroke (see Exercise 11.1.7). Patients were classified into the following groups according to the perceived cause of their dementia: unknown cause, with normal angiogram, with tandem arterial pathology, cardiogenic embolism, atherothrombotic, lacunes. There were 168 dementia patients in the study who presented a history of stroke. These 168 patients were grouped as follows: unknown cause, 61; normal angiogram, 8; with tandem arterial pathology, 8; cardiogenic embolism, 33; atherothrombotic, 18; lacunes, 40. Is the given classification scheme for patients with dementia exhaustive and mutually exclusive?

7. (Continued from Problem 6) The classification pattern for dementia patients with no history of stroke was as follows: unknown, .341; with normal angiogram, .034; with tandem arterial pathology, .057; cardiogenic embolism, .174; atherothrombotic, .059; and lacunes, .335. The numbers given are proportions; for example, the proportion of nonstroke patients classified into the lacunes group is .335 (33.5%).

   a. Is the classification pattern for dementia patients with a history of stroke consistent with the given classification pattern for dementia patients without stroke?

   b. Is the classification pattern for dementia patients with a history of stroke consistent with the idea that these patients are evenly distributed throughout the various groups?

8. Problem 5.1.4 gave the results of a computer simulation of 100 families, each having five children. Let X denote the number of girls in a family of five children. Are the results consistent with the binomial model $X = \text{Bino}(5, .5)$?

Problems 9–12 are based on research by Thompson et al, who studied the occurrence of acute myocardial infarction (MI) in relation to the day of the week. Thompson et al wondered whether an acute MI was independent of the day of the week or whether an acute MI was more likely to occur on a particular day of the week. The study encompassed 2254 patients admitted to a coronary care unit in the United Kingdom over a 10-year period. Note that if acute MI is uniformly distributed over the days of the week, then the proportion of MIs for any given day of the week is 1/7. For Problems 9–12, test the null hypothesis that acute MI is uniformly distributed over the days of the week. If the uniform distribution hypothesis is rejected, which days of the week are overrepresented or underrepresented for acute MI?

9. The distribution of 2254 acute MIs over the days of the week was Monday, 363; Tuesday, 277; Wednesday, 324; Thursday, 330; Friday, 308; Saturday, 337; and Sunday, 315.

10. The distribution of 1743 acute MIs for men over the days of the week was Monday, 280; Tuesday, 206; Wednesday, 258; Thursday, 249; Friday, 231; Saturday, 271; and Sunday, 248.

11. The distribution of 511 acute MIs for women over the days of the week was Monday, 83; Tuesday, 71; Wednesday, 66; Thursday, 81; Friday, 77; Saturday, 66; and Sunday, 67.

12. The distribution of 244 acute MIs for women under 65 years of age over the days of the week was Monday, 39; Tuesday, 32; Wednesday, 27; Thursday, 51; Friday, 33; Saturday, 19; and Sunday, 43.

13. Chapman and Duff studied glove perforations associated with selected obstetric procedures (see Problems 10.1.21–24). The 52 perforations in a glove worn on the left hand occurred as follows: thumb, 13; index finger, 21; middle finger, 12; ring finger, 0; little finger, 1; and palm, 5. Conduct a chisquared goodness of fit test to determine whether or not perforation is equally likely at the indicated sites.

14. Chapman and Duff studied glove perforations associated with selected obstetric procedures (see Problems 10.1.21–24). The 78 perforations occurred in the following glove sites: left thumb, 13; left index finger, 21; left middle finger, 12; left ring finger, 0; left little finger, 1; left palm, 5; right thumb, 11; right index finger, 3; right middle finger, 7; right ring finger, 1; right little finger, 2; and right palm, 2. Conduct a chisquared goodness of fit test to determine whether or not perforation is equally likely at the indicated sites.

SECTION 13.2

Independence of Attributes

OBJECTIVES This section will

1 Construct a contingency table for data obtained from a random sample in which the design of the study contains two multiattribute factors.

2 Conduct a chisquared test of hypothesis for independence of attributes when provided with an appropriate health sciences problem.

In an actual health science study, the investigator makes several observations of a given subject; that is, there are several random variables (RVs) observed simultaneously. Thus far we have been studying a population by examining just one RV of interest. Even when several RVs were presented, we studied them one at a time.

The health sciences, however, are much more complex. The status of a given patient is not dependent on just one condition. Usually one must consider not only several conditions but also how these conditions interact. For example, in considering risk factors for predicting a cardiac event, one must be aware that elevated cholesterol interacts with smoking to produce a greater risk than elevated cholesterol or smoking considered individually. The effectiveness of a drug regime depends not only on the given drugs but on how they may interact.

In this section we consider interaction effects when two factors are considered simultaneously. Data from a study involving two factors are presented effectively by means of a two-factor frequency distribution table.

Two-Factor Frequency Distribution Tables

In a study design involving two factors, the sample data are nicely organized and presented by means of a **two-factor frequency distribution table**.

EXAMPLE 13.2.1 Murph et al studied occupational risk for cytomegalovirus (CMV) at three midwestern day-care centers. The researchers particularly noted that CMV

- Is the world's most common agent of congenital viral infection;
- Affects about 1% to 2% of all newborns in the United States. Of these, about 10% suffer consequences to hearing, vision, and mental development;
- Is commonly transmitted in group child-care environments, especially among toddlers;
- Places parents and adult child care workers at risk.

The investigators classified toddlers from the following two-factor viewpoint at enrollment:

Factor	Attributes
Age at entry	< 2, 2, 3, ≥ 4
Day-care center	A, B, C

Note that both attribute lists are exhaustive and mutually exclusive. Each child in the CMV study is classified with precisely one age at entry and is enrolled at exactly one day-care center.

The associated two-factor frequency distribution table is shown in Table 13.2.1.

TABLE **13.2.1**
Two-factor frequency distribution table for the Murph et al day care study.

Age at Entry	DAY-CARE CENTER			Total
	A	B	C	
<2	29	35	10	74
2	14	6	3	23
3	18	11	21	50
≥ 4	29	9	34	72
Total	90	61	68	219

In a two-factor frequency distribution table, the table layout presents one of the factors in the rows, the other factor in the columns. Table 13.2.1 is referred to as a "4-by-3 table" since the table presents 4 row attributes (age at entry) and 3 column attributes (day-care center). In general, one displays an *r* by *c* table, where *r* is the number of row attributes and *c* is the number of column attributes.

A position in the table located by a given row and column is called a **cell**. Since there are 4 age at entry attributes and 3 day-care center attributes, there are $4 \times 3 = 12$ cells in the age at entry versus day-care center frequency distribution table. The (age < 2, center B) cell has a frequency of 35, as indicated by the shading in Table 13.2.1.

Note that there are three kinds of totals (also called marginal sums) in Table 13.2.1:

1. *Row totals*, giving the total number of children at each age;
2. *Column totals*, giving the total number of children at each day-care center;
3. *Grand total*, giving the total number of children in the study.

EXAMPLE 13.2.2 The researchers were also interested in the number of children excreting CMV at the time of entry into the study. For all day-care centers combined, the 4-by-2 frequency distribution table is shown in Table 13.2.2.

TABLE **13.2.2**
Two-factor frequency distribution table for age at entry versus excreting CMV from the Murph et al day care study.

Age at Entry	EXCRETING CMV		Total
	Yes	No	
< 2	16	58	74
2	8	15	23
3	6	44	50
≥ 4	2	70	72
Total	32	187	219

Table 13.2.2 classifies each child using the factors age at entry and excreting CMV:

Factor	Attributes
Age at entry	< 2, 2, 3, ≥ 4
Excreting CMV	Yes, no

When two factors are imposed on a population of interest, one wonders whether the factors interrelate or act independently. If factors act independently, then one may simplify the analysis of the data by considering each factor separately. When factors act independently, the distribution of the attributes of one factor is the same among the various attributes of the other factor. If the factors interact, then a serious study must take the interaction into account and study both factors as they work in tandem.

One tests for interaction between two factors by applying a test of hypothesis for **independence of attributes**. The appropriate hypotheses are

H_0: The given factors are independent of each other.
H_a: The given factors interact with each other.

Comment Technically, a test for independence of attributes is a test of hypothesis about proportions. Specifically, the null hypothesis states that the proportion of any given attribute in one factor is the same across all attributes of the other factor. For example, the full statement in terms of proportions of the null and alternate hypotheses for the age at entry versus day-care center (Example 13.2.1) is

$$H_0: p_{<2|\text{center A}} = p_{<2|\text{center B}} = p_{<2|\text{center C}}$$
$$p_{2|\text{center A}} = p_{2|\text{center B}} = p_{2|\text{center C}}$$
$$p_{3|\text{center A}} = p_{3|\text{center B}} = p_{3|\text{center C}}$$
$$p_{\geq 4|\text{center A}} = p_{\geq 4|\text{center B}} = p_{\geq 4|\text{center C}}$$

H_a: the proportions are otherwise.

The first line in this formalized null hypothesis says that the children under 2 years of age are distributed in the same fashion among the three day-care centers; that is, the fraction of children under 2 years of age is the same at centers A, B, and C.

The most common test for independence is the chisquared test for independence of attributes. In order to conduct a chisquared test, one must calculate an expected frequency to accompany each observed frequency. A two-factor table that augments each cell's observed frequency with its expected frequency is called a contingency table.

Contingency Tables

A **contingency table** is a two-factor frequency distribution table in which each observed frequency is accompanied by its expected frequency. Each expected frequency is calculated contingent on the assumption that the null hypothesis of independence of attributes is true; hence, the name contingency table. A contingency table is needed for calculating the sample chisquared value in a chisquared test for independence of attributes.

In general, assuming independence of attributes, the **expected frequency** for the cell in row i and column j is given by

$$\text{expected frequency for cell in row } i, \text{ column } j = \frac{(\text{rowsum } i) \times (\text{columnsum } j)}{(\text{grand total})}$$

EXAMPLE 13.2.3 Consider the CMV study, age at entry versus day-care center (Table 13.2.1). The observed frequency for age < 2 at center A is 29. This frequency is located in row 1, column 1 of the given frequency distribution table. The expected frequency for the cell under the assumption of independence of attributes is

$$\text{expected frequency for cell in row 1, column 1} = \frac{\text{rowsum 1} \times \text{columnsum 1}}{\text{grand total}} = \frac{74 \times 90}{219} = 30.41$$

Similarly, the observed frequency for 3-year-olds at center B is 11. This observation is located in row 3, column 2. Hence,

$$\text{expected frequency for cell in row 3, column 2} = \frac{\text{rowsum 3} \times \text{columnsum 2}}{\text{grand total}} = \frac{50 \times 61}{219} = 13.93$$

The expected frequency for a given cell is placed underneath the cell observed frequency. The resulting two-factor frequency distribution table in which each cell is augmented with its expected frequency, where the expectation is based on the independence of the two given sets of attributes, is called a contingency table.

EXAMPLE 13.2.4 The 4-by-3 contingency table for the age at entry versus day-care center from Murph et al (Example 13.2.1) is given in Table 13.2.3.

TABLE **13.2.3** A 4-by-3 contingency table for the Murph et al study, day care center versus age at entry.

Age at Entry	DAY-CARE CENTER			Total
	A	B	C	
< 2	29 30.41	35 20.61	10 22.98	74
2	14 9.45	6 6.41	3 7.14	23
3	18 20.55	11 13.93	21 15.53	50
≥ 4	29 29.59	9 20.05	34 22.36	72
Total	90	61	68	219

EXAMPLE 13.2.5 The 4-by-2 contingency table for age at entry versus excreting CMV from Murph et al (Example 13.2.2) is given in Table 13.2.4.

TABLE **13.2.4** A 4-by-2 contingency table for the Murph et al day care study, excreting CMV versus age at entry.

Age at Entry	EXCRETING CMV		Total
	Yes	No	
< 2	16 10.81	58 63.19	74
2	8 3.36	15 19.64	23
3	6 7.31	44 42.69	50
≥ 4	2 10.52	70 61.48	72
Total	32	187	219

Chisquared Test for Independence of Attributes

Once a contingency table is presented, the immediate question is, Is this a good fit? Are the observed frequencies consistent with the expected frequencies? Of course, the observed values are different than the expected values. This is no surprise. The situation is analogous to flipping a fair coin 100 times and observing 53 heads and 47 tails. The results are not exactly fifty-fifty, but they are close enough; that is, the results are consistent with the fair-coin hypothesis. A common statistical test to determine whether the observed values in a contingency table are consistent with the expected values is the **chisquared test for independence of attributes**.

EXAMPLE 13.2.6 We conduct a chisquared test of hypothesis to determine whether the attributes for age at entry and day-care center are independent of each other (Example 13.2.1). Formally,

H_0: Age at entry and day-care center are independent factors.
H_a: Age at entry and day-care center interact.

Since the computations needed for construction of a contingency table are somewhat extensive, we gratefully engage Minitab. Minitab's output for this chisquared test is given in Figure 13.2.1.

To apply the chisquared test for independence of attributes in Minitab, first enter the two-factor frequency table; second, PRINT the data and check them for accuracy; then issue the CHISQUARED command. For example, the chisquare test for Example 13.2.6 is carried out in Minitab as follows:

```
MTB > NAME C1 'A', C2 'B', C3 'C'
MTB > READ C1 - C3
DATA> 29 35 10
DATA> 14 6 3
DATA> 18 11 21
DATA> 29 9 34
DATA> END OF DATA
MTB > PRINT C1 - C3
MTB > CHISQUARED C1 - C3
```

In examining Minitab's output in Figure 13.2.1, notice that all expected cell frequencies are greater than 5. Hence, the sample size is sufficiently large to apply the chisquared test. Further, since the p-value is so very small, we can immediately announce the following conclusion:

Based on the given data, we reject H_0: Age at entry and day care center are independent. The age distribution of the children differs from center to center ($\chi^2 = 37.1, df = 6, p = .000002$).

Because of some unexplainable lapse, Minitab fails to automatically provide the p-value for the chisquared test for independence of attributes. Fortunately, it is not a difficult task to obtain the p-value. One applies the four commands after "NOTE p-value" in Figure 13.2.1. In the CDF command, use the sample ChiSq value from Minitab's chisquared output (here, 37.086). Follow the CDF command with a semi-colon. In the CHIS subcommand, use the degrees of freedom from the chisquared output (here, $df = 6$). Round the computer's output to give a humane answer; here, $p = .000002$ will do. For some problems, Minitab will simply print a p-value of 0. In that event, the first nine decimal places are all zero! You may report $p < .0000000005$, $p \approx 0$, or even $p < .001$.

FIGURE **13.2.1**
Minitab session for the
chisquared test for
independence of
attributes for the age
at entry versus
day-care center for the
CMV study (Examples
13.2.1, 3, 4, and 6).

```
MTB > CHISQUARED C1 - C3

Expected counts are printed below observed counts

                A         B         C      Total
     1         29        35        10         74
             30.41     20.61     22.98

     2         14         6         3         23
              9.45      6.41      7.14

     3         18        11        21         50
             20.55     13.93     15.53

     4         29         9        34         72
             29.59     20.05     22.36

  Total        90        61        68        219

ChiSq =    0.065 + 10.044 +  7.329 +
           2.188 +  0.026 +  2.402 +
           0.316 +  0.615 +  1.931 +
           0.012 +  6.094 +  6.064 = 37.086
df = 6

MTB > NOTE p-value
MTB > CDF 37.086 K1;
SUBC> CHIS 6.
MTB > LET K1 = 1 - K1
MTB > PRINT K1 #K1 contains the p-value.
K1       0.000001669
```

In Example 13.2.6, we reject the null hypothesis that the attributes are independent. Consequently, the proportion of children of a given age is not the same between day-care centers. A natural follow-up inquiry is, Where are the discrepancies? What age-group is overrepresented or underrepresented at what day-care center? For insight into such an inquiry, we examine the meaning of chisquared.

A cell's chisquared value is a measure of the "statistical distance" between the observed and expected frequencies. A small chisquared value indicates that the observed and expected frequencies are close together. A large chisquared value indicates that the observed and expected frequencies are far apart. The (total) sample chisquared value then gives a composite "goodness of fit" measure for the whole study.

When is a sample chisquared value large enough to indicate a mismatch between the observed and expected frequencies? That's where the level of significance (LOS) comes in. Let's continue our analysis of Example 13.2.6 (Figure 13.2.1) at the usual 5% LOS. The test critical value is obtained from Table 12 (Appendix). Using the 5% LOS and $df = 6$, we obtain the critical chisquared value of 12.5916. Since the sample chisquared value of 37.086 exceeds the test critical value of 12.5916, we reject the null hypothesis of independence of attributes. Much like ANOVA, the chisquared test for independence of attributes can identify that a dependency (interaction, relationship) occurs, but does not specify exactly which attributes are involved.

For guidance as to what attributes are involved when factors are found to interact, we reexamine Minitab's output (Figure 13.2.1). In particular, we focus on the ChiSq computation cell by cell, looking for those cells with the largest ChiSq values. Most noticeable are cells 2 and 3 in row 1 (with ChiSq values of 10.044 and 7.329), and cells 2 and 3 in row 4 (with ChiSq values of 6.094 and 6.064).

Although no one cell has a cell chisquared value exceeding the critical value 12.5916, note that cells 2 and 3 in row 1 have a combined chisquared value of 10.044 + 7.329 = 17.373. These two cells by themselves are enough to reject the null hypothesis of independence of attributes. Altogether, at a minimum, one would need to remove cells 2 and 3 in row 1, and cells 2 and 3 in row 4 in order to bring the sample chisquared value down below the critical value. We conclude that day-care center A has more children than expected under the age of 2 years, while day-care center C has fewer such children than expected. Similarly, center B has fewer children than expected of age 4 or older, while center C has more such children than expected.

EXAMPLE 13.2.7 We conduct a chisquared test of hypothesis to determine whether the attributes for age at entry and excreting CMV are independent of each other (Examples 13.2.2 and 5). Specifically, we inquire whether the proportion of children excreting CMV is the same in all four of the age-groups. Formally,

H_0: Age at entry and excreting CMV are independent factors.
H_a: Age at entry and excreting CMV interact.

Minitab's output for this chisquared test is given in Figure 13.2.2.

The sample size is sufficiently large. All expected frequencies are greater than 1, and only one cell of eight (12.5%) has an expected frequency less than 5. Since all expected frequencies are at least 1 and the proportion of cells with an expected frequency less than 5 is under 20%, we may proceed with the chisquared test for independence of attributes.

FIGURE **13.2.2**
Minitab output for the chisquared test for independence of attributes for the age at entry versus excreting CMV factors in the CMV study (Examples 13.2, 5, and 7).

```
MTB > CHISQUARED C1 C2

Expected counts are printed below observed counts

              Yes        No      Total
     1         16        58        74
            10.81     63.19

     2          8        15        23
             3.36     19.64

     3          6        44        50
             7.31     42.69

     4          2        70        72
            10.52     61.48

Total         32       187       219

ChiSq =   2.488 +  0.426 +
          6.404 +  1.096 +
          0.233 +  0.040 +
          6.901 +  1.181 = 18.769
df = 3
1 cells with expected counts less than 5.0

MTB > NOTE    p-value
MTB > CDF  18.769  K1;
SUBC> CHIS 3.
MTB > LET K1 = 1 - K1
MTB > PRINT K1    #K1 contains the p-value.
K1        0.000305355
```

Since the p-value is very small, we announce the conclusion. The formal statistical conclusion is that based on the given data, at the 5% level of significance we reject H_0: Age at entry and excreting CMV are independent. Of greater relevance is the corresponding health sciences conclusion:

The proportion of children excreting CMV is different among age-groups ($\chi^2 = 18.8$, $df = 3$, $p = .0003$). In particular, a larger proportion than expected of 2-year-old children are excreting CMV. Conversely, a smaller proportion of 4-year-old children are excreting CMV.

A program for effectively controlling CMV by age-group in day-care centers needs to set the highest priority on 2-year-olds and the lowest priority on 4-year-olds. Since the computations for a chisquared test for independence of attributes can be quite extensive, we engaged Minitab to do them for us. An industrious student may want to perform some tests by hand with a calculator to become thoroughly familiar with the calculations. To perform a chisquared test for independence of attributes by hand, first construct the contingency table. For example, Table 13.2.3 displays the contingency table for day-care center versus age at entry (Example 13.2.4). Then compute the chisquared value for each cell in the contingency table:

$$\text{cell chisquared} = \frac{(\text{observed} - \text{expected})^2}{\text{expected}}$$

The sum of all the cell chisquared values yields the sample chisquared value for the independence of attributes test. The test critical value is obtained from Table 12 (Appendix). The degrees of freedom (df) are obtained as follows. Let r be the number of rows and c the number of columns in the contingency table; then

$$df = (r - 1) \times (c - 1)$$

For example, Table 13.2.3 is a 4-by-3 table (4 rows and 3 columns); hence

$$df = (r - 1) \times (c - 1) = (4 - 1) \times (3 - 1) = 3 \times 2 = 6$$

This matches Minitab's output in Figure 13.2.1 that $df = 6$. From Table 12, at the 5% LOS and $df = 6$, the critical chisquared value is 12.5916. We reject the null hypothesis of independence of attributes if the sample chisquared value is greater than 12.5916. For convenience, we have included Chart 7, which presents the chisquared test for independence of attributes in the usual test of hypothesis format.

EXERCISES 13.2

**Warm-ups
13.2**

Chyou et al studied the risk of cancer and cigarette smoking. A smoking history was obtained from a large sample of Japanese-American men during a 22-year period. These men were born during 1900–1919 and were living on Oahu (Hawaiian Islands) at the time of enrollment into the Honolulu Heart Program in 1965. Data on cancer versus cigarette smoking are shown in Table 13.2.5. Smoking is measured in pack-years (one pack-year is the equivalent of smoking a pack of cigarettes per day for 1 year). The data include cases of cancer from time of enrollment to May 1990. A light smoker is defined as a smoker with less than 31 pack-years of smoking; medium smoker, between 31 and 45 pack-years (inclusively); heavy smoker, more than 45 pack-years.

TABLE **13.2.5** Data
from Chyou et al.

Cancer Site	SMOKING HISTORY				Total
	Never	Light	Medium	Heavy	
Lung	12	33	44	92	
Oral-bladder	37	37	42	36	
Other cancer	270	138	182	136	
No cancer	2025	996	880	738	
Total					

1. What are the two factors of interest displayed in Table 13.2.5?

2. State the attribute list for each factor.

3. Determine the marginal totals for Table 13.2.5.

4. What proportion of the study group never smoked?

5. What proportion of the study group developed cancer during the study period?

Figure 13.2.3 displays Minitab's output for a chisquared independence of attributes test on the data shown in Table 13.2.5.

6. State a suitable null and alternate hypothesis for the chisquared independence of attributes test.

FIGURE **13.2.3** Minitab session for a chisquared independence of attributes test on the Chyou smoking data (Table 13.2.5).

```
MTB > CHISQUARED C1 - C4

Expected counts are printed below observed counts

            Never    Light   Medium    Heavy    Total
      1        12       33       44       92      181
             74.46    38.25    36.47    31.83

      2        37       37       42       36      152
             62.53    32.12    30.62    26.73

      3       270      138      182      136      726
            298.66   153.41   146.27   127.67

      4      2025      996      880      738     4639
           1908.36   980.23   934.64   815.77

Total      2344     1204     1148     1002     5698

ChiSq = 52.392 +  0.719 +  1.556 +113.750 +
        10.423 +  0.742 +  4.226 +  3.215 +
         2.750 +  1.547 +  8.728 +  0.544 +
         7.130 +  0.254 +  3.194 +  7.415 = 218.584
df = 9

MTB > NOTE   The p-value:
MTB > CDF 218.584 K1;
SUBC> CHIS 9.
MTB > LET K1 = 1 - K1
MTB > PRINT K1
K1        0
```

7. What is the observed frequency of oral-bladder cancers among medium smokers?

8. An expected frequency is determined contingent on the null hypothesis that cancer and smoking history are independent. The expected frequency of oral-bladder cancers among medium smokers is calculated by

expected frequency

$$= \frac{\text{(oral-bladder row total)} \times \text{(medium smokers column total)}}{\text{grand total}}$$

$$= \frac{(152) \times \square}{\square} = \underline{\quad}$$

9. What is the expected frequency of oral-bladder cancers among medium smokers displayed in Minitab's output (Figure 13.2.3)?

10. In your judgment, do the observed and expected frequencies shown in Minitab's output look significantly different?

11. What is the sample chisquared value for medium smokers with oral-bladder cancer?

12. What is the sample chisquared value?

13. How many degrees of freedom are there in this statistical design?

14. What is the p-value for the chisquared independence of attributes test?

15. At the 5% LOS, what is the critical value for the test (Appendix, Table 12)?

16. Which groups are overrepresented?

17. Which groups are underrepresented?

18. Is smoking bad for you? Justify your response on the basis of the contingency table displayed in Figure 13.2.3 and the results of the chisquared test.

Problems 13.2

1. Ratner et al presented the data shown in Table 13.2.6 regarding 117 patients at a geriatric nursing facility.

TABLE **13.2.6** Data from Ratner et al.

GALLSTONE DISEASE	SEX		Total
	Male	Female	
Yes	28	17	
No	54	18	
Total			

   a. Complete the two-factor frequency distribution table by presenting the marginal totals and the grand total.
      i. How many males are in the study?
      ii. How many females are in the study?
      iii. How many patients in the study have gallstone disease?
      iv. How many patients in the study do not have gallstone disease?
      v. What is the total number of patients in the study?

   b. Determine the expected frequencies assuming independence of attributes. Present the results in the form of a 2-by-2 contingency table.

   c. Conduct a chisquared test for independence of attributes at the 5% LOS.

2. Ratner et al (see Exercise 13.2.1) also presented the data displayed in Table 13.2.7 concerning age and gallstones in women. At the 5% LOS, are these factors independent?

TABLE **13.2.7** Data from Ratner et al contrasting age and gallstones in women.

GALLSTONE DISEASE	AGE CLASS			Total
	50–79	80–89	≥ 90	
Yes	12	22	20	54
No	9	14	5	28
Total	21	36	25	82

3. Ratner et al (see Exercise 13.2.1) also presented the data displayed in Table 13.2.8 concerning age and gallstones in men. At the 5% LOS, are these factors independent?

TABLE **13.2.8** Data from Ratner et al contrasting age and gallstones in men.

GALLSTONE DISEASE	AGE CLASS		Total
	50–79	≥ 80	
Yes	5	13	18
No	7	10	17
Total	12	23	35

4. (Continued from Problems 2 and 3) Is the proportion of women of aged ≥ 80 with gallstone disease greater than the proportion of men of aged ≥ 80 with gallstone disease?

5. Held et al presented the data shown in Table 13.2.9. Conduct a chisquared test at the 5% LOS to determine whether the factors of duration of dialysis and race are independent.

TABLE **13.2.9** Data from Held et al concerning race and duration of dialysis.

Race	DURATION OF DIALYSIS			Total
	Short	Conventional	Long	
White	74	319	26	419
Black	39	102	8	149
Other	8	29	1	38
Total	121	450	35	606

6. Held et al presented the data shown in Table 13.2.10. Conduct a chisquared test to determine whether the factors of duration of dialysis and nausea are independent.

TABLE **13.2.10** Data from Held et al concerning nausea and duration of dialysis.

Nausea	DURATION OF DIALYSIS			Total
	Short	Conventional	Long	
Yes	43	104	3	150
No	78	346	32	456
Total	121	450	35	606

7. Chavigny and Fischer studied infection in patients with long hospital stays. A convenience sample of 762 patients from two hospitals was studied (Table 13.2.11). Based on the following data, is there any significant difference in infection between the two hospitals?

TABLE *13.2.11* Data from Chavigny and Fischer on infections in two hospitals.

	Contracted Infection	No Contract of Infection
Hospital A	130	210
Hospital B	142	280

   a. Justify your answer by conducting a z-test for comparison of proportions for two populations.

   b. Justify your answer using a chisquared test for independence of attributes.

8. Kline presented a description of the effectiveness of tissue plasminogen activator (tPA) and streptokinase therapies for treatment of myocardial infarction. The article presents the data shown in Table 13.2.12 regarding incidence of bleeding episodes in patients under the two modes of therapy. Conduct a chisquared independence of attributes test to determine whether the factors of mode of therapy and bleeding episode are independent.

TABLE *13.2.12* Data from Kline.

Bleeding Episode	MODE OF THERAPY	
	tPA	Streptokinase
Major	22	23
Minor	25	23
Transfusion	32	29
None	64	71

9. In a study by Cyganski et al of heparin versus saline flushes for heparin lock patency, the number of infiltrations from a 50U heparin wash given q8h was 8 out of 25 washes; whereas, the number of infiltrations from a saline flush given q8h was 5 out of 34 washes. The researchers wondered if there is any significant difference in infiltrations between the two wash methods in heparin lock patency.

   a. Compare the two methods by conducting an appropriate z-test for comparison of proportions between two populations.

   b. Describe the relevant factors with their list of attributes appropriate for this study.

   c. Construct a two-factor frequency table to display the data.

   d. Construct a contingency table based on the factors described in (c).

   e. Perform a chisquared analysis for the study based on the contingency table constructed in (d).

10. Funk et al studied lower limb ischemia related to use of the intra-aortic balloon pump. They reported that of 72 women in the study, 46 presented lower limb ischemia; of 168 men, 68 reported lower limb ischemia. We inquire whether the occurrence of lower limb ischemia in intra-aortic balloon pump patients is related to gender.

   a. Conduct an analysis based on conducting an appropriate z-test for comparison of proportions between two populations.

   b. Conduct an analysis based on the chisquared test for independence of attributes.

   c. What do you think: Is the occurrence of lower limb ischemia in intra-aortic balloon pump patients related to gender?

Problems 11–15 are based on research by Rovner et al, who studied depression among patients in nursing homes (see Example 13.1.2). They contrasted depression against a number of factors, including race, gender, presence of dementia, past mental health care, and 1-year mortality. In each problem, conduct a chisquared test for independence of attributes to determine whether the depression factor is related to the other factor.

11. The data for depression and race are displayed in Table 13.2.13.

TABLE *13.2.13* Data from Rovner et al contrasting depression with race.

Race	Depression Disorder	Depression Symptoms	No Depression
White	52	77	299
Nonwhite	5	5	16

12. The data for depression and gender are displayed in Table 13.2.14.

TABLE *13.2.14* Data from Rovner et al contrasting depression with gender.

Gender	Depression Disorder	Depression Symptoms	No Depression
Female	44	61	46
Male	13	21	69

13. The data for depression and dementia are displayed in Table 13.2.15.

TABLE **13.2.15** Data from Rovner et al contrasting depression with dementia.

Dementia	Depression Disorder	Depression Symptoms	No Depression
Yes	35	45	227
No	22	37	88

14. The data for depression and a history of past mental health care are displayed in Table 13.2.16.

TABLE **13.2.16** Data from Rovner et al contrasting depression with history of past mental health care.

Past Mental Health Care	Depression Disorder	Depression Symptoms	No Depression
Yes	18	20	50
No	39	62	265

15. The data for depression and 1-year survivorship are displayed in Table 13.2.17.

TABLE **13.2.17** Data from Rovner et al contrasting depression with 1-year survivorship.

1-Year Survival	Depression Disorder	Depression Symptoms	No Depression
Yes	27	20	94
No	30	62	221

16. Klerman et al provided the data shown in Table 13.2.18 in reporting their research on panic attacks in the community. The panic factor contained four groups (attributes). The first group included all subjects diagnosed with a panic disorder at some time in their lives. The second group contained subjects who had panic attacks without meeting the criteria for panic disorder. The third group contained subjects who had psychiatric disorders other than panic disorder or panic attacks. The fourth group contained subjects who had none of these disorders. Is the panic factor related to site?

17. Clochesy et al reported on their study of electrode site preparation techniques. They compared the offset potential across electrode pairs using four different skin preparation techniques (SPTs). A decrease in offset potential from the controlled to the prepared site was considered beneficial. There were 30 subjects in each of four treatment groups. The data are shown in Table 13.2.19. For example, of the 30 subjects using skin preparation technique 1 (SPT-1), 5 subjects showed no decrease and 25 subjects a decrease in offset potential. Is the proportion of subjects showing a decrease in offset potential independent of the SPT used?

TABLE **13.2.19** Data from Clochesy et al.

Offset Potential	TREATMENT GROUP				
	SPT-1	SPT-2	SPT-3	SPT-4	Total
No decrease	5	12	7	21	45
Decrease	25	18	23	9	75
Total	30	30	30	30	120

18. Shaffer et al studied adolescent suicide attempts. Several high schools participated in the study. Usable results were obtained from 1048 ninth- and tenth-grade students. At introduction to the study, students were given a questionnaire. Items surveyed included race (white, black, other) and an inquiry about whether the student had ever attempted suicide (yes, no). After presentation of a suicide prevention program, students were given a follow-up questionnaire in which the suicide inquiry was repeated. Consequently, students' responses fell into four groups: no-no, yes-yes, yes-no, and no-yes. For example, a student fell in the yes-no group if he or she answered yes on the initial questionnaire but answered no on the follow-up questionnaire. The

TABLE **13.2.18**
Data from Klerman et al.

Site	Panic Disorder	Panic Attacks	Other Disorder	No Disorder	Total
New Haven, CT	60	190	897	3731	4878
Baltimore, MD	47	128	1137	1975	3287
St. Louis, MO	48	84	852	1965	2949
Durham, NC	50	132	1066	2561	3809
Los Angeles, CA	49	133	905	2001	3088
Total	254	667	4857	12233	18011

results are displayed in Table 13.2.20. Are the questionnaire responses independent of race?

TABLE *13.2.20* Data from Shaffer et al.

Race	QUESTIONNAIRE RESPONSES				Total
	No-No	Yes-Yes	Yes-No	No-No	
White	711	49	22	28	810
Black	138	5	7	8	158
Other	61	9	5	5	80
Total	910	63	34	41	1048

19. The preliminary report on the incidence of cancer in 1988 for three northern California counties (Del Norte, Humboldt, and Lake counties) included the data shown in Table 13.2.21 regarding the primary site of the cancer. Based on the given data, is the primary site of cancer independent of county?

TABLE *13.2.21* Cancer in three northern California counties.

Primary Site	COUNTY		
	Del Norte	Humboldt	Lake
Digestive system	20	118	48
Respiratory	24	102	84
Breast	6	68	28
Genitals	8	88	54
Urinary tract	2	56	26
Other	2	106	52
Total	62	538	292

Problems 20–23 are based on research by Klatsky et al, who studied the records of 101,774 people who received health examinations at the Oakland and San Francisco facilities of the Kaiser Permanente Medical Care Program from January 1978 through December 1985. Subjects were followed from the time of their initial physical examination until either (1) the subject left the health plan, (2) the subject was hospitalized for a coronary disease, or (3) December 1986, when the study ended. The median time of study per subject was about 5 years. During that time there were 99,860 noncases (the subject was not admitted to the hospital for a coronary disease) and 1914 subjects admitted to the hospital for a coronary disease.

Of the 1914 admissions for coronary disease, there were 740 admissions for infarction and 1174 for other coronary cases. Of the 99,860 noncases, 9986 (10%) were randomly selected for analysis. Subjects in the study were thus

assigned a coronary classification of either noncase, infarction, or other coronary. This coronary classification was studied against a variety of factors, including gender, coffee consumption, tea consumption, and alcohol consumption.

20. Data for the factors of coronary classification and gender are shown in Table 13.2.22. Are these factors independent?

TABLE *13.2.22* Data from Klatsky et al for coronary classification and gender.

Gender	CORONARY CLASSIFICATION		
	Noncase	Infarction	Other Coronary
Men	4300	513	736
Women	5686	227	438
Total	9986	740	1174

21. Data for the factors of coronary classification and coffee consumption (cups per day) are shown in Table 13.2.23. Are these factors independent?

TABLE *13.2.23* Data from Klatsky et al for coronary classification and level of coffee consumption.

Coffee Consumption	CORONARY CLASSIFICATION		
	Noncase	Infarction	Other Coronary
0	2738	109	236
<1	1384	61	140
1–3	4142	363	536
4–6	1283	153	188
>6	439	54	74
Total	9986	740	1174

22. Data for the factors of coronary classification and tea consumption (cups per day) are shown in Table 13.2.24. Are these factors independent?

TABLE *13.2.24* Data from Klatsky et al for coronary classification and level of tea consumption.

Tea Consumption	CORONARY CLASSIFICATION		
	Noncase	Infarction	Other Coronary
0	5400	422	670
<1	2803	178	258
1–3	1537	121	208
4–6	180	11	25
>6	66	8	13
Total	9986	740	1174

23. Data for coronary classification and alcohol consumption (drinks per day) are shown in Table 13.2.25. Are these factors independent?

TABLE *3.2.25* Data from Klatsky et al for coronary classification and level of alcohol consumption.

Alcohol Consumption	CORONARY CLASSIFICATION		
	Noncase	Infarction	Other Coronary
Never	923	107	162
Former	309	54	78
<3	7895	525	825
≥3	859	54	109
Total	9986	740	1174

Problems 24–25 are based on research by Clapp, who studied delivery among two groups of women. The study enrolled 131 women who were either recreational runners (67) or aerobic dancers (64). All subjects had been exercising regularly for at least 6 months before conception. The women self-divided into two groups. Group A consisted of 87 women (46 runners and 41 aerobic dancers) who continued to exercise at or above 50% of their preconceptual level throughout pregnancy. Group B consisted of the other 44 women (21 runners and 23 aerobic dancers), who stopped their regular exercise routine by the end of the first trimester.

24. Data on the method of delivery are shown in Table 13.2.26. Is there a difference in the method of delivery between the two groups?

TABLE *3.2.26* Data from Clapp for method of delivery.

Method of Delivery	Group A	Group B
Spontaneous	77	22
Forceps	5	9
Cesarean	5	13
Total	87	44

25. Among the 87 women in group A, 82 gave vaginal birth. Of these 82 women, 38 had an episiotomy.

Among the 44 women in group B, 31 gave vaginal birth. Of these 31 women, 25 had an episiotomy. Is there a significant difference between the two groups in the proportion of women giving vaginal birth who have an episiotomy?

26. Coates et all reported the data displayed in Table 13.2.27 concerning breast cancer in black and white American women. Is there a significant difference in stage of cancer at the time of diagnosis between black and white American women? Cancer development is classified from stage I, the least advanced, through stage IV, the most advanced, state of tumor development.

TABLE *13.2.27* Data from Coates et al.

Race	STAGE OF CANCER				
	I	II(N0)	II(N1)	III	IV
Black	63	89	130	87	27
White	95	64	96	44	10

27. Tatemichi et al (continued from Problem 11.1.7) studied the prevalence of dementia in patients, aged ≥60 years, with acute ischemic stroke. There were 610 patients in the study who were testable for the presence or absence of dementia. The researchers classified patients according to age and dementia as shown in Table 13.2.28.

  a. Complete Table 13.2.28.

  b. Is age class related to presence of dementia in patients aged ≥60 who have suffered acute ischemic stroke?

Problems 28 and 29 are based on the gallstones study by Sackman et al (see the introduction to Chapter 12 and Problems 12.2.1–3). Sackman et al studied the long-term results of three types of shock wave treatments for gallstones. The three treatment levels were defined as shown in Table 13.2.29.

TABLE *13.2.28* Data from Tatemichi et al.

Dementia	60–64	65–69	70–74	75–79	80–84	≥85	Total
Yes	13	18	24	25	22	14	
No							
Total	117	145	139	93	67	49	610

TABLE **13.2.29** Treatment groups in the Sackman et al gallstones study.

Group	n	Treatment
A	184	Model GM 1 lithotroper equipped with a water tank; patient partially immersed
B	242	Model MPL9000 with water cushion; low-energy shock wave
C	285	Model MPL9000 with water cushion; high-energy shock wave

The data included the information shown in Table 13.2.30.

TABLE **13.2.30** Data from Sackman et al.

	Group A	Group B	Group C
Women/men (%)	71/29	68/32	68/32
Single/multiple stones (%)	84/16	74/26	87/16

28. Determine whether or not there is there a statistically significant difference between the three groups in gender makeup. Note that in group A there are 71% men and 29% women.

29. Determine whether or not there is there a statistically significant difference between the three groups in single versus multiple stones. Note that in group A, 84% of the patients had a single gallstone and 16% of the patients had multiple gallstones.

30. D'Agostino et al reported on the use of aspirin as a primary prevention of cardiovascular disease (CVD) in a letter to the *Journal of the American Medical Association*. During a regular physical examination, each subject in the study was found to be free of CVD. Aspirin use was noted for 2 years, as was the occurrence of a CVD event. The resulting data are summarized in Table 13.2.31.

TABLE **13.2.31** Data from D'Agostino et al.

Number of Aspirin/Week	Number of Subjects	Number of CVD Events
0	1018	133
1–6	237	20
≥7	170	18
Total	1425	171

a. Construct a two-factor frequency distribution table for aspirin use versus CVD event.

b. Conduct a chisquared independence of attributes test to determine whether aspirin use and CVD events are independent.

c. What do you think; that is, how are aspirin use and CVD events related?

Summary

Chisquared tests are applied for testing a variety of goodness of fit situations. The simple **goodness of fit** test is applied to one-population, one-factor problems. The **independence of attributes** test is applied to one-population, two-factor problems.

In a simple chisquared goodness of fit test, one is supplied with a hypothesized set of factor proportions (**model**). Applying the model to a sample, one obtains a set of expected frequencies to compare with the frequencies observed in the sample. An attribute's chisquared value is computed by (observed − expected)^2/expected. This attribute chisquared value measures the statistical distance between the **observed frequency** and the **expected frequency**. The **sample chisquared value** is the sum of all the attribute chisquared values and is a measure of the goodness of fit between the observed and expected frequencies.

In a chisquared independence of attributes test, one is supplied with two **factors** of interest. The main inquiry is whether the factors are independent or interact in some way. Independent factors can be studied separately. Dependent factors work together and need to be studied together.

A chisquared independence of attributes test is conducted by expanding the original data set from a **two-factor frequency distribution table** into a **contingency table**. A contingency table displays both the observed and the expected frequencies for each cell. The expected value is calculated contingent on the null hypothesis of independence of attributes. Once the contingency table is constructed, the independence of attributes test reduces to a chisquared goodness of fit test.

When the null hypothesis in a goodness of fit test is rejected, although one is informed that a good fit does not exist, one is not informed where the fit breaks down. For analysis into where the fit breaks down, one needs the chisquared critical value associated with a given level of significance. Individual attribute or cell chisquared values are then compared against the critical value in order to sleuth where the fit breaks down.

Keywords

attribute
cell
chisquared test
  goodness of fit
  independence of
    attributes
contingency table
exhaustive list of attributes
expected frequency
factor
goodness of fit

independence of attributes
model
mutually exclusive list of
  attributes
observed frequency
population
proportion
sample size
test of hypothesis
two-factor frequency
  distribution table

References

Chapman S and Duff P: Frequency of glove perforations and subsequent blood contact in association with selected obstetric surgical procedures. *Am J Obstet Gynecol* 168, no. 5 (May 1993): 1354.

Chavigny K and Fischer J: A method of selecting a sample of long-staying hospitalized patients with nosocomial infections as the outcome event. *Heart Lung* 12, no. 1 (January 1983): 15.

Clapp J: The course of labor after endurance exercise during pregnancy. *Am J Obstet Gynecol* 163, no. 6, pt. 1 (December 1990): 1799.

Clochesy J et al: Electrode site preparation techniques: A follow-up study. *Heart Lung* 20, no. 1 (January 1991): 27.

Coates R et al: Differences between black and white women with breast cancer in time from symptom recognition to medical consultation. *J Natl Cancer Inst* 84, no. 12 (17 June 1992): 938.

Cyganski J et al: The case for the saline flush. *Am J Nurs* 87, no. 6 (June 1987): 796.

D'Agostino R et al: Aspirin use and cardiovascular disease in women (letters). *JAMA* 267, no. 3 (15 January 1992): 364.

Funk M et al: Lower limb ischemia related to use of the intraaortic balloon pump. *Heart Lung* 18, no. 6 (November 1989): 542.

Held P et al: Mortality and duration of hemodialysis treatment. *JAMA* 265, no. 7 (20 February 1991): 871.

Keeton W: *Biological Science*. New York: W. W. Norton, 1967.

Klatsky A et al: Coffee use prior to myocardial infarction restudied: Heavier intake may increase the risk. *Am J Epidemiol* 132, no. 3 (September 1990): 479.

Klerman G et al: Panic attacks in the community. *JAMA* 256, no. 6 (13 February 1991): 742.

Kline E: Management of bleeding in the patient receiving thrombolytic therapy for acute myocardial infarction: A nursing perspective. *Heart Lung* 17, no. 6, pt. 2 (November 1988): 771.

Murph J et al: The occupational risk of cytomegalovirus infection among day-care providers. *JAMA* 265, no. 5 (6 February 1991): 603.

Ratner J et al: The prevalence of gallstone disease in very old institutionalized persons. *JAMA* 265, no. 7 (20 February 1991): 902.

Rovner B et al: Depression and mortality in nursing homes. *JAMA* 265, no. 8 (27 February 1991): 993.

Sackman M et al: The Munich Gallbladder Lithotripsy Study. *Ann Intern Med* 114, no. 4 (15 February 1991): 290.

Shaffer D et al: Adolescent suicide attempters: Response to suicide prevention programs. *JAMA* 264, no. 24 (26 December 1990): 3151.

Tatemichi T et al: Dementia in stroke survivors in the Stroke Data Bank cohort. *Stroke* 21, no. 6 (June 1990): 858.

Thompson D et al: Acute myocardial infarction and day of the week. *Am J Cardiol* 69, no. 3 (15 January 1992): 266.

Correlation and Regression

In Chapters 1 through 12 we dealt with univariate statistics; that is, we considered only one random variable (RV) acting on a given population. Even when several RVs were presented, we treated them one at a time. In Section 12.3 and Chapter 13 we began to consider interactions between RVs. Specifically, Section 13.2 studied interaction between two *categorical* RVs (factors) by applying the chisquared test for independence of attributes. In Section 12.3, two-way ANOVA considers the interaction of two categorical RVs with a normal RV. In Chapter 14 we consider interaction between two *continuous* RVs.

When presented with two continuous RVs defined on a population of interest, we make two inquiries:

■ Is there an interaction between the two variables?
■ If so, then what is the nature of that interaction?

Chapter 14 responds to these two questions when there is a linear association between two given variables. Section 14.1 inquires whether or not there is *linear* interaction. Section 14.2 discusses how to determine the equation describing the nature of linear interaction.

Taking measurements is expensive in both time and resources. If we can establish that one measurement is related to another by means of a simple formula, then we can simplify the process of making assessments. Instead of measuring all variables, we may take fewer measurements and then simply calculate the other variables of interest.

In our final chapter we illustrate the concepts needed to study interaction between two variables by working through examples. One set of examples studies two important blood measurements: hemoglobin content and packed cell volume. An inquiry is made whether these two measurements are related in some simple and straightforward fashion. Because of the complexity (and tediousness) of the computations, we invoke Minitab's assistance from the start.

The last set of examples pays a final tribute to the Daily and Mersch cardiac output study. Most of our chapters have exploited this study from one point of view or another—which brings us to a final point to be made. There is no one "right" statistical method to apply to any study. Each of the statistical tools applied to the Daily and Mersch cardiac output study has lent some insight into the problem of accuracy of cardiac output measurements and choice of instrumentation for taking those measurements. As most students have probably discovered along the line during this course, the "math" is the easy part of statistical analysis. The hard part is answering the question, What does it all mean for providing the best care? We hope you find that the statistical tools found in this text provide a valuable resource for providing better care.

Comment ANOVA and regression are intimately related. In fact, ANOVA can be considered to be a special case of regression. For a readable presentation of the details in a health sciences setting, we recommend Glantz and Slinker.

SECTION 14.1

Correlation

OBJECTIVES This section will

1 Describe a paired-data, random effects design.

2 Conduct a correlation analysis when provided with data from a health sciences study that uses a paired-data, random effects design.

Many studies in the health sciences are concerned with how two RVs of interest interact with each other.

EXAMPLE 14.1.1 Bridges et al tested a new instrumentation system for obtaining blood measurements. A convenience sample of 14 female blood bank donors yielded the measurements shown in Table 14.1.1 for blood hemoglobin (Hb) and packed cell volume (PCV).

TABLE **14.1.1**
Data from Bridges et al.

Hb Data	PCV Data
15.5	0.450
13.6	0.420
13.5	0.440
13.0	0.395
13.3	0.395
12.4	0.370
11.1	0.390
13.1	0.400
16.1	0.445
16.4	0.470
13.4	0.390
13.2	0.400
14.3	0.420
16.1	0.450

We inquire about whether or not there is an interaction between the two given variables Hb and PCV when considered in the female population. In this chapter we will be able to assess interaction in a study that incorporates a paired-data, random effects design.

Paired-Data, Random Effects Design

Bridges et al (Example 14.1.1) start with a population of interest (females) and a pair of RVs (Hb, PCV). We present the variables as the ordered pair (Hb, PCV) to stress that both measurements are taken on each subject in the sample. Hence, each subject in the study yields a data pair. Both Hb and PCV are continuous RVs (their measurements are decimal numbers), neither of which is controlled by the researcher. One summarizes these features by saying that the study uses a paired-data, random effects design.

Paired-Data Design

A **paired-data design** is a study design in which two RVs are considered on each member of the population of interest. Consequently, when a random sample is obtained from the population, each subject in the study yields a pair of measurements; hence the term *paired data*. In this chapter we restrict our attention to quantitative RVs (categorical variables were studied in Section 13.2). We will be particularly interested when both variables are continuous (the data sets are made up of decimal numbers). For convenience, we simply refer to a continuous RV as a *variate*.

In Section 7.2 and Section 10.3 we examined paired-data studies that were paired-difference compatible. In those studies it made sense to subtract the two measurements associated with a given member of the study. This subtraction yielded a paired-data difference that was useful in analyzing certain studies, like before and after studies or method A versus method B studies. However, not all quantitative data pairs are paired-difference compatible. In Example 14.1.1 it makes no sense to subtract Hb and PCV. Consequently, we need new techniques for analyzing general paired-data studies.

Random Effects Design

A **random effects design** is a study design in which the researcher does not exercise any control over the variables in the study. In the Bridges et al study (Example 14.1.1), both Hb and PCV are randomly presented by any subject in the study. In contrast, a **fixed treatments design** is a study design in which the researcher fixes the value of one (or more) variable(s) and then records the response of the other variable(s). A study in which a researcher fixes the value of a variable and measures the response in another variable is called an **experiment**. For example, a researcher can conduct an experiment by randomizing a convenience sample into three treatment groups, giving each group a carefully prescribed diet that differs only in a prescribed amount of dietary fat over a fixed time period, and then measuring serum triglycerides. The experimenter is interested in knowing how serum triglycerides are affected by a fixed amount of fat in the diet.

In this section we assess the presence of interaction between two variates in a study using a random effects, paired-data design. As usual, we recall the first rule of applied statistics: Look at the data. The main tool for looking at paired variates is the scatterplot.

The Scatterplot

The injunction to "look at the data" involves more than staring at columns of numbers. Since an investigation about an association between two variates is computer intensive, we invoke Minitab from the start. Of course, the first chore is to enter and check the data. After data entry, we start the investigation by obtaining a scatterplot of the data. A **scatterplot** is a graph of a paired-data sample.

To initialize the process for the (Hb, PCV) study (Example 14.1.1) in Minitab, we first appropriately NAME two columns (here, column C1 and column C2), enter the data (Table 14.1.1) by READing them into those columns, then PRINT and check the data for accuracy. Once the data are entered and checked, request a PLOT. Minitab's output is displayed in Figure 14.1.1.

```
MTB > NAME C1 'Hb Data', C2 'PCV Data'
MTB > READ C1 C2
DATA> 15.5 .45
DATA> 13.6 .42
DATA>  .  .  .
DATA> 16.1.45
DATA> END OF DATA
MTB > PRINT C1 C2
MTB > PLOT C2 VS C1
```

Comment In issuing the PLOT command in Minitab, one must accompany the keyword PLOT with two columns of data of equal length. The first column specifies the vertical, the second column specifies the horizontal. Minitab automatically selects the scaling of the axes. The user may override the automatic features and control several aspects of the presentation of a PLOT. For details, ask for help: MTB > HELP PLOT. If one is working on a computer with graphics capabilities (e.g., a laser

FIGURE **14.1.1**
Minitab's PLOT
of the (Hb, PCV)
data (Example
14.1.1).

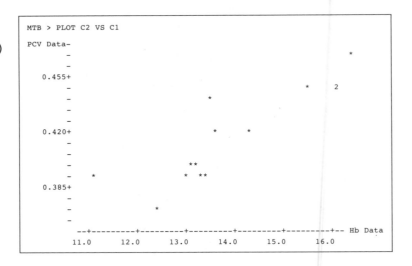

printer is attached) then one may be interested in using the GPLOT (graphics plot) command. Incidentally, the "2" in the data field in the PLOT in Figure 14.1.1 indicates that two points are plotted in the same location.

The scatterplot in Figure 14.1.1 begins to tell an obvious story. PCV is positively related to Hb in that, in general, the larger the Hb, the larger the PCV. As one scans horizontally from left to right, the points in the plot show an upward trend.

In looking at a scatterplot, we inquire whether it seems reasonable to draw a straight line through the field of data points as a general description of the relationship between PCV and Hb. A straight line describes the simplest relationship that can occur between two variates. Can you visualize a straight line representing in general the data on the scatterplot in Figure 14.1.1? To assist in answering this question, it often helps to study an associated centered graphic, the mean enhanced scatterplot.

Mean Enhanced Scatterplot

To get a better sight on the relationship that may exist between the two variates, we enhance the scatterplot by including the mean point $(\bar{x}, \bar{y})$ in the graph. This point is made up of the mean of each data column; hence, the point locates the center of the data points. A graph of the original data along with the mean point is called the **mean enhanced scatterplot**.

To obtain the mean enhanced scatterplot, first COPY the original data into two other columns, then enhance those columns by attaching their respective means. We need to retain the original (unenhanced) data set for other purposes. For example, the following sequence of instructions creates a mean enhanced scatterplot for the Bridges et al data (Example 14.1.1). The output is displayed in Figure 14.1.2.

```
MTB > NAME C11 'Hb', C12 'PCV'
MTB > COPY C1 - C2 INTO C11 - C12
MTB > LET C11(15) = MEAN(C1)
MTB > LET C12(15) = MEAN(C2)
MTB > PRINT C11 C12
MTB > PLOT C12 VS C11
```

Columns C11 and C12 contain the raw data with the mean Hb attached as the last entry in C11 and the mean PCV attached as the last entry in C12. This new data set is called the *mean enhanced data set* since it is composed of the original data set where the sample for each variate is enhanced by its mean value.

Locate the enhanced point on the new scatterplot (Figure 14.1.2) and circle it. Circling the point identifies it as a nondata point inserted by the user for enhancement. Using a straightedge, draw a horizontal line and a vertical line through the mean enhanced point. Both lines should extend through the entire data field. This set of lines imposes a rifle scope on the data with a bull's-eye at the center of the data field. If there is a descriptive straight line for the data, it will pass through the bull's-eye.

It is important to appeal to intuition to feel comfortable with data and for insights to pose questions of interest. In statistics, however, one eventually must apply tests of hypothesis to support or contraindicate those insights. The specific problem posed for

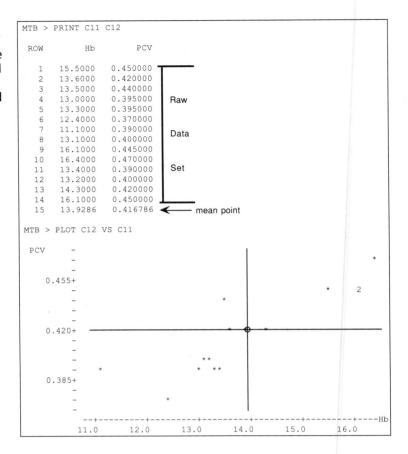

FIGURE **14.1.2**
Minitab's PRINT and PLOT of the (Hb, PCV) blood measurement mean enhanced data set.

```
MTB > PRINT C11 C12

 ROW        Hb         PCV

   1     15.5000    0.450000   ⌐
   2     13.6000    0.420000   │
   3     13.5000    0.440000   │
   4     13.0000    0.395000   │ Raw
   5     13.3000    0.395000   │
   6     12.4000    0.370000   │
   7     11.1000    0.390000   │ Data
   8     13.1000    0.400000   │
   9     16.1000    0.445000   │
  10     16.4000    0.470000   │
  11     13.4000    0.390000   │ Set
  12     13.2000    0.400000   │
  13     14.3000    0.420000   │
  14     16.1000    0.450000   └
  15     13.9286    0.416786   ◄─── mean point

MTB > PLOT C12 VS C11

 PCV     -
         -
         -
 0.455+                                              *
         -
         -                          *            *     2
         -                        *
         -
 0.420+  ───────────────────────────⊕──*──────
         -
         -                      * *
         -                   *   * *
 0.385+
         -
         -              *
         -
         --+---------+---------+---------+---------+---------+----Hb
          11.0      12.0      13.0      14.0      15.0      16.0
```

us here is whether or not a straight line can act as a general representation for the data. Is the straight line we see real? Or perhaps our vision isn't sharp enough to see clearly. We need a technical measure that can assess the straightness of the points in a scatterplot. The simplest such measure is correlation.

Sample Correlation

Correlation is a statistical measure of the strength of a *linear* relationship between paired data. We investigate this relationship as it applies to the sample (the given data). Correlation in a sample of paired data is called the **sample correlation**. One obtains the sample correlation in Minitab by issuing the CORRELATION command. To obtain the sample correlation for the Bridges et al data (Example 14.1.1),

```
MTB > CORRELATION C1 AND C2
```

In response, Minitab displays the sample (Hb, PCV) correlation:

Correlation of Hb data and PCV data $= .877$

The number .877 is the sample (Hb, PCV) correlation. It is a measure of the linear relationship between the (Hb, PCV) data pairs. The sample correlation is usually denoted by *r*. Here, $r = .877$.

Correlation may be thought of as a special ruler that measures straightness in a scatterplot. The ruler extends from -1 to $+1$ inclusively (correlation is always between -1 and 1). The measure of straightness implied by *r* for a general pair of variates (X, Y) is: if

$r = 1$, then there is a perfect positive linear relation;
$0 < r < 1$, then *Y* tends to increase as *X* increases;
$r = 0$, then *Y* and *X* are not linearly related;
$-1 < r < 0$, then *Y* tends to decrease as *X* increases;
$r = -1$, then there is a perfect negative linear relation.

When $r = 1$, then there is a perfect positive linear relation; that is, all the data points fit exactly on a straight line that slopes upward. When $r = -1$, then there is a perfect negative linear relation; that is, all the data points fit exactly on a straight line that slopes downward. The more compactly the data points lie about a straight line, the closer the magnitude of *r* is to 1; the more scattered the points, the closer *r* is to 0. The general nature of correlation is portrayed in Figure 14.1.3.

Comment An industrious student may want to calculate a sample correlation by hand. In general, suppose one is given a data set for the pair (X, Y) of variates. The formula for calculating the sample correlation *r* is

$$r = \frac{n\Sigma xy - \Sigma x \Sigma y}{\sqrt{[n\Sigma x^2 - (\Sigma x)^2][n\Sigma y^2 - (\Sigma y)^2]}}$$

In order to organize the calculation for *r*, we recommend the student use the worksheet displayed in Table 14.1.2. The *x* and *y* columns represent the given data set. The other columns need to be computed. The various sums are then substituted into the formula to calculate *r*.

TABLE **14.1.2**
Worksheet template for computing the sample when given a data set of paired data.

x	y	xy	x^2	y^2
Σx	Σy	Σxy	Σx^2	Σy^2

As with all cases, a statistic (number based on a sample, like *r*) is a point estimate of a corresponding parameter (measure in the population as a whole, like ρ). We now inquire what the sample correlation allows us to infer about the population correlation.

Population Correlation

The purpose of studying a sample is to allow us to make inferences about the population as a whole. The **population correlation** is simply the correlation in the population. The sample correlation, *r*, is a point estimate of the population correlation based on the sample. The population correlation is denoted by ρ (rho, the Greek *r*).

FIGURE **14.1.3** (a)
Perfect positive linear
correlation; all points
lie exactly on an
upward-sloping
straight line. (b)
Positive linear
correlation; *y* tends to
increase as *x* increases.
(c) Zero linear
correlation; it would
take more arrogance
than intelligence to
force a representative
straight line through
this complete scatter
of points. (d) Zero
linear correlation; the
points fit perfectly on
a nonlinear curve. (e)
Perfect negative linear
correlation; all points
lie exactly on a
downward straight
line. (f) Negative linear
correlation; *y* tends to
decrease as *x*
increases.

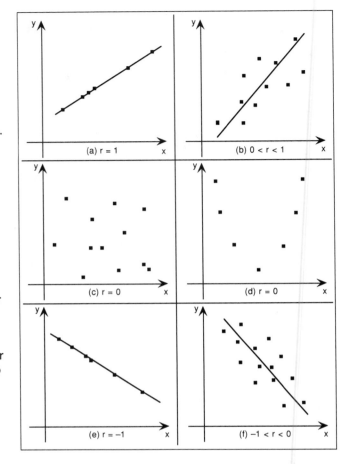

If $\rho = 0$, then there is no linear correlation in the population as a whole. Hence, the natural technical inquiry, Is the sample correlation significantly different from zero? If no, then the sample is unable to detect a linear relationship between the two given variates. If yes, then the sample is detecting linearity in the population at large.

To determine whether an inference of linear correlation in the population is reasonable based on the given data, we test the hypothesis $H_0: \rho = 0$ versus $H_a: \rho \neq 0$. If the null hypothesis is rejected, then the sample provides evidence for linear correlation between the variates of interest. The formal protocol for this test is presented in Chart 9 (Appendix). For example, the (Hb, PCV) data provide evidence for positive linear correlation ($r = .877, p < .01$). A formal write-up for the (Hb, PCV) data is given in Figure 14.1.4.

Comment The technical preliminary assumption for our correlation test of hypothesis is that the paired variates possess what is called a "bivariate normal distribution," which is a three-dimensional analogue of a normal distribution. However, there is no test for bivariate normality. When a pair of variates is bivariate normal, then each

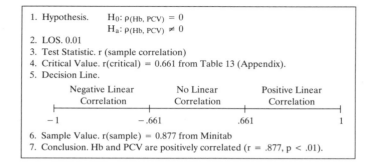

FIGURE **14.1.4** Test of hypothesis for a linear relationship for (Hb, PCV).

1. Hypothesis. $H_0: \rho_{(Hb, PCV)} = 0$
               $H_a: \rho_{(Hb, PCV)} \neq 0$
2. LOS. 0.01
3. Test Statistic. r (sample correlation)
4. Critical Value. r(critical) = 0.661 from Table 13 (Appendix).
5. Decision Line.

Negative Linear Correlation	No Linear Correlation	Positive Linear Correlation

-1 $-.661$ $.661$ 1

6. Sample Value. r(sample) = 0.877 from Minitab
7. Conclusion. Hb and PCV are positively correlated (r = .877, p < .01).

variate individually is normal. Hence, we will be content with a preliminary testing of each variate for normality. If both variates pass normality, then announce that you are assuming a bivariate normal distribution. If one (or both) of the variates is nonnormal, then the test presented in Chart 9 should not be applied. In Figure 14.1.4, both the Hb and PCV have been previously shown to be consistent with normality. Hence, we assume that (Hb, PCV) has a bivariate normal distribution.

In a health sciences study, one seldom measures just one variate on a subject; more frequently, several variates are measured. Which variates are related? One obtains insights with correlation analysis. The prospect, however, of performing correlation analysis on just two variates at a time seems intimidating. For example, if a study has five variates of interest, then there are ten possible pairwise combinations (C(5, 2) = 10). Fortunately, the correlation command in Minitab accomplishes all this at once.

EXAMPLE 14.1.2 Diesel et al studied patients with end-stage renal disease receiving hemodialysis. They reported data (Table 14.1.3) from a convenience sample of ten patients on several variates, including height (m), weight (kg), hemoglobin (g/liter), hematocrit (%), and total hemoglobin content (THC, g).

TABLE **14.1.3** Data from Diesel et al.

Height	Weight	Hemoglobin	Hematocrit	THC
1.55	58.2	83	26	386
1.59	57.0	82	24	374
1.64	56.8	75	23	341
1.64	62.2	75	21	373
1.60	61.3	78	23	383
1.52	51.8	86	26	398
1.64	62.1	91	26	452
1.55	45.1	46	12	166
1.68	59.4	86	25	409
1.51	44.8	110	30	394

A Minitab session giving all ten sample pairwise correlations is displayed in Figure 14.1.5.

FIGURE **14.1.5**
Minitab session for the
Diesel et al data
(Example 14.1.2).

```
MTB > PRINT C1 - C5

ROW   Height   Weight      Hb     Hct      THC

  1     1.55     58.2      83      26      386
  2     1.59     57.0      82      24      374
  3     1.64     56.8      75      23      341
  4     1.64     62.2      75      21      373
  5     1.60     61.3      78      23      383
  6     1.52     51.8      86      26      398
  7     1.64     62.1      91      26      452
  8     1.55     45.1      46      12      166
  9     1.68     59.4      86      25      409
 10     1.51     44.8     110      30      394

MTB > NAME C11 'Nscores'
MTB > NSCORES C1 INTO C11
MTB > CORRELATION C1 AND C11

Correlation of Height and Nscores = 0.987

MTB > NSCORES C2 INTO C11
MTB > CORRELATION C2 AND C11

Correlation of Weight and Nscores = 0.928

MTB > NSCORES C3 AND C11
MTB > CORRELATION C3 AND C11

Correlation of Hb and Nscores = 0.934

MTB > NSCORES C4 AND C11
MTB > CORRELATION C4 AND C11

Correlation of Hct and Nscores = 0.914

MTB > NSCORES C5 AND C11
MTB > CORRELATION C5 AND C11

Correlation of THC and Nscores = 0.828

MTB > CORRELATION C1 - C5

            Height   Weight       Hb      Hct
Weight       0.751
Hb          -0.124    0.065
Hct         -0.094    0.179    0.968
THC          0.255    0.573    0.833    0.884
```

Note the output for CORRELATION C1–C5 in Figure 14.1.5. All ten sample pairwise correlations are neatly displayed. For example, the sample correlation between hemoglobin (Hb) and hematocrit (Hct) is .968. The sample correlation between height and Hb is $-.124$, indicating a negative correlation in the sample; that is, the taller the dialysis patient, the lower the Hb as a rough general tendency. Although this negative correlation occurs in the sample, we cannot infer such a negative correlation for the entire population of end-stage renal disease patients receiving hemodialysis. For a sample of size ten, at the 1% level of significance (LOS) the correlation critical value is .765 (Appendix, Table 13). Since THC is inconsistent with normality, we eliminate this variate from further consideration. Hence, we conclude there is a positive correlation between Hb and Hct. The sample does not provide sufficient evidence for correlation between any of the other variates.

If one retains the null hypothesis $H_0: \rho = 0$, then the analysis at this time is complete. One simply announces that on the basis of the evidence presented by the sample, there is no evidence for a linear association between the given variates. When a sample provides evidence for a relationship, it is then natural to inquire about the precise nature of that relationship. The determination of that linear relationship is made by regression analysis, which is the topic of the next section.

Figure 14.1.6 displays a Minitab session for the Daily and Mersch cardiac output study. In particular, a correlation analysis is conducted between the variates room-temperature cardiac output (RTCO) and Fick (cardiac output measured by the Fick method). The session determines the sample nscores correlations, a scatterplot, the sample means, a mean enhanced scatterplot, and the sample correlation.

Do the Daily and Mersch data for cardiac output comparing RTCO with Fick cardiac output satisfy each of the requirements for correlation analysis specified in Warm-ups 1–5?

1. Paired data

2. Random effects

3. Random sample

4. Normal distributions

5. Bivariate normal distribution

6. Using your intuition, in the scatterplot in Figure 14.1.6, draw a straight line that represents the data.

7. What is the mean RTCO?

8. What is the mean Fick cardiac output?

9. The mean point is (____, ____).

10. Circle the mean point in the mean enhanced scatterplot in Figure 14.1.6.

11. Draw a rifle scope through the mean point in the mean enhanced scatterplot.

12. In the mean enhanced scatterplot, draw a straight line that passes through the bull's-eye and represents the data.

13. What is the sample (RTCO, Fick) correlation?

14. $r = $ ____?

15. $\rho = $ ____?

16. The sample correlation is .842 means

   a. Fick $= .842 \times$ RTCO.

   b. Fick $= .842 +$ RTCO.

   c. Since $.842 < 1$, there is no relationship between Fick and RTCO.

   d. Usually, the larger the RTCO, the larger the Fick cardiac output.

   e. Usually, the larger the RTCO, the smaller the Fick cardiac output.

17. Why does one test $H_0: \rho = 0$ versus $H_a: \rho \neq 0$?

18. At the 1% LOS, what is the critical value for the test in Warm-up 17?

19. Construct the decision line.

20. Based on the given data, what conclusions can you draw about the population correlation, ρ?

Problems 14.1

1. Match the following list of sample correlation values with the graphs displayed in Figure 14.1.7: $r = -1, -.145, .748, .926, 1$.

For the data sets specified in Problems 2–26,

   a. **Construct a scatterplot.**

   b. **Construct a mean enhanced scatterplot and draw in a straight line that appears to describe the paired data.**

   c. **Determine the sample correlation between the given variables.**

   d. **If appropriate, test the null hypothesis H_0: $\rho = 0$.**

2. The Daily and Mersch cardiac output study (Appendix, Data Set 1), iced versus Fick. In the scatterplot, put iced on the horizontal axis and Fick on the vertical axis.

FIGURE **14.1.6**
Minitab session for
correlation analysis of
room-temperature
injectate versus Fick
cardiac output from
the Daily and Mersch
study (Appendix, Data
Set 1). RTCO is con-
tained in column C1
and Fick in column C3.

```
MTB > NSCORES C1 INTO C11
MTB > CORRELATION C1 AND C11

Correlation of RTCO and Nscores = 0.984

MTB > NSCORES C3 INTO C11
MTB > CORRELATION C3 AND C11

Correlation of FICK and Nscores = 0.990

MTB > PLOT C3 VS C1

        7.5+
           -                                         *
    FICK   -                                                  *
           -                                 *
           -                                        *
        6.0+                          *      *
           -                                          2
           -                            *      **
           -          *      *                *
           -                 *                *
        4.5+               *    *    *         *
           -
           -   *        *
           -         *   *        *
           -      *      *
        3.0+   *      *
           -
           +---------+---------+---------+---------+---------+------RTCO
          2.40      3.20      4.00      4.80      5.60      6.40

MTB > LET K1 = MEAN(C1)
MTB > LET K3 = MEAN(C3)
MTB > PRINT K1 K3
K1      4.49621
K3      4.83793
MTB > NAME C5 'Room CO', C6 'Fick CO'
MTB > COPY C1 C3 INTO C5 C6
MTB > LET C5(30) = K1
MTB > LET C6(30) = K3
MTB > PLOT C6 C5

        7.5+
    FICK CO -                                 *            *
           -                                 *
           -                                          *
        6.0+                          *      *
           -                                          2
           -                            *      **
           -          *      *                *
           -                 *    *           *
        4.5+               *    *    *         *
           -
           -   *        *
           -         *   *        *
           -      *      *
        3.0+   *      *
           -
           +---------+---------+---------+---------+---------+------Room CO
          2.40      3.20      4.00      4.80      5.60      6.40

MTB > CORRELATION C1 AND C3

Correlation of RTCO and FICK = 0.842
```

FIGURE **14.1.7**
Five scatterplots are
depicted in graphs
(a)–(e).

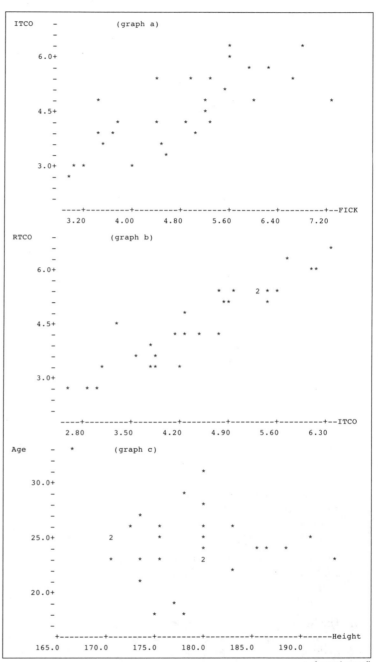

(continued)

FIGURE **14.1.7** (continued)

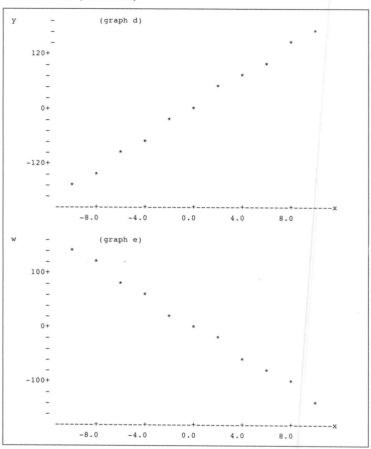

3. The Barcelona et al cardiac output study (Appendix, Data Set 2), prefilled syringes, iced versus room. In the scatterplot, put room on the horizontal axis and iced on the vertical axis.

4. The Barcelona et al cardiac output study (Appendix, Data Set 2), Co-Set, iced versus room. In the scatterplot, put room on the horizontal axis and iced on the vertical axis.

5. The Molyneaux et al coagulation study (Appendix, Data Set 3), 1.6-mL discard, arterial versus venous. In the scatterplot, put arterial on the horizontal axis and venous on the vertical axis.

6. The Molyneaux et al coagulation study (Appendix, Data Set 3), 3.2-mL discard, arterial versus venous.

In the scatterplot, put arterial on the horizontal axis and venous on the vertical axis.

7. The Molyneaux et al coagulation study (Appendix, Data Set 3), 4.8-mL discard, arterial versus venous. In the scatterplot, put arterial on the horizontal axis and venous on the vertical axis.

In Problems 8–16, put start on the horizontal axis.

8. The Bodai et al suctioning study (Appendix, Data Set 4), group 2, routine suctioning (control), start versus end.

9. The Bodai et al suctioning study (Appendix, Data Set 4), group 2, routine suctioning (control), start versus 5 minutes.

10. The Bodai et al suctioning study (Appendix, Data Set 4), group 2, routine suctioning (control), start versus 1 minute.

11. The Bodai et al suctioning study (Appendix, Data Set 4), group 2, oxygen insufflation alone, start versus end.

12. The Bodai et al suctioning study (Appendix, Data Set 4), group 2, oxygen insufflation alone, start versus 5 minutes.

13. The Bodai et al suctioning study (Appendix, Data Set 4), group 3, control, start versus end.

14. The Bodai et al suctioning study (Appendix, Data Set 4), group 3, control, start versus 5 minutes.

15. The Bodai et al suctioning study (Appendix, Data Set 4), group 3, oxygen insufflation with valve adapter, start versus end.

16. The Bodai et al suctioning study (Appendix, Data Set 4), group 3, oxygen insufflation with valve adapter, start versus 5 minutes.

In Problems 17–20, put the 0 time on the horizontal axis.

17. The Shively bed positioning study (Appendix, Data Set 5), group 1, RL 0′ versus RL 1°.

18. The Shively bed positioning study (Appendix, Data Set 5), group 1, S45 0′ versus S45 1°.

19. The Shively bed positioning study (Appendix, Data Set 5), group 2, RL 0′ versus RL 2°.

20. The Shively bed positioning study (Appendix, Data Set 5), group 2, S45 0′ versus S45 2°.

21. The Clark and Hoffer metabolism study (Appendix, Data Set 6), age versus height.

22. The Clark and Hoffer metabolism study (Appendix, Data Set 6), age versus weight.

23. The Clark and Hoffer metabolism study (Appendix, Data Set 6), age versus BMI.

24. The Clark and Hoffer metabolism study (Appendix, Data Set 6), height versus weight.

25. The Clark and Hoffer metabolism study (Appendix, Data Set 6), height versus BMI.

26. The Clark and Hoffer metabolism study (Appendix, Data Set 6), weight versus BMI.

SECTION 14.2

Linear Regression

OBJECTIVES This section will

1 Conduct a linear regression analysis when provided with a sample obtained in a health sciences study based on a paired-data, random effects design.

2 Apply a linear regression equation to predict the output variable when given a value for the input variable.

3 Apply linear regression analysis to resolve a method A versus method B paired-data study in the health sciences.

Correlation analysis establishes whether or not there is a linear association between two given variates. If a linear association is indicated, then the next step is to determine the exact nature of that relationship. The process used to determine the nature of a linear relationship based on data is called regression analysis.

Regression Analysis

When a sample offers evidence that paired variates are linearly related, the next step is to specify the exact nature of that linear relationship. **Regression analysis** is the process of obtaining, displaying, and applying a linear relationship based on a random sample with independent observations. We initiate regression analysis by (1) obtaining the regression equation and (2) imposing the regression line on a scatterplot of the data.

The straight line that best fits a set of paired data as presented in a scatterplot is called the **regression line**. The regression line is the line of best fit in the sense that the variation of the data points about the regression line is a minimum. Variation of the data points about any other straight line will be larger. The equation of the regression line is called the **regression equation**. To conduct regression analysis, we first obtain the regression equation. Once we have the regression equation, we impose the regression line onto the scatterplot by graphing the regression equation.

The regression equation is easily obtained in Minitab by using the REGRESS command. For example, we have already determined that in the Bridges et al blood measurements study (Example 14.1.1), the variables of blood hemoglobin (Hb) and packed cell volume (PCV) are highly correlated (Example 14.1.2). To begin regression analysis based on the (Hb, PCV) data (Table 14.1.1), we issue the following command in Minitab:

```
MTB > REGRESS C2 ON 1 VARIABLE IN C1
```

The resulting output is displayed in Figure 14.2.1.

The regression equation is the first item of output from the REGRESS command. For the (Hb, PCV) data, from Figure 14.2.1 we obtain

PCV data = .183 + .0168 Hb data

This equation is the equation of the straight line that best fits and describes the sample (Hb, PCV) linear relationship.

FIGURE 14.2.1
Minitab's REGRESSion output for the (Hb, PCV) blood measurement data set (Example 14.2.1).

```
MTB > REGRESS  C2  ON  1  VARIABLE IN  C1

The regression equation is
PCV Data = 0.183 + 0.0168 Hb Data

Predictor      Coef       Stdev      t-ratio        p
Constant     0.18318     0.03716        4.93    0.000
Hb Data     0.016772    0.002652        6.32    0.000

s = 0.01489      R-sq = 76.9%      R-sq(adj) = 75.0%

Analysis of Variance

SOURCE         DF         SS          MS         F        p
Regression      1    0.0088686   0.0088686     39.98    0.000
Error          12    0.0026618   0.0002218
Total          13    0.0115304

Unusual Observations
Obs. Hb Data  PCV Data       Fit Stdev.Fit  Residual   St.Resid
  3     13.5   0.44000   0.40960   0.00414    0.03040      2.13R

R denotes an obs. with a large st. resid.
```

We now superimpose the regression line represented by the regression equation onto the scatterplot of the raw data. Recall that in order to plot a straight line, one only needs to obtain two points known to lie on the line. Then, using a straightedge, draw the straight line through those two points. Inspect the original scatterplot along with the data set to locate where two new enhanced points would be easy to spot. If reasonable, *select points just within the left and right edge of the field of data*. Examining the (Hb, PCV) scatterplot in Figure 14.1.1 in tandem with the raw data in Table 14.1.1, we see that extra points located at Hb = 11.5 and Hb = 16.3 would be easy to recognize.

Minitab's given regression equation for the (Hb, PCV) data

$$PCV = .183 + .0168 \times Hb$$

is mainly for display purposes. For purposes of computing, in order to avoid round-off error, use Minitab's full report of the linear coefficients (see Coef column in the regression output in Figure 14.2.1). Hence,

$$PCV = .18318 + .016772 \times Hb$$

is the equation to use for computational needs. Accordingly, we now enhance columns C11 and C12, the columns containing the mean enhanced data set for (Hb, PCV) (see Figure 14.1.2), as follows. The output is displayed in Figure 14.2.2.

```
MTB > LET C11(16) = 11.5
MTB > LET C12(16) = .18318 + .016772*11.5
MTB > LET C11(17) = 16.3
MTB > LET C12(17) = .18318 + .016772*16.3
MTB > PLOT C12 VS C11
```

The PLOT in Figure 14.2.2 displays an *enhanced data set*, that is, a data set augmented with additional points. Here, we enhanced with two points that lie on the regression line at Hb = 11.5 and Hb = 16.3. In addition, the regression line always passes through the mean enhanced point. Circle all enhanced points in the scatterplot as shown in Figure 14.2.2. Using a straightedge through the enhanced points, draw a straight line that fully encompasses the data field. Finally, label the straight line with the regression equation and place the sample correlation in the graphic.

For the Bridges et al blood measurements study, we label the regression line with its display equation, PCV = .183 + .0168Hb. The plot in Figure 14.2.2 summarizes the correlation and regression analysis. The final graphic should display a scatterplot with the regression line imposed on the data, the regression line should be labeled with its equation, and the sample correlation should be conveniently displayed. The resulting graphic clearly shows the positive linear correlation between Hb and PCV.

Comment In Figure 14.2.2, the three enhanced points actually all lie on the regression line. The apparent miss for the mean enhanced point is an artifact of Minitab's default printing mode in a line printer format, in which only lines of characters are printed. Characters cannot be accommodated in spaces between lines. That is why, for example, "straight" lines on some computer screens have a zigzag, lightning-bolt appearance. One can overcome this deficiency with the GPLOT command (GPLOT

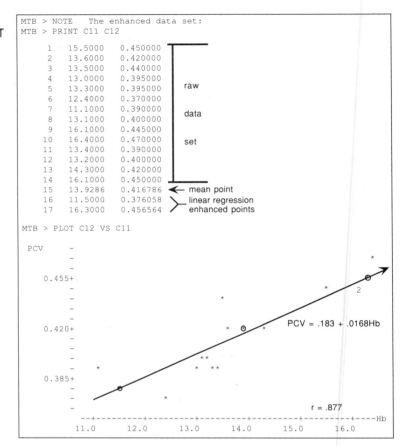

FIGURE **14.2.2**
PRINT and PLOT
of the linearly
enhanced (Hb,
PCV) blood
measurement
data set. The
regression line
is imposed on
the scatterplot
of the data.

means *Graphics PLOT*). However, one needs a printer with graphics capabilities in order to get a high-quality printout. GPLOT output from Minitab using a Macintosh computer with a laser printer is displayed in Figure 14.2.3. The GPLOT command only yields the scatterplot. The straight line, circling of the enhanced points, regression equation, and correlation were imposed on the scatterplot using a drawing program.

FIGURE **14.2.3**
Graphics plot
(GPLOT) for the
(Hb, PCV)
regression
analysis.

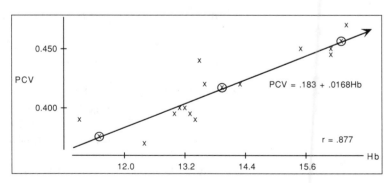

Calculator enthusiasts may want to determine the equation of a regression line by hand. When given a data set for paired variates (X, Y), the equation of the regression line has the form $Y = a + bX$, where a and b are calculated as follows:

$$b = \frac{n\Sigma xy - \Sigma x \Sigma y}{n\Sigma x^2 - (\Sigma x)^2} \qquad a = \bar{y} - b\bar{x} \qquad \text{where } (\bar{x}, \bar{y}) \text{ is the mean point}$$

We recommend the student utilize the worksheet displayed in Table 14.1.2 in carrying out these computations by hand.

Once regression analysis is started, one can further apply the (Hb, PCV) regression equation to predict (calculate) PCV values when given an appropriate Hb value.

Predicting with the Regression Equation

When given a linearly correlated pair of variates (X, Y), a regression of Y against X yields a regression equation of the form $Y = a + bX$, where a and b are the regression **coefficients**. The coefficient a is called the **constant** term; geometrically, it is the vertical intercept of the regression line. The coefficient b is simply called the **coefficient of** X; geometrically, it is the slope of the regression line. Note that in the general equation $Y = a + bX$, one inputs a value for X and calculates the associated value of Y.

For example, in the (Hb, PCV) case, the regression equation applied at Hb = 13.6 yields

$$\text{PCV(Hb} = 13.6) = .18318 + .016772 \times 13.6$$
$$= .411$$

This calculated value for PCV at Hb = 13.6 compares quite favorably with the observed data value of .420 when Hb = 13.6 (see Table 14.1.1, second entry).

Applied at Hb = 16.1, the regression equation yields

$$\text{PCV(Hb} = 16.1) = .18318 + .016772 \times 16.1$$
$$= .453$$

The calculated value .453 compares favorably with the data *mean* PCV of .4475 when Hb = 16.1. In Table 14.1.1, there are two data entries where Hb = 16.1. In the sample data, the (Hb, PCV) value for subject 9 is (16.1, .445); for subject 14, (16.1, .450). The mean of the PCV values for Hb = 16.1 is (.445 + .450)/2 = .4475.

When Hb = 15.0, the regression equation predicts

$$\text{PCV(Hb} = 15.0) = .18318 + .016772 \times 15.0$$
$$= .435$$

This calculation tells us that when a female subject presents Hb = 15.0, we predict by calculation that her measured PCV would be .435. Technically, .435 is the mean PCV of all subjects who have an Hb = 15.0. Not all females with Hb = 15.0 will have PCV = .435. However, the distribution of PCV for Hb = 15.0 is a normal distribution with a (predicted) mean of .435. The word *predicted* here means calculated and based on the given data.

A prediction calculation may be done in Minitab by attaching the PREDICT subcommand to the main REGRESS command. For example, Figure 14.2.4 displays Minitab's output to predict PCV at Hb values 15.0, 13.6, 16.1, and 14.0.

In contrast to the REGRESSion output (Figure 14.2.1), each PREDICT subcommand adds an additional line of output. Now consider the last four lines of output in Figure 14.2.4. These four lines are in response to the four PREDICT subcommands. There are two columns of interest: Fit and 95% prediction interval (PI). The Fit column provides us with the calculated predicted values. In our first PREDICT subcommand, we requested PCV for Hb = 15. The calculated (fitted) PCV is .43476 from Minitab's output. We round to the precision of the given data set; hence, PCV(Hb = 15) = .435. Similarly, PCV(Hb = 13.6) = .411, PCV(Hb = 16.1) = .453, and PCV(Hb = 14) = .418.

The predicted value PCV(Hb = 15) = .435 does not tell us that a particular female subject whose Hb is 15 must have a PCV of .435. The PCV value of .435 represents the *mean* PCV of females whose Hb is 15. For information about an individual female subject with Hb = 15, we report the 95% PI, (.400, .469). In general, a 95% **prediction interval** for Y is the estimated range where 95% of all individual values for Y will occur for a specified (fixed) value of X, based on the given (X, Y) data set. Based on the Bridges et al (Hb, PCV) data set, 95% of all female subjects with Hb = 15 will have a PCV between .400 and .469.

FIGURE **14.2.4**
Minitab output illustrating the PREDICT subcommand.

```
MTB > REGRESS C2 1 C1;
SUBC> PREDICT 15;
SUBC> PREDICT 13.6;
SUBC> PREDICT 16.1;
SUBC> PREDICT 14.

The regression equation is
PCV Data = 0.183 + 0.0168 Hb Data

Predictor       Coef       Stdev    t-ratio         p
Constant     0.18318     0.03716       4.93     0.000
Hb Data     0.016772    0.002652       6.32     0.000

s = 0.01489     R-sq = 76.9%     R-sq(adj) = 75.0%

Analysis of Variance

SOURCE        DF          SS          MS         F         p
Regression     1   0.0088686   0.0088686     39.98     0.000
Error         12   0.0026618   0.0002218
Total         13   0.0115304

Unusual Observations
Obs. Hb Data  PCV Data       Fit Stdev.Fit   Residual    St.Resid
  3     13.5   0.44000   0.40960   0.00414    0.03040       2.13R

R denotes an obs. with a large st. resid.

    Fit  Stdev.Fit         95% C.I.           95% P.I.
0.43476    0.00489   (0.42410,0.44541)   (0.40059,0.46892)

0.41128    0.00407   (0.40239,0.42016)   (0.37762,0.44493)

0.45320    0.00700   (0.43795,0.46846)   (0.41734,0.48907)

0.41798    0.00398   (0.40930,0.42667)   (0.38438,0.45158)
```

There are many details displayed in Minitab's output to the REGRESS command, most of which are of interest primarily to biostatisticians. One item of particular interest is s, which is the sample's estimate of the standard deviation in Y given a particular value of X. One of the consequences of the bivariate normal assumption in correlation analysis is that the standard deviation for Y given a value for X is constant; that is, the amount of variation in Y given a value for X is independent of that value of X. Hence, for any fixed value of X, the distribution of Y is normal with mean as given by the regression equation and standard deviation estimated by s.

For the (Hb, PCV) example, $s = 0.01489$ as reported by Minitab (Figure 14.2.1); that is, $s = 0.015$ rounded to three places like the (Hb, PCV) data. Clinically, this tells us that there is not much variation in (Hb, PVC) points about the regression line. It may be clinically reasonable simply to estimate a healthy female's PCV based on a regression equation, rather than to go through the time and expense of laboratory work for PCV.

The regression equation for the Bridges et al (Hb, PCV) data is a *sample* regression equation. The sample regression equation is the equation for the sample regression line, the straight line that best fits the sample data. Of course, different samples have different regression lines. The main utility of a sample regression line is to serve as an estimate of the population regression line. The population regression line is simply the regression line for the entire population. How much confidence can one put in a sample regression line?

The situation is akin to estimating a population mean μ with a sample mean, $\bar{x}$. The sample mean is a point estimate for μ. A better estimate for μ is a confidence interval estimate, which provides an interval ballpark where μ resides (with a given level of confidence). Analogous to the confidence interval used to estimate μ, one can display a pair of bands around a sample regression line. The bands define a confidence region for the population regression line. Just as the confidence interval for μ is centered around the sample mean $\bar{x}$, the confidence region for the population regression line is centered around the sample regression line. Unfortunately, Minitab does not have a command for constructing a graphic that displays these bands. Figure 14.2.5 displays a confidence band graphic for the Bridges et al (Hb, PCV) data that was created with the assistance of a MyStat statistical package on a Macintosh computer.

Confidence bands are curves that mark the boundary of a confidence region for the population regression line. The bands displayed in Figure 14.2.5 are the 95% confidence bands for the population regression line. Among all possible samples of paired data drawn from the population, 95% of those samples will yield bands that actually contain the population regression line. As always, the associated 5% risk is a natural accompaniment of making an inference about a population based on a sample. A professionally presented graphic of a regression line often displays the 95% confidence bands in the scatterplot.

There are many applications of regression in the health sciences. One application is to relate a pair of otherwise incompatible variates, like PCV to Hb. Another major application occurs in paired-data studies using difference-compatible variates obtained in method A versus method B studies.

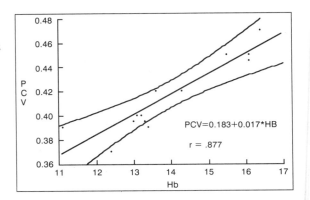

FIGURE **14.2.5**
Confidence band graphic for the Bridges et al (Hb, PCV) data.

PCV=0.183+0.017*HB

r = .877

Regression in Method A versus Method B Studies

Taking measurements is vital in assessing the condition of any patient: Age, height, weight, temperature, pulse, blood pressure, hematocrit, hemoglobin, serum cholesterol, cardiac output only initiate an encyclopedia of possible variates of interest. Measurements are often difficult to obtain. They take time and instrumentation. They can be costly and uncomfortable.

A common study in the health sciences is to determine whether some promising new method can give measurements as accurate as those obtained by some acceptable method. The new method may be simpler in time and mechanics for caregivers, more comfortable and less costly for the patient. The design of choice for researching whether to convert to a new method is the method A versus method B design. The Daily and Mersch cardiac output study (Appendix, Data Set 1) exemplifies this classic design.

Although Daily and Mersch studied three cardiac output methods, we focus on two: Fick and room temperature (RTCO). An ice-temperature injectate is less desirable than a room-temperature injectate from the standpoint of patient comfort, potential for contamination, and ease of administration (accuracy, however, is another matter). The Fick method was defined as the **gold standard**, a method assumed to give an accurate measurement. Accuracy studies frequently choose a method A versus method B design featuring a gold standard versus the new method.

Although considered the gold standard, the Fick method has several disadvantages; it is laboratory intensive, time-consuming, and expensive. By comparison, RTCO can be managed at the bedside by an attending nurse, its results are immediate, and it is less expensive. RTCO is considerably more convenient than the Fick method for hemodynamic monitoring, for both the patient and the caregiver.

To compare Fick versus RTCO, Daily and Mersch engaged a classic paired-data design. They used a convenience sample of 29 cardiac patients for whom cardiac outputs were ordered. Each patient had cardiac output measured by both methods. Hence, each patient yields a pair of measurements, (RTCO, Fick). This design produces a set of paired data obtained from a random sample with independent observations.

In Sections 7.2 (confidence intervals) and 10.3 (tests of hypothesis), we determined that the mean cardiac output determined by the two methods was significantly different. In particular, RTCO in general underestimates cardiac output according to the Fick gold standard. Since the two methods yield measurements that are significantly different, it may seem that RTCO must be rejected as inaccurate. However, this verdict is premature. Perhaps a simple adjustment in the RTCO reading will rescue the method. Accordingly, we apply a correlation and regression analysis. The correlation analysis was conducted in Warm-ups 14.1, where we discovered significant linear correlation between RTCO and Fick (Figure 14.1.6, $r = .842$).

Since RTCO and Fick are linearly correlated, we conduct a regression analysis. In our Minitab worksheet, the RTCO data are in column C1; Fick, column C3. It is extremely important to note that the regression is carried out on Fick versus RTCO (not RTCO versus Fick)! We want to be able to apply an equation that converts a given RTCO to a Fick. An equation for calculating RTCO from a given Fick would be clinically useless (in fact, backward from our clinical need). Hence, we issue

```
MTB > REGRESS C3 ON 1 VARIATE IN C1
```

An edited Minitab output is displayed in Figure 14.2.6.

Although RTCO in general is significantly different from Fick, the regression equation provides a simple equation by which an adjustment can be made. A clinical products manufacturer would apply the regression equation by merely programming the equation into the RTCO monitor, so all the work is done automatically. Based on a correlation and regression analysis, Daily and Mersch concluded, "This study indicates that RT injectate can be accurately used to determine cardiac output, at least in the range studied."

There is an additional point, however, that must be made. At this juncture in our analysis, the regression equation provides a mechanism by which RTCO can be converted to a corresponding Fick measurement. We apply the regression equation to the RTCOs in column C1 to obtain the fitted values in column C5. Column C6 is obtained by subtracting the fitted RTCO from the Fick values to see how much each patient's adjusted RTCO misses the gold standard value (error = Fick − adjusted RTCO). Clinically, one would like a cardiac output reading accurate to within .5. An examination of column C6 reveals the disappointing result that 8 of 29 patients (28%) have an adjusted RTCO that exceeds the .5 tolerance. It is the variation in the error that is causing concern here. The magnitude of the variation in error is indicated by $s = .6505$; that is, the standard deviation of Fick values for a given RTCO appears a bit too large for clinical comfort.

Comment The Daily and Mersch article appeared in *Heart and Lung* in May 1987. Since then, instrumentation for cardiac output has advanced considerably. Currently, room-temperature injectate is the method of choice for determining cardiac output. Recent advances are making notable progress in this area. Two methods are worth special mention. One uses an indwelling cardiac catheter to take *continuous* measurements (measurements can be read every minute). This saves considerable application time and bypasses the difficulties inherent with manual bolus injections. For example, Interflo (Plano, TX) currently markets the *Vigilance* monitor and *IntelliCath*

FIGURE **14.2.6**
Edited Minitab
regression
output for the
Daily and Mersch
cardiac output
study, Fick versus
RTCO.

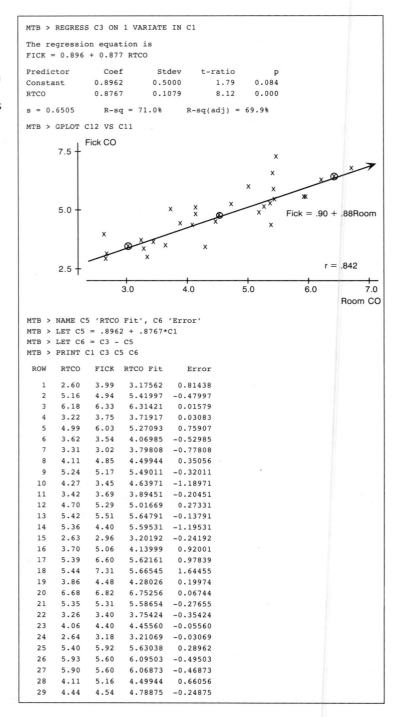

```
MTB > REGRESS C3 ON 1 VARIATE IN C1

The regression equation is
FICK = 0.896 + 0.877 RTCO

Predictor      Coef      Stdev    t-ratio        p
Constant     0.8962     0.5000       1.79    0.084
RTCO         0.8767     0.1079       8.12    0.000

s = 0.6505      R-sq = 71.0%     R-sq(adj) = 69.9%

MTB > GPLOT C12 VS C11
```

Fick CO

Fick = .90 + .88Room

r = .842

Room CO

```
MTB > NAME C5 'RTCO Fit', C6 'Error'
MTB > LET C5 = .8962 + .8767*C1
MTB > LET C6 = C3 - C5
MTB > PRINT C1 C3 C5 C6

 ROW    RTCO    FICK   RTCO Fit      Error

   1    2.60    3.99    3.17562    0.81438
   2    5.16    4.94    5.41997   -0.47997
   3    6.18    6.33    6.31421    0.01579
   4    3.22    3.75    3.71917    0.03083
   5    4.99    6.03    5.27093    0.75907
   6    3.62    3.54    4.06985   -0.52985
   7    3.31    3.02    3.79808   -0.77808
   8    4.11    4.85    4.49944    0.35056
   9    5.24    5.17    5.49011   -0.32011
  10    4.27    3.45    4.63971   -1.18971
  11    3.42    3.69    3.89451   -0.20451
  12    4.70    5.29    5.01669    0.27331
  13    5.42    5.51    5.64791   -0.13791
  14    5.36    4.40    5.59531   -1.19531
  15    2.63    2.96    3.20192   -0.24192
  16    3.70    5.06    4.13999    0.92001
  17    5.39    6.60    5.62161    0.97839
  18    5.44    7.31    5.66545    1.64455
  19    3.86    4.48    4.28026    0.19974
  20    6.68    6.82    6.75256    0.06744
  21    5.35    5.31    5.58654   -0.27655
  22    3.26    3.40    3.75424   -0.35424
  23    4.06    4.40    4.45560   -0.05560
  24    2.64    3.18    3.21069   -0.03069
  25    5.40    5.92    5.63038    0.28962
  26    5.93    5.60    6.09503   -0.49503
  27    5.90    5.60    6.06873   -0.46873
  28    4.11    5.16    4.49944    0.66056
  29    4.44    4.54    4.78875   -0.24875
```

catheter with continuous monitoring capabilities. Gillman, in a recent survey of the current situation, notes that there are five different invasive methods of continuous cardiac monitoring at various stages of development in the United States. Another method uses a bioimpedance approach. Both Renaissance Technologies and Sorba Medical Systems are marketing equipment for *noninvasive* hemodynamic surveillance based on this technology. Accurate noninvasive techniques should yield massive improvements in patient care of coronary patients in need of cardiac output measurements. Statistics guides the development and implementation of new technology.

EXERCISES 14.2

Warm-ups 14.2

Figure 14.2.7 displays a Minitab session for the Daily and Mersch cardiac output study. The session conducts a correlation and regression analysis for Fick cardiac output versus ice-temperature cardiac output (ITCO). From previous work, we assume that Fick and ITCO satisfy the normality assumption. Accordingly, we assume that (ITCO, Fick) has a bivariate normal distribution.

1. What is the critical correlation from Table 13 (Appendix)?

2. Display the correlation decision line.

3. What is the sample (ITCO, Fick) correlation?

4. Do the data indicate significant positive linear correlation?

5. Is linear regression justified?

6. What is the equation of the sample regression line?

7. Why are some points in the scatterplot circled?

8. What Fick cardiac output would you expect for a patient who has an ITCO of 3.26?

9. What Fick cardiac output would you expect for a patient who has an ITCO of 5?

10. In the regression output, s stands for the sample's estimate of the standard deviation of the Fick values given a fixed ITCO. Here, $s =$ ___.

11. Based on the Daily and Mersch data, does ITCO appear to be a suitable replacement for the Fick method of determining cardiac outputs? Explain.

Problems 14.2

1. Conduct a regression analysis for each of the problems you worked in Problems 14.1.

2. Schols et al (see Section 11.2) studied body composition by bioelectrical impedance analysis in patients with chronic obstructive pulmonary disease. For the 32 patients in the study, the authors obtained the regression equation

$$y = 7.17 + .52x$$

where y is total body water in liters and $x =$ Ht^2/res, Ht = body height, and res = electrical body resistance. The sample correlation between x and y was $r = .93$.

a. Test H_0: $\rho_{(X, Y)} = 0$.

b. If $Ht^2/res = 50$, what value would you expect for total body water?

3. Melchior et al studied resting energy expenditures (REE) in 50 malnourished patients with AIDS. A linear regression analysis was performed to determine REE as a function of fat-free mass (FFM).

a. The sample correlation was .72. Test H_0: $\rho_{(FFM, REE)} = 0$.

b. The sample regression equation was REE = 1366 + 126FFM. What is the expected REE of a malnourished AIDS patient with a FFM of 50 kg?

Problems 4–9 are based on data from Tarasuk and Beaton. They reported the data shown in Table 14.2.1 describing a convenience sample of 14 female subjects in their study.

FIGURE 14.2.7
Minitab session for correlation and regression analysis of the Daily and Mersch cardiac output study for (ITCO, Fick).

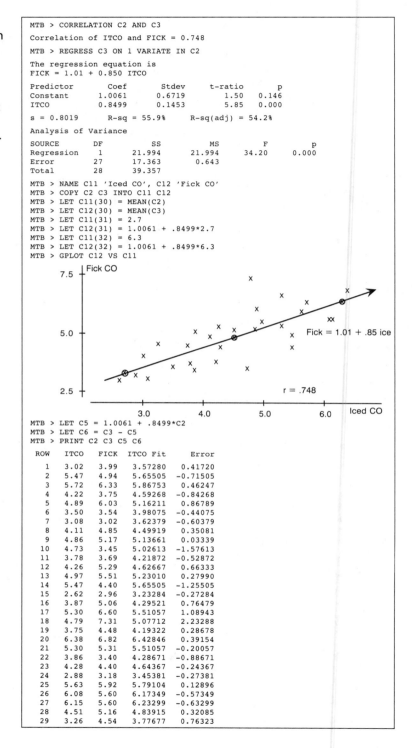

```
MTB > CORRELATION C2 AND C3

Correlation of ITCO and FICK = 0.748

MTB > REGRESS C3 ON 1 VARIATE IN C2

The regression equation is
FICK = 1.01 + 0.850 ITCO

Predictor      Coef        Stdev      t-ratio        p
Constant     1.0061       0.6719        1.50      0.146
ITCO         0.8499       0.1453        5.85      0.000

s = 0.8019      R-sq = 55.9%      R-sq(adj) = 54.2%

Analysis of Variance

SOURCE         DF          SS          MS         F          p
Regression      1      21.994      21.994     34.20      0.000
Error          27      17.363       0.643
Total          28      39.357

MTB > NAME C11 'Iced CO', C12 'Fick CO'
MTB > COPY C2 C3 INTO C11 C12
MTB > LET C11(30) = MEAN(C2)
MTB > LET C12(30) = MEAN(C3)
MTB > LET C11(31) = 2.7
MTB > LET C12(31) = 1.0061 + .8499*2.7
MTB > LET C11(32) = 6.3
MTB > LET C12(32) = 1.0061 + .8499*6.3
MTB > GPLOT C12 VS C11
```

Fick CO

Fick = 1.01 + .85 ice

r = .748

Iced CO

```
MTB > LET C5 = 1.0061 + .8499*C2
MTB > LET C6 = C3 - C5
MTB > PRINT C2 C3 C5 C6

ROW    ITCO    FICK    ITCO Fit      Error

  1    3.02    3.99    3.57280     0.41720
  2    5.47    4.94    5.65505    -0.71505
  3    5.72    6.33    5.86753     0.46247
  4    4.22    3.75    4.59268    -0.84268
  5    4.89    6.03    5.16211     0.86789
  6    3.50    3.54    3.98075    -0.44075
  7    3.08    3.02    3.62379    -0.60379
  8    4.11    4.85    4.49919     0.35081
  9    4.86    5.17    5.13661     0.03339
 10    4.73    3.45    5.02613    -1.57613
 11    3.78    3.69    4.21872    -0.52872
 12    4.26    5.29    4.62667     0.66333
 13    4.97    5.51    5.23010     0.27990
 14    5.47    4.40    5.65505    -1.25505
 15    2.62    2.96    3.23284    -0.27284
 16    3.87    5.06    4.29521     0.76479
 17    5.30    6.60    5.51057     1.08943
 18    4.79    7.31    5.07712     2.23288
 19    3.75    4.48    4.19322     0.28678
 20    6.38    6.82    6.42846     0.39154
 21    5.30    5.31    5.51057    -0.20057
 22    3.86    3.40    4.28671    -0.88671
 23    4.28    4.40    4.64367    -0.24367
 24    2.88    3.18    3.45381    -0.27381
 25    5.63    5.92    5.79104     0.12896
 26    6.08    5.60    6.17349    -0.57349
 27    6.15    5.60    6.23299    -0.63299
 28    4.51    5.16    4.83915     0.32085
 29    3.26    4.54    3.77677     0.76323
```

TABLE **14.2.1** Data from Tarasuk and Beaton.

Subject	Age (years)	Height (cm)	Weight (kg)
1	21	165	56
2	21	150	46
3	39	160	56
4	35	158	49
5	35	171	70
6	39	157	50
7	24	166	68
8	38	164	59
9	47	165	70
10	25	162	55
11	42	157	50
12	41	160	106
13	21	158	46
14	20	151	49

4. Check age, height, and weight for normality.

5. Determine the mean ± standard deviation for each variate.

6. Determine a 95% confidence interval for each variate.

7. Conduct a correlation and regression analysis on age versus height.

8. Conduct a correlation and regression analysis on age versus weight.

9. Conduct a correlation and regression analysis on height versus weight.

Problems 10–14 are based on research by Bashir et al. Data were obtained from a convenience sample of 18 patients requiring an intracardiac electrophysiological examination as part of a routine investigation of rhythm disorders. All subjects had normal ventricular function. The following data report systolic and diastolic blood pressures:

140/90	110/70	160/90	150/100	130/90
130/80	130/100	120/70	125/70	110/60
130/80	100/70	130/80	140/70	130/70
115/75	120/80	125/70		

10. Check both systolic and diastolic blood pressure for normality.

11. Determine the mean ± standard deviation for each variate.

12. Determine a 95% confidence interval for each variate.

13. Conduct a correlation and regression analysis on systolic versus diastolic blood pressure.

14. Based on these data, how reasonable do you feel it would be to calculate diastolic pressure based on the systolic pressure?

15. Medley et al studied thermodilution cardiac output. The pulmonary artery catheter provides the access for most cardiac output measurements. Common catheters have a variety of lumens (small tubes leading into the heart) for various functions. For example, the Swan-Ganz VIT thermodilution pulmonary artery catheter features a proximal injectate lumen and a proximal infusion lumen. The proximal injectate lumen is there specifically to act as the infusion port for the bolus injectate for cardiac output determinations. However, on occasion, this lumen may become occluded or pre-empted for infusion of medications. Medley et al inquired whether under such circumstances the proximal infusion lumen could serve as a satisfactory substitute for the proximal injectate lumen.

Incorporating a paired-data design, Medley et al used a convenience sample of 21 critically ill patients who already had a Swan-Ganz VIP thermodilution pulmonary artery catheter in place. Cardiac outputs were obtained using an ice-temperature injectate for both lumens in each of the 21 patients in the study. The results are displayed in Table 14.2.2. Based on this study, would you recommend the proximal infusion lumen as a suitable substitute for the proximal injectate lumen for the purpose of cardiac output determination?

TABLE **14.2.2** Data from Medley et al on cardiac output (liters/minute) in critically ill patients.

Patient	Injectate Lumen	Infusion Lumen
1	9.85	9.21
2	5.15	5.20
3	10.39	11.36
4	4.58	4.78
5	4.21	4.39
6	6.79	6.04
7	11.98	11.72
8	4.35	4.58
9	10.76	11.76
10	5.69	5.52
11	7.82	6.54
12	9.37	10.37
13	6.93	7.32
14	15.95	13.43
15	7.93	8.82
16	6.18	5.72
17	6.35	5.85
18	2.41	3.10
19	4.40	4.07
20	5.84	5.52
21	8.67	9.24

Summary

When presented with two continuous random variables (**variates**) of interest on a given population, one inquires whether there is an association between them. In particular, can knowledge of the value of one variate be used to calculate the value of the other variate? The simplest relationship between two variates occurs when they are linearly related; that is, one variable is a linear function of the other. Analysis to determine whether two variates are linearly related is called **correlation analysis**.

Correlation is a population parameter that measures the degree of linear association between variates in members of the population. One estimates the population correlation by obtaining a random sample with independent paired observations and calculating the sample correlation. The sample correlation is simply a measure of linearity in the sample. One performs a test of hypothesis to determine whether the amount of correlation in the sample is statistically significant.

Paired variates (X, Y) can be visualized in a scatterplot. A **scatterplot** is a graph of a paired data set. One examines the scatterplot for a sense of correlation. Zero correlation means that there is no *straight line* (linear) relationship between the given variates. When the paired data points lie perfectly on a straight line, then correlation is 1 for perfect positive linear correlation and -1 for perfect negative linear correlation. The variates (X, Y) are said to be **positively correlated** when, in general, Y tends to increase as X increases. The variates (X, Y) are said to be **negatively correlated** when, in general, Y tends to decrease as X increases.

When paired variates (X, Y) are correlated, they can be related by means of a linear equation: $Y = a + bX$. The numbers a and b are called **coefficients** in the equation. The linear equation $Y = a + bX$ is called the **regression equation**. The graph of the regression equation is a straight line called the **regression line**. The sample regression line is that straight line which best fits and describes the linear association present in a paired data set. The sample regression line always passes through the mean point of the data set. The project of obtaining, displaying, and applying the regression line is called **regression analysis**.

Correlation and regression analysis may be conducted on a data set obtained from a random sample with independent observations within a study using a **paired-data, random effects design**, where the pair of variates follow a bivariate normal distribution. A **bivariate normal distribution** is a three-dimensional analogue of a normal distribution.

Correlation and regression analysis have many applications in the health sciences. Such analysis is especially applicable in studies involving a **method A versus method B study**. A decision regarding whether or not to adopt a new technique for making measurements frequently is made on the basis of correlation and regression analysis.

Keywords

bivariate normal distribution	negative linear correlation
coefficient	normal distribution
confidence bands	paired-data design
constant term	population correlation
continuous random variable	positive linear correlation
correlation	prediction interval
experiment	random effects design
fixed treatments design	regression
gold standard	analysis
linear correlation	equation
mean enhanced	line
data set	sample correlation
scatterplot	scatterplot
method A versus method	variate
B study	

References

Bashir Y et al: The electrophysiological effects of flosequinan. *Eur Heart J* 12, no. 12 (December 1991): 1288.

Bridges N et al: Evaluation of a new system for hemoglobin measurement. *Am Clin Prod Rev* (April 1987): 22.

Daily E and Mersch J: Thermodilution cardiac outputs using room and ice temperature injectate: Comparison with the Fick method. *Heart Lung* 16, no. 3 (May 1987): 294.

Diesel W et al: Isokinetic muscle strength predicts maximum exercise tolerance in renal patients on chronic hemodialysis. *Am J Kidney Dis* 16, no. 2 (August 1990): 109.

Gillman P: Continuous measurement of cardiac output: A milestone in hemodynamic monitoring. Focus on Critical Care 19, no. 2 (April 1992): 155.

Glantz S and Slinker B: *Primer of Applied Regression and Analysis of Variance*. New York: McGraw-Hill, 1990.

Medley R: Comparability of the thermodilution cardiac output method: Proximal injectate versus proximal infusion lumens. *Heart Lung* 21, no. 1 (January 1992): 12.

Melchior J et al: Resting energy expenditure is increased in stable, malnourished HIV infected patients. *Am J Clin Nutr* 53 (February 1991): 437.

Tarasuk V and Beaton G: Menstrual cycle patterns in energy and macronutrient intake. *Am J Clin Nutr* 53 (February 1991): 442.

An Orientation to Multi-Faceted Statistics
A REVIEW

Commonplace questions in the health sciences not only present major areas of current research but also touch areas of interest in individual practice.

- Is susceptibility to various bacterial infections related to a certain genetic defect?
- Are serious side effects of drug therapy related to abnormal plasma chemistry?
- Is iron deficiency in infants related to infant formulas used in standard feeding regimens?
- Is 5-year survivorship in lung cancer patients related to ABO blood type?
- Is survivorship in aged burn patients related to the percent of body surface area involved in the burn?

The previous five questions all have something in common: Research motivated by obtaining answers to them is concerned with several items simultaneously.

- There are several bacterial infections of concern (Mediterranean spotted fever, typhoid, meningitis).
- Plasma chemistry may need to take into account the relationship between free and total carnitine in patients on valproic acid therapy.
- Iron deficiency may need to be considered for babies receiving unfortified cow's milk, fortified cow's milk, human milk, or injection supplements.
- There are four ABO blood types: O, A, B, and AB.
- Survivorship may be classified as immediate mortality (≤ 3 days), intermediate mortality (3–48 days), or survive (> 48 days).

Questions involving multiple variates or relationships between them are analyzed by techniques in multifaceted statistics. Part III presents an orientation to three major topics in multifaceted statistics: analysis of variance (ANOVA), chisquared, and regression. These topics are extensions of ideas introduced in Part II: An Orientation to Inferential Statistics.

ANOVA allows one to compare the means of several levels simultaneously. One applies ANOVA to compare a single variate in several populations, or to compare the effect of several treatments in a single population. The keyword here is *several*. A companion to ANOVA is the Mood test for comparison of medians.

Chisquared tests are concerned with proportions. Two standard applications of chisquared tests are goodness of fit and independence of attributes. In goodness of fit tests we inquire whether the attribute list for a factor fits some hypothesized distribution. In independence of attribute tests we inquire whether two given factors act independently of each other. The independence of attributes test is somewhat of a threshold—it is the first time we seriously considered *interaction* between two random variables.

Linear regression studies interaction between two continuous random variables (variates). One inquires how the variates interact or influence each other. The inquiry begins by conducting a correlation analysis to determine whether or not the variates are linearly related. If so, one performs a linear regression analysis to obtain the equation (model) that precisely describes that linear relationship.

We invite you to apply these multifaceted techniques to investigate the questions of concern introduced at the start of this review. Details are provided in the review problems.

PART III Review Problems

Problems 1–8 are based on research by Meloni et al, who studied bacterial infections in people with glucose-6-phosphate dehydrogenase (G6PD) deficiency. This inherited enzymatic defect occurs frequently on the island of Sardinia, where bacterial infections are endemic. From 1976 to 1988, there were 458 children with bacterial infections admitted to the pediatric department of the University of Sassai, the only pediatric hospital in the district serving a population of about 250,000. Of these 458 children with infection, 248 (132 boys) had Mediterranean spotted fever (MSF), 149 (86 girls) had typhoid (T), and 61 (31 boys) had meningitis (M).

1. Construct a frequency distribution table for bacterial infections in northern Sardinian children. Accompany the table with a suitable graphic.
2. Conduct a chisquared independence of attributes test to determine whether the bacterial disease is related to gender.
3. The proportion of G6PD-deficient males in the general population in northern Sardinia is 7.37%. Among the 226 boys with bacterial infections, 17 had G6PD-deficiency. Let p be the proportion of G6PD-deficient cases among boys with bacterial infections. Test the hypothesis $H_0: p = .0737$ versus $H_a: p \neq .0737$.
4. The proportion of G6PD-deficient females in the general population in northern Sardinia is 14.20%. Among the 232 girls with bacterial infections, 28 were G6PD-deficient. Let p be the proportion of G6PD-deficient cases among girls with bacterial infections. Test the hypothesis $H_0: p = .1420$ versus $H_a: p \neq .1420$.
5. Of the 226 boys with bacterial infections, 17 had G6PD deficiency. Of the 232 girls with bacterial infections, 28 had G6PD deficiency. Let p_1 be the proportion of boys with bacterial infections who have G6PD deficiency and p_2 the proportion of girls with bacterial infections who have G6PD deficiency. Test the hypothesis $H_0: p_1 \leq p_2$ versus $H_a: p_1 > p_2$.
6. A two-factor frequency distribution table for G6PD deficiency versus bacterial disease in boys is provided in Table III-1. Conduct a chisquared independence of attributes test to determine whether bacterial disease is related to G6PD deficiency in boys.
7. A two-factor frequency distribution table for G6PD deficiency versus bacterial disease in girls is provided in Table III-2. Conduct a chisquared

independence of attributes test to determine whether bacterial disease is related to G6PD deficiency in girls.
8. What do you think: Are northern Sardinian children with G6PD deficiency at greater risk for bacterial infection than the general population?

Problems 9–18 are based on research by Shapira and Gutman, who studied muscle carnitine deficiency in patients using valproic acid (VPA). Shapira and Gutman were concerned since a major side effect of long-term VPA therapy is an illness similar to Reye's syndrome associated with serum carnitine deficiency. Free and total carnitine for seven patients with seizures treated with VPA therapy are given in Table III-3.

TABLE **III-3** Data from Shapira and Gutman of free and total carnitine levels.

Patient	Free	Total
1	24	31
2	23	28
3	31	35
4	17	25
5	35	44
6	43	55
7	32	48

9. Test free carnitine for normality.
10. Test total carnitine for normality.
11. Determine the sample legend for free carnitine.
12. Determine the sample legend for total carnitine.
13. Determine a 95% confidence interval for free carnitine.
14. Determine a 95% confidence interval for total carnitine.
15. Based on the confidence intervals in Problems 13 and 14, what can you say about comparing the mean values of free and total carnitine?
16. Conduct a paired-difference test to determine whether total carnitine is significantly greater than free carnitine.
17. Conduct a correlation analysis between free and total carnitine.
18. Conduct an appropriate linear regression analysis.

Problems 19–21 are based on research by Pizarro et al, who studied iron status with different infant feeding regimens. Data were collected in Chile from 1975 to 1986 to evaluate the need for iron fortification of the infant formula distributed nationally, but in an unfortified form. The status of 854 nine-month-old infants using three different feeding regimens and another regimen of

TABLE **III-1** Data from Meloni et al for G6PD deficiency versus bacterial desease in boys.

G6PD Deficiency	BOYS		
	MSF	T	M
No	132	63	31
Yes	10	5	2

TABLE **III-2** Data from Meloni et al for G6PD deficiency versus bacterial disease in girls.

G6PD Deficiency	GIRLS		
	MSF	T	M
No	101	74	30
Yes	15	9	4

TABLE III-4 Data from Pizarro et al (mean ± standard deviation).

	Unfortified Cow Milk Formula (n = 405)	Iron Fortified Cow Milk Formula (n = 310)	Human Milk (n = 102)	Iron Dextrose Injection (n = 77)
Hemoglobin	114 ± 11	123 ± 9	117 ± 10	124 ± 7
Erythrocyte protoporphyrin	111 ± 49	87 ± 20	101 ± 36	82 ± 32
Transferrin saturation	10.6 ± 5.6	15.4 ± 7.0	12.9 ± 7.2	20.1 ± 8.2

iron dextrose injection was determined. The data are displayed in Table III-4. Variates measured included blood hemoglobin (g/liter), erythrocyte protoporphyrin (μg/dL RBC), and transferrin saturation.

19. Is there a significant difference in the mean levels of hemoglobin between the four groups?

20. Is there a significant difference in the mean levels of erythrocyte protoporphyrin between the four groups?

21. Is there a significant difference in the mean levels of transferrin saturation between the four groups?

Problems 22–27 are based on research by Miyake et al on the 5-year survivorship of patients with lung cancer. Tissue sections from 149 patients with primary lung cancer were treated with a stain (MIA-15–5). The tissue showed either a positive (MIA+) or negative (MIA−) reactivity to the stain. Each patient was classified according to two factors: MIA activity (MIA+ or MIA−) and ABO blood type (O, A, B, AB). The data are displayed in Table III-5.

TABLE III-5 Data from Miyake et al for ABO blood type versus MIA reactivity.

MIA Reactivity	ABO BLOOD TYPE				Total
	O	A	B	AB	
MIA+	32	35	19	5	
MIA−	11	25	15	7	
Total					

22. Complete Table III-5 by filling in the marginal totals.
23. How many patients in the study had blood type A?
24. How many patients in the study were MIA+ ?
25. Conduct a chisquared test for independence of attributes between ABO blood type and MIA reactivity.
26. Of the 35 MIA+ patients with blood type A, 6 survived at least 5 years. Of the 25 MIA− patients with blood type A, 17 survived at least 5 years. Is there a statistically significant difference in the 5-year survival rate between the two groups?

27. Of 91 MIA+ patients, 19 survived 5 years. Of 58 MIA− patients, 34 survived 5 years.

a. Conduct a z-test for comparison of proportions to determine whether there is a significant difference in the 5-year survival rate between the two groups.

b. Conduct a chisquared test for independence of attributes to determine whether there is a significant difference in the 5-year survival rate between the two groups.

c. How do the results of the z-test and chisquared test compare?

Problems 28 and 29 are based on research by Scholes et al, who inquired about an association between pelvic inflammatory disease (PID) and cigarette smoking. The study included 131 women with PID enrolled in a health maintenance organization (HMO). Controls (n = 294), women with no history of PID, were randomly selected from the HMO files.

28. Scholes et al reported, "More case patients (43.5%) than control patients (25.6%) were current smokers."

a. Construct a two-factor frequency distribution table for PID versus current smoker by completing Table III-6.

TABLE III-6 Data from Scholes et al.

	CURRENT SMOKER		
	Yes	No	Total
PID			131
No PID			294
Total			

b. Test the authors' claim by conducting a z-test for comparison of proportions.

c. Test the authors' claim by conducting a chisquared test for independence of attributes.

d. Does smoking cause PID?

29. Data for PID versus smoking history are given in Table III-7. In the smoking history factor, < 10 represents a current smoker who smokes under 10 cigarettes a day, and ≥ 10 represents a current smoker who smokes 10 or more cigarettes per day.

TABLE *III-7* Data from Scholes et al on PID versus smoking history.

PID	SMOKING HISTORY				Total
	Never	Former	< 10	≥ 10	
Yes	54	11	46	20	131
No	171	21	55	47	294
Total	225	32	101	67	425

a. Conduct a chisquared test for independence of attributes between PID and smoking history.

b. What conclusions can you draw from this chisquared test?

30. (Project) Templin et al conducted a study similar to the Molyneaux study (Appendix, Data Set 3). On each of 30 patients, venous and arterial blood draws were taken in three modes: dead space with no discard volume (DS), dead space with 2-mL discard (DS + 2), and dead space with 4-mL discard (DS + 4). Blood activated partial thromboplastin time (aPPT, a blood-clotting time measurement) was measured for each sample.

Each patient had an A-line (arterial catheter) already in place. Researchers wanted to know if blood drawn from the A-line would provide accurate aPTT measurements. They were concerned that heparin used to keep the A-line patent would interfere with the blood-clotting time measurements. Based on past research (Molyneax, for example), they thought that blood drawn from an A-line to include the dead space plus a discard volume may provide accurate aPTT measurements in comparison with blood drawn from a venipuncture (venous). A venous draw would involve another needle stick, which, of course, it would be desirable to avoid if possible.

Templin et al presented the data displayed in Table III-8. Analyze the data. Based on the given data, what blood-sampling protocol would you

TABLE *III-8* Data from Templin et al.

Patient	DS V	DS A	DS + 2 V	DS + 2 A	DS + 4 V	DS + 4 A
1	67.9	86.9	62.8	73.8	62.4	86.4
2	116.3	130.6	91.5	91.9	80.7	85.8
3	81.8	84.9	88.9	101.1	77.2	92.5
4	59.7	69.4	61.4	63.3	56.7	61.6
5	83.3	90.9	75.4	75.3	80.2	79.4
6	84.8	100.5	82.8	88.4	62.4	63.0
7	69.1	84.9	70.8	60.3	65.7	72.7
8	52.4	77.4	56.3	63.0	57.8	57.0
9	120.1	132.8	80.4	98.7	106.8	114.7
10	61.3	71.9	76.3	79.0	75.8	80.7
11	79.7	103.0	46.5	49.5	57.4	58.6
12	87.0	108.8	73.2	79.0	75.5	82.1
13	103.3	80.4	78.8	82.4	61.3	62.3
14	75.7	84.8	97.1	103.2	75.3	81.4
15	70.4	81.8	62.8	65.8	67.3	66.2
16	130.9	144.9	102.4	111.8	110.0	112.4
17	81.3	106.0	102.4	118.5	86.7	86.1
18	60.7	79.4	80.5	87.2	66.0	75.3
19	64.1	84.1	93.5	104.7	62.5	65.0
20	106.0	130.8	113.1	123.1	130.4	122.5
21	87.5	106.5	86.4	89.0	119.1	118.4
22	44.1	43.3	41.2	42.5	79.3	95.7
23	51.4	52.5	44.4	45.6	61.0	58.2
24	88.3	110.9	86.6	96.4	86.3	106.0
25	97.9	124.1	103.6	113.4	110.1	150.0
26	91.6	111.0	77.6	84.8	83.7	94.1
27	71.4	73.1	75.9	74.5	75.8	76.1
28	116.3	133.7	134.7	126.9	108.8	131.4
29	96.1	117.0	95.6	103.9	112.7	121.2
30	117.7	131.0	100.3	97.7	114.6	119.0

recommend? Justify your recommendation with appropriate statistical presentations.

31. (Project) Anous and Heimbach studied the survivorship in burn patients aged ≥ 60 years. Patients were classified into one of three groups. Group 1 consisted of those patients who died within 3 days. Group 2 consisted of those patients who survived 3 days but died within 5 to 48 days. Group 3 consisted of patients who survived beyond 48 days. Table III-9 displays the amount of burn sustained as measured by percent of body surface area burned. Analyze the data. In particular, is survival from being burned in a patient aged ≥ 60 years related to percent of body surface area burned? Justify your conclusions with appropriate statistical presentations.

References

Anous M and Heimbach O: Causes of death and predictors in burned patients more than 64 years of age. *J Trauma* 26 (1986): 135.

Meloni T et al: Glucose-6-phosphate dehydrogenase deficiency and bacterial infections in northern Sardinia. *J Pediatr* 118, no. 6 (June 1991): 909.

TABLE III-9 Data from Anous and Heimbach on percent of body surface area burned in three groups of patients.

Group 1	Group 2		Group 3
65	10	15	30
53	17	17	18
48	20	38	17
71	35	25	17
50	23	56	41
36	38	50	15
60	36	30	24
30	36	11	22
50	30	60	20
74	42	35	19
80			34

Miyake M et al: Correlation of expression of H/Le^y/Le^b antigens with survival in patients with carcinoma of the lung. *N Engl J Med* 327, no. 1 (2 July 1992): 14.

Pizarro F et al: Iron status with different infant feeding regimens: Relevance to screening and prevention of iron deficiency. *J Pediatr* 118, no. 4 (May 1991): 687.

Scholes D et al: Current cigarette smoking and risk of acute pelvic inflammatory disease. *Am J Public Health* 82, no. 10 (October 1992): 1352.

Shapira Y and Gutman A: Muscle carnitine deficiency in patients using valproic acid. *J Pediatr* 118, no. 4, pt. 1 (April 1991): 646.

Templin K et al: Accuracy of drawing coagulation samples from heparinized arterial lines. *Am J Crit Care* 2, no. 1 (January 1993): 88.

APPENDIX

1. Daily E and Mersch J: Thermodilution cardiac outputs using room and ice temperature injectate: Comparison with the Fick method. *Heart Lung* 16, no. 3 (May 1987): 294.

      Each patient had cardiac output determined by three different methods: (1) room-temperature injectate, (2) ice-temperature injectate, and (3) the Fick method.

2. Barcelona M et al: Cardiac output determined by the thermodilution method: Comparison of ice temperature injectates versus room temperature injectates contained in prefilled syringes or a closed injectate delivery system. *Heart Lung* 14, no. 3 (May 1985): 232.

      Patients were divided into two groups: prefilled syringes group and Co-Set group.

3. Molyneaux R et al: Coagulation studies and the indwelling catheter. *Heart Lung* 16, no. 1 (January 1987): 20.

      Each patient had both an arterial and a venous blood sample taken at (1) 1.6-mL, (2) 3.2-mL, and (3) 4.8-mL discard. The data present aPTT, a blood-clotting time.

4. Bodai B et al: A clinical evaluation of an oxygen insufflation/suction catheter. *Heart Lung* 16, no. 1 (January 1987): 39.

      Ventilatory-dependent patients were randomized into three groups representing three different suctioning methods. The research studied the effect of suctioning on PaO_2 (a blood gas measurement) by both a routine method and an oxygenation method applied to each patient in the study.

5. Shively M: Effect of position change on mixed venous oxygen saturation in coronary artery bypass surgery patients. *Heart Lung* 17, no. 1 (January 1988): 51.

      Coronary patients were randomized into two groups. The research studied the effect of position change by monitoring blood oxygen saturation (a blood gas measurement). One group was turned every hour; the other group, every two hours.

6. Clark H and Hoffer L: Reappraisal of the resting metabolic rate of normal young men. *Am J Clin Nutr* 53, no. 1 (January 1991): 21.

      Background data are presented on each subject in a metabolism study.

7. Winklhofer-Roob B et al: Short-term changes in erythrocyte α-tocopherol content of vitamin E–deficient patients with cystic fibrosis. *Am J Clin Nutr* 55, no. 1 (January 1992): 100.

      The researchers studied vitamin E deficiency in a sample of ten children with cystic fibrosis.

DATA SET 1: Daily and Mersch Cardiac Output Study

BACKGROUND. A convenience sample of 34 patients scheduled for cardiac catheterization was recruited into the study. Five patients were excluded from analysis due to suspected technical failure of equipment for taking their cardiac output measurements. Hence, data were obtained from 29 patients. Each patient had cardiac output measured by three different methods: thermodilution using a room-temperature injectate, thermodilution using an ice-temperature injectate, and the Fick method. For the thermodilution methods, cardiac output was recorded as the average (mean) of three successive determinations. Cardiac output was measured as liters/minute. Normal range for cardiac output is 4–6 liters/minute.

Patient	RTCO	ITCO	Fick
1	2.60	3.02	3.99
2	5.16	5.47	4.94
3	6.18	5.72	6.33
4	3.22	4.22	3.75
5	4.99	4.89	6.03
6	3.62	3.50	3.54
7	3.31	3.08	3.02
8	4.11	4.11	4.85
9	5.24	4.86	5.17
10	4.27	4.73	3.45
11	3.42	3.78	3.69
12	4.70	4.26	5.29
13	5.42	4.97	5.51
14	5.36	5.47	4.40
15	2.63	2.62	2.96
16	3.70	3.87	5.06
17	5.39	5.30	6.60
18	5.44	4.79	7.31
19	3.86	3.75	4.48
20	6.68	6.38	6.82
21	5.35	5.30	5.31
22	3.26	3.86	3.40
23	4.06	4.28	4.40
24	2.64	2.88	3.18
25	5.40	5.63	5.92
26	5.93	6.08	5.60
27	5.90	6.15	5.60
28	4.11	4.51	5.16
29	4.44	3.26	4.54

RTCO means room-temperature cardiac output
ITCO means ice-temperature cardiac output
Fick CO means Fick cardiac output (used as gold standard).

DATA SET 2: Barcelona et al Cardiac Output Study

BACKGROUND. A convenience sample of 21 patients in the cardiac intensive care unit was studied in two successive groups. Group 1 consisted of 10 patients; group 2, of 11 patients. In group 1, cardiac outputs were determined by using a room- or ice-temperature injectate contained in prefilled syringes and given in random sequence. In group 2, cardiac outputs were determined by using an ice-temperature injectate in prefilled syringes or a room-temperature injectate from the Co-Set apparatus. There were 41 cardiac output sessions recorded for each group. CAUTION: This data set was not obtained from a random sample with independent observations. In several examples in the text, for *purposes of illustration*, we took the liberty of adjusting the assumptions to fit the discussion. In particular, we viewed the data *as if* they were obtained from a random sample with 41 independent observations. In reality, this was not the case. Since several measurements were taken on the same individual, repeated measures analysis should have been applied. However, the presentation of the data did not identify which measurements were taken on which patient.

Prefilled Syringes		Co-Set	
Iced	Room	Iced	Room
3.8	3.7	5.2	4.9
3.8	3.7	4.7	4.5
3.2	3.2	4.5	2.5
3.5	3.2	5.3	5.3
4.0	3.9	3.0	3.4
3.8	4.1	3.9	5.9
4.0	3.9	5.6	4.6
3.9	3.8	4.7	4.4
3.1	3.2	4.1	3.7
3.8	3.8	3.7	3.6
3.4	4.2	5.7	5.9
3.8	3.2	6.1	5.7
3.4	3.0	5.8	6.4
3.3	3.4	3.0	2.7
3.7	3.5	5.0	4.4
3.5	3.8	4.2	4.2
3.5	3.5	4.3	4.3
3.2	3.5	5.0	2.4
3.4	3.6	3.8	2.8
3.5	3.8	2.5	3.9

Prefilled Syringes		Co-Set	
Iced	Room	Iced	Room
4.5	4.8	4.4	5.3
4.6	4.1	4.1	3.7
4.2	3.9	4.4	3.8
5.0	5.5	4.2	3.6
5.3	5.3	4.4	4.0
4.7	4.3	3.2	2.9
4.8	4.0	2.6	2.7
2.8	2.8	3.3	2.9
2.2	2.3	3.2	2.8
2.7	2.5	5.3	4.0
6.2	6.9	6.4	5.3
6.7	6.7	7.3	6.1
7.2	6.1	4.8	4.3
5.7	6.0	3.7	3.7
3.0	2.8	4.3	4.1
3.7	2.7	4.0	3.5
3.4	3.3	3.5	3.4
2.4	2.5	3.7	3.3
2.9	2.5	3.9	3.1
2.7	2.8	3.9	3.9
3.8	4.2	3.5	4.1

DATA SET 3: Molyneaux et al Clotting Time Study

BACKGROUND. A convenience sample of 24 patients was recruited into the study. Four patients who were immunosuppressed were excluded from analysis (AIDS, leukemia, chemotherapy, and radiation therapy patients were excluded). All patients in the study had an indwelling catheter in place, which was kept patent with a heparin wash. The heparin contaminates blood samples drawn from the arterial line. This heparin contamination interferes with blood-clotting measurements (aPTT, measured in seconds). The research was undertaken to determine if blood drawn from the arterial line could give reliable aPTT measurements after an initial discard. The heparin wash was turned off, an initial amount was discarded to free the catheter from heparin, and a sample of blood was then drawn for aPTT measurements. A simultaneous arterial blood sample and a sample taken by venipuncture were obtained from each of 20 patients using (1) 1.6-mL discard, (2) 3.2-mL discard, and (3) 4.8-mL discard. The "deadspace" volume of the catheter was 0.8 mL; hence, the 1.6-mL increments used in the study. Molyneaux et al concluded:

We recommend that a minimal discard volume of six times the deadspace volume of the catheter be withdrawn before sampling blood for aPTT determinations from heparinized intraarterial lines.

Patient	1.6-mL discard		3.2-mL discard		4.8-mL discard	
	Arterial	Venous	Arterial	Venous	Arterial	Venous
1	33.1	31.6	29.1	29.7	34.1	33.2
2	30.2	31.5	30.2	29.9	27.9	27.5
3	34.6	34.3	29.7	26.9	24.8	23.8
4	32.2	30.2	28.8	29.8	30.5	30.7
5	26.0	26.5	29.3	31.5	29.9	31.4
6	41.8	31.2	29.6	29.8	25.0	25.2
7	30.5	27.4	45.5	43.5	30.0	30.2
8	41.2	39.1	41.2	36.1	35.0	35.5
9	29.3	28.3	54.8	52.4	29.0	29.4
10	29.7	30.3	38.1	37.5	26.4	25.9
11	30.5	29.7	64.0	59.7	26.4	26.0
12	32.9	29.1	36.6	41.3	38.9	39.5
13	36.4	32.3	46.4	44.6	43.5	44.4
14	26.5	20.1	56.0	49.5	28.1	31.7
15	33.7	33.4	27.4	27.1	41.9	41.8
16	34.3	34.4	27.9	26.6	32.3	32.2
17	31.4	30.3	26.1	24.9	45.6	45.5
18	119.3	120.8	31.0	30.5	28.9	29.5
19	50.8	46.7	30.7	31.1	35.8	36.3
20	48.7	44.7	44.7	46.6	28.8	27.7

DATA SET 4: Bodai et al Suction Study

BACKGROUND. A convenience sample of 24 respiratory failure, ventilator-dependent patients was randomly assigned to one of three study groups. The purpose of the study was to evaluate the effectiveness of a double-lumen catheter system, which allowed oxygen insufflation during the suctioning procedure in three different clinical settings. Arterial blood gases (ABGs) were sampled at the start, end, 1 minute after, and 5 minutes after suctioning using the two specified methods for each patient within each group. For each ABG, partial pressures of oxygen (PaO_2) in mm Hg were measured. Group 1 compared routine preoxygenation/hyperinflation and suction with and without oxygenation insufflation. Group 2 compared preoxygenation/hyperinflation and suction with oxygen insufflation/suction alone. Group 3 compared suctioning with and without oxygen insufflation within a valve system that allowed for continuous ventilation. The assignment of suctioning protocol (control or oxygenated) was made randomly. After data were collected, patients with presuction PaO_2 were excluded from the analysis.

Group 1 (n = 4)

Routine suctioning (control)				Routine suctioning with insufflation catheter			
Start	End	1 min	5 min	Start	End	1 min	5 min
65	88	80	73	67	103	83	69
56	60	57	61	53	65	63	59
71	86	68	72	70	122	74	74
83	72	89	111	91	122	105	99

Group 2 (n = 6)

Routine suctioning (control)				Oxygen insufflation alone			
Start	End	1 min	5 min	Start	End	1 min	5 min
90	67	73	122	83	80	120	84
78	86	82	78	71	63	71	70
90	57	63	83	88	77	98	90
69	40	54	59	80	41	54	56
70	59	100	130	93	63	73	82
84	114	74	73	86	118	88	90

Group 3 (n = 6)

Standard suction with valve adapter (control)				Oxygen insufflation with valve adapter			
Start	End	1 min	5 min	Start	End	1 min	5 min
74	60	58	62	50	54	57	59
65	62	67	64	70	65	68	74
85	80	75	85	78	85	79	82
72	73	93	107	63	84	81	79
91	83	82	84	89	89	89	92
92	86	94	92	84	94	103	86

DATA SET 5: Shively et al Positioning Study

BACKGROUND. In 1980 the American Association of Critical Care Nurses commissioned a study to identify research priorities for critical care. Among the top 15 priorities was: What are the effects of patient positioning on cardiovascular and pulmonary functioning of various types of critically ill patients? In response, Shively wanted to determine the effect of (1) position change on oxygenation in patients after coronary artery bypass graft surgery and (2) frequency of position change on oxygenation in those patients.

Oxygenation was measured by monitoring mixed venous oxygen saturation, $S\bar{v}O_2$. Such monitoring provides assessment of oxygenation at the patient's bedside. Normal is 75%; normal range, 68% to 77%.

A convenience sample of 30 patients was randomized into two groups of 15 patients each. Selection criteria included adult, undergoing coronary artery bypass surgery within 24 hours, extubated, and hemodynamically stable. Patients with chronic pulmonary disease were excluded. Patients in group 1 were turned every hour; group 2, every 2 hours. All patients were turned through the same sequence of positions. The data set includes $S\bar{v}O_2$ measurements taken while the patient was in the right lateral (RL) position, where the bed was elevated 20 degrees, and supine, with the head of the bed elevated 45 degrees (S45). Measurements were taken at the start of the study (baseline). Measurements were taken at the start (0′) of a turning session and at 15 minutes (15′), 1 hour (1°), and for group 2, at 2 hours (2°).

Group 1 (n = 15)

ID	Baseline	RL 0′	RL 15′	RL 1°	RL 2°	S45 0′	S45 15′	S45 1°	S45 2°
2	63	63	68	66	—	56	67	64	—
6	75	67	74	75	—	74	76	72	—
7	73	68	72	74	—	71	74	72	—
8	56	50	55	57	—	53	53	55	—
10	69	51	73	72	—	58	70	69	—
13	73	53	70	71	—	67	71	69	—
14	71	65	71	70	—	71	72	70	—
16	69	58	68	69	—	64	65	69	—
17	70	75	79	79	—	69	70	64	—
18	65	58	69	69	—	66	72	69	—
20	67	56	65	67	—	60	64	65	—
21	69	63	71	71	—	69	68	69	—
22	71	61	67	65	—	63	66	69	—
23	68	61	66	68	—	59	67	65	—
24	61	56	59	58	—	54	56	58	—

Group 2 (n = 15)

ID	Baseline	RL 0′	RL 15′	RL 1°	RL 2°	S45 0′	S45 15′	S45 1°	S45 2°
1	64	56	65	64	64	54	65	64	60
3	72	73	74	73	73	70	74	60	66
4	73	66	68	72	69	60	67	68	64
5	57	44	58	60	57	38	54	56	54
9	67	64	65	62	65	59	65	67	65
11	60	50	63	60	62	58	62	62	63
12	66	43	69	68	66	50	62	62	58
15	74	63	73	74	73	67	72	74	70
19	67	53	66	66	61	62	65	65	65
25	72	72	74	75	73	71	72	75	72
26	73	74	74	71	72	66	72	74	75
27	66	55	65	69	70	63	66	65	65
28	70	67	68	68	70	67	69	68	69
29	78	67	74	77	75	65	75	75	72
30	77	72	76	76	77	74	77	73	78

Data Set 6: Clark and Hoffer Metabolism Study

BACKGROUND. A convenience sample of 29 male subjects was recruited into a research program to study metabolism. Several baseline variates were measured in each subject. The study was restricted to healthy, nonsmoking, weight-stable men aged 18–33 years. Professional or competitive athletes, and those with a perforated eardrum, recent weight change, using drugs or medications, or unusual diets were excluded from the study.

Subject	Age (years)	Height (cm)	Weight (kg)	Body Mass Index (kg/m²)
1	23	193	75	20.1
2	24	180	63	19.4
3	24	186	84	42.3
4	26	183	78	23.3
5	23	180	73	22.5
6	33	166	62	22.5
7	23	175	70	22.9
8	25	175	82	26.8
9	26	180	80	24.7
10	26	172	77	26.0
11	23	170	69	23.9
12	22	183	86	25.7
13	27	173	72	24.1
14	24	185	69	20.2
15	19	177	71	22.7
16	28	180	63	19.4
17	23	173	67	22.4
18	26	175	61	19.9
19	24	188	65	18.4
20	23	180	67	20.7
21	31	180	76	23.5
22	21	173	74	24.7
23	25	180	74	22.8
24	25	191	111	30.4
25	18	178	70	22.1
26	25	170	69	23.9
27	18	175	68	22.2
28	25	170	80	27.7
29	29	178	72	22.7

Data Set 7: Winklhofer-Roob Cystic Fibrosis Study

BACKGROUND. A convenience sample of ten children with cystic fibrosis was recruited into the study. Of these, five children had cholestatic liver disease (CLD). Vitamin E deficiency is a common condition in children with cystic fibrosis (Cf). The patients fasted overnight, and then erythrocyte and serum vitamin E levels (μmol/liter) were measured. Each patient was then given an oral dose of 100-mg vitamin E per kilogram of body weight. Erythrocyte and serum vitamin-E measurements were again taken at 1, 3, 6, 9, 12, and 24 hours.

Level of erythrocyte vitamin-E (μmol/liter)

Patient	CLD	Start	1 hr	3 hrs	6 hrs	9 hrs	12 hrs	24 hrs
1	yes	1.50	2.30	3.40	4.10	5.40	4.30	6.20
2	yes	4.10	4.80	4.00	3.70	7.80	9.20	6.50
3	yes	1.00	1.30	1.20	2.40	3.30	3.30	4.10
4	yes	3.50	4.10	4.90	5.80	5.90	7.30	4.60
5	yes	1.90	2.00	1.70	3.00	3.10	3.30	3.70
6	no	2.10	2.10	3.80	4.40	5.60	5.80	6.20
7	no	2.30	2.60	3.10	5.10	8.10	7.60	7.40
8	no	1.50	1.70	1.80	3.30	6.70	7.00	7.80
9	no	3.10	3.50	5.20	4.60	3.90	4.30	3.90
10	no	1.70	1.60	1.90	3.00	6.00	5.40	6.40

Level of serum vitamin-E (μmol/liter)

Patient	CLD	Start	1 hr	3 hrs	6 hrs	9 hrs	12 hrs	24 hrs
1	yes	7.43	6.96	12.07	22.98	24.84	20.20	16.95
2	yes	17.65	17.41	20.20	41.09	29.02	27.17	21.59
3	yes	8.59	8.36	10.68	25.31	23.68	20.90	17.88
4	yes	11.84	11.84	14.63	24.84	23.45	21.82	17.41
5	yes	5.11	5.34	6.27	12.07	11.38	10.45	8.59
6	no	9.75	10.68	33.67	35.29	35.99	31.58	26.00
7	no	5.80	4.18	10.45	20.20	19.97	19.73	16.95
8	no	8.13	8.13	14.63	24.38	25.77	24.61	16.48
9	no	17.18	16.72	26.00	27.17	23.68	22.29	20.66
10	no	5.57	5.80	7.20	18.34	29.95	23.45	19.73

STATISTICAL TABLES

Table 1: Values for C(n, k).

n	\multicolumn{9}{c}{k}

n	2	3	4	5	6	7	8	9	10
2	1								
3	3	1							
4	6	4	1						
5	10	10	5	1					
6	15	20	15	6	1				
7	21	35	35	21	7	1			
8	28	56	70	56	28	8	1		
9	36	84	126	126	84	36	9	1	
10	45	120	210	252	210	120	45	10	1
11	55	165	330	462	462	330	165	55	11
12	66	220	495	792	924	792	495	220	66
13	78	286	715	1287	1716	1716	1287	715	286
14	91	364	1001	2002	3003	3432	3003	2002	1001
15	105	455	1365	3003	5005	6435	5005	3003	1365
16	120	560	1820	4368	8008	11440	12870	11440	8008
17	136	680	2380	6188	12376	19448	24310	24310	19448
18	153	816	3060	8568	18564	31824	43758	48620	43758
19	171	969	3876	11628	27132	50388	75582	92378	92378
20	190	1140	4845	15504	38760	77520	125970	167960	184756

For any whole number n,
  $C(n, 0) = 1$ and $C(n, n) = 1$
  $C(n, 1) = n$ and $C(n, n - 1) = n$
  $C(n, k) = C(n, n - k)$

For example,
  $C(7, 0) = 1$ and $C(7, 7) = 1$
  $C(9, 1) = 9$ and $C(9, 8) = 9$
  $C(15, 12) = C(15, 15 - 12) = C(15, 3) = 455$

Table 2: Cumulative Binomial Probabilities.

The table gives the cumulative probability for up to x successes in a binomial experiment consisting of n independent Bernoulli trials, where each trial has probability of success p.

$n = 5$; column heading $= p$; $x =$ number of successes in 5 trials

x	.10	.20	.25	.30	.40	.50	.60	.70	.75	.80	.90
0	0.59049	0.32768	0.23730	0.16807	0.07776	0.03125	0.01024	0.00243	0.00098	0.00032	0.00001
1	0.91854	0.73728	0.63281	0.52822	0.33696	0.18750	0.08704	0.03078	0.01563	0.00672	0.00046
2	0.99144	0.94208	0.89648	0.83692	0.68256	0.50000	0.31744	0.16308	0.10352	0.05792	0.00856
3	0.99954	0.99328	0.98437	0.96922	0.91296	0.81250	0.66304	0.16308	0.10352	0.05792	0.00856
4	0.99999	0.99968	0.99902	0.99757	0.98976	0.96875	0.92224	0.83193	0.76270	0.67232	0.40951
5	1.00000	1.00000	1.00000	1.00000	1.00000	1.00000	1.00000	1.00000	1.00000	1.00000	1.00000

$n = 10$; column heading $= p$; $x =$ number of successes in 10 trials

x	.10	.20	.25	.30	.40	.50	.60	.70	.75	.80	.90
0	0.34868	0.10737	0.05631	0.02825	0.00605	0.00098	0.00010	0.00001	0.00000	0.00000	0.00000
1	0.73610	0.37581	0.24403	0.14931	0.04636	0.01074	0.00168	0.00014	0.00003	0.00000	0.00000
2	0.92981	0.67780	0.52559	0.38278	0.16729	0.05469	0.01229	0.00159	0.00042	0.00008	0.00000
3	0.98720	0.87913	0.77588	0.64961	0.38228	0.17187	0.05476	0.01059	0.00351	0.00086	0.00001
4	0.99837	0.96721	0.92187	0.84973	0.63310	0.37695	0.16624	0.04735	0.01973	0.00637	0.00015
5	0.99985	0.99363	0.98027	0.95265	0.83376	0.62305	0.36690	0.15027	0.07813	0.03279	0.00163
6	0.99999	0.99914	0.99649	0.98941	0.94524	0.82812	0.61772	0.35039	0.22412	0.12087	0.01280
7	1.00000	0.99992	0.99958	0.99841	0.98771	0.94531	0.83271	0.61722	0.47441	0.32220	0.07019
8	1.00000	1.00000	0.99997	0.99986	0.99832	0.98926	0.95364	0.85069	0.75597	0.62419	0.26390
9	1.00000	1.00000	1.00000	0.99999	0.99990	0.99902	0.99395	0.97175	0.94369	0.89263	0.65132
10	1.00000	1.00000	1.00000	1.00000	1.00000	1.00000	1.00000	1.00000	1.00000	1.00000	1.00000

$n = 15$; column heading $= p$; $x =$ number of successes in 15 trials

x	.10	.20	.25	.30	.40	.50	.60	.70	.75	.80	.90
0	0.20589	0.03518	0.01336	0.00475	0.00047	0.00003	0.00000	0.00000	0.00000	0.00000	0.00000
1	0.54904	0.16713	0.08018	0.03527	0.00517	0.00049	0.00003	0.00000	0.00000	0.00000	0.00000
2	0.81594	0.39802	0.23609	0.12683	0.02711	0.00369	0.00028	0.00001	0.00000	0.00000	0.00000
3	0.94444	0.64816	0.46129	0.29687	0.09050	0.01758	0.00193	0.00009	0.00001	0.00000	0.00000
4	0.98728	0.83577	0.68649	0.51549	0.21728	0.05923	0.00935	0.00067	0.00012	0.00001	0.00000
5	0.99775	0.93895	0.85163	0.72162	0.40322	0.15088	0.03383	0.00365	0.00079	0.00011	0.00000
6	0.99969	0.98194	0.94338	0.86886	0.60981	0.30362	0.09505	0.01524	0.00419	0.00078	0.00000
7	0.99997	0.99576	0.98270	0.94999	0.78690	0.50000	0.21310	0.05001	0.01730	0.00424	0.00003
8	1.00000	0.99922	0.99581	0.98476	0.90495	0.69638	0.39019	0.13114	0.05662	0.01806	0.00031
9	1.00000	0.99989	0.99921	0.99635	0.96617	0.84912	0.59678	0.27838	0.14837	0.06105	0.00225
10	1.00000	0.99999	0.99988	0.99933	0.99065	0.94077	0.78272	0.48451	0.31351	0.16423	0.01272
11	1.00000	1.00000	0.99999	0.99991	0.99807	0.98242	0.90950	0.70313	0.53871	0.35184	0.05556
12	1.00000	1.00000	1.00000	0.99999	0.99972	0.99631	0.97289	0.87317	0.76391	0.60198	0.18406
13	1.00000	1.00000	1.00000	1.00000	0.99997	0.99951	0.99483	0.96473	0.91982	0.83287	0.45096
14	1.00000	1.00000	1.00000	1.00000	1.00000	0.99997	0.99953	0.99525	0.98664	0.96482	0.79411
15	1.00000	1.00000	1.00000	1.00000	1.00000	1.00000	1.00000	1.00000	1.00000	1.00000	1.00000

n = 20; column heading = p; x = number of successes in 20 trials

x	.10	.20	.25	.30	.40	.50	.60	.70	.75	.80	.90
0	0.12158	0.01153	0.00317	0.00080	0.00004	0.00000	0.00000	0.00000	0.00000	0.00000	0.00000
1	0.39175	0.06918	0.02431	0.00764	0.00052	0.00002	0.00000	0.00000	0.00000	0.00000	0.00000
2	0.67693	0.20608	0.09126	0.03548	0.00361	0.00020	0.00001	0.00000	0.00000	0.00000	0.00000
3	0.86705	0.41145	0.22516	0.10709	0.01596	0.00129	0.00005	0.00000	0.00000	0.00000	0.00000
4	0.95683	0.62965	0.41484	0.23751	0.05095	0.00591	0.00032	0.00001	0.00000	0.00000	0.00000
5	0.98875	0.80421	0.61717	0.41637	0.12560	0.02069	0.00161	0.00004	0.00000	0.00000	0.00000
6	0.99761	0.91331	0.78578	0.60801	0.25001	0.05766	0.00647	0.00026	0.00003	0.00000	0.00000
7	0.99958	0.96786	0.89819	0.77227	0.41589	0.13159	0.02103	0.00128	0.00018	0.00002	0.00000
8	0.99994	0.99002	0.95907	0.88667	0.59560	0.25172	0.05653	0.00514	0.00094	0.00010	0.00000
9	0.99999	0.99741	0.98614	0.95204	0.75534	0.41190	0.12752	0.01714	0.00394	0.00056	0.00000
10	1.00000	0.99944	0.99606	0.98286	0.87248	0.58810	0.24466	0.04796	0.01386	0.00259	0.00001
11	1.00000	0.99990	0.99906	0.99486	0.94347	0.74828	0.40440	0.11333	0.04093	0.00998	0.00006
12	1.00000	0.99998	0.99982	0.99872	0.97897	0.86841	0.58411	0.22773	0.10181	0.03214	0.00042
13	1.00000	1.00000	0.99997	0.99974	0.99353	0.94234	0.74999	0.39199	0.21422	0.08669	0.00239
14	1.00000	1.00000	1.00000	0.99996	0.99839	0.97931	0.87440	0.58363	0.38283	0.19579	0.01125
15	1.00000	1.00000	1.00000	0.99999	0.99968	0.99409	0.94905	0.76249	0.58516	0.37035	0.04317
16	1.00000	1.00000	1.00000	1.00000	0.99995	0.99871	0.98404	0.89291	0.77484	0.58855	0.13295
17	1.00000	1.00000	1.00000	1.00000	0.99999	0.99980	0.99639	0.96452	0.90874	0.79392	0.32307
18	1.00000	1.00000	1.00000	1.00000	1.00000	0.99998	0.99948	0.99236	0.97569	0.93082	0.60825
19	1.00000	1.00000	1.00000	1.00000	1.00000	1.00000	0.99996	0.99920	0.99683	0.98847	0.87842
20	1.00000	1.00000	1.00000	1.00000	1.00000	1.00000	1.00000	1.00000	1.00000	1.00000	1.00000

n = 25; column heading = p; x = number of successes in 25 trials

x	.10	.20	.25	.30	.40	.50	.60	.70	.75	.80	.90
0	0.07179	0.00378	0.00075	0.00013	0.00000	0.00000	0.00000	0.00000	0.00000	0.00000	0.00000
1	0.27121	0.02739	0.00702	0.00157	0.00005	0.00000	0.00000	0.00000	0.00000	0.00000	0.00000
2	0.53709	0.09823	0.03211	0.00896	0.00043	0.00001	0.00000	0.00000	0.00000	0.00000	0.00000
3	0.76359	0.23399	0.09621	0.03324	0.00237	0.00008	0.00000	0.00000	0.00000	0.00000	0.00000
4	0.90201	0.42067	0.21374	0.09047	0.00947	0.00046	0.00001	0.00000	0.00000	0.00000	0.00000
5	0.96660	0.61669	0.37828	0.19349	0.02936	0.00204	0.00005	0.00000	0.00000	0.00000	0.00000
6	0.99052	0.78004	0.56110	0.34065	0.07357	0.00732	0.00028	0.00000	0.00000	0.00000	0.00000
7	0.99774	0.89088	0.72651	0.51185	0.15355	0.02164	0.00121	0.00002	0.00000	0.00000	0.00000
8	0.99954	0.95323	0.85056	0.67693	0.27353	0.05388	0.00433	0.00010	0.00001	0.00000	0.00000
9	0.99992	0.98267	0.92867	0.81056	0.42462	0.11476	0.01317	0.00045	0.00004	0.00000	0.00000
10	0.99999	0.99445	0.97033	0.90220	0.58577	0.21218	0.03439	0.00178	0.00021	0.00001	0.00000
11	1.00000	0.99846	0.98927	0.95575	0.73228	0.34502	0.07780	0.00599	0.00092	0.00008	0.00000
12	1.00000	0.99963	0.99663	0.98253	0.84623	0.50000	0.15377	0.01747	0.00337	0.00037	0.00000
13	1.00000	0.99992	0.99908	0.99401	0.92220	0.65498	0.26772	0.04425	0.01073	0.00154	0.00000
14	1.00000	0.99999	0.99979	0.99822	0.96561	0.78782	0.41422	0.09780	0.02967	0.00555	0.00001
15	1.00000	1.00000	0.99996	0.99955	0.98683	0.88524	0.57538	0.18944	0.07133	0.01733	0.00008
16	1.00000	1.00000	0.99999	0.99990	0.99567	0.94612	0.72647	0.32307	0.14944	0.04677	0.00046
17	1.00000	1.00000	1.00000	0.99998	0.99879	0.97836	0.84645	0.48815	0.27349	0.10912	0.00226
18	1.00000	1.00000	1.00000	1.00000	0.99972	0.99268	0.92643	0.65935	0.43890	0.21996	0.00948
19	1.00000	1.00000	1.00000	1.00000	0.99995	0.99796	0.97064	0.80651	0.62172	0.38331	0.03340
20	1.00000	1.00000	1.00000	1.00000	0.99999	0.99954	0.99053	0.90953	0.78626	0.57933	0.09799
21	1.00000	1.00000	1.00000	1.00000	1.00000	0.99992	0.99763	0.96676	0.90379	0.76601	0.23641
22	1.00000	1.00000	1.00000	1.00000	1.00000	0.99999	0.99957	0.99104	0.96789	0.90177	0.46291
23	1.00000	1.00000	1.00000	1.00000	1.00000	1.00000	0.99995	0.99843	0.99298	0.97261	0.72879
24	1.00000	1.00000	1.00000	1.00000	1.00000	1.00000	1.00000	0.99987	0.99925	0.99622	0.92821
25	1.00000	1.00000	1.00000	1.00000	1.00000	1.00000	1.00000	1.00000	1.00000	1.00000	1.00000

TABLE 3: CDF for the Standard Normal Distribution (left-tail areas).

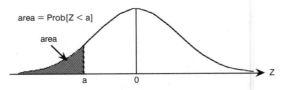

area = Prob[Z < a]

z	0.00	0.01	0.02	0.03	0.04	0.05	0.06	0.07	0.08	0.09
−3.4	0.000337	0.000325	0.000313	0.000302	0.000291	0.000280	0.000270	0.000260	0.000251	0.000242
−3.3	0.000483	0.000467	0.000450	0.000434	0.000419	0.000404	0.000390	0.000376	0.000362	0.000350
−3.2	0.000687	0.000664	0.000641	0.000619	0.000598	0.000577	0.000557	0.000538	0.000519	0.000501
−3.1	0.000968	0.000935	0.000904	0.000874	0.000845	0.000816	0.000789	0.000762	0.000736	0.000711
−3.0	0.001350	0.001306	0.001264	0.001223	0.001183	0.001144	0.001107	0.001070	0.001035	0.001001
−2.9	0.001866	0.001807	0.001750	0.001695	0.001641	0.001589	0.001538	0.001489	0.001441	0.001395
−2.8	0.002555	0.002477	0.002401	0.002327	0.002256	0.002186	0.002118	0.002052	0.001988	0.001926
−2.7	0.003467	0.003364	0.003264	0.003167	0.003072	0.002980	0.002890	0.002803	0.002718	0.002635
−2.6	0.004661	0.004527	0.004396	0.004269	0.004145	0.004025	0.003907	0.003793	0.003681	0.003573
−2.5	0.006210	0.006037	0.005868	0.005703	0.005543	0.005386	0.005234	0.005085	0.004940	0.004799
−2.4	0.008198	0.007976	0.007760	0.007549	0.007344	0.007143	0.006947	0.006756	0.006569	0.006387
−2.3	0.010724	0.010444	0.010170	0.009903	0.009642	0.009387	0.009137	0.008894	0.008656	0.008424
−2.2	0.013903	0.013553	0.013209	0.012874	0.012545	0.012224	0.011911	0.011604	0.011304	0.011011
−2.1	0.017864	0.017429	0.017003	0.016586	0.016177	0.015778	0.015386	0.015003	0.014629	0.014262
−2.0	0.022750	0.022216	0.021692	0.021178	0.020675	0.020182	0.019699	0.019226	0.018763	0.018309
−1.9	0.028717	0.028067	0.027429	0.026803	0.026190	0.025588	0.024998	0.024419	0.023852	0.023295
−1.8	0.035930	0.035148	0.034379	0.033625	0.032884	0.032157	0.031443	0.030742	0.030054	0.029379
−1.7	0.044565	0.043633	0.042716	0.041815	0.040929	0.040059	0.039204	0.038364	0.037538	0.036727
−1.6	0.054799	0.053699	0.052616	0.051551	0.050503	0.049471	0.048457	0.047460	0.046479	0.045514
−1.5	0.066807	0.065522	0.064255	0.063008	0.061780	0.060571	0.059380	0.058208	0.057053	0.055917
−1.4	0.080757	0.079270	0.077804	0.076359	0.074934	0.073529	0.072145	0.070781	0.069437	0.068112
−1.3	0.096801	0.095098	0.093418	0.091759	0.090123	0.088508	0.086915	0.085343	0.083793	0.082264
−1.2	0.115070	0.113140	0.111233	0.109349	0.107488	0.105650	0.103835	0.102042	0.100273	0.098525
−1.1	0.135666	0.133500	0.131357	0.129238	0.127143	0.125072	0.123024	0.121001	0.119000	0.117023
−1.0	0.158655	0.156248	0.153864	0.151505	0.149170	0.146859	0.144572	0.142310	0.140071	0.137857
−0.9	0.184060	0.181411	0.178786	0.176185	0.173609	0.171056	0.168528	0.166023	0.163543	0.161087
−0.8	0.211855	0.208970	0.206108	0.203269	0.200454	0.197663	0.194894	0.192150	0.189430	0.186733
−0.7	0.241964	0.238852	0.235762	0.232695	0.229650	0.226627	0.223627	0.220650	0.217695	0.214764
−0.6	0.274253	0.270931	0.267629	0.264347	0.261086	0.257846	0.254627	0.251429	0.248252	0.245097
−0.5	0.308538	0.305026	0.301532	0.298056	0.294599	0.291160	0.287740	0.284339	0.280957	0.277595
−0.4	0.344578	0.340903	0.337243	0.333598	0.329969	0.326355	0.322758	0.319178	0.315614	0.312067
−0.3	0.382089	0.378281	0.374484	0.370700	0.366928	0.363169	0.359424	0.355691	0.351973	0.348268
−0.2	0.420740	0.416834	0.412936	0.409046	0.405165	0.401294	0.397432	0.393580	0.389739	0.385908
−0.1	0.460172	0.456205	0.452242	0.448283	0.444330	0.440382	0.436441	0.432505	0.428576	0.424655
−0.0	0.500000	0.496011	0.492022	0.488033	0.484047	0.480061	0.476078	0.472097	0.468119	0.464144

CDF = one tailed table
- minitab CDF = left side
- Rt tail = (1 − left tail)

Table 4: Standard Normal Distribution (right-tail areas).

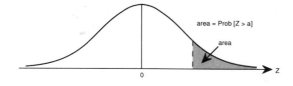

area = Prob [Z > a]

z	0.00	0.01	0.02	0.03	0.04	0.05	0.06	0.07	0.08	0.09
0.0	0.500000	0.496011	0.492022	0.488033	0.484047	0.480061	0.476078	0.472097	0.468119	0.464144
0.1	0.460172	0.456205	0.452242	0.448283	0.444330	0.440382	0.436441	0.432505	0.428576	0.424655
0.2	0.420740	0.416834	0.412936	0.409046	0.405165	0.401294	0.397432	0.393580	0.389739	0.385908
0.3	0.382089	0.378281	0.374484	0.370700	0.366928	0.363169	0.359424	0.355691	0.351973	0.348268
0.4	0.344578	0.340903	0.337243	0.333598	0.329969	0.326355	0.322758	0.319178	0.315614	0.312067
0.5	0.308538	0.305026	0.301532	0.298056	0.294599	0.291160	0.287740	0.284339	0.280957	0.277595
0.6	0.274253	0.270931	0.267629	0.264347	0.261086	0.257846	0.254627	0.251429	0.248252	0.245097
0.7	0.241964	0.238852	0.235762	0.232695	0.229650	0.226627	0.223627	0.220650	0.217695	0.214764
0.8	0.211855	0.208970	0.206108	0.203269	0.200454	0.197663	0.194894	0.192150	0.189430	0.186733
0.9	0.184060	0.181411	0.178786	0.176185	0.173609	0.171056	0.168528	0.166023	0.163543	0.161087
1.0	0.158655	0.156248	0.153864	0.151505	0.149170	0.146859	0.144572	0.142310	0.140071	0.137857
1.1	0.135666	0.133500	0.131357	0.129238	0.127143	0.125072	0.123024	0.121001	0.119000	0.117023
1.2	0.115070	0.113140	0.111233	0.109349	0.107488	0.105650	0.103835	0.102042	0.100273	0.098525
1.3	0.096801	0.095098	0.093418	0.091759	0.090123	0.088508	0.086915	0.085343	0.083793	0.082264
1.4	0.080757	0.079270	0.077804	0.076359	0.074934	0.073529	0.072145	0.070781	0.069437	0.068112
1.5	0.066807	0.065522	0.064256	0.063008	0.061780	0.060571	0.059380	0.058208	0.057053	0.055917
1.6	0.054799	0.053699	0.052616	0.051551	0.050503	0.049471	0.048457	0.047460	0.046479	0.045514
1.7	0.044565	0.043633	0.042716	0.041815	0.040929	0.040059	0.039204	0.038364	0.037538	0.036727
1.8	0.035930	0.035148	0.034379	0.033625	0.032884	0.032157	0.031443	0.030742	0.030054	0.029379
1.9	0.028717	0.028067	0.027429	0.026803	0.026190	0.025588	0.024998	0.024419	0.023852	0.023295
2.0	0.022750	0.022216	0.021692	0.021178	0.020675	0.020182	0.019699	0.019226	0.018763	0.018309
2.1	0.017864	0.017429	0.017003	0.016586	0.016177	0.015778	0.015386	0.015003	0.014629	0.014262
2.2	0.013903	0.013553	0.013209	0.012874	0.012545	0.012224	0.011911	0.011604	0.011304	0.011011
2.3	0.010724	0.010444	0.010170	0.009903	0.009642	0.009387	0.009137	0.008894	0.008656	0.008424
2.4	0.008198	0.007976	0.007760	0.007549	0.007344	0.007143	0.006947	0.006756	0.006569	0.006387
2.5	0.006210	0.006037	0.005868	0.005703	0.005543	0.005386	0.005234	0.005085	0.004940	0.004799
2.6	0.004661	0.004527	0.004396	0.004269	0.004145	0.004025	0.003907	0.003793	0.003681	0.003573
2.7	0.003467	0.003364	0.003264	0.003167	0.003072	0.002980	0.002890	0.002803	0.002718	0.002635
2.8	0.002555	0.002477	0.002401	0.002327	0.002256	0.002186	0.002118	0.002052	0.001988	0.001926
2.9	0.001866	0.001807	0.001750	0.001695	0.001641	0.001589	0.001538	0.001489	0.001441	0.001395
3.0	0.001350	0.001306	0.001264	0.001223	0.001183	0.001144	0.001107	0.001070	0.001035	0.001001
3.1	0.000968	0.000935	0.000904	0.000874	0.000845	0.000816	0.000789	0.000762	0.000736	0.000711
3.2	0.000687	0.000664	0.000641	0.000619	0.000598	0.000577	0.000557	0.000538	0.000519	0.000501
3.3	0.000483	0.000467	0.000450	0.000434	0.000419	0.000404	0.000390	0.000376	0.000362	0.000350
3.4	0.000337	0.000325	0.000313	0.000302	0.000291	0.000280	0.000270	0.000260	0.000251	0.000242

Table 5: Test for Normal Distribution.

The table gives the critical value for Minitab's nscores correlation test for a normal distribution at three levels of significance. The table is based on information contained in Technical Reports, Minitab, Inc., November 1990 (Ryan and Joiner, Technical Report 1: Normal Probability Plots and Tests for Normality, 1976). In the first column, n denotes sample size.

	Level of Significance (α)		
n	.10	.05	.01
5	.8951	.8804	.8320
10	.9347	.9180	.8804
15	.9506	.9383	.9110
20	.9600	.9503	.9290
25	.9662	.9582	.9408
30	.9707	.9639	.9490
40	.9767	.9715	.9597
50	.9807	.9764	.9664
60	.9835	.9799	.9710
75	.9865	.9835	.9757

Comment. In conducting a preliminary test for normality, use the .01 level of significance. The critical values for LOS .05 and .10 are provided for convenience in reporting a p-value for normality.

Comment. For sharper results, the following approximation formulas may be used for interpolation to obtain the critical value cv(n) for a sample of intermediate size n.

$$\alpha = .01: \text{cv}(n) = 0.9963 - \frac{0.0211}{\sqrt{n}} - \frac{1.4106}{n} + \frac{3.1791}{n^2}$$

$$\alpha = .05: \text{cv}(n) = 1.0063 - \frac{0.1288}{\sqrt{n}} - \frac{0.6118}{n} + \frac{1.3505}{n^2}$$

$$\alpha = .10: \text{cv}(n) = 1.0071 - \frac{0.1371}{\sqrt{n}} - \frac{0.3682}{n} + \frac{0.7780}{n^2}$$

For example, at $\alpha = .01$, an approximate nscores correlation critical value for a sample of size 29 is

$$\text{cv}(29) = 0.9963 - \frac{0.0211}{\sqrt{n}} - \frac{1.4106}{n} + \frac{3.1791}{n^2}$$

$$= 0.9963 - \frac{0.0211}{\sqrt{29}} - \frac{1.4106}{29} + \frac{3.1791}{29^2}$$

$$= 0.9475$$

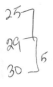

Table 6: t-Table for Confidence Intervals.

Assumption: Normal Distribution

	Level of Confidence (percent)					
df	80	90	95	98	99	99.9
1	3.07768	6.31375	12.7062	31.8206	63.6570	636.607
2	1.88562	2.91999	4.3027	6.9646	9.9248	31.598
3	1.63778	2.35341	3.1825	4.5407	5.8410	12.924
4	1.53320	2.13184	2.7764	3.7470	4.6041	8.610
5	1.47589	2.01505	2.5706	3.3649	4.0321	6.869
6	1.43977	1.94317	2.4469	3.1427	3.7075	5.959
7	1.41493	1.89456	2.3646	2.9980	3.4995	5.408
8	1.39685	1.85953	2.3060	2.8965	3.3554	5.041
9	1.38303	1.83313	2.2622	2.8215	3.2498	4.781
10	1.37215	1.81244	2.2281	2.7638	3.1693	4.587
11	1.36342	1.79588	2.2010	2.7181	3.1058	4.437
12	1.35621	1.78228	2.1788	2.6810	3.0545	4.318
13	1.35019	1.77094	2.1604	2.6503	3.0123	4.221
14	1.34502	1.76133	2.1448	2.6245	2.9768	4.140
15	1.34060	1.75307	2.1315	2.6025	2.9467	4.073
16	1.33677	1.74587	2.1199	2.5835	2.9208	4.015
17	1.33338	1.73962	2.1098	2.5669	2.8982	3.965
18	1.33036	1.73407	2.1009	2.5524	2.8784	3.922
19	1.32775	1.72911	2.0930	2.5395	2.8610	3.883
20	1.32533	1.72474	2.0860	2.5280	2.8453	3.849
21	1.32320	1.72074	2.0796	2.5176	2.8314	3.819
22	1.32125	1.71715	2.0739	2.5083	2.8187	3.792
23	1.31944	1.71389	2.0687	2.4999	2.8074	3.768
24	1.31783	1.71087	2.0639	2.4921	2.7969	3.745
25	1.31636	1.70813	2.0595	2.4851	2.7874	3.725
26	1.31497	1.70563	2.0556	2.4786	2.7787	3.707
27	1.31369	1.70326	2.0519	2.4727	2.7707	3.690
28	1.31253	1.70112	2.0484	2.4671	2.7633	3.674
29	1.31142	1.69911	2.0452	2.4620	2.7564	3.659
30	1.31038	1.69724	2.0423	2.4573	2.7500	3.646
40	1.30308	1.68386	2.0211	2.4232	2.7045	3.551
50	1.29868	1.67589	2.0085	2.4033	2.6778	3.496
60	1.29581	1.67065	2.0003	2.3902	2.6604	3.460
70	1.29376	1.66692	1.9944	2.3808	2.6480	3.435
80	1.29222	1.66413	1.9901	2.3739	2.6387	3.416
90	1.29103	1.66196	1.9867	2.3685	2.6316	3.402
100	1.29007	1.66024	1.9840	2.3642	2.6259	3.391
∞	1.28155	1.64485	1.9600	2.3264	2.5758	3.291

The t-value for any level of confidence (c) and degrees of freedom (df) can be obtained in Minitab as follows:

GENERAL
```
MTB > LET K1 = (c + 100)/200
MTB > INVCDF K1 K2;
SUBC> T df.
MTB > PRINT K2
K2    [ t-value ]
```

EXAMPLE (92%, df = 13)
```
MTB > LET K1 = (92 + 100)/200
MTB > INVCDF K1 K2;
MTB > PRINT K2
K2    [ 1.89888 ]
```

Table 7: z-Table for Confidence Intervals.

Confidence (Percent)	z
80	1.282
90	1.645
95	1.960
98	2.326
99	2.576
99.8	3.090
99.9	3.291
99.99	3.891
99.999	4.491

The z-value for a given $c\%$ level of confidence may be obtained in Minitab by

```
MTB > LET K1 = (100 + c)/200
MTB > INVCDF K1 K2;
SUBC> NORMAL 0 1.
MTB > PRINT K2
K2 X      z-value
```

For example, to obtain the z-value for 85% confidence,

```
MTB > LET K1 = (85 + 100)/200
MTB > INVCDF  K1  K2;
SUBC> NORMAL  0  1.
MTB > PRINT  K2
K2      1.43953
```

Hence, to five places past the decimal point, the z-value needed to construct an 85% confidence interval is 1.43953.

The z-value for a z-test of hypothesis may be obtained in Minitab as follows:

1. One-tailed test.

General Algorithm (S% LOS)
```
MTB > LET K1 = (100 − S)/100
MTB > INVCDF K1 K2;
SUBC> NORMAL 0 1.
MTB > PRINT K2
K2       z-value
```

Example (4% LOS)
```
MTB > LET K1 = (100 − 4)/100
MTB > INVCDF K1 K2;
SUBC> NORMAL 0 1.
MTB > PRINT K2
K2      1.75069
```

2. Two-tailed test.

General Algorithm (S% LOS)
```
MTB > LET K1 = (100 − S/2)/100
MTB > INVCDF K1 K2;
SUBC> NORMAL 0 1.
MTB > PRINT K2
K2  z-value
```

Example (4% LOS)
```
MTB > LET K1 = (100 − 4/2)/100
MTB > INVCDF K1 K2;
SUBC> NORMAL 0 1.
MTB > PRINT K2 K2   2.05375
```

Hence, to five places past the decimal point, at the 4% level of significance the critical z-value for a one-tailed z-test is 1.75069; for a two-tailed z-test, 2.05375.

Table 8: Test of Hypothesis z-Table.

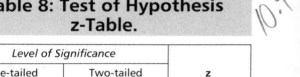

Level of Significance		z
One-tailed	Two-tailed	
.10	.20	1.282
.05	.10	1.645
.025	.05	1.960
.01	.02	2.326
.005	.01	2.567
.001	.002	3.090
.0005	.001	3.291
.00005	.0001	3.891
.000005	.00001	4.491

as z↓ Los↑.

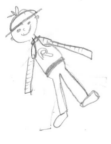

Table 9: Test of Hypothesis t-Table.

Assumption: Normal Distribution

df	Level of Significance for one-tailed test					
	.10	.05	.025	.01	.005	.0005
	Level of Significance for two-tailed test					
	.20	.10	.05	.02	.01	.001
1	3.07768	6.31375	12.7062	31.8206	63.6570	636.607
2	1.88562	2.91999	4.3027	6.9646	9.9248	31.598
3	1.63778	2.35341	3.1825	4.5407	5.8410	12.924
4	1.53320	2.13184	2.7764	3.7470	4.6041	8.610
5	1.47589	2.01505	2.5706	3.3649	4.0321	6.869
6	1.43977	1.94317	2.4469	3.1427	3.7075	5.959
7	1.41493	1.89456	2.3646	2.9980	3.4995	5.408
8	1.39685	1.85953	2.3060	2.8965	3.3554	5.041
9	1.38303	1.83313	2.2622	2.8215	3.2498	4.781
10	1.37215	1.81244	2.2281	2.7638	3.1693	4.587
11	1.36342	1.79588	2.2010	2.7181	3.1058	4.437
12	1.35621	1.78228	2.1788	2.6810	3.0545	4.318
13	1.35019	1.77094	2.1604	2.6503	3.0123	4.221
14	1.34502	1.76133	2.1448	2.6245	2.9768	4.140
15	1.34060	1.75307	2.1315	2.6025	2.9467	4.073
16	1.33677	1.74587	2.1199	2.5835	2.9208	4.015
17	1.33338	1.73962	2.1098	2.5669	2.8982	3.965
18	1.33036	1.73407	2.1009	2.5524	2.8784	3.922
19	1.32775	1.72911	2.0930	2.5395	2.8610	3.883
20	1.32533	1.72474	2.0860	2.5280	2.8453	3.849
21	1.32320	1.72074	2.0796	2.5176	2.8314	3.819
22	1.32125	1.71715	2.0739	2.5083	2.8187	3.792
23	1.31944	1.71389	2.0687	2.4999	2.8074	3.768
24	1.31783	1.71087	2.0639	2.4921	2.7969	3.745
25	1.31636	1.70813	2.0595	2.4851	2.7874	3.725
26	1.31497	1.70563	2.0556	2.4786	2.7787	3.707
27	1.31369	1.70326	2.0519	2.4727	2.7707	3.690
28	1.31253	1.70112	2.0484	2.4671	2.7633	3.674
29	1.31142	1.69911	2.0452	2.4620	2.7564	3.659
30	1.31038	1.69724	2.0423	2.4573	2.7500	3.646
40	1.30308	1.68386	2.0211	2.4232	2.7045	3.551
50	1.29868	1.67589	2.0085	2.4033	2.6778	3.496
60	1.29581	1.67065	2.0003	2.3902	2.6604	3.460
70	1.29376	1.66692	1.9944	2.3808	2.6480	3.435
80	1.29222	1.66413	1.9901	2.3739	2.6387	3.416
90	1.29103	1.66196	1.9867	2.3685	2.6316	3.402
100	1.29007	1.66024	1.9840	2.3642	2.6259	3.391
∞	1.28155	1.64485	1.9600	2.3264	2.5758	3.291

Minitab critical t-value for any given LOS α and *df* is obtained as follows:

one-tailed test
MTB > LET K1 = 1 − α
MTB > INVCDF K1 K2;
SUBC> T df.
MTB > PRINT K2
K2 [t-value]

two-tailed test
MTB > LET K1 = 1 − α/2
MTB > INVCDF K1 K2;
SUBC> T df.
MTB > PRINT K2
K2 [t-value]

Table 10a: F-Table (LOS = .01).

rowdf	column df										
	1	2	3	4	5	6	7	8	9	10	11
2	98.5057	99.0001	99.1692	99.2495	99.2982	99.3317	99.3545	99.3772	99.3896	99.4035	99.4069
3	34.1169	30.8156	29.4571	28.7099	28.2374	27.9105	27.6723	27.4889	27.3453	27.2289	27.1327
4	21.1977	18.0000	16.6946	15.9771	15.5215	15.2071	14.9757	14.7987	14.6591	14.5460	14.4522
5	16.2579	13.2739	12.0600	11.3920	10.9670	10.6721	10.4556	10.2893	10.1577	10.0512	9.9626
6	13.7452	10.9246	9.7796	9.1482	8.7460	8.4661	8.2601	8.1016	7.9762	7.8740	7.7896
7	12.2462	9.5464	8.4514	7.8465	7.4605	7.1913	6.9929	6.8400	6.7187	6.6201	6.5382
8	11.2587	8.6490	7.5909	7.0061	6.6319	6.3707	6.1777	6.0289	5.9106	5.8144	5.7344
9	10.5614	8.0215	6.9920	6.4221	6.0570	5.8018	5.6128	5.4671	5.3512	5.2565	5.1779
10	10.0443	7.5594	6.5523	5.9944	5.6363	5.3858	5.2001	5.0566	4.9424	4.8492	4.7715
11	9.6460	7.2057	6.2167	5.6683	5.3160	5.0692	4.8861	4.7445	4.6315	4.5393	4.4625
12	9.3302	6.9267	5.9525	5.4119	5.0643	4.8206	4.6395	4.4994	4.3875	4.2961	4.2198
13	9.0737	6.7010	5.7394	5.2053	4.8616	4.6204	4.4410	4.3021	4.1911	4.1002	4.0245
14	8.8616	6.5150	5.5639	5.0354	4.6950	4.4558	4.2778	4.1400	4.0297	3.9394	3.8640
15	8.6831	6.3589	5.4169	4.8932	4.5556	4.3183	4.1415	4.0044	3.8948	3.8050	3.7299
16	8.5310	6.2263	5.2922	4.7726	4.4374	4.2017	4.0260	3.8896	3.7804	3.6909	3.6161
17	8.3998	6.1121	5.1850	4.6690	4.3359	4.1015	3.9267	3.7909	3.6822	3.5931	3.5185
18	8.2854	6.0128	5.0919	4.5790	4.2478	4.0146	3.8406	3.7054	3.5971	3.5082	3.4338
19	8.1850	5.9259	5.0102	4.5003	4.1708	3.9386	3.7653	3.6305	3.5225	3.4338	3.3596
20	8.0960	5.8489	4.9382	4.4307	4.1027	3.8714	3.6987	3.5644	3.4567	3.3682	3.2941
21	8.0166	5.7804	4.8740	4.3688	4.0422	3.8117	3.6396	3.5056	3.3981	3.3098	3.2359
22	7.9453	5.7189	4.8166	4.3134	3.9880	3.7583	3.5867	3.4530	3.3458	3.2576	3.1837
23	7.8812	5.6636	4.7649	4.2636	3.9392	3.7102	3.5390	3.4057	3.2986	3.2106	3.1368
24	7.8229	5.6137	4.7180	4.2184	3.8951	3.6667	3.4959	3.3629	3.2560	3.1681	3.0944
25	7.7698	5.5679	4.6754	4.1774	3.8550	3.6272	3.4568	3.3239	3.2172	3.1294	3.0558
26	7.7213	5.5263	4.6366	4.1400	3.8183	3.5911	3.4210	3.2884	3.1818	3.0941	3.0206
27	7.6767	5.4881	4.6009	4.1057	3.7848	3.5580	3.3882	3.2558	3.1494	3.0618	2.9882
28	7.6357	5.4530	4.5681	4.0740	3.7539	3.5275	3.3581	3.2259	3.1196	3.0320	2.9585
29	7.5977	5.4204	4.5378	4.0449	3.7254	3.4995	3.3303	3.1982	3.0920	3.0045	2.9311
30	7.5625	5.3904	4.5097	4.0179	3.6990	3.4735	3.3045	3.1726	3.0665	2.9791	2.9057
40	7.3141	5.1786	4.3126	3.8283	3.5138	3.2910	3.1237	2.9930	2.8876	2.8005	2.7273
50	7.1705	5.0566	4.1993	3.7195	3.4077	3.1865	3.0202	2.8900	2.7850	2.6981	2.6250
60	7.0771	4.9774	4.1259	3.6490	3.3389	3.1187	2.9530	2.8233	2.7185	2.6317	2.5587
75	6.9854	4.8998	4.0540	3.5801	3.2716	3.0524	2.8874	2.7581	2.6534	2.5668	2.4938
100	6.8952	4.8239	3.9837	3.5127	3.2059	2.9877	2.8233	2.6943	2.5898	2.5033	2.4302

Table 10a, continued: F-Table (LOS = .01).

rowdf	column df									
	12	13	14	15	20	25	30	40	50	100
2	99.4132	99.4260	99.4311	99.4288	99.4444	99.4585	99.4689	99.4708	99.4837	99.4890
3	27.0510	26.9824	26.9244	26.8723	26.6907	26.5783	26.5052	26.4109	26.3539	26.2405
4	14.3736	14.3066	14.2485	14.1982	14.0199	13.9107	13.8379	13.7453	13.6899	13.5768
5	9.8882	9.8250	9.7700	9.7221	9.5527	9.4492	9.3793	9.2911	9.2377	9.1299
6	7.7182	7.6575	7.6049	7.5591	7.3958	7.2960	7.2285	7.1433	7.0915	6.9867
7	6.4691	6.4100	6.3590	6.3144	6.1555	6.0580	5.9920	5.9084	5.8577	5.7547
8	5.6667	5.6088	5.5589	5.5151	5.3590	5.2631	5.1981	5.1156	5.0654	4.9634
9	5.1114	5.0545	5.0052	4.9621	4.8080	4.7131	4.6486	4.5666	4.5168	4.4149
10	4.7058	4.6496	4.6008	4.5581	4.4054	4.3110	4.2469	4.1653	4.1155	4.0137
11	4.3974	4.3416	4.2932	4.2508	4.0991	4.0051	3.9411	3.8595	3.8097	3.7077
12	4.1552	4.0998	4.0518	4.0097	3.8584	3.7647	3.7008	3.6192	3.5692	3.4668
13	3.9603	3.9052	3.8573	3.8154	3.6646	3.5710	3.5071	3.4253	3.3752	3.2723
14	3.8001	3.7452	3.6975	3.6557	3.5052	3.4116	3.3476	3.2656	3.2153	3.1118
15	3.6663	3.6115	3.5640	3.5222	3.3719	3.2782	3.2141	3.1319	3.0813	2.9772
16	3.5527	3.4981	3.4507	3.4090	3.2587	3.1650	3.1007	3.0182	2.9675	2.8626
17	3.4552	3.4007	3.3533	3.3117	3.1615	3.0676	3.0033	2.9205	2.8694	2.7639
18	3.3706	3.3162	3.2689	3.2273	3.0771	2.9831	2.9185	2.8354	2.7842	2.6779
19	3.2965	3.2422	3.1949	3.1533	3.0031	2.9089	2.8442	2.7608	2.7093	2.6023
20	3.2311	3.1769	3.1296	3.0880	2.9378	2.8434	2.7785	2.6947	2.6430	2.5353
21	3.1730	3.1187	3.0715	3.0299	2.8796	2.7851	2.7199	2.6359	2.5839	2.4755
22	3.1209	3.0667	3.0195	2.9780	2.8275	2.7328	2.6675	2.5831	2.5308	2.4217
23	3.0740	3.0199	2.9727	2.9311	2.7805	2.6856	2.6202	2.5355	2.4829	2.3732
24	3.0316	2.9775	2.9303	2.8887	2.7380	2.6429	2.5773	2.4923	2.4395	2.3291
25	2.9931	2.9389	2.8917	2.8502	2.6993	2.6041	2.5383	2.4530	2.4000	2.2888
26	2.9578	2.9037	2.8565	2.8150	2.6640	2.5686	2.5026	2.4170	2.3637	2.2519
27	2.9256	2.8715	2.8243	2.7827	2.6316	2.5360	2.4699	2.3840	2.3304	2.2180
28	2.8959	2.8418	2.7946	2.7530	2.6018	2.5060	2.4397	2.3535	2.2997	2.1867
29	2.8685	2.8144	2.7672	2.7256	2.5742	2.4783	2.4118	2.3253	2.2714	2.1577
30	2.8431	2.7890	2.7418	2.7002	2.5487	2.4526	2.3860	2.2992	2.2450	2.1307
40	2.6648	2.6107	2.5634	2.5216	2.3689	2.2714	2.2034	2.1142	2.0581	1.9383
50	2.5625	2.5083	2.4609	2.4190	2.2652	2.1667	2.0976	2.0066	1.9490	1.8248
60	2.4961	2.4419	2.3944	2.3523	2.1978	2.0984	2.0285	1.9360	1.8772	1.7493
75	2.4312	2.3769	2.3292	2.2870	2.1316	2.0312	1.9604	1.8663	1.8060	1.6738
100	2.3676	2.3132	2.2654	2.2230	2.0666	1.9652	1.8933	1.7972	1.7353	1.5977

Table 10b: F-Table (LOS = .05).

rowdf	1	2	3	4	5	6	7	8	9	10	11
						column df					
2	18.5121	19.0000	19.1634	19.2468	19.2971	19.3294	19.3533	19.3716	19.3854	19.3959	19.4042
3	10.1282	9.5522	9.2769	9.1169	9.0135	8.9405	8.8867	8.8450	8.8122	8.7854	8.7634
4	7.7086	6.9443	6.5913	6.3881	6.2559	6.1632	6.0942	6.0412	5.9989	5.9643	5.9359
5	6.6079	5.7860	5.4094	5.1923	5.0502	4.9503	4.8758	4.8184	4.7724	4.7351	4.7040
6	5.9874	5.1431	4.7570	4.5337	4.3874	4.2839	4.2067	4.1468	4.0990	4.0599	4.0275
7	5.5913	4.7373	4.3469	4.1203	3.9715	3.8660	3.7870	3.7258	3.6767	3.6365	3.6030
8	5.3176	4.4590	4.0661	3.8379	3.6876	3.5806	3.5004	3.4382	3.3881	3.3472	3.3130
9	5.1174	4.2566	3.8625	3.6331	3.4816	3.3738	3.2928	3.2296	3.1789	3.1373	3.1024
10	4.9646	4.1029	3.7083	3.4780	3.3259	3.2172	3.1355	3.0717	3.0204	2.9783	2.9430
11	4.8442	3.9822	3.5874	3.3567	3.2039	3.0947	3.0123	2.9480	2.8962	2.8536	2.8179
12	4.7472	3.8853	3.4903	3.2592	3.1059	2.9961	2.9134	2.8486	2.7964	2.7534	2.7173
13	4.6673	3.8055	3.4105	3.1792	3.0254	2.9153	2.8321	2.7669	2.7144	2.6710	2.6347
14	4.6001	3.7388	3.3439	3.1123	2.9582	2.8478	2.7642	2.6986	2.6458	2.6022	2.5655
15	4.5432	3.6823	3.2874	3.0556	2.9013	2.7905	2.7066	2.6408	2.5876	2.5437	2.5068
16	4.4940	3.6338	3.2389	3.0069	2.8524	2.7413	2.6572	2.5911	2.5377	2.4935	2.4564
17	4.4512	3.5915	3.1968	2.9647	2.8100	2.6987	2.6143	2.5480	2.4943	2.4499	2.4125
18	4.4140	3.5545	3.1599	2.9278	2.7729	2.6613	2.5767	2.5102	2.4563	2.4117	2.3741
19	4.3807	3.5219	3.1274	2.8951	2.7401	2.6283	2.5436	2.4768	2.4227	2.3780	2.3402
20	4.3513	3.4928	3.0984	2.8661	2.7109	2.5989	2.5140	2.4471	2.3928	2.3479	2.3100
21	4.3249	3.4668	3.0725	2.8401	2.6848	2.5727	2.4876	2.4204	2.3660	2.3209	2.2829
22	4.3010	3.4433	3.0491	2.8168	2.6613	2.5490	2.4638	2.3965	2.3419	2.2967	2.2585
23	4.2794	3.4221	3.0280	2.7955	2.6400	2.5277	2.4422	2.3748	2.3201	2.2747	2.2364
24	4.2597	3.4029	3.0088	2.7763	2.6207	2.5082	2.4226	2.3551	2.3002	2.2548	2.2163
25	4.2417	3.3852	2.9912	2.7587	2.6030	2.4904	2.4048	2.3371	2.2821	2.2365	2.1979
26	4.2253	3.3690	2.9752	2.7426	2.5868	2.4741	2.3883	2.3205	2.2654	2.2197	2.1810
27	4.2101	3.3541	2.9603	2.7278	2.5719	2.4591	2.3732	2.3053	2.2501	2.2043	2.1655
28	4.1959	3.3404	2.9467	2.7141	2.5581	2.4453	2.3592	2.2913	2.2360	2.1900	2.1512
29	4.1829	3.3277	2.9341	2.7014	2.5454	2.4324	2.3463	2.2783	2.2229	2.1768	2.1379
30	4.1709	3.3159	2.9223	2.6896	2.5336	2.4205	2.3343	2.2662	2.2107	2.1646	2.1256
40	4.0847	3.2317	2.8387	2.6060	2.4494	2.3359	2.2490	2.1802	2.1240	2.0773	2.0376
50	4.0343	3.1826	2.7900	2.5572	2.4004	2.2865	2.1992	2.1299	2.0733	2.0261	1.9861
60	4.0012	3.1504	2.7581	2.5252	2.3683	2.2541	2.1665	2.0970	2.0401	1.9926	1.9522
75	3.9686	3.1186	2.7266	2.4937	2.3366	2.2221	2.1343	2.0644	2.0073	1.9594	1.9188
100	3.9361	3.0873	2.6955	2.4626	2.3053	2.1906	2.1025	2.0323	1.9748	1.9267	1.8857

Table 10b, continued: F-Table (LOS = .05).

rowdf	column df									
	12	13	14	15	20	25	30	40	50	100
2	19.4124	19.4190	19.4243	19.4287	19.4466	19.4557	19.4626	19.4711	19.4752	19.4861
3	8.7448	8.7288	8.7149	8.7028	8.6601	8.6339	8.6163	8.5943	8.5809	8.5537
4	5.9118	5.8912	5.8732	5.8578	5.8025	5.7688	5.7460	5.7170	5.6995	5.6640
5	4.6776	4.6552	4.6358	4.6189	4.5582	4.5210	4.4957	4.4637	4.4444	4.4050
6	3.9999	3.9763	3.9559	3.9380	3.8743	3.8348	3.8082	3.7743	3.7537	3.7117
7	3.5747	3.5504	3.5293	3.5108	3.4445	3.4036	3.3758	3.3405	3.3189	3.2749
8	3.2839	3.2590	3.2374	3.2183	3.1503	3.1081	3.0794	3.0428	3.0204	2.9746
9	3.0730	3.0476	3.0254	3.0061	2.9365	2.8932	2.8637	2.8259	2.8029	2.7555
10	2.9130	2.8871	2.8647	2.8450	2.7740	2.7298	2.6996	2.6608	2.6371	2.5884
11	2.7875	2.7614	2.7386	2.7186	2.6465	2.6014	2.5705	2.5309	2.5066	2.4566
12	2.6867	2.6602	2.6371	2.6168	2.5436	2.4977	2.4663	2.4259	2.4010	2.3498
13	2.6037	2.5769	2.5536	2.5331	2.4589	2.4123	2.3803	2.3392	2.3138	2.2614
14	2.5342	2.5073	2.4837	2.4630	2.3879	2.3407	2.3082	2.2664	2.2405	2.1870
15	2.4753	2.4481	2.4244	2.4035	2.3275	2.2798	2.2468	2.2043	2.1780	2.1234
16	2.4247	2.3972	2.3733	2.3522	2.2755	2.2272	2.1938	2.1507	2.1240	2.0685
17	2.3807	2.3531	2.3290	2.3077	2.2304	2.1815	2.1477	2.1040	2.0769	2.0204
18	2.3421	2.3143	2.2900	2.2686	2.1907	2.1413	2.1071	2.0629	2.0354	1.9780
19	2.3080	2.2800	2.2556	2.2340	2.1555	2.1057	2.0712	2.0264	1.9986	1.9403
20	2.2776	2.2495	2.2249	2.2033	2.1241	2.0739	2.0391	1.9938	1.9656	1.9065
21	2.2503	2.2221	2.1975	2.1757	2.0960	2.0454	2.0103	1.9645	1.9360	1.8761
22	2.2258	2.1975	2.1727	2.1508	2.0707	2.0196	1.9842	1.9380	1.9092	1.8486
23	2.2036	2.1752	2.1502	2.1282	2.0476	1.9963	1.9606	1.9139	1.8848	1.8234
24	2.1834	2.1548	2.1298	2.1077	2.0267	1.9750	1.9389	1.8919	1.8625	1.8005
25	2.1649	2.1362	2.1111	2.0889	2.0075	1.9554	1.9192	1.8718	1.8421	1.7794
26	2.1479	2.1192	2.0940	2.0716	1.9898	1.9375	1.9010	1.8532	1.8233	1.7599
27	2.1323	2.1035	2.0781	2.0558	1.9736	1.9210	1.8842	1.8361	1.8059	1.7419
28	2.1179	2.0889	2.0636	2.0411	1.9585	1.9057	1.8687	1.8203	1.7898	1.7251
29	2.1045	2.0755	2.0500	2.0275	1.9446	1.8915	1.8543	1.8055	1.7748	1.7096
30	2.0921	2.0630	2.0374	2.0148	1.9317	1.8783	1.8409	1.7918	1.7609	1.6950
40	2.0035	1.9737	1.9476	1.9245	1.8389	1.7835	1.7444	1.6928	1.6600	1.5892
50	1.9515	1.9214	1.8949	1.8714	1.7841	1.7273	1.6872	1.6337	1.5995	1.5249
60	1.9174	1.8870	1.8602	1.8364	1.7480	1.6902	1.6492	1.5943	1.5590	1.4814
75	1.8836	1.8530	1.8259	1.8018	1.7121	1.6532	1.6112	1.5548	1.5183	1.4371
100	1.8503	1.8193	1.7919	1.7675	1.6764	1.6163	1.5733	1.5151	1.4772	1.3917

Table 11: F_{max} Table.

n	LOS	Number of levels							
		3	4	5	6	7	8	9	10
5	.05	15.5	20.6	25.2	29.5	33.6	37.5	41.1	44.6
	.01	37	49	59	69	79	89	97	106
6	.05	10.8	13.7	16.3	18.7	20.8	22.9	24.7	26.5
	.01	22	28	33	38	42	46	50	54
7	.05	8.38	10.4	12.1	13.7	15.0	16.3	17.5	18.6
	.01	15.5	19.1	22	25	27	30	32	34
8	.05	6.94	8.44	9.70	10.8	11.3	12.7	13.5	14.3
	.01	12.1	14.5	16.5	18.4	20	22	23	24
9	.05	6.00	7.18	8.12	9.03	9.78	10.5	11.1	11.7
	.01	9.9	11.7	13.2	14.5	15.8	16.9	17.9	18.9
10	.05	5.34	6.31	7.11	7.80	8.41	8.95	9.45	9.91
	.01	8.5	9.9	11.1	12.1	13.1	13.9	14.7	15.3
11	.05	4.85	5.67	6.34	6.92	7.42	7.87	8.28	8.66
	.01	7.4	8.6	9.6	10.4	11.1	11.8	12.4	12.9
13	.05	4.16	4.79	5.30	5.72	6.09	6.42	6.72	7.00
	.01	6.1	6.9	7.6	8.2	8.7	9.1	9.5	9.9
16	.05	3.54	4.01	4.37	4.68	4.95	5.19	5.40	5.59
	.01	4.9	5.5	6.0	6.4	6.7	7.1	7.3	5.5
21	.05	2.95	3.29	3.54	3.76	3.94	4.10	4.24	4.37
	.01	3.8	4.3	4.6	4.9	5.1	5.3	5.5	5.6
31	.05	2.40	2.61	2.78	2.91	3.02	3.12	3.21	3.29
	.01	3.0	3.3	3.4	3.6	3.7	3.8	3.9	4.0
61	.05	1.85	1.96	2.04	2.11	2.17	2.22	2.26	2.30
	.01	2.2	2.3	2.4	2.4	2.5	2.5	2.6	2.6

n = sample size, LOS = level of significance

Comment. For a preliminary test for homoscedasticity, use LOS = .01; LOS = .05 is provided for convenience in reporting a p-value for the F_{max} test.

This table is adapted from David HA: *Biometrika* 219, (1952): 422.

Table 12: Chisquared Table.

df	.99	.95	.90	.50	.25	.10	.05	.01	.005
							Level of Significance		
1	0.0002	0.0039	0.0158	0.4549	1.3233	2.7055	3.8415	6.6349	7.8795
2	0.0201	0.1026	0.2107	1.3863	2.7726	4.6052	5.9915	9.2103	10.5966
3	0.1148	0.3518	0.5844	2.3660	4.1083	6.2514	7.8147	11.3449	12.8382
4	0.2971	0.7107	1.0636	3.3567	5.3853	7.7794	9.4877	13.2767	14.8603
5	0.5543	1.1455	1.6103	4.3515	6.6257	9.2364	11.0705	15.0863	16.7496
6	0.8721	1.6354	2.2041	5.3481	7.8408	10.6446	12.5916	16.8119	18.5476
7	1.2390	2.1674	2.8331	6.3458	9.0371	12.0170	14.0671	18.4753	20.2778
8	1.6465	2.7326	3.4895	7.3441	10.2189	13.3616	15.5073	20.0902	21.9550
9	2.0879	3.3251	4.1682	8.3428	11.3888	14.6837	16.9190	21.6660	23.5893
10	2.5582	3.9403	4.8652	9.3418	12.5489	15.9872	18.3070	23.2093	25.1882
11	3.0535	4.5748	5.5778	10.3410	13.7007	17.2750	19.6751	24.7250	26.7569
12	3.5706	5.2260	6.3038	11.3403	14.8454	18.5493	21.0261	26.2170	28.2996
13	4.1069	5.8919	7.0415	12.3398	15.9839	19.8119	22.3620	27.6882	29.8194
14	4.6604	6.5706	7.7895	13.3393	17.1169	21.0641	23.6848	29.1413	31.3194
15	5.2293	7.2609	8.5468	14.3389	18.2451	22.3071	24.9958	30.5779	32.8013
16	5.8122	7.9616	9.3122	15.3385	19.3689	23.5418	26.2963	32.0001	34.2674
17	6.4078	8.6718	10.0852	16.3382	20.4887	24.7690	27.5871	33.4085	35.7182
18	7.0149	9.3905	10.8649	17.3379	21.6049	25.9894	28.8693	34.8053	37.1564
19	7.6327	10.1170	11.6509	18.3377	22.7178	27.2036	30.1435	36.1907	38.5820
20	8.2604	10.8508	12.4426	19.3374	23.8277	28.4120	31.4104	37.5662	39.9968
21	8.8972	11.5913	13.2396	20.3372	24.9348	29.6151	32.6706	38.9322	41.4011
22	9.5425	12.3380	14.0415	21.3370	26.0393	30.8133	33.9245	40.2895	42.7960
23	10.1957	13.0905	14.8480	22.3369	27.1413	32.0069	35.1724	41.6382	44.1808
24	10.8564	13.8484	15.6587	23.3367	28.2412	33.1962	36.4150	42.9798	45.5586
25	11.5240	14.6114	16.4734	24.3366	29.3389	34.3816	37.6525	44.3144	46.9285
26	12.1981	15.3792	17.2919	25.3365	30.4346	35.5632	38.8852	45.6419	48.2903
27	12.8785	16.1514	18.1139	26.3363	31.5284	36.7412	40.1133	46.9631	49.6452
28	13.5647	16.9279	18.9392	27.3362	32.6205	37.9159	41.3372	48.2783	50.9936
29	14.2565	17.7084	19.7677	28.3361	33.7109	39.0875	42.5570	49.5881	52.3360
30	14.9535	18.4927	20.5992	29.3360	34.7997	40.2560	43.7730	50.8922	53.6720

Table 13: Critical Correlation Values.

This table provides the critical correlation (critical r) at the 1% level of significance.

Technical note: The computations are based on the fact that the distribution of sample correlations from a bivariate normal distribution follows the statistic

$$T_{n-2} = \frac{r\sqrt{n-2}}{\sqrt{1-r^2}}$$

which has a T distribution with $n-2$ degrees of freedom.

n	critical r
5	0.959
6	0.917
7	0.875
8	0.834
9	0.798
10	0.765
11	0.735
12	0.708
13	0.684
14	0.661
15	0.641
16	0.623
17	0.606
18	0.590
19	0.575
20	0.561
21	0.549
22	0.537
23	0.526
24	0.515
25	0.505
26	0.496
27	0.487
28	0.479
29	0.471
30	0.463
31	0.456
32	0.449
33	0.442
34	0.436
35	0.430
36	0.424
37	0.418
38	0.413
39	0.408
40	0.403
41	0.398
42	0.393
43	0.389
44	0.384
45	0.380
46	0.376
47	0.372
48	0.368
49	0.365
50	0.361

Table14: The Greek Alphabet.

Letter name	lower case	CAPITAL
alpha	α	A
beta	β	B
gamma	γ	Γ
delta	δ	Δ
epsilon	ϵ	E
zeta	ζ	Z
eta	η	H
theta	θ	Θ
iota	ι	I
kappa	κ	K
lambda	λ	Λ
mu	μ	M
nu	ν	N
xi	ζ	Z
omicron	o	O
pi	π	Π
rho	ρ	P
sigma	ς	Σ
tau	τ	T
upsilon	υ	Y
phi	ϕ	Φ
chi	χ	X
psi	ψ	Ψ
omega	ω	Ω

TEST OF HYPOTHESIS CHARTS

General Format

Use the Test of Hypothesis Charts as a guide to write up your solution in the seven-step test of hypothesis protocol (see Section 9.1 for general outline of the seven-step protocol). The only exception is Chart 2C, since the s-test (Section 10.2) has its own procedure. In each test of hypothesis chart, only the first five steps are provided. Steps 6 and 7 are as follows.

Step 6. Sample value. Compute the sample value based on the test statistic provided in step 3 and the sample data. Include the appropriate sample legend if the raw data set is not provided.

Step 7. Conclusion. The decision should state the statistical conclusion of the test in one of the two following forms:

    a. If the computed value falls in the "do not reject H_0" region of the decision line, then:
    Based on the given data, at the a level of significance do not reject H_0.

    b. If the computed value falls in the "reject H_0" region of the decision line, then:
    Based on the given data, at the α level of significance reject H_0 and accept H_a.

In addition to the statistical conclusion, an appropriate clinical interpretation should also be given (i.e., what does it all mean?).

After Section 10.4, the p-value should also be stated in step 7. In the literature, often the entire computational part of a test of hypothesis is reduced to merely reporting the p-value for the test.

Standard test of hypothesis symbols include:

H_0:	null hypothesis
H_a:	alternate hypothesis
μ	population mean
p	population proportion
LOS	level of significance
n	sample size

I. Preliminary. $np_0 \geq 5$ and $n(1 - p_0) \geq 5$ where
n = sample size
p_0 = test reference value

10.1

II. Main Test of Hypothesis.

1. Hypothesis. p_0 = test reference value

     Test Alternate: (a)   (b)   (c)

                     $H_0: p = p_0$ $H_0: p \geq p_0$ $H_0: p \leq p_0$

                     $H_a: p \neq p_0$ $H_a: p < p_0$ $H_a: p > p_0$

2. LOS. α

3. Test Statistic. $\dfrac{\hat{p} - p_0}{\sqrt{\dfrac{p_0(1 - p_0)}{n}}}$ where $\hat{p}$ = sample proportion

4. Critical Value. Obtain z from Z-Table (Appendix, Table 8).

Test Alternate	Z-Table Column Heading
(a)	LOS for two-tailed test
(b) or (c)	LOS for one-tailed test

5. Decision Line. z is the critical value from step 4.

Test Alternate	Decision Line
(a)	Reject H_0 Do Not Reject H_0 $-z$ Reject H_0 z Z
(b)	Reject H_0 Do Not Reject H_0 $-z$ Z
(c)	Do Not Reject H_0 Reject H_0 z Z

≠ or =

>

≥

≤

CHART 2: TEST OF HYPOTHESIS FOR AN AVERAGE VALUE, SINGLE POPULATION.

Background. One may conduct a test of hypothesis for an average using this chart when provided with a data set obtained from a random sample with independent observations. The data set must consist of interval numbers.

I. Raw Data Given

1. Normal distribution.
   Apply the t-test for the mean (Chart 2A).
2. Large sample size ($n > 30$).
   Apply the z-test for the mean (Chart 2B).
3. s-Test for the median (Chart 2C).

II. Sample Legend (size, mean, standard deviation) Given

1. Large sample size ($n > 30$).
   Apply the z-test for the mean (Chart 2B).
2. Continuous data (decimal numbers).
   Assume normal distribution.
   Apply the t-test for the mean (Chart 2A).
3. Otherwise, insufficient information for analysis.

CHART 2A: TEST OF HYPOTHESIS FOR THE MEAN, ONE POPULATION, NORMAL RANDOM VARIABLE.

assuming normality.

1. Hypothesis. μ_0 = test reference number

   Test Alternate: (a)   (b)   (c)

(a)	(b)	(c)
$H_0: \mu = \mu_0$	$H_0: \mu \geq \mu_0$	$H_0: \mu \leq \mu_0$
$H_a: \mu \neq \mu_0$	$H_a: \mu < \mu_0$	$H_a: \mu > \mu_0$

2. LOS. α $\approx .05$

3. Test Statistic. $\dfrac{\overline{X} - \mu_0}{(s/\sqrt{n})}$

   test reference mean

4. Critical Value.   Obtain t from T-Table (Appendix, Table 9)
   where $df = n - 1$ (n = sample size), and

Test Alternate	T-Table Column Heading
(a)	LOS for two-tailed test
(b) or (c)	LOS for one-tailed test

5. Decision Line. t is the critical value obtained in step 4.

Test Alternate	Decision Line
(a)	Reject H_0 Do Not Reject H_0 $-t$ Reject H_0 t T_{n-1}
(b)	Reject H_0 Do Not Reject H_0 $-t$ T_{n-1}
(c)	Do Not Reject H_0 Reject H_0 t T_{n-1}

1. Hypothesis. μ_0 = test reference number

     Test Alternate:

(a)	(b)	(c)
$H_0: \mu = \mu_0$	$H_0: \mu \geq \mu_0$	$H_0: \mu \leq \mu_0$
$H_a: \mu \neq \mu_0$	$H_a: \mu < \mu_0$	$H_a: \mu > \mu_0$

2. LOS. α

3. Test Statistic. $\dfrac{\overline{X} - \mu_0}{(s/\sqrt{n})}$

4. Critical Value. Obtain z from Z-Table (Appendix, Table 8)

Test Alternate	Z-Table Column Heading
(a)	LOS for two-tailed test
(b) or (c)	LOS for one-tailed test

5. Decision Line. z is the critical value obtained in step 4.

Test Alternate	Decision Line
(a)	
(b)	
(c)	

1. Hypothesis $\quad\quad\quad \eta_0 =$ test reference number

      Test Alternate: (a)   (b)   (c)

                       $H_0: \eta = \eta_0 \quad H_0: \eta \geq \eta_0 \quad H_0: \eta \leq \eta_0$

                       $H_a: \eta \neq \eta_0 \quad H_a: \eta < \eta_0 \quad H_a: \eta > \eta_0$

2. LOS. α

3. Minitab.   MTB > SET C
                    DATA > enter data
                    MTB > END OF DATA
                    MTB > STEST η_0 C;
                    SUBC> ALTERNATE K.

NOTE. In a problem you must specify a column C and use the test reference value, η_0. The alternate K is coded in Minitab as either 0, -1, or 1, respectively, according to the test alternate (a), (b), or (c) identified in the hypothesis in step 1.

    For example, to test $H_0: \eta \geq 50$ versus $H_a: \eta < 50$,

```
MTB > STEST  50 C1;
SUBC> ALTERNATE -1.
```

4. Conclusion.

    a. Do not reject H_0 if p-value $\geq \alpha$, where α is the LOS specified in step 2.

    b. Reject H_0 and accept H_a if p-value $< \alpha$.

PAIRED-DIFFERENCE t-TEST

1. Hypothesis. $0 = $ test reference number

   Test Alternate:

(a)	(b)	(c)
$H_0: \mu_D = 0$	$H_0: \mu_D \geq 0$	$H_0: \mu_D \leq 0$
$H_a: \mu_D \neq 0$	$H_a: \mu_D < 0$	$H_a: \mu_D > 0$

2. LOS. α

3. Test Statistic. $\dfrac{\overline{D}}{(s_d/\sqrt{n})}$

4. Critical Value.   Obtain t from T-Table (Appendix, Table 9) where $df = n - 1$ ($n =$ sample size), and

Test Alternate	T-Table Column Heading
(a)	LOS for two-tailed test
(b) or (c)	LOS for one-tailed test

5. Decision Line. t is the critical value obtained in step 4.

Test Alternate	Decision Line
(a)	Reject H_0 — Do Not Reject H_0 — Reject$_0$ $-t$ t T_{n-1}
(b)	Reject H_0 — Do Not Reject H_0 $-t$ T_{n-1}
(c)	Do Not Reject H_0 — Reject H_0 t T_{n-1}

Note. If D is not consistent with normality, but n is large ($n > 30$), then apply Chart 2B to D, using a test reference value of 0.

CHART 4: COMPARISON OF PROPORTIONS, TWO POPULATIONS.

I. Preliminary Criterion (adequacy of sample sizes). Let

m = size of sample 1 (from population 1);
x = number in sample 1 with attribute of interest;
n = size of sample 2 (from population 2);
y = number in sample 2 with attribute of interest;
$\hat{p} = \frac{x+y}{m+n}$
$\hat{q} = 1 - \hat{p}$

Then, the samples are adequate if $m\hat{p}, m\hat{q}, n\hat{p}$, and $n\hat{q}$ are all ≥ 5.

II. Main Test of Hypothesis.

1. Hypothesis.

Test Alternate:

	(a)	(b)	(c)
	$H_0: p_1 = p_2$	$H_0: p_1 \geq p_2$	$H_0: p_1 \leq p_2$
	$H_a: p_1 \neq p_2$	$H_a: p_1 < p_2$	$H_a: p_1 > p_2$

2. LOS. α

3. Test Statistic. $\dfrac{\frac{x}{m} - \frac{y}{n}}{\sqrt{\hat{p}\hat{q}\left(\frac{1}{m} + \frac{1}{n}\right)}}$

4. Critical Value. Obtain z from Z-Table (Appendix, Table 8).

Test Alternate	Z-Table Column Heading
(a)	LOS for two-tailed test
(b) or (c)	LOS for one-tailed test

5. Decision Line. z is the critical value from step 4.

Test Alternate	Decision Line
(a)	Reject H_0 Do Not Reject H_0 $-z$ Reject H_0 z Z
(b)	Reject H_0 Do Not Reject H_0 $-z$ Z
(c)	Do Not Reject H_0 Reject H_0 z Z

CHART 5: COMPARISON OF AVERAGES FOR TWO POPULATIONS, INTERVAL DATA.

1. **Normal Distributions**
   If both distributions are normal, either by testing the raw data or by assumption from the data legend, then next test for homoscedasticity.
   a. If homoscedastic, then apply the pooled t-test for comparison of means (Chart 5A).
   b. If heteroscedastic, then apply the Smith-Satterthwaite t-test for comparison of means (Chart 5B).

2. **Large Sample Sizes**
   If both sample sizes are large (both greater than 30), then apply the large-samples z-test for comparison of means (Chart 5C).

3. **Mann-Whitney Test in Minitab**
   Suppose that the raw data set is given. Then apply Minitab to conduct a Mann-Whitney test for comparison of medians.

CHART 5A: POOLED t-TEST FOR COMPARISON OF MEANS.

1. Hypothesis.

	(a)	(b)	(c)
Test Alternate:	$H_0: \mu_1 = \mu_2$	$H_0: \mu_1 \geq \mu_2$	$H_0: \mu_1 \leq \mu_2$
	$H_a: \mu_1 \neq \mu_2$	$H_a: \mu_1 < \mu_2$	$H_a: \mu_1 > \mu_2$

2. LOS. α

3. Test Statistic.

$$\frac{\overline{X}_1 - \overline{X}_2}{\sqrt{s_p^2\left(\frac{1}{n_1} + \frac{1}{n_2}\right)}}$$

$$\text{where } s_p^2 = \frac{(n_1 - 1)s_1^2 + (n_2 - 1)s_2^2}{n_1 + n_2 - 2}$$

4. Critical Value. Obtain t from T-Table (Appendix, Table 9) where $df = n_1 + n_2 - 2$ and

Test Alternate	T-Table Column Heading
(a)	LOS for two-tailed test
(b) or (c)	LOS for one-tailed test

5. Decision Line. t is the critical value obtained in step 4.

Test Alternate	Decision Line
(a)	Reject H_0 — Do Not Reject H_0 — Reject H_0; $-t$, t, T_{n-1}
(b)	Reject H_0 — Do Not Reject H_0; $-t$, T_{n-1}
(c)	Do Not Reject H_0 — Reject H_0; t, T_{n-1}

CHART 5B: SMITH-SATTERTHWAITE t-TEST FOR COMPARISON OF MEANS (two-sample t-test without pooling).

1. Hypothesis.

    Test Alternate: $\qquad$ (a) $\qquad$ (b) $\qquad$ (c)

    $H_0: \mu_1 = \mu_2 \qquad H_0: \mu_1 \geq \mu_2 \qquad H_0: \mu_1 \leq \mu_2$

    $H_a: \mu_1 \neq \mu_2 \qquad H_a: \mu_1 < \mu_2 \qquad H_a: \mu_1 > \mu_2$

2. LOS. α

3. Test Statistic. $\dfrac{\overline{X}_1 - \overline{X}_2}{\sqrt{\dfrac{s_1^2}{n_1} + \dfrac{s_2^2}{n_2}}}$

4. Critical Value. Obtain t from T-Table (Appendix, Table 9) where

$$df = \frac{[s_1^2/n_1 + s_2^2/n_2]^2}{\left[\dfrac{(s_1^2/n_1)^2}{n_1 - 1} + \dfrac{(s_2^2/n_2)^2}{n_2 - 1} \right]} \text{ integer part only}$$

    simply discard the decimal part of the answer; do not round.

Test Alternate	T-Table Column Heading
(a)	LOS for two-tailed test
(b) or (c)	LOS for one-tailed test

5. Decision Line. t is the critical value obtained in step 4.

Test Alternate	Decision Line
(a)	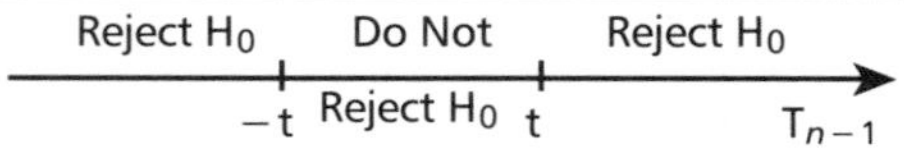 Reject H_0 $\quad$ Do Not $\quad$ Reject H_0 $\longrightarrow$ $-t$ $\quad$ Reject H_0 $\quad$ t $\qquad$ T_{n-1}
(b)	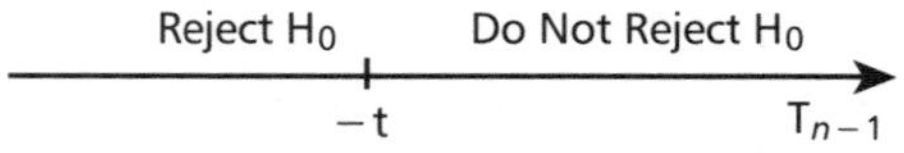 Reject H_0 $\qquad$ Do Not Reject H_0 $\longrightarrow$ $-t$ $\qquad\qquad$ T_{n-1}
(c)	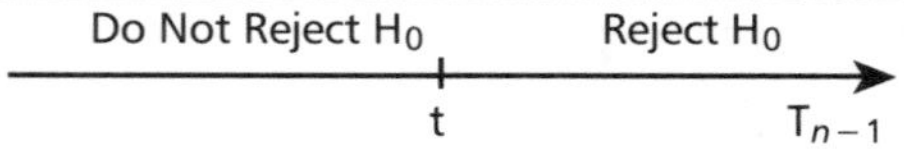 Do Not Reject H_0 $\qquad$ Reject H_0 $\longrightarrow$ t $\qquad\qquad$ T_{n-1}

CHART 5C: LARGE-SAMPLES Z-TEST FOR COMPARISON OF MEANS, TWO POPULATIONS (continuous random variable, both sample sizes greater than 30).

1. Hypothesis.

	(a)	(b)	(c)
Test Alternate:	$H_0: \mu_1 = \mu_2$	$H_0: \mu_1 \geq \mu_2$	$H_0: \mu_1 \leq \mu_2$
	$H_a: \mu_1 \neq \mu_2$	$H_a: \mu_1 < \mu_2$	$H_a: \mu_1 > \mu_2$

2. LOS. α

3. Test Statistic.
$$\frac{\overline{X}_1 - \overline{X}_2}{\sqrt{\frac{s_1^2}{n_1} + \frac{s_2^2}{n_2}}}$$

4. Critical Value. Obtain z from Z-Table (Appendix, Table 8).

Test Alternate	Z-Table Column Heading
(a)	LOS for two-tailed test
(b) or (c)	LOS for one-tailed test

5. Decision Line. z is the critical value from step 4.

Test Alternate	Decision Line
(a)	Reject H_0 Do Not Reject H_0 $-z$ Reject H_0 z Z
(b)	Reject H_0 Do Not Reject H_0 $-z$ Z
(c)	Do Not Reject H_0 Reject H_0 z Z

CHART 6: Analysis of Variance (ANOVA), Comparison of Means for Several Levels.

I. Preliminaries. a. Fixed treatments
b. Random and independent samples
c. Normal distribution in each level
d. Homoscedasticity

Comment. ANOVA is robust. Up to moderate violations of normality or homoscedasticity, apply ANOVA and report the p-value as approximate.

II. The Main Test.

1. Hypothesis. H_0: $\mu_1 = \mu_2 = \cdots = \mu_n$
H_a: means otherwise

2. LOS. α

3. Test Statistic. F-ratio

4. Critical Value. Obtain f from F-Table (Table 10a for a $= .01$, Table 10b for a $= .05$). The column and row headings are the first two numbers in the DF column in the ANOVA table, respectively. The column and row df are calculated by column $df = k - 1$ and row $df = N - k$ (k = number of levels, N = grand sample size).

5. Decision Line. f is the critical value obtained in Step 4.

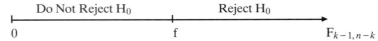

6. Sample Value.
   a. Minitab using the raw data set:
   MTB > SET level data into columns C1 through Ck
   MTB > PRINT C1 − Ck
   MTB > AOVONEWAY C1 − Ck
   b. Minitab using the sample legend:
   MTB > SET sample legend in C1 (sizes), C2 (means), C3 (SDs)
   MTB > EXECUTE 'ANOVALEGEND'

   The sample value is the number below F in Minitab's ANOVA table.

   c. Calculator ANOVA using the sample legend:
   see Section 12.2 for computational details.

CHART 7: CHISQUARED TEST FOR GOODNESS OF FIT.

I. Preliminaries.
    1. Each expected frequency is at least 1.
    2. At most 20% of the expected frequencies are less than 5.

II. The Main Test.
    1. Hypothesis.

$$H_0: p_1 = a_1, p_2 = a_2, \cdots, p_n = a_k$$
$$H_a: \text{the proportions are otherwise}$$

where $\{a_1, a_2, \cdots, a_k\}$ is a hypothesized set of proportions for the factor attributes. Note that $\Sigma a_i = 1$.

    2. LOS. α

    3. Test Statistic. $\Sigma(\text{Observed} - \text{Expected})^2/\text{Expected}$
    where the sum is taken over each attribute specified in the null hypothesis.

    4. Critical Value. χ^2 obtained from Table 12 with $df = k - 1$
    where k is the number of factor attributes.

       5. Decision Line.

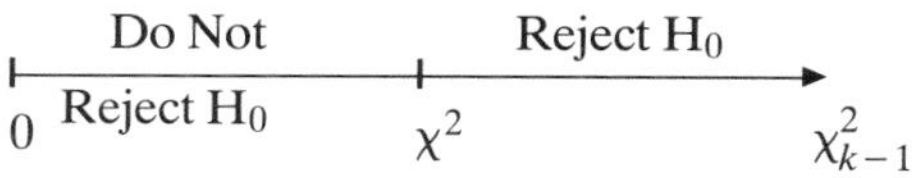

CHART 8: CHISQUARED TEST FOR INDEPENDENCE OF ATTRIBUTES.

I. Preliminaries.
    1. Each expected frequency is at least 1.
    2. At most 20% of the cells in the contingency table contain an expected frequency less than 5.

II. The Main Test
    1. Hypothesis. H_0: The given factors are independent.
                           H_a: The given factors interact.
    2. LOS. α

    3. Test Statistic. $\Sigma(\text{Observed} - \text{Expected})^2/\text{Expected}$

    4. Critical Value. χ^2 obtained from Appendix Table 12, where
            $df = (r - 1)(c - 1)$
            r = number of given row attributes
            c = number of given column attributes.
    5. Decision Line.

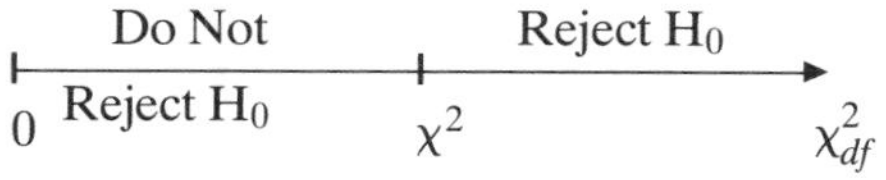

CHART 9: TEST FOR LINEAR CORRELATION.

I. Preliminaries. The following test is valid assuming that (X, Y) has a bivariate normal distribution. There is no statistical test, however, to test this assumption. We do test the samples for the random variables X and Y individually for normality. If either sample for X or Y (or both) shows an inconsistency with normal, then (X, Y) cannot be bivariate normal; hence, the following test should not be done. If both X and Y are consistent with normality, then make a statement assuming a bivariate normal distribution for (X, Y) and proceed.

II. The Main Test.

1. Hypothesis. $H_0: \rho(X, Y) = 0$
$H_a: \rho(X, Y) \neq 0$

2. LOS. α

3. Test Statistic. r (sample correlation)

4. Critical Value. r(critical) is obtained from Table 13.

5. Decision Line.

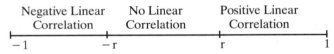

where r is the critical value obtained in step 4.

Minitab Computer Laboratory

An Overview of Minitab
LAB 1: Introduction to Minitab
LAB 2: Basic Descriptive Statistics
LAB 3: Minitab as Spreadsheet
LAB 4: Probability and Simulation
LAB 5: Binomial Experiments
LAB 6: The Normal Distribution
LAB 7: Confidence Intervals
LAB 8: t-Test of Hypothesis for the Mean
LAB 9: t-Tests for Comparison of Means
LAB 10: Analysis of Variance
LAB 11: Tables from Categorical Data
Minitab Command Glossary

An Overview of Minitab

When one accesses Minitab, one gets two things: a **worksheet** and a **slave**.

Minitab's *worksheet* has two components: a **spreadsheet** and a **pad**.

The *spreadsheet* is a large electronic "sheet of paper" arranged in 1000 **columns**. Initially,

- the spreadsheet is blank;
- the columns are generically named C1, C2, C3, . . . , C1000;
- each column can hold up to 1000 entries.

The *pad* is an electronic "pad of paper" containing 1000 "pages" called **constant boxes**. The constant boxes are generically called K1, K2, K3, . . . , K1000. Only a single number can be placed in a constant box (in contrast to a column, which can hold up to 1000 numbers). Initially, the first 998 constant boxes are blank, K999 contains the mathematical constant *e* (2.71828), and K1000 contains the number π (3.14159).

The initial state of Minitab's worksheet is:

```
                  MINITAB WORKSHEET
                    SPREADSHEET              PAD
         ┌──┬──┬──┬─────┬──────┐     ┌─────────┬──────┐
         │C1│C2│C3│ --- │C1000 │     │         │ K1   │
   row 1 │  │  │  │     │      │     │         │ K2   │
       2 │  │  │  │     │      │     │         │ K3   │
       3 │  │  │  │     │      │     │         │      │
     ... │  │  │  │     │      │     │         │ ...  │
     999 │  │  │  │     │      │     │ 2.71828 │ K999 │
    1000 │  │  │  │     │      │     │ 3.14159 │ K1000│
         └──┴──┴──┴─────┴──────┘     └─────────┴──────┘
```

When accessing Minitab, in addition to the initial Minitab worksheet as diagramed above, one also gets the immediate services of Minitab's slave. The slave performs chores according to your command.

> Computers never do what you *want* them to do, they only do what you *tell* them to do.
> Murphy's Law

Once you have accessed Minitab, you know that the slave is waiting for your direction by display of Minitab's prompt

    MTB >

You command the slave to do something by entering a Minitab **keyword** (a chore) along with any columns and/or constant boxes where the work is to be done. By using the generic worksheet diagramed above, you can keep track of the job being ordered.

Chores include entering data, processing data, and outputting results. The function of the computer laboratories is to show you how to instruct Minitab's slave to enter data into columns and/or constant boxes, process the data according to some plan you have in mind, and obtain the results. Minitab's chief service to you is to spare you the drudgery of tedious and time-consuming computations.

Introduction to Minitab

In statistics one must make several numerical computations. Fortunately, the computer can assume most of the drudgery of this task and relieve the user of the fear of computational errors. In this capacity, however, the computer is only a tool. Like any tool, we must learn how to use it.

One interacts with a computer at a **terminal**. A terminal is a station for entering information into and obtaining information from a computer. Each station contains a keyboard, a viewing screen, and a printer access.

In this computing session we learn how to:

1. access the computer,
2. obtain Minitab,
3. use Minitab,
4. exit Minitab, and
5. exit the computer.

> "If you use it, put it back where you found it in a condition you would like to find it."
> Ann Landers

Minitab is an easy to learn and use computer package that can do most statistical computations.

PART I   LAB PRACTICE

Accessing the Computer System

Every computer system is different. Some of you may be using a mainframe computer such as a Vax. A mainframe serves several users simultaneously; each user interacts with the computer through a computer terminal. Some of you may be using a personal computer such as an IBM-PC or a Macintosh.

Regardless of what kind of computer system one is using, one must be able to make the computer available for use. The process of accessing a computer for one's own use in a network environment is called *logging on*. Most university and agency computer systems are networked so that they are available to several people authorized to use the computer system. The process of leaving the computer in an appropriate condition for the next user is called *logging off*. One should never just walk away from a computer on a network while one's account is still active.

If you are using a network system, your instructor will show you how to logon and logoff your system. Most systems require an access code (password) for security or authorization purposes. Your instructor will also show you how to access Minitab once you have logged on.

Using Minitab

1. Logon to your computer system and obtain Minitab. Your cue that you have successfully accessed Minitab is the appearance of Minitab's prompt on the screen

```
MTB >
```

When you see Minitab's prompt, then Minitab is ready to serve you.

2. Enter the following sequence of instructions (don't type the MTB > which is Minitab prompting you for instructions) and observe what happens on the screen. Remember to depress the RETURN key at the end of each line. After you do this, we will reenter the commands and examine them carefully one at a time.

```
MTB > SET C1
DATA> 29 7 6 6 4
DATA> 2 7
DATA> END OF DATA
MTB > PRINT C1
MTB > NAME C1 'FREQ'
MTB > PRINT C1
MTB > NAME C2 'REL FREQ', C3 '%RELFREQ'
MTB > LET C2 = C1/SUM(C1)
MTB > LET C3 = C2*100
MTB > PRINT C1 - C3
```

A relative frequency table appears on the screen (if not, repeat the sequence of commands).

We now review the commands one at a time to see what is going on. This time, enter the commands as directed and visualize what is happening in the Minitab worksheet.

```
MTB > SET C1
DATA>
```

The command SET C1 informs Minitab that you want to enter data into column C1 of the Minitab spreadsheet. In response, Minitab changes the prompt from MTB > to DATA> to inform you that Minitab is ready to receive your data.

```
DATA> 29 7 6 6 4
DATA> 2 7
DATA> END OF DATA
```

You may enter data as long as the DATA> prompt is in effect. Individual numbers must be separated either by a space or a comma (warning: for example, Minitab interprets 3,147 as the two numbers 3 and 147). We recommend that you do not enter more than five individual numbers on a given DATA> line. The command END OF DATA informs Minitab that you are done entering data into the specified column. Hence, to "set up" any column of numbers in the spreadsheet, use the SET and END OF DATA commands.

```
MTB > PRINT C1
```

The command PRINT C1 displays the contents of the requested column C1 on the screen. The column entries are displayed across the screen for human convenience in reading the data contained in a single column. Good computer work demands that the user display data and check the column entries to ensure that the data you see are the data you want to work with. PRINT any column after entering data in it. If you detect any errors, you may reSET the column.

```
MTB > NAME C1 'FREQ'
MTB > PRINT C1
```

The command NAME C1 lets you give any heading (name) you want to the column C1. The name of your choice must be enclosed in single quotes. The name may use up to eight characters, except that neither the first nor the last character may be a blank. Note that before you NAMEd C1, the column was PRINTed with the generic heading of C1. After NAMEing, the column of data is printed using the given column NAME.

We now (a) compute the relative frequencies of the entries in column C1 and put them into column C2, and (b) compute the percent relative frequencies of the entries in column C1 and put them into column C3. In anticipation of these computations, we first appropriately name C2 and C3.

```
MTB > NAME C2 'REL FREQ', C3 '%RELFREQ'
MTB > LET C2 = C1/SUM(C1)
```

The LET command performs major computations in a single command line. In general, the LET command creates a new column of numbers (here C2) by doing arithmetic on the numbers in another column (here C1). In the above LET command, each number in the column C1 is divided by the SUM of the numbers in C1 (here, the sum of the numbers in column C1 is 61). In Minitab, the arithmetic operations of addition, subtraction, multiplication, and division are denoted by $+$, $-$, $*$, $/$ respectively. Note that a star, $*$, must be used for multiplication. Column C2 now contains the relative frequencies corresponding to the absolute frequencies set in column C1.

```
MTB > LET C3 = C2*100
```

This LET command computes the percent relative frequencies corresponding to the relative frequencies in column C2. Recall that to convert relative frequency to percent relative frequency, merely multiply by 100. Note the power of the above LET command. You do not have to multiply every individual relative frequency by 100. With the LET command, you can do arithmetic on an entire column of numbers in a single command line. In the previous LET command, a new column C3 of numbers is created by multiplying each entry in column C2 by 100.

Finally, to see the contents of the three columns C1 through C3 inclusively on the screen, we PRINT them. The final frequency distribution table is displayed by

```
MTB > PRINT C1 - C3
```

Notice that when you PRINT a single column

```
MTB > PRINT C1
```

Minitab presents the column horizontally (the way you usually read a script). However, when you PRINT several columns simultaneously, Minitab presents them in a columnwise (downward) fashion for the sake of easy comparisons between columns.

```
MTB > PRINT C1 - C3
```

3. In order to get some help on any command in Minitab, you can have the computer come to your aid. For example, to obtain help with the SET command:

```
MTB > HELP SET
```

In general, MTB > HELP command, where you specify the command you want help with, will give you a short description of how to use the command. If the prompt More? is given, type YES or NO depending on whether or not you would like more explanation, sometimes including examples.

The HELP procedure sometimes contains helpful hints. HELP SET contains shortcuts on entering certain patterned types of data; for example, if one is to enter consecutive integers. For example, to enter the integers from 0 to 9 inclusively

```
MTB > SET C5
DATA> 0:9
DATA> END OF DATA
MTB > PRINT C5
```

4. To prepare for a printed copy of the three-column table you constructed in step 2, we create a *stored program* of what we want to print on paper. Do the following and observe what happens.

```
MTB > STORE 'EX1'        STORE 'A:EX1'
STOR> NAME C1 'FREQ', C2 'RELFREQ', C3
      '%RELFREQ'
STOR> SET C1
STOR> 29 7 6 6 4
STOR> 2 7
STOR> LET C2 = C1/SUM(C1)
STOR> LET C3 = C2*100
STOR> PRINT C1 - C3
STOR> END OF PROGRAM
MTB > EXECUTE 'EX1'       MTB > STORE 'A:EX1'
                       MTB > EXECUTE 'A:EX1'
```

Observe that the STORE command changes the prompt from MTB > to STOR>. The instructions following STOR> are not carried out immediately after RETURN, as they are with the MTB > prompt, but are "stored up" to be executed later. When you command EXECUTE 'EX1', the commands stored under the program labeled 'EX1' are then executed. If all goes well, you will see the desired frequency distribution table displayed on the screen; otherwise, go back and repeat step 4. When you are sure that the STOREd program EXECUTEs what you want, then you are ready to obtain a copy of the results on paper.

The STOREd program is a nice way to compactly and concisely show your work. The STOREd program should contain just the commands needed to do a job. Before writing a STOREd program, however, it is important to practice; that is, enter commands one line at a time to see the immediate feedback.

> WARNING: When entering data into a column via the SET command within a STOREd program, do not include the END OF DATA. Minitab would interpret this as END (of program!). Minitab will automatically supply the END OF DATA when entering data within a STOREd program. Use

END (of anything) only to END the STOREd program itself.

5. In preparation for final printed copy, create a headline banner that will identify the printout.

```
MTB > STORE 'HEADLINE'     MTB > STORE 'A: HEADLINE'
STOR> NOTE your name
STOR> NOTE today's date
STOR> NOTE Health Sciences Statistics
STOR> NOTE Lab 1 Exercise
STOR> END OF PROGRAM
MTB > EXECUTE 'HEADLINE'    MTB > EXECUTE 'A: Headline'
```

The NOTE command allows you to write any notes for your Minitab output. This is useful for commentary and documenting work. Upon EXECUTEing 'HEADLINE', if you got *ERROR* messages, they are probably caused by a failure to use the keyword NOTE in one of your command lines. Simply reSTORE your headline program and reEXECUTE.

6. We are now ready for a paper printout ("hard copy").

If you are using a network, your instructor will show you how to activate and deactivate use of a printer so that you can get a copy of your results on paper. Once the printer is accessed,

```
MTB > EXECUTE 'HEADLINE'
MTB > EXECUTE 'EX1'
```

After printing is complete, disengage your terminal from the printer. Take your printed output back to your workstation. Inform anyone waiting to use the printer that you are now done with it.

Practice this laboratory session until you feel comfortable with logging on and off the computer system, accessing Minitab, and getting a paper printout of your work.

> The hardest part of any project is getting started.
>
> Biles's Laws

7. Unaccessing Minitab

When you are finished with your Minitab session, to leave Minitab

```
MTB > STOP
```

Once you have STOPped Minitab, then logoff if you are working on a computer network. After logoff, you are free to leave your workstation. If you are using a network terminal, be sure to leave the workstation in good order for the next user.

Comment Personal computer users may be interested in the following method of obtaining hard copy, especially users who are acquainted with a word processing program (e.g., Word, WordPerfect, MacWrite) and perhaps a drawing program (e.g., Super Paint, Harvard Graphics). After you have practiced the various items in the Lab Practice and you are ready to create your hard copy, then

```
MTB > OUTFILE 'thisfile'
```

After the OUTFILE command is issued, everything seen on the screen is also sent to an external file. Minitab gives this external file the name "thisfile.lis" (or whatever name you happen to give the file). The appendage ".lis" identifies the file as a "list" file. Such files can be imported into word processing programs. When you are done sending output to the outfile, then

```
MTB > NOOUTFILE
```

When you STOP Minitab, you return to the desktop. You can then access your favorite word processing program and open thisfile.lis in the word processing program. Once thisfile.lis is opened in your word processing program, you can edit your output, delete errors, add commentary, import graphics, or add page layout features to your hard copy.

PART II HOMEWORK

Using Minitab, produce a table that gives the temperature in degrees Fahrenheit from 85° to 105° and the equivalent temperature in degrees Celsius. To convert from degrees Fahrenheit to degrees Celsius, first subtract 32, then multiply this result by 5, then divide this result by 9; that is,

$$°C = (°F - 32)*5/9.$$

1. Create a STOREd program that will print an appropriate HEADLINE for your homework paper.
2. Create a STOREd program that will create and print your temperature conversion table.
3. Obtain a paper printout of your final checked-out results (the final product should be *ERROR* free).

Comment Just before turning on the printer to obtain your hard copy:

```
MTB > OH = 0   (letter-o letter-h equals number-zero)
```

This maneuver will get rid of the prompt Continue? which is useful during a practice session but annoying on a final product. To restore the Continue? prompt,

```
MTB > OH = 24
```

The reason for the 24 is that a terminal usually displays 24 lines of output on the screen before scrolling off the screen.

Minitab command summary for Lab 1.

SET	NOTE
END OF DATA	HELP
PRINT	STORE
NAME	END OF PROGRAM
LET	EXECUTE
	OH = 0

Comment You can obtain a virtual course in Minitab by MTB > HELP OVERVIEW.

LAB 2

Basic Descriptive Statistics

The new Minitab commands for this lab are

INFORMATION	SAVE	RETRIEVE
MEAN MEDIAN	STANDARD DEVIATION	RANGE
DESCRIBE	SORT	DOTPLOT

Recall that to get HELP with any Minitab command, use the HELP command; for example, MTB > HELP MEAN.

PART I LAB PRACTICE

Data Entry

1. *Logon and access Minitab.*
2. *Enter the data.* A northern California corporation sponsored a program of fitness and health for its permanent employees. To pilot test the program, a group of 19 employees volunteered for the program for 6 months. Several variables were measured, including serum cholesterol.

```
MTB > NAME C1 'CHOLEST'
MTB > SET C1
DATA> 395 251 296 249 182
DATA> 205 240 263 238 253
DATA> 167 156 222 230 255
DATA> 230 292 221 275
DATA> END OF DATA
MTB > PRINT C1
```

The numbers are SET down the specified column C1 in the order in which you entered them: 395 is the first number in C1, 251 the second number, 296 the third number, and so forth. When asked to PRINT a single column, Minitab displays the numbers in horizontal lines on the screen in the same way you would read a book.

3. *Check and edit the data.* Examine the data for any data entry errors. Suppose you mistyped the seventh entry as 204. To correct the error, enter the correct number of 240 into row 7 of column C1 by

```
MTB > LET C1(7) = 240
MTB > PRINT C1
```

Do not proceed until you have checked the entered data for accuracy and any data entry errors are corrected. If the whole data set is messed up, simply reSET the data.

4. *SAVE the checked data set.* A real data set usually gets reworked and analyzed on several occasions, not just during a single computer session. You won't want to reenter a data set each time you want to study it. Hence, after entering a real data set and checking it for accuracy, SAVE it:

```
MTB > INFORMATION
MTB > SAVE 'CHOLDATA'
```

The INFORMATION command gives a status report on the Minitab worksheet, informing the user what parts of the worksheet are occupied with data.

The SAVE command orders the computer to make a copy of the Minitab worksheet. Any part of the worksheet (columns or constant boxes) that contains data will be SAVEd into a permanent file for you. The name for the file must be contained in single quotes. Although different computer systems have somewhat different filename specifications, a safe guide is to use only alphanumeric characters (only letters and/or numbers); do not use a punctuation or special symbol like a dash, period, semicolon, # or @.

Any data file that has been SAVEd can be later RETRIEVEd during the current or any future computer session.

```
MTB > RETRIEVE 'CHOLDATA'
MTB > INFORMATION
```

Descriptive Statistics

1. *Sort (order) the data.* The most basic rule for analyzing any data set is to look at it.

```
MTB > PRINT C1
```

In its raw, unprocessed form, a data set at first looks like a bewildering sea of numbers. To begin to hear the story told by a data set, we first SORT the data.

```
MTB > SORT C1 INTO C1
MTB > PRINT C1
```

Observe that the original data are now sorted (ordered) from smallest to largest. Now for a visual graphic of the sorted data:

```
MTB > DOTPLOT C1
```

2. *Descriptive statistics.* The following commands are self-explanatory. Carry out the Minitab commands and observe the results on the screen.

```
MTB > MEAN C1
MTB > MEDIAN C1
MTB > RANGE C1
MTB > STANDARD DEVIATION C1
```

You can get a full summary of the descriptive statistics by

```
MTB > DESCRIBE C1
```

For a detailed description of the output for the DE-SCRIBE command

```
MTB > HELP DESCRIBE
```
[handwritten: PAPER / NO PAPER]

Obtaining the Results

1. *STOREing the results.* After practicing with the data, one develops a sense of what information is useful to obtain from the data. These useful items are collected together and organized in a presentable fashion, like a final report. For this purpose one creates a STOREd program that contains one's organized processing of the data. The STOREd program is very useful for obtaining a nice paper copy of desired results. The STOREd program also allows the presenter to show one's work; that is, it displays the individual steps used in describing or analyzing a given data set.

For a hard copy of desired results, we create a STOREd program, which we will EXECUTE later for the actual paper copy.

[handwritten left margin: HARD COPY]

```
MTB > STORE 'BASICS'
STOR> NOTE Basic Descriptive Statistics
STOR> PRINT C1
STOR> MEAN C1
STOR> MEDIAN C1
STOR> RANGE C1
STOR> STANDARD DEVIATION C1
STOR> DESCRIBE C1
```

```
STOR> END OF PROGRAM
MTB > EXECUTE 'BASICS'
```

If the STOREd program EXECUTEd OK, we are ready to proceed; otherwise, reSTORE the 'BASICS' program.

Comment The commands STORE and EXECUTE go together. STORE and EXECUTE apply only to a "processing program," a collection of Minitab commands grouped together in a given program file. Once a STOREd program has been created, it can be EXECUTEd at any time, including future computer sessions. Once STOREd, in order for 'BASICS' to work, one only needs data in column C1. 'BASICS' will provide the basic descriptive statistics for any data set SET in C1.

[handwritten right margin: DATA MUST BE IN C1]

Comment The commands SAVE and RETRIEVE go together. SAVE and RETRIEVE apply only to a Minitab worksheet, a data set contained in Minitab's columns and constant boxes.

Hence, one may SAVE and RETRIEVE data worksheets that contain data. Or one may STORE and EXECUTE programs which process data. You will get an error message if you try to RETRIEVE a STOREd program.

2. *Headlines.* A paper printout from the computer is often called *hard copy*. We want our hard copy to contain not just the immediate statistical results but also documentation of what these results are all about and what they apply to. Hence, before accessing the printer, we create a STOREd 'HEADLINE' program.

```
MTB > STORE 'HEADLINE'
STOR> NOTE your name
STOR> NOTE today's date
STOR> NOTE Health Sciences Statistics
STOR> NOTE Lab 2
STOR> NOTE anything else you want to say
STOR> END OF PROGRAM
MTB > EXECUTE 'HEADLINE'
```
[handwritten: HEDLL]

Of course, you may insert any other NOTEs that you would like to assist in identifying or documenting the output you are about to obtain. If the 'HEADLINE' program EXECUTEd properly, we are ready for the printer.

3. *Hard copy.* If necessary, access the printer. Then *[handwritten: PAPER]*

```
MTB > EXECUTE 'HEADLINE'
MTB > EXECUTE 'BASICS'
```

Then pick up the paper copy of your work (and disengage from the printer, if necessary).

4. *Summary.* Once you have entered a data set into column(s), printed it, examined it, corrected any input errors, and you are satisfied that the data set is correct, you probably will not want to repeat that process

[handwritten bottom: Execute HEADL. / Retrieve Choldata / Execute Basics]

again. Hence, *after entering a data set, SAVE the worksheet*. For practice, we will enter and save the Sands age data from Problem 1.2.4.

```
MTB > NAME C1 'AGES'
MTB > SET C1
DATA> 16 25 26 50 51
DATA> 55 62 63 67 78
DATA> END OF DATA
MTB > PRINT C1
```

After examining the output for accuracy,

```
MTB > SAVE 'SANDS'
```

The data set is now permanently saved. At any future time, you only need to RETRIEVE 'SANDS'.

Now suppose that we want to process Sands age data by finding the mean, median, range, and standard deviation. Notice that these are exactly the same commands that we included in our BASICS program that we STOREd (i.e., created) earlier. Since our Age data are located in column C1 and the BASICS program processes data in C1, we merely need to EXECUTE it:

```
MTB > EXECUTE 'BASICS'
```

Here is the wonderful feature of a STOREd program. Once it has been STOREd, we do not have to recreate it every time we want to use it; we merely need to EXECUTE it. One may EXECUTE a STOREd program at any time, including future Minitab sessions.

In order to process both the Cholesteroldata and the Sandsdata in one sitting:

```
MTB > RETRIEVE 'CHOLDATA'
MTB > EXECUTE 'BASICS'
MTB > RETRIEVE 'SANDS'
MTB > EXECUTE 'BASICS'
```

In summary, BASICS processes whatever data set you happen to SET into column C1.

PART II LAB HOMEWORK

Using Minitab, determine the mean, median, range, and standard deviation for each of the following data sets. Include a PRINT of the data set.

1. The temperature data set given in Problem 1.2.2.
2. The room-temperature cardiac output data set (Appendix, Data Set 1). Retrieve Daily *Problem*.
3. The Brandstetter et al PaO_2 data set 1.2.5. Include the first PaO_2, second PaO_2, and the change.

LAB 3

Minitab as Spreadsheet

The new Minitab commands for this lab are

READ   PARSUM
HISTOGRAM (subcommands: START, INCREMENT)

Recall that to get HELP with any Minitab command, use the HELP command; for example, MTB > HELP PARSUM.

PART I LAB PRACTICE

A **spreadsheet** is a large sheet of paper arranged in columns. The key utility of a spreadsheet is that one can work with several columns of data simultaneously, like an accounting ledger. We illustrate Minitab as spreadsheet by constructing a frequency distribution table for the cholesterol data set first introduced in Lab 2.

1. Logon the computer and access Minitab.
2. Retrieve the cholesterol data set:

```
MTB > RETRIEVE 'CHOLDATA'
MTB > INFORMATION
MTB > SORT C1 INTO C1
MTB > PRINT C1
```

3. A frequency distribution table. Using pencil and paper and applying Sturges's Rule, we obtain the following class limits for the cholesterol data:

Class	Limits	
	Lower	Upper
1	156	203
2	204	251
3	252	299
4	300	347
5	348	395

One must use pencil and paper to construct at least this much for a frequency distribution table; after that, we can use Minitab for the computations in completing the table. Notice that the class width is 48.

a. READ in the class limits.

```
MTB > NAME C11 'LOWLIM', C12 'UPLIM'
MTB > READ C11 C12
DATA> 156 203
DATA> 204 251
DATA> 252 299
DATA> 300 347
DATA> 348 395
```

```
DATA> END OF DATA
MTB > PRINT C11 C12
```

The READ command allows one to enter several columns of data at the same time, whereas, SET allows one to input only one column of data.

b. Class marks. The class mark is the midpoint of the class.

```
MTB > NAME C13 'MARK'
MTB > LET C13 = (C11 + C12)/2
MTB > PRINT C11 - C13
```

Observe that the first class mark is at 179.5.

c. Class frequencies.

```
MTB > HISTOGRAM C1;        #use the raw data
SUBC> START 179.5;         #first class mark
SUBC> INCREMENT 48.        #class width
```

Notice the structure of this usage of the HISTOGRAM command. To get the information we want, we need to tell Minitab the first class mark and the class width. We do this by use of *subcommands* to the main HISTOGRAM command. Notice that the main command

```
MTB > HISTOGRAM C1;
```

ends with a semicolon. The semicolon informs Minitab that the main command is to be augmented with further direction. Notice next that the Minitab prompt changes to SUBC>. The first subcommand ends with a semicolon, indicating that we want to continue augmenting the main HISTOGRAM command. One ends the last subcommand with a period (note the period at the end of the last subcommand). The # symbol is like the command NOTE; that is, the # symbol and what follows it are not part of the command, but allow the user to make notes about what one is doing (these notes are optional and are inserted at the discretion of the user).

The reason for using the subcommand structure here is that Minitab does not automatically make use of Sturges's Rule but chooses default class limits by another criterion. For the HISTOGRAM command, the subcommand START allows the user to specify where the first class mark is located; the subcommand INCREMENT allows the user to specify the class width to be used. Compare

```
MTB > HISTOGRAM C1
```

and

```
MTB > HISTOGRAM C1;
SUBC> START 179.5;
SUBC> INCREMENT 48.
```

The HISTOGRAM output provides us with the class frequencies.

```
MTB > NAME C14 'FREQ'
MTB > SET C14 #enter the class frequencies
DATA> 3 9 6 0 1
DATA> END OF DATA
MTB > PRINT C11 C12 C14 #frequency table
```

4. The complete frequency distribution table. We now make columns for relative frequency, percent relative frequency, cumulative frequency, cumulative relative frequency, and cumulative percent relative frequency and compute these quantities. This activity should clearly illustrate Minitab as spreadsheet.

The command PARSUM creates a cumulative column. For example,

```
MTB > PARSUM C14 INTO C17
MTB > PRINT C14 C17
```

computes the cumulative sums from column C14 and puts the results into column C17. Notice that the first entries in both columns are the same. The second entry in C17 is the sum of the first two entries in C14, the third entry in C17 is the sum of the first three entries in C14, the fourth entry in C17 is the sum of the first four entries in C14, and so forth. Hence, C17 contains the cumulative frequencies of the individual class frequencies contained in C14. The command PARSUM stands for *partial sums*, another term for cumulative sums.

```
MTB > NAME C15 'RELFREQ', C16 '%RELFREQ'
MTB > NAME C17 'CUMUL F', C18 'CUMUL RF'
MTB > NAME C19 'CUMUL%RF'
MTB > LET C15 = C14/SUM(C14)
MTB > LET C16 = C15*100
MTB > PARSUM C14 INTO C17
MTB > PARSUM C15 INTO C18
MTB > PARSUM C16 INTO C19
MTB > PRINT C11 C12 C14 - C16
MTB > PRINT C11 C12 C17 - C19
```

If the frequency distribution table looks OK, we will create a small STOREd program to obtain a paper copy.

```
MTB > STORE 'DISTTABS'
STOR> PRINT C1 #The Cholesterol Raw Data Set
STOR> NOTE  Frequency Distribution Table
STOR> PRINT C11 C12 C14 - C16
STOR> NOTE Cumulative Frequency Distribution
   Table
STOR> PRINT C11 C12 C17 - C19
STOR> END OF PROGRAM
MTB > EXECUTE 'DISTTABS'
```

5. Paper copy.

Before accessing the printer, create a STOREd headline program.

```
MTB > STORE 'HEADLINE'
STOR> NOTE your name
STOR> NOTE today's date
STOR> NOTE Health Sciences Statistics
STOR> NOTE Lab 3
STOR> END OF PROGRAM
MTB > EXECUTE 'HEADLINE'
```

If the headline program went well, we are ready for the printer. First, access the printer, if necessary. Then,

```
MTB > EXECUTE 'HEADLINE'
MTB > EXECUTE 'DISTTABS'
```

Then pick up your paper copy as practiced in Lab 1.

PART II LAB HOMEWORK

Using the data from the Daily and Mersch room-temperature cardiac output study (Appendix), (Data Set 1), apply Minitab to construct the following:

1. A frequency distribution table that includes the class limits, frequency, relative frequency, and percent relative frequency;

2. A cumulative frequency distribution table that includes frequency, cumulative frequency, cumulative relative frequency, and cumulative percent relative frequency.

LAB 4

Probability and Simulation

The new Minitab commands for this lab are

```
RANDOM (subcommands: INTEGER, DISCRETE)
TALLY (subcommand: PERCENT)
SAMPLE PLOT
```

To get help on any Minitab command: MTB > HELP command

PART I LAB PRACTICE

RANDOM (subcommand: INTEGER)

In Minitab, the way to randomly sample from a set of consecutive integers is

```
MTB > RANDOM K OBSERVATIONS INTO C;
SUBC> INTEGER K TO K.
```

For example,

```
MTB > RANDOM 25 OBSERVATIONS INTO C1;
SUBC> INTEGER 1 TO 6.
MTB > PRINT C1
```

In response to these commands, Minitab randomly chooses 25 numbers, all between 1 and 6, and puts them in C1 (in order to see the numbers chosen, you must ask for a PRINT). You can think of rolling a single die 25 times and recording the numbers that turn up. Or, you can think of *sampling with replacement*. Put six slips of paper, numbered 1 through 6, into a hat. Then draw a slip at random and record the number. Put the slip back into the hat, mix well, and draw again (hence, drawing with replacement) until you have 25 draws.

1. Observe the results of the following commands:

```
MTB > RANDOM 25 INTEGERS INTO C1;
SUBC> INTEGER 1 6.
MTB > PRINT C1
MTB > TALLY C1
```

The TALLY command will make a frequency distribution table for a column of integers. You can get a relative frequency table (tally) by using the PERCENTS subcommand.

```
MTB > TALLY C1;
SUBC> PERCENTS.
```

Appeal to HELP TALLY for further details.

2. To simulate 25 tosses of a fair coin (0 = tails, 1 = heads):

```
MTB > RANDOM 25 C1;
SUBC> INTEGER 0 1.
MTB > PRINT C1
MTB > TALLY C1
```

How many of your 25 tosses came up heads?

3. To simulate the birth of 50 infants in the nursery with 1 = girl and 0 = boy:

```
MTB > RANDOM 50 C1;
SUBC> INTEGER 0 1.
MTB > TALLY C1
```

How many girls were born in your simulation? How many boys?

4. Will 2 people in a group (say a group of 30 people) have the same birthday? Suppose there are 365 days in the year and number them consecutively from 1 to 365. Suppose the probability of being born on any given day is the same, 1/365.

```
MTB > RANDOM 30 C1;
SUBC> INTEGER 1 365.
MTB > PRINT C1
```

This command chooses 30 numbers at random between 1 and 365 (with replacement). This simulates choosing 30 people at random and obtaining their birthdays. Do any 2 people have the same birthday? By looking at the output on the screen, it is not immediately apparent whether 2 people have the same birthday or not. To make this determination easy:

```
MTB > SORT C1 INTO C2
MTB > PRINT C2
```

Now, do at least 2 people have the same birthday?

To examine five different groups where each individual group has 30 people, run the following:

```
MTB > STORE 'BDAY'
STOR> RANDOM 30 PUT IN C1;
STOR> INTEGER 1 365.
STOR> SORT C1 INTO C1
STOR> PRINT C1
STOR> END OF PROGRAM
MTB > EXECUTE 'BDAY' 5 TIMES
```

How many of your five groups of 30 people had at least 2 people with the same birthday?

SAMPLE

1. The RANDOM with INTEGER subcommand samples with replacement. To sample without replacement (i.e., a number once drawn is not put back in the hat) from an equiprobable space (each item has an equal chance of being drawn), use the SAMPLE command. Before using SAMPLE, however, you must first set up the "hat."

```
MTB > NAME C1 'Hat', C2 'The Draw'
MTB > SET C1
DATA> 1:20
DATA> END OF DATA
MTB > PRINT C1
```

The general form of the SAMPLE command is

```
MTB > SAMPLE K ITEMS FROM C PUT IN C
```

Now run

```
MTB > SAMPLE 5 ITEMS FROM C1 PUT IN C2
MTB > PRINT C2
```

Five numbers have been randomly selected from C1. Once a number is drawn, it cannot be redrawn; hence, there are no repeats (i.e., we SAMPLEd without replace-

ment). The numbers drawn were recorded in C2 as specified. To see this, we PRINT C2.

2. There are 23 students currently enrolled in this class. Let's number them from 1 to 23:

```
MTB > NAME C1 'Student'
MTB > SET C1
DATA> 1:23
DATA> END
MTB > PRINT C1
```

Suppose we want to randomly select a committee of 3 students to carry a complaint to the professor. To form the committee:

```
MTB > SAMPLE 3 STUDENTS FROM C1 INTO C2
MTB > PRINT C2
```

Which students are on the complaint committee?

RANDOM (subcommand: DISCRETE)

The purpose of the RANDOM with DISCRETE subcommand is to enable simulation of sampling with replacement for a nonequiprobable space. To set the stage, we must enter two columns of background information: first, the items that can be chosen and, second, the probability with which they can be chosen.

1. Family gender simulation study. The following sets up the probability of having a certain number of girls in a family with six children. Note that in a family of six children, there may be zero to six girls inclusively. We assume a one-to-one sex ratio; that is, the probability that a newborn is female is .5.

```
MTB > NAME C1 'GIRLS', C2 'PROB'
MTB > READ C1 C2
DATA> 0 .0156
DATA> 1 .0938
DATA> 2 .2344
DATA> 3 .3125
DATA> 4 .2344
DATA> 5 .0938
DATA> 6 .0156
DATA> END OF DATA
MTB > PRINT C1 C2
```

The probabilities in C2 are theoretical probabilities (we'll cover that later). We simulate what would happen in a field study of 20 randomly selected families where each family has six children:

```
MTB > NAME C3 'STUDY'
MTB > RANDOM 20 PUT IN C3;
SUBC> DISCRETE C1 C2.
```

```
MTB > PRINT C3
MTB > TALLY C3
```

This command selects 20 families at random from C1, with corresponding probability of being selected in C2. The results are recorded in C3 and, upon request, are PRINTed and TALLYed. The TALLY command output gives you the observed frequencies.

The results of the study can now be summarized as follows:

```
MTB > NAME C11 'OBSERVED', C12 'EXPECTED'
MTB > LET C12 = C2*20  #expected frequencies
MTB > SET C11
DATA> enter the observed frequencies from the output of
      TALLY C3
DATA> END OF DATA
MTB > PRINT C1 C11 C12
```

The resulting table that appears on the screen summarizes the results of this simulation. In particular, one can compare the observed frequencies (what one actually obtained in the study or simulation) with the expected frequencies, where the expectation is based on the column of theoretical probabilities. What do you think? Do you feel that the observed frequencies are consistent with the expected frequencies?

2. Winning/losing streaks simulation study. Gamblers, sports fans, and investors claim there are times when they have a streak of good luck or a streak of bad luck. We use simulation to show that such luck may be nothing more than chance variation.

Consider the following simple gambling game. You and your opponent each bet a dollar. Then you toss a fair coin. If it comes up tails, you win one dollar; if heads, you lose your dollar. If you play a long game, will you have any hot or cold streaks? Let's simulate a game. The following program simulates a game with 50 plays.

```
MTB > NAME C1 'COIN', C2 'PROB', C3 'RESULT'
MTB > READ C1 C2   #Give Minitab a Coin.
DATA>  -1    .5
DATA>  +1    .5
DATA> END OF DATA
MTB > SET C5         #Get set for 50 tosses.
DATA> 1:50
DATA> END
MTB > NAME C4 'Winnings', C5 'Toss'
MTB > STORE 'STREAK'
STOR> RANDOM 50 PLAYS IN C3;
STOR> DISCRETE C1 C2.
STOR> PRINT C3
STOR> PARSUM C3 PUT CUMULATIVE SUMS IN C4
```

```
STOR> PLOT C4 VS C5
STOR> END OF PROGRAM
MTB > EXECUTE 'STREAK'
```

When I ran this simulation, my first five results were: -1, 1, -1, -1, 1. This means I lost on the first, third, and fourth plays and won on the second and fifth tosses. So after one play I was behind $1; after two plays, even; after three plays, behind $1; after four plays, behind $2; after five plays, behind $1. These cumulative winnings are in C4. We could PRINT C4 to see the full story of the progress of the game. It is very convenient, however, to PLOT the results so we can see the game visually. For full visual effect, on a paper copy of your plot, connect the dots (you'll have to do this by hand since Minitab cannot do it for you). From the PLOT, not only can you see the game at a glance, but you can pick out the winning and losing streaks. This gambler's scenario is often called "Gambler's Ruin." Notice that the game is over if you lose all your money. This is more fun than the lottery!

Comment In population ecology, this scenario is called "critter extinction." Here you start with an initial population. A toss is a simulation of a vital event, which could be either a birth (heads) or a death (tails). One then wonders if the critters go extinct. This simulation could also represent births in a nursery, where $+1$ represents a girl and -1 represents a boy.

PART II LAB HOMEWORK

1. Run the birthday simulation for ten different groups of 30 people each (see Lab Practice [Random subcommand: Integer], item 4). For each group, indicate 2 (or more) people having the same birthday by circling the equal numbers. How many of your groups contained at least 2 people with the same birthday?

2. A hat contains 20 slips of paper numbered 1 through 20.
   a. Suppose you draw 5 slips with replacement. How would you simulate this using Minitab?
   b. Suppose you draw 5 slips without replacement. How would you simulate this using Minitab?

For a and b, include the printout of your simulation. What numbers were selected in your draws? Be sure to indicate on your printout which draw is with replacement and which draw is without replacement.

3. Consider the family gender simulation study (see Lab Practice RANDOM [subcommand: DISCRETE], item 1). Conduct a simulation with 100 families. Make a frequency distribution table for the results that includes both observed and expected frequencies (use absolute frequencies, not relative or percent relative frequencies). How do you think the observed frequencies compare with the expected frequencies?

4. Run the program for winning/losing streaks (see Lab Practice item C2) three times. Include your PLOTs. On each of your PLOTs, *connect the dots using a ruler.* Also, draw a horizontal line through 0 on the vertical (this line represents the baseline or break-even line). Describe your final winnings for each game. How'd you do?

Birthday Probability Table

N = number of people in a random group
p = probability that at least two people in the group will have the same birthday

N	p	N	p	N	p
10	.1169	24	.5383	38	.8641
11	.1411	25	.5687	39	.8782
12	.1670	26	.5982	40	.8912
13	.1944	27	.6269	41	.9032
14	.2231	28	.6545	42	.9140
15	.2529	29	.6810	43	.9239
16	.2836	30	.7063	44	.9329
17	.3150	31	.7305	45	.9410
18	.3469	32	.7533	46	.9483
19	.3791	33	.7750	47	.9548
20	.4114	34	.7953	48	.9606
21	.4437	35	.8144	49	.9658
22	.4757	36	.8322	50	.9704
23	.5073	37	.8487		

LAB 5

Binomial Experiments

The new Minitab commands for this lab are

RANDOM (subcommands: BERNOULLI, BINOMIAL)
PDF   CDF

To get HELP on any Minitab command: MTB > HELP command
To get HELP on any subcommand: MTB > HELP command subcommand

PART I LAB PRACTICE

The primary new Minitab skill in this laboratory practice is how to use either BERNOULLI or BINOMIAL as a subcommand for the RANDOM command to simulate binomial experiments.

One Binomial Experiment

The general way to simulate a single binomial experiment consisting of N independent and identical Bernoulli trials each with probability P is:

```
MTB > RANDOM N BERNOULLI TRIALS INTO C;
SUBC> BERNOULLI P.
```

Example:
```
MTB > RANDOM 50 C1;
SUBC> BERNOULLI 0.6.
MTB > PRINT C1
MTB > TALLY C1
```

This command performs one binomial experiment that consists of 50 independent Bernoulli trials in which the probability of success for each Bernoulli trial is .6. The results "success" (which Minitab denotes by 1) and "failure" (which Minitab denotes by 0) are stored in C1. The TALLY command summarizes the results.

Binomial Probability Density Function Tables

First we illustrate how to obtain a copy of either a probability density function (PDF) table or a cumulative density function (CDF) table. Consider a binomial experiment where $n = 4$ and $p = .85$; that is, Bino(4, .85).

To obtain a PDF (probability density function) table:

```
MTB > PDF;
SUBC> BINOMIAL  4  .85.
```

To obtain a CDF (cumulative density function) table:

```
MTB > CDF;
SUBC> BINOMIAL  4  .85.
```

In addition, we may need to construct the full table with the results put in specified columns where we can access the probabilities for further calculations. For practice, we construct a full density table for a binomial experiment where $n = 15$ and $P = .6$; that is, Bino(15, .6).

```
MTB > STORE 'TABLE'
STOR> SET C1
STOR> 0:15
STOR> NAME C1 'X', C2 'PDF(X)', C3 'CDF(X)'
STOR> PDF C1 INTO C2;
STOR> BINOMIAL 15 .6.
STOR> PARSUM C2 INTO C3
STOR> PRINT C1 - C3
STOR> END OF PROGRAM
MTB > EXECUTE 'TABLE'
```

The table printed is the desired probability function table for the given binomial random variable.

Binomial Experiments

The RANDOM command with the BINOMIAL subcommand will perform several runs of a given binomial experiment. The general form is:

MTB > RANDOM K EXPERIMENTS INTO C;
SUBC> BINOMIAL N P.

This command performs K binomial experiments, in contrast to BERNOULLI, which performs only one binomial experiment. Here, each of the K binomial experiments has N independent Bernoulli trials in which the probability of success of each Bernoulli trial is P. The number of successes for each of the K experiments is put in column C.

Example.
```
MTB > RANDOM  50  C1;
SUBC> BINOMIAL  10  .5.
MTB > PRINT C1
MTB > TALLY C1;
SUBC> PERCENTS.
```

The commands in the preceding example perform 50 binomial experiments. Each of the binomial experiments consists of ten Bernoulli trials. In each trial the probability of success is .5. For example, this simulates the tossing of ten fair coins where on each toss you record the number of heads; you repeat the toss of the ten coins 50 times. The results are put in the specified column C1. TALLY produces a frequency distribution table for the results of your simulation.

Comment Practice the preceding lab until you feel comfortable with the commands and what they do. After that, go home and think about the homework problems. Write up your programs to solve the homework problems on paper. Then come in to the lab at another time and complete the homework exercises.

PART II LAB HOMEWORK

Your solutions to these lab homework exercises should include appropriate use of NOTEs and STOREd programs. Be sure to use a HEADLINE to identify your output.

1. Suppose X is the binomial random variable with $n = 5$ and $p = .5$. Use Minitab to construct a probability density function table for X. Your table should have three columns: x, f(x), and F(x); that is, a combined PDF and CDF.

2. A binomial experiment consists of having a family with five children and observing the number of girls in the family.

a. Simulate this experiment 100 times (i.e., consider a study where you observe the number of girls in 100 families of five children).

b. Complete the following table:

Number of Girls	Observed Frequency	Expected Frequency
0		
1		
2		
3		
4		
5		

Use the table obtained in lab homework exercise 1 to obtain the expected frequencies. Record the absolute frequencies (counts), not the relative frequencies.

c. How often did a family in your simulation have all girls? How often would you expect this event to occur in the 100 simulations based on classical (theoretical) probabilities?

d. How often did you get more girls than boys in a family? How often would you expect this event to occur in the 100 simulations?

e. How often did you get three girls and two boys? How often would you expect this event to occur in the 100 simulations?

The Normal Distribution

The new Minitab commands for this lab are

RANDOM (subcommand: NORMAL) TINTERVAL

To obtain HELP on any Minitab command: MTB > HELP command

PART I LAB PRACTICE

Simulation

In this lab we will take a sample of size 50 from a large population. We will consider a random variable X, which in the general population has a normal distribution with mean 100 and standard deviation 15. The goal of the simulation is to see how well sample data reflect the reality of the population.

In order to simulate taking a sample from such a population, use the RANDOM command with the NORMAL subcommand. The general form is

```
MTB > RANDOM K OBSERVATIONS INTO C;
SUBC> NORMAL M S.
```

This command simulates taking a simple random sample (each member of the population has an equal chance of being selected) of K members from a large population. Each member is measured for the random variable of interest which has a normal distribution with mean M and standard deviation S. The sample data are put in the specified column C. For example,

```
MTB > RANDOM  50  C1;
SUBC> NORMAL  100  15.
MTB > PRINT C1
```

obtains a simple random sample of size 50 from a normally distributed population that has a mean of 100 and a standard deviation of 15. We now study the sample data to see if the sample reflects the population.

Be aware of the fact that we are looking at a sample whose size is very small in comparison to the whole population. Our sample has only 50 observations in it. Our hope, however, is that the sample can give us good clues about the nature of the underlying population. Fortunately, with computers we can conduct simulations. In this case, we *know* that the underlying population has a normal distribution with a population mean of 100 and a population standard deviation of 15. How well does our sample reflect this reality?

Exploratory Data Analysis

Before starting a formal analysis, get acquainted with the sample data with some introductory exploratory data analysis (EDA).

```
MTB > HISTOGRAM C1
MTB > DOTPLOT C1
MTB > BOXPLOT C1
```

Do the graphics give a visual sense of a normal distribution? Do the quick histogram and dotplot give a sense of a bell-shaped curve? Is the boxplot symmetrical, with the median in the middle of the box and whiskers about of equal length?

Normality

We now formally check to see if the sample is indicative of being drawn from a normal distribution; that is, we check the sample data for consistency with a normal distribution.

```
MTB > NAME C1 'DATA', C30 'NSCORES'
MTB > NSCORES C1 INTO C30
MTB > CORRELATION C1 AND C30
```

The critical nscores correlation for a sample of size 50 is .9664. If the sample nscores correlation is ≥ .9664, the sample is consistent with a normal distribution. If the sample nscores correlation is < .9664, then the sample is indicating that it is not the kind of sample that one usually gets from a normal distribution. Is your sample consistent with normality?

Comment Of all possible samples of size 50 that can be drawn from a normal distribution, 99% of them yield a sample nscores correlation ≥ .9664; only 1% of them will yield a sample nscores correlation < .9664. Only about 1 time out of 100 will you by the luck of the draw get a sample atypical of the normality quality of the parent population.

Statistics

How do the sample mean and sample standard deviation compare with the population mean and population standard deviation? Our sample was obtained from a normal distribution with population mean 100 and standard deviaiton 15. To obtain the sample statistics,

```
MTB > MEAN C1
MTB > STANDARD DEVIATION C1
```

	Population	Sample
Mean	100	
SD	15	

Is your sample mean exactly equal to the population mean of 100? Is your sample standard deviation exactly equal to the population standard deviation of 15? How can you explain these discrepancies? Are the population and sample means close?

A normal distribution is symmetrical about the mean. Symmetry is indicated when the mean and the median are equal. The sample median is obtained by

```
MTB > MEDIAN C1
```

Are your sample mean and median about the same? Why wouldn't you expect them to be exactly the same when the mean and median are equal in the population at large?

The Empirical Rule

Recall that in a normal distribution about 68% of the data fall within one standard deviation (SD) of the mean. We inquire whether or not our sample reflects this fact. We look through the sample's 1 SD window to see whether it will show about 68% of the data.

```
MTB > LET K1 = MEAN(C1) - STAN(C1)
MTB > LET K2 = MEAN(C1) + STAN(C1)
MTB > PRINT K1 K2
MTB > SORT C1 PUT IN C2
MTB > NAME C2 'Sortdata'
MTB > PRINT C2
```

Count the number of observations that fall between K1 and K2. We expect about 34 such observations (68% of 50 is 34). How many sample observations are contained in the sample's 1 SD window?

We also expect about 95% of the data to fall within 2 standard deviations of the mean.

```
MTB > LET K1 = MEAN(C1) - 2*STAN(C1)
MTB > LET K2 = MEAN(C1) + 2*STAN(C1)
MTB > PRINT K1 K2
MTB > PRINT C2
```

Count the observations that fall between K1 and K2. We expect about 47 or 48 (95% or 50 is 47.5). How many sample observations are contained in the sample's 2SD window?

Finally, an interval within 3 standard deviations of the mean should account for about 99.7% of the data.

```
MTB > LET K1 = MEAN(C1) - 3*STAN(C1)
MTB > LET K2 = MEAN(C1) + 3*STAN(C1)
MTB > PRINT K1 K2
MTB > PRINT C2
```

Summarize by completing the following table:

Window	Expected	Observed	% Expected	% Observed
$\bar{x} \pm s$	34.1		68.26	
$\bar{x} \pm 2s$	47.8		95.44	
$\bar{x} \pm 3s$	49.9		99.74	

In actual practice you don't know anything about the nature of a random variable X in the general population in advance. That's why you do a study. For practical reasons you take a sample of the population to study. You obtain the sample mean, $\bar{x}$. But the real question is: What is the population mean, μ? You don't know! All you know is $\bar{x}$. Knowing $\bar{x}$, though, you should be able to say something about what μ is. You can

```
MTB > TINTERVAL 90 C1
```

Notice Minitab's automatic feedback to the TINTERVAL command: sample size, sample mean, sample standard deviation, and a 90% C.I. (confidence interval) for the population mean. This means you have 90% confidence that the population mean μ lies inside that **t-interval** somewhere. Among all the random samples

that could possibly be drawn, 90% of the resulting t-intervals will in fact contain μ (unluckily, the other 10% won't—it's the natural risk inherent with sampling).

Each sample begets its own t-interval. What is the t-interval associated with your sample? Does the t-interval contain the population mean $\mu = 100$? Was your sample among the 90% of the lucky samples, or among the 10% of the unlucky samples?

Minitab will provide everybody with a different sample. Most will get good agreement between the sample and the population; a few won't. Whether or not you get good agreement between your sample and the population is just the luck of the draw. Hence, go through this lab practice at least twice (you will get a different sample each time).

PART II LAB HOMEWORK

1. Obtain a sample of size 50 from a population in which we consider a normal random variable X, which has a mean of 16 and a standard deviation of 3. Intraocular eye pressure in the general U.S. population has these characteristics. Glaucoma is a disease of the eye manifested by high intraocular pressure. Turn in a printout of your sample.
2. Is the sample consistent with normality?
3. What is your sample mean and sample median?
4. What is your sample standard deviation?
5. Determine the 1SD, 2SD, and 3SD windows.
6. Print the sorted data set and display the 1SD, 2SD, and 3SD windows on the data.
7. Complete the table:

Window	Expected	Observed
$\bar{x} \pm s$		
$\bar{x} \pm 2s$		
$\bar{x} \pm 3s$		

8. What do you think: Does your sample reflect a normal distribution with mean 16 and standard deviation 3? Explain your answer.
9. What is your 90% t-interval? Does your t-interval contain the population mean $\mu = 16$?
10. (Optional) Make a relative frequency distribution table for grouped data for your sample. Use Sturges's Rule to determine the number of classes for your data set. Construct a relative frequency histogram based on class boundaries. Does the distribution portrayed by the histogram look normal; i.e., does it have the general look of a normal distribution?

Confidence Intervals

The new Minitab commands for this laboratory are

RETRIEVE INFO SAVE ECHO NOECHO

For HELP on any Minitab command: MTB > HELP command

PART I LAB PRACTICE

1. Confidence interval for the mean. In the general U.S. population, serum cholesterol level (mg/dL) is (approximately) normally distributed, with a mean of 214.8 and a standard deviation of 34.2. We draw a sample of 35 from the population.

```
MTB > NAME C1 'DATA'
MTB > RANDOM 35 C1;
SUBC> NORMAL 214.8 34.2.
MTB > PRINT C1
```

The sample data are now displayed on the screen and also put in the specified column, C1. A 90% confidence interval for the population mean is obtained by

```
MTB > TINTERVAL 90 C1
```

Minitab responds to the TINTERVAL command by displaying the sample size, sample mean, sample standard deviation, standard error of the mean, and the 90% confidence interval for μ. Did your confidence interval actually contain the population mean $\mu = 214.8$?

If you do not want the sample data displayed on the screen as a result of the RANDOM command, then don't request the PRINT.

```
MTB > RANDOM 35 C1;
SUBC> NORMAL 214.8 34.2.
MTB > TINTERVAL 90 C1
```

This procedure provides you with the bottom line, the desired statistical information, without displaying the actual sample data. How was your luck with this confidence interval (did it contain $\mu = 214.8$)?

2. Confidence interval for the mean difference of paired data. We illustrate with the Daily and Mersch cardiac output data. (If you do not have the Daily and Mersch cardiac output data set [see Appendix, Data Set 1] in a SAVEd data file, then you will need to enter the room-temperature cardiac outputs in C1 and the ice-temperature cardiac outputs in C2.)

```
MTB > RETRIEVE 'DAILY'
MTB > INFO
MTB > NAME C5 'ROOM-ICE'
MTB > LET C5 = C1 - C2
MTB > PRINT C1 C2 C5
MTB > TINTERVAL 90 C5
```

What do you think? Is there a statistically significant difference between these two methods of measuring cardiac output?

3. Confidence interval for an average, nonnormal distribution. When dealing with a normal distribution, one constructs a t-interval for the mean. When dealing with a large sample size ($n > 30$), one may construct a z-interval for the mean without regard to the nature of the distribution (normal or not). If the distribution is nonnormal and the sample size is not large, construct an s-interval for the median.

We have not studied specific nonnormal distributions. One of the more common types of nonnormal distribution is an exponential distribution. For example, an exponential model is used to describe the concentration of a drug in the bloodstream through time. We will sample from an exponential distribution; first using a large sample size of $n = 50$, then a small sample size of $n = 20$. (We are not concerned here with the details of an exponential distribution—only that it is a common nonnormal distribution. An exponential distribution is mathematically equal to a chisquared—pronounced "kie [rhymes with pie] squared" distribution.)

The following command draws a sample of size 50 from an exponential distribution (a nonnormal distribution) with a population mean of 2 ($\mu = 2$).

```
MTB > RANDOM 50 C1;
SUBC> CHISQUARED 2.
```

To get a feel for the nature of the distribution of the data, we do some EDA.

```
MTB > HISTOGRAM C1
MTB > BOXPLOT C1
```

Notice the skewed nature of the distribution. The distribution "tails off" toward the right.

We now check for normality. The critical nscores correlation in the test for normality is .9664 for sample size 50.

```
MTB > NSCORES C1 INTO C2
MTB > CORRELATION C1 AND C2
```

Place the sample nscores correlation on the following decision graphic:

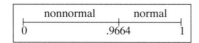

Did your sample pass normal? Most samples will indicate a nonnormal distribution.

We drew a sample of size 50 from a chisquared distribution where $\mu = 2$. Let's see how well the sample reflects this.

```
MTB > DESCRIBE C1
```

Did the sample mean come close to the population mean? We can formally check this out since we have a large sample size.

```
MTB > LET K1 = STDEV(C1)
MTB > ZINTERVAL 95 K1 C1
```

The above ZINTERVAL command constructs a 95% confidence z-interval for the mean using the standard deviation in constant box K1. Does your z-interval contain the population mean $\mu = 2$? If so, then one can say that the sample mean is close to the population mean, at least from a statistical point of view given the sample size.

We now consider a smaller sample drawn from the same chisquared distribution with mean 2.

```
MTB > RANDOM 20 C1;
SUBC> CHISQUARED 2.
MTB > HISTOGRAM C1
MTB > BOXPLOT C1
```

We check the sample for normality.

```
MTB > NSCORES C1 INTO C2
MTB > CORRELATION C1 AND C2
```

Place the sample nscores correlation on the following decision line:

nonnormal	normal
0	.9290	1

Most samples will "flunk" the test for normality. A t-interval for the mean is not appropriate here since the distribution of the random variable in the population is nonnormal. We construct an s-interval for the median. In a skewed distribution such as the chisquared-2 distribution, the mean and the median are different.

```
MTB > SINTERVAL 95 C1
```

We inquire whether this interval contains the population median.

```
MTB > LET K1 = 2*LOGE(2)
MTB > PRINT K1
```

The number in K1 is the population median, η. What is η? Does the s-interval contain η? Does the s-interval contain $\mu = 2$?

PART II LAB HOMEWORK

1. The following program will give you 20 confidence intervals for the mean serum cholesterol level determined by 20 different samples of size 35 from the U.S. population.

```
MTB > ERASE C1 - C20
MTB > STORE 'CONFINT'
STOR> RANDOM   35  C1 - C20;
STOR> NORMAL   214.8   34.2.
STOR> TINTERVAL   90   C1 - C20
STOR> END OF PROGRAM
MTB > EXECUTE  'CONFINT'
MTB > ECHO
```

Turn in a printout of the output of the above program and make a chart like in the figure below for your confidence intervals.

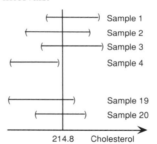

Carefully draw your figure to scale using a metric ruler. Draw in the vertical line at the mean, 214.8. Note how most of the confidence intervals "capture" the population mean of 214.8. HOW MANY OF YOUR CONFIDENCE INTERVALS CONTAIN THE POPULATION MEAN SERUM CHOLESTEROL LEVEL ($\mu = 214.8$)?

2. Draw a sample of size 25 from a normal distribution with mean 215 and standard deviation 35.
   a. Submit a printout of your data set.
   b. Is your sample consistent with normality?
   c. What is your sample mean?
   d. What is the population mean, μ?
   e. Construct 80%, 90%, 95%, 99%, and 99.9% confidence intervals for μ.
   f. Do your confidence intervals contain μ?
   g. What is the effect on the confidence intervals of increasing the level of confidence?

3. Consider a chisquared-2 distribution. Draw a sample of size 40.
   a. Submit a printout of your data set.
   b. Is your sample consistent with normality?
   c. What is your sample mean?
   d. What is the population mean, μ?
   e. Construct a 95% confidence z-interval for μ.
   f. Does your confidence z-interval contain μ?
   g. What is the sample median?
   h. What is the population median?
   i. Construct a 95% confidence s-interval for the population median.
   j. Does your confidence s-interval contain the population median?
   k. What do you think—does your sample reflect the general nature of the population?
4. Consider the chisquared-2 distribution. Draw a sample of size 20.
   a. Submit a copy of your sample.
   b. Check the sample for normality.
   c. What is the sample median?
   d. What is the population median?
   e. Construct a 95% s-interval for the median.
   f. Does the s-interval contain the population median?
   g. What do you think—does your sample reflect the general nature of the population?

LAB 8

t-Test of Hypothesis for the Mean

New Minitab command: MTB > TTEST;
      Subcommand: SUBC> ALTERNATE

For HELP on any Minitab command: MTB > HELP command

For HELP on any subcommand: MTB > HELP command subcommand

PART I LAB PRACTICE

1. Two-tailed test for the mean, one population. The height of women in the United States has a distribution that is approximately normal, with a mean of 64 inches and standard deviation of 3 inches. We draw a simple random sample of 16 women and measure their heights.

```
MTB > NAME C1 'HEIGHT'
MTB > RANDOM 16 C1;
SUBC> NORMAL 64 3.
MTB > PRINT C1
```

Is the sample consistent with normality?

```
MTB > NAME C11 'Nscores'
MTB > NSCORES C1 INTO C11
MTB > CORRELATION C1 AND C11
```

We assume that the sample passes the check for normalcy (if not, draw another sample).

To see whether our sample reflects reality, we perform a test of hypothesis, H_0: mu = 64 versus H_a: mu N.E. 64 (N.E. means "not equal").

```
MTB > TTEST 64 C1;
SUBC> ALTERNATE 0.
```

Observe Minitab's automatic printout. A trial run of this command produced the following output (warning: your numbers will be different since your sample is different):

```
MTB > TTEST 64 C1;
SUBC> ALTERNATE 0.

TEST OF MU = 64.000 VS MU N.E. 64.000

            N     MEAN   STDEV  SE MEAN       T   P VALUE
HEIGHT     16   63.206   2.377    0.594   -1.34      0.20
```

What a nice result! The output contains all the information we need to write up a test of hypothesis. All the necessary calculations are done!

2. p-value. The importance of the **p-value** in the context of the previous example is that
   a. if LOS ≤ .20, then do not reject H_0;
   b. if LOS > .20, then reject H_0 and accept H_a.

At the 5% or 10% LOS (level of significance) in the example you would not reject H_0; but at the much riskier 25% LOS you reject H_0 and accept H_a.

The p-value can be looked at from two different perspectives:
   a. the p-value is the largest LOS at which one can accept the null hypothesis;
   b. the p-value is the smallest LOS at which one can reject the null hypothesis and accept the alternate hypothesis.

Now you do it:

```
MTB > RANDOM 16 C1;
SUBC> NORMAL 64 3.
MTB > TTEST 64 C1;
SUBC> ALTERNATE 0.
```

Pause to answer each of the following:
- *a.* What is the sample size? Mean? Standard deviation?
- *b.* What test of hypothesis was performed?
- *c.* What is the sample t-value for this test?
- *d.* What is the decision at the 5% LOS?
- *e.* What is the *p*-value for this test? In your own words, what is the meaning of this *p*-value?

3. One-sided test of hypothesis, one population.
   For H_0: mu = M versus H_a: mu > M, use

```
MTB > TTEST M C;
SUBC> ALTERNATE 1.
```

Here, M is our reference value for the mean. The subcommand ALTERNATE 1 for the TTEST command informs Minitab that you want to perform a *right*-tailed test on the sample data stored in column C. A right-tailed test is a test of alternate (c) in our test of hypothesis charts (Appendix).
   For H_0: mu = M versus H_a: mu < M, use

```
MTB > TTEST M C;
SUBC> ALTERNATE -1.
```

Again, M is our reference value for the mean. The subcommand ALTERNATE −1 for the TTEST command informs Minitab that you want to perform a *left*-tailed test on the sample data stored in column C. A left-tailed test is a test of alternate (b) in our charts. For illustration we conduct the test H_0:mu = 4 versus H_a:mu < 4 using the following data:

```
MTB > NAME C1 'DATA'
MTB > SET C1
DATA> 3.9 3.8 3.5 4.1 3.2
DATA> 3.5 3.6 3.7 3.8 3.7
DATA> 4.2 3.4 4.0 4.0 3.6
DATA> 4.3
DATA> END OF DATA
MTB > TTEST 4 C1;
SUBC> ALTERNATE = -1.
```

The output should read:

```
MTB > TTEST 4 C1;
SUBC> ALTERNATE = -1.

TTEST OF MU = 4.0000 VS. MU L.T. 4.0000 (L.T. means Less Than)

            N    MEAN    STDEV   SE MEAN     T   P VALUE
FIREFLY    16  3.7687   0.3027   0.0757  -3.06   0.0040
```

Since the *p*-value (to four decimal places) is .0040,
- *a.* if LOS < .0040, then do not reject H_0;
- *b.* if LOS > .0040, then reject H_0 and accept H_a.
Here, the evidence from the sample is very strong that the null hypothesis is false. If H_0 were in reality true, then the

chance of drawing a simple random sample like ours would be less that one chance in 100 (more precisely, 4 chances in 1000). If the null hypothesis were in fact true, then only .4% of all possible samples will have t-value ≤ -3.06.

PART II LAB HOMEWORK

Draw a random sample of size 20 from a normal distribution with mean 100 and standard deviation of 13.

1. Submit a copy of the data set.
2. What is the sample mean?
3. What is the population mean?
4. Is the sample mean equal to the population mean?
5. Test the sample for normality.
6. Display a 95% confidence interval for the population mean, μ. Is μ in the interval?
7. Based on your sample, test H_0:μ = 100 versus H_a: $\mu \neq 100$.
8. Based on your sample, test H_0:μ = 110 versus H_a: $\mu < 100$.
9. Based on your sample, test H_0:μ = 90 versus H_a: $\mu > 100$.
10. What do you think? How well does your sample reflect the reality of the population?

LAB 9

t-Tests for Comparison of Means

New Minitab commands for this laboratory are

TWOSAMPLE (subcommands: ALTERNATE, POOLED)

For HELP on any Minitab command: MTB > HELP command

For HELP on any subcommand: MTB > HELP command subcommand

PART I LAB PRACTICE

In this laboratory you will conduct t-tests of hypothesis comparing the means of two populations. The new Minitab command to learn is TWOSAMPLE. This main command has two subcommands: ALTERNATE (to specify the test alternate) and POOLED (to conduct a pooled test when the data are consistent with equality of variances).

The general form for the TWOSAMPLE command is

```
MTB > TWOSAMPLE [CONF] C C;
SUBC> ALTERNATE K.
```

The TWOSAMPLE command will conduct a Smith-Satterthwaite t-test for comparison of means. A pooled t-test for comparison of means is conducted by adding the subcommand POOLED. The general form is

```
MTB > TWOSAMPLE [CONF] C C;
SUBC> ALTERNATE = K;
SUBC> POOLED.
```

The specific details of the for the TWOSAMPLE command include:

a. ALTERNATE K specifies a one-tailed test of hypothesis when K is -1 or $+1$. Use ALTERNATE $= -1$ when you want to specify a left-tailed test H_0: mu1 = mu2 versus H_a: mu1 < mu2. Use ALTERNATE $= 1$ when you want to specify a right-tailed test H_0: mu1 = mu2 versus H_a: mu1 > mu2. For a two-tailed test, specify ALTERNATE 0. By default Minitab uses ALTERNATE 0 when the ALTERNATE subcommand is missing.

In comparison with our test of hypothesis charts (Appendix), Minitab codes the test alternate as follows: alternate (a), 0; alternate (b), -1; alternate (c), 1.

b. POOLED instructs Minitab to conduct a pooled test for comparison of means.

c. [CONF] is an option whereby you can specify the level of confidence for a CI for the difference between the two means; otherwise, by default, Minitab computes a 95% confidence interval for the difference of the two means.

d. C C denotes two columns where the two samples are located.

The POOLED subcommand assumes that the variances of the background random variables in the two populations are equal. Hence, a POOLED test should be accompanied by a preliminary test that the data are consistent with an assumption of equality of variances.

Example.
```
MTB > TWOSAMPLE 90 C1 C2;
SUBC> ALTERNATE 0;
SUBC> POOLED.
```
performs a two-tailed test, H_0: mu1 = mu2 vs H_a: mu1 N.E. mu2, on sample data given in C1 and C2. A 90% confidence interval for the difference between the two population means, mu1–mu2, is also given.

Example.
```
MTB > TWOSAMPLE C1 C6;
SUBC> ALTERNATE 1;
SUBC> POOLED.
```
performs a one-tailed test, H_0: mu1 = mu2 versus H_a: mu1 > mu2, on sample data given in C1 and C6. A 95% confidence interval for the difference between the two population means, mu1–mu2, is also given.

For practice, we first use Minitab to obtain some samples for us.

```
MTB > RANDOM 20 C1;
SUBC> NORMAL 15 3.
MTB > RANDOM 30 C2;
SUBC> NORMAL 15 3.
MTB > DESCRIBE C1 C2
MTB > DOTPLOT C1 C2;
SUBC> SAME.
```

The two RANDOM commands select two simple random samples of sizes 20 and 30, respectively, from a normal distribution with mean $\mu = 15$ and standard deviation $\sigma = 3$. The DESCRIBE and DOTPLOT commands provide a quick graphic look at the samples. Do the samples look like they were drawn from the same normal distribution? Since we know that the samples were drawn from a normal distribution, we forgo the check for normality. In order to compare the two samples:

```
MTB > TWOSAMPLE 92 C1 C2;
SUBC> ALTERNATE 0.

MTB > TWOSAMPLE 92 C1 C2;
SUBC> ALTERNATE 0;
SUBC> POOLED.
```

The first TWOSAMPLE command performs the Smith-Satterthwaite comparison of means, whereas the second TWOSAMPLE conducts a pooled t-test. Note the output and compare the confidence intervals and the p-values provided by these two tests.

PART II LAB HOMEWORK

1. Consider a normal distribution with a mean of 100 and a standard deviation of 13. Apply the RANDOM command to select a simple random sample of size 15 and another sample of size 23. Apply the TWOSAMPLE command with the POOLED subcommand to test equality of means.

2. Apply the RANDOM command to select a sample of size 17 from a normal distribution with mean 100 and standard deviation 13. Then select a sample of size 17 from a normal distribution with mean 125 and standard deviation 13. Apply the TWOSAMPLE command with the POOLED subcommand to test (a) equality of means, and (b) that the mean of the first population is smaller than the mean of the second population.

3. Apply the RANDOM command to select a sample of size 17 from a normal distribution with mean 100 and standard deviation 10. Then select a sample of size 17 from a normal distribution with mean 100 and standard deviation of 50. Obtain quick histograms and boxplots for each sample. Apply the f-test for homoscedasticity. Apply the TWOSAMPLE command (without pooling) to test equality of population means.

4. Apply the RANDOM command to select two samples of size 17 from an exponential distribution with mean 3. Apply the Mann-Whitney test to test equality of means.

LAB 10

Analysis of Variance

New Minitab commands for this laboratory are

    AOVONEWAY   MOOD   ONEWAY

    STACK (subcommand: SUBSCRIPTS)

For HELP on any Minitab command: MTB > HELP command

For HELP on any subcommand: MTB > HELP command subcommand

PART I LAB PRACTICE

We will utilize simulation to demonstrate ANOVA. We consider two scenarios.

Normal Distributions, Same Means

Our first scenario considers the situation in which all means are in reality the same. Suppose that in an untreated population, vitamin X is normally distributed with a mean of 100 and a standard deviation of 15. Two possible treatments are considered. In reality, the treatments do not do any good; that is, they really don't affect vitamin X. A study is conducted in which a convenience sample of

60 recruits is randomized into three groups. Each group receives 20 subjects. The groups are defined as follows.

    Group 1: Control group (no treatment)
    Group 2: Treatment A
    Group 3: Treatment B

We simulate the sampling design

```
MTB > NAME C1 'Control', C2 'A', C3 'B'
MTB > RANDOM 20 C1 - C3;
SUBC> NORMAL 100 15.
MTB > PRINT C1 - C3
```

The preceding commands obtain three random samples, each containing 20 subjects. Each sample is drawn from a normal distribution with mean 100 and standard deviation 15. Note that in reality the population mean and standard deviation are the same for all three groups. Each group represents a random sample of size 20 drawn from the same normal distribution. We now inquire whether the samples are statistically significantly different from others.

We first STACK the data set. Some analysis is more conveniently done in Minitab in the STACKed form.

```
MTB > NAME C5 'Data', C6 'Level'
MTB > STACK C1 - C3 INTO C5;
SUBC> SUBSCRIPTS INTO C6.
MTB > PRINT C5 C6
```

We now conduct some exploratory data analysis (EDA) to look at the data. In particular, we inquire whether our sample data basically reflect the fact that the distribution in all three groups is the same.

```
MTB > DESCRIBE C1 - C3
MTB > DOTPLOT C1 - C3;
SUBC> SAME.
```

We augment the DOTPLOT command with the SAME subcommand so that each of the three dotplot graphics is displayed on the same scale. The same technique will not work for boxplots. To have boxplots all displayed on the same scale, we must engage the stacked data set.

```
MTB > BOXPLOT C5;
SUBC> BY C6.
```

We can also obtain the dotplots on the same scale using this format on the stacked data.

```
MTB > DOTPLOT C5;
SUBC> BY C6.
```

What do you think? Do your three samples seem to indicate that they were all drawn from the same distribution? For the acid test, we apply ANOVA. We first check the preliminaries.

```
MTB > NAME C11 'Nscores'
MTB > NSCORES C1 INTO C11
MTB > CORRELATION C1 AND C11
MTB > NSCORES C2 INTO C11
MTB > CORRELATION C2 AND C11
MTB > NSCORES C3 INTO C11
MTB > CORRELATION C3 AND C11
```

For a sample of size 20, the critical nscores correlation is .929. Hence, if the sample nscores correlation is $\geq .929$, then the sample is consistent with normality. Are your three samples consistent with normality?

The next consideration is to determine whether the three samples indicate that they are all drawn from distributions that all have the same standard deviation. The following trick will allow you to obtain the sample f_{max}-value for the homoscedasticity test without having to inspect the sample standard deviations to see which is larger.

```
MTB > NAME C12 'SD'
MTB > LET C12(1) = STDEV(C1)
MTB > LET C12(2) = STDEV(C2)
MTB > LET C12(3) = STDEV(C3)
MTB > LET K1 = (MAXI(C12)/MINI(C12))**2
MTB > PRINT K1
```

The printed value from constant box K1 contains the sample f_{max}-value. Using Appendix Table 11, the critical f_{max}-value for three levels for a sample of size 16 is 6.1; for a sample of size 21, it is 4.9. Hence, if the sample f_{max}-value is less than 4.9, the samples are consistent with homoscedasticity. If the sample f_{max}-value is greater than 6.1, the samples are inconsistent with homoscedasticity. If the sample f_{max}-value is between 4.9 and 6.1, the result is inconclusive.

Do your samples pass the preliminary tests for normality and homoscedasticity? We expect that they should. However, whenever we make decisions about a population based on a sample, there is always a risk. In this case, about 2 times in 100 we will, by the luck of the draw, obtain samples that are not consistent with normality or not consistent with homoscedasticity.

We now conduct analysis of variance to determine whether, on average, the mean vitamin X levels observed in the three groups are significantly different from each other. We conduct the analysis using both the stacked and the unstacked form of the data for the purpose of illustration. The AOVONEWAY command conducts ANOVA on an unstacked data set; ONEWAY, a stacked data set.

```
MTB > AOVONEWAY C1 - C3
MTB > ONEWAY C5 C6
```

Does your analysis of variance indicate that all three means are equal? If not, it is not because you did something wrong! It is merely the result of the luck of the draw.

Also for illustration, we conduct the so-called nonparametric test for comparing averages. In the text, we recommend the Mood test. Some abbreviated versions (e.g., the Student Edition) of Minitab do not support the Mood command but instead support another common test for comparison of medians called the Kruskal-Wallis test. We perform both of these tests for the sake of illustration. Both the Mood test and the Kruskal-Wallis test must be conducted on the stacked data set.

```
MTB > MOOD C5 C6
MTB > KRUSKAL-WALLIS C5 C6.
```

Do your samples indicate that the medians are all equal? Compare the output from the Mood test and the Kruskal-Wallis test.

Normal Distributions, Different Means

We repeat the preceding simulation with one modification. Suppose that, in reality, vitamin X is raised by treatment B.

```
MTB > RANDOM 20 C1 C2;
SUBC> NORMAL 100 15.
MTB > RANDOM 20 C3;
SUBC> NORMAL 120 15.
```

We inquire whether the sample in column C3 detects the upward shift in the mean. Conduct an EDA and ANOVA analysis similar to the previous section. What do you think? Does the analysis of the sample data reflect that the mean of the treatment B group is statistically significantly greater than the mean of the control group and treatment A group?

Part II Lab Homework

Draw a random sample of size 25 for each of four groups where group 1 is drawn from a normal distribution with mean 90 and standard deviation 10; groups 2 and 3 are drawn from a normal distribution with mean 100 and standard deviation 10; and group 4 is drawn from a normal distribution with a mean of 105 and standard deviation of 10. Analyze the samples for comparison of average values. Do your samples reflect the reality of the populations?

LAB 11

Tables from Categorical Data

The new Minitab commands for this laboratory is TABLE.

Subcommands: ALL, CHISQUARE, COUNTS,
CUMCOUNTS, CUMPERCENTS,
PERCENTS, STORE

For HELP on any Minitab command: MTB > HELP command

For HELP on any subcommand: MTB > HELP command subcommand

PART I LAB PRACTICE

One-Way Tables

In the text, Example 1.1.9 presents data from a study by Simpson et al. Patients recalled various technical care actions 24 to 48 hours after discharge from a critical care setting as follows:

29 Medication (1)
7 Specialized care (2)
6 Fluids (3)
6 Respiratory (4)
4 Nursing care (5)
2 Surgery (6)
7 Special procedures (7)

We recognize the single factor "technical care" with attributes: medication, specialized care, fluids, respiratory, nursing care, surgery, and special procedures. To apply Minitab, we first code these attributes with nominal numbers (any integer coding scheme will do). For convenience, we choose 1 = medication, 2 = specialized care, 3 = fluids, 4 = respiratory, 5 = nursing care, 6 = surgery, and 7 = special procedures.

The one-way raw (i.e., one-factor) data set is entered into Minitab's worksheet.

```
MTB > NAME C1 'Data'
MTB > SET C1
DATA> 29(1), 7(2), 6(3), 6(4), 4(5),
2(6), 7(7)
DATA> END OF DATA
MTB > PRINT C1
```

To obtain the frequency distribution, apply the TALLY command:

```
MTB > TALLY C1
```

To obtain a frequency distribution table,

```
MTB > TALLY C1;
SUBC> COUNTS;
SUBC> PERCENTS.
```

To include a cumulative frequency distribution table,

```
MTB > TALLY C1;
SUBC> COUNTS;
SUBC> PERCENTS;
SUBC> CUMCOUNTS;
SUBC> CUMPERCENTS.
```

For convenience, one may obtain the entire frequency with cumulative frequency table by

```
MTB > TALLY C1;
SUBC> ALL.          STOP.
```

Although the TALLY command creates and displays a frequency distribution table, the results are not automatically retained. To retain any result, use the STORE subcommand (do not confuse with the STORE command for an executable list of commands).

```
MTB > NAME C5 'TechCare', C6 'Freq',
C7 '%Freq'
MTB > NAME C8 'Cumul F', C9 '%Cumul F'
MTB > TALLY C1;
SUBC> COUNTS;
SUBC> PERCENTS;
SUBC> CUMCOUNTS;
SUBC> CUMPERCENTS;
SUBC> STORE C5 - C9.
MTB > PRINT C5 - C9
```

The number of columns listed with the STORE subcommand must equal the number of columns displayed by the main TALLY command.

Two-Way Tables

In the text, Example 13.2.2 presents data from Murph et al regarding cytomegalovirus among children in day care centers. We adopt the following coding scheme for recording the two-factor data.

Age at Entry	Excreting CMV
1 = <2 years	0 = No
2 = 2 years	1 = Yes
3 = 3 years	
4 = ≥ 4 years	

The raw data set is entered into Minitab's worksheet.

```
MTB > NAME C1 'AGE', C2 'CMV'
MTB > SET C1
DATA> 74(1), 23(2), 50(3), 72(4)
DATA> END OF DATA
MTB > SET C2
DATA> 16(1), 58(0), 8(1), 15(0), 6(1)
DATA> 44(0), 2(1), 70(0)
DATA> END OF DATA
MTB > PRINT C1 C2
```

Minitab has extensive capabilities to produce two-way tables. For the full story, MTB > HELP TABLE. The TABLE command can compile summary information on both categorical and continuous data. Examine the output of the TABLE command with the following subcommands. First, the TABLE command constructs a basic two-factor frequency distribution table. The subcommand ALL includes the marginal totals for the specified columns. One may also include cell row percentages and/or cell column percentages. In addition, one may conduct a chisquared analysis.

```
MTB > TABLE C1 C2

MTB > TABLE C1 C2;
SUBC> ALL C1 C2.

MTB > TABLE C1 C2;
SUBC> ROWPERCENTS.

MTB > TABLE C1 C2;
SUBC> ROWPERCENTS;
SUBC> COLPERCENTS;
SUBC> ALL C1 C2.

MTB > TABLE C1 C2;
SUBC> CHISQUARED.
```

The TABLE command is very useful for tabulating the results of surveys.

PART II LAB HOMEWORK

1. We consider the binomial random variable $X =$ Bino(6, .5).

  a. Obtain a random sample of 200 from this distribution:

```
MTB > NAME C1 'Data'
MTB > RANDOM 200 C1;
SUBC> BINO 6 .5.
```

  Print your data set.

  b. Use the TALLY command with appropriate subcommands to make a frequency distribution table and a cumulative frequency distribution table.

  c. Construct appropriate graphics for your tables.

2. Simulate the distribution of two factors as follows. Factor A has 3 attributes and Factor B has 4 attributes.

```
MTB > NAME C1 'Factor A', C2 'Factor B'
MTB > RANDOM 75 C1;
SUBC> INTEGER 1 3.
MTB > RANDOM 75 C2;
SUBC> INTEGER 1 4.
```

  a. Display a two-factor frequency distribution table for the data that includes the marginal sums.

  b. Conduct a chiquared test for independence of attributes. Are the two factors independent?

  c. What percent of the sample has factor A, attribute 2?

  d. What percent of the sample has factor B, attribute 3?

  e. What percent of the sample has factor A, attribute 2, and factor B, attribute 3?

GLOSSARY of COMMANDS

ANOVA response = patient factor;
  RANDOM patient.

Performs an analysis of variance for the specified model on a balanced data set presented in stacked form. Used particularly for one-way repeated measures ANOVA.

Example.

```
MTB > ANOVA output = patient method;
SUBC> RADDOM patient.
```

AOVONEWAY C C-C

Performs an analysis of variance (ANOVA) on the data in the specified columns.

Example.

```
MTB > AOVONEWAY C1 - C3
```

BOXPLOT C

Constructs a boxplot for the data in the specified column. For comparison purposes, to plot boxplots on the same axes when the data are in stacked form, use the BY subcommand. To display a 95% confidence interval for the median, use the NOTCH subcommand.

Examples.

```
MTB > BOXPLOT C1
MTB > BOXPLOT C1;
SUBC> NOTCH.
MTB > BOXPLOT C11;# stacked data in C11
SUBC> BY C12;# levels in C12
SUBC> NOTCH.
```

CDF;

Constructs a cumulative density function table.

Example.

```
MTB > CDF;
SUBC> BINOMIAL 6 0.5.
```

CHISQUARED C C - C

Conducts a chisquared test for independence of attributes on the data in the specified columns.

Example.

```
MTB > CHISQUARE C1 - C4
```

COPY C INTO C

Copies the numbers in the first specified column into the second specified column.

Examples.

```
MTB > COPY C11 INTO C12
MTB > COPY C1-C3 INTO C11-C13
```

CORRELATION C C

Computes and displays the correlation between two specified columns of numbers.

Examples.

```
MTB > CORRELATION C1 C2
MTB > CORR C4 C17
```

DESCRIBE C

Gives the main descriptive statistics of the specified column, including the mean, median, standard deviation, and others, for the specified column(s).

Examples.

```
MTB > DESCRIBE C1
MTB > DESCRIBE C1 - C3
```

DOTPLOT C

Displays a horizontal graphic for the distribution of a numerical data set. When requesting a DOTPLOT for the data in several columns at once (unstacked data), use the SAME command to have each axis scaled in the same way. For the data in stacked form, use the BY subcommand.

Examples.

```
MTB > DOTPLOT C3
MTB > DOTPLOT C1 - C3;
SUBC> SAME.
MTB > DOTPLOT C11; # stacked data in C11
SUBC> BY C12.      # levels in C12
```

ECHO

Turns on the ECHO mode whereby commands EXECUTEd in a STOREd program are printed. In the NOECHO mode, the printing of the individual commands and any comments designated by # are not printed.

Example.

```
MTB > ECHO
```

END
Signifies END OF DATA for the SET or READ commands. Also signifies END OF PROGRAM for a STOREd program. Warning: Do not include an END OF DATA in a stored program. Minitab will interpret any END statement in a stored program as END OF PROGRAM.

EXECUTE 'programname'
Executes the sequence of instructions exactly as specified in the STOREd program created under the label 'programname'. If an error message occurs while executing, then redo the STOREd program.

Examples.
```
MTB > EXECUTE 'LAB1'
MTB > EXECUTE 'BDAY' 5 TIMES
```

GBOXPLOT Gives graphics capabilities to the BOX-
GHISTOGRAM PLOT, HISTOGRAM, and PLOT
GPLOT commands. Use these commands if you have a laser printer attached to your computer.

GLM response = general linear model;
MEANS factor1 factor2.
Performs ANOVA on a stacked data set.

Example.
```
MTB > GLM heartwt = gender race gender*race;
SUBC> MEANS gender race.
```

HELP command
Gives some on-line assistance about using a specified Minitab command or subcommand.

Examples.
```
MTB > HELP NAME
MTB > HELP SET
MTB > HELP RANDOM NORMAL
```

HISTOGRAM C
Displays a frequency "histogram" in the form of a bar diagram. The diagram shows the class marks (midpoints) and the class frequencies.

Examples.
```
MTB > HISTOGRAM C1

MTB > HISTOGRAM C1;
SUBC> START 179.5;     #first class mark
SUBC> INCREMENT 48.    #class width
```

INFO
Gives a status report of the current Minitab worksheet. The report lists the columns occupied, their count, and NAME. Any occupied constant boxes are also listed.

Example.
```
MTB > INFO
```

INVCDF;
Performs the inverse (reverse) operation of CDF.

Example.
```
MTB > INVCDF .95 K1;
SUBC> NORMAL 0 1.
```

KRUSKIL-WALLIS C C
Performs a Kruskil-Wallis test for comparison of medians. The Kruskil-Wallis test is an alternative to the Mood test. Like the Mood test, the data must be in stacked form.

Example.
```
MTB > KRUSKIL-WALLIS C1 C2
```

LET C = algebraic expression
Creates a new spreadsheet column of numbers by doing arithmetic on the numbers in another column(s) as directed in the algebraic expression.

Example.
```
MTB > LET C5 = (C1 + C2)*C3/C4
```

MANN-WHITNEY [conf] C C;
ALTERNATE K.
Conducts a Mann-Whitney test for the comparison of medians on the two samples specified in the given two columns. The [conf] specifies the level of confidence for a confidence interval for the difference between the medians. If no [conf] is specified, 95% is used by default.

Example.
```
MTB > MANN-WHITNEY 90 C1 C2;
SUBC> ALTERNATE 1.
```

MEAN C
Displays the mean of the specified column.

Example.
```
MTB > MEAN C4
```
Example.
```
MTB > LET K1 = MEAN(C4)
MTB > PRINT K1
```

MEDIAN C
Displays the median of the specified column.

Example.
```
MTB > MEDIAN C3
```

MOOD C C

Conducts a Mood test for comparison of level medians. The data must be presented in stacked form. The first specified column contains the data; the second column, the levels. Data can be stacked with the STACK command.

Example.
```
MTB > MOOD C1 C2
```

NAME C 'colname'

Names the column specified by C with the specified 'colname'. The column name must be enclosed in single quotes and cannot exceed eight characters. Only columns can be NAMEd; constant boxes cannot.

Examples.
```
MTB > NAME C1 'TEMP', C2 'Degrees'
MTB > NAME C3 '%RF90@3'
```

NOECHO

Turns off the ECHO mode. In the NOECHO mode, commands EXECUTEd in a STOREd program are not printed. Also, any notes indicated by # are not printed. The NOECHO mode is useful for obtaining the printed output of thoroughly checked-out programs to save computer paper.

Example.
```
MTB > NOECHO
MTB > EXECUTE 'BDAY' 10 TIMES
MTB > ECHO
```

NOTE message

Allows you to include any documentation, annotation, or explanation with your work. If your message results in an *ERROR*, you probably forgot the command keyword NOTE.

Example.
```
NOTE Lyda Caine
NOTE Assignment 1    12/25/90
```

NSCORES C INTO C

Calculates the nscores for each item in a quantitative data set. Used in a test for normality in conjunction with the CORRELATION command.

Example.
```
MTB > NSCORES C1 INTO C11
MTB > CORRELATION C1 AND C2
```

ONEWAY C C

Conducts an ANOVA on data in a stacked format.

Example.
```
MTB > ONEWAY C1 C2
```

OW

Sets output width (number of characters printed in a line of type) for a line printer.

Example.
```
MTB > OW 65
```

PARSUM C INTO C

Computes the cumulative sums of the first specified column and puts the results into the second specified column.

Example.
```
MTB > PARSUM C14 INTO C17
```

PDF;

Constructs a probability density function (PDF) Table.

Example.
```
MTB > PDF;
SUBC> BINOMIAL 4 0.85.
```

PLOT C VS C

Constructs a two-dimensional graph (plot). The first specified column is plotted on the vertical axis; the second specified column is plotted on the horizontal.

Example.
```
MTB > PLOT C4 VS C5
```

PRINT C K

Displays the contents of any specified column(s) or constant box(es) in the worksheet.

Examples.
```
MTB > PRINT C3
MTB > PRINT C1   C5-C8   K3   K7-K10
MTB > PRINT K2
```

RANDOM K INTO C;

Selects K observations at random and puts them into the specified column C. The RANDOM command must be augmented by a subcommand to specify the underlying probability distribution from which the random selections are made. Available subcommands are BERNOULLI, BINOMIAL, DISCRETE, INTEGER, NORMAL.

Examples.
```
MTB > RANDOM 25 INTO C1;
SUBC> INTEGER 1 TO 6.

MTB > RANDOM 20 INTO C3;
SUBC> DISCRETE C1 C2.

MTB > RANDOM 50 INTO C2;
SUBC> BERNOULLI 0.5.
```

```
MTB > RANDOM 30 INTO C1;
SUBC> BINOMIAL 10 0.5.

MTB > RANDOM 50 INTO C1;
SUBC> NORMAL 100 15.

MTB > RANDOM 20 INTO C1 - C5;
SUBC> NORMAL 100 15.
```

RANGE C

Computes the range of the specified column.

Example.
```
MTB > RANGE C3
```

READ C C C

Allows the user to enter data into several specified columns simultaneously.

Example.
```
MTB > READ C1 C2 C5-C7
DATA> 3   17   4.1   6.2   -3.57
DATA> 5   13   3.6   5.8   -4.72
DATA> 2   15   5.3   2.7    8.96
DATA> END OF DATA
```

REGRESS C 1 C

Performs a linear regression analysis on the y-values contained in the first specified column against the x-values contained in the second specified column.

Example.
```
MTB > REGRESS C12 1 C11
```

RETRIEVE 'filename'

Recalls any previously SAVEd Minitab worksheet.

Examples.
```
MTB > RETRIEVE 'CARDIAC'
MTB > INFO

MTB > RETR '[SCIENCE.BILESC] CARDIAC.MTW'
MTB > INFO
MTB > SAVE 'CARDIAC'
```

SAMPLE K FROM C INTO C

Selects K numbers at random from the first specified column and puts those selections into the second specified column.

Example.
```
MTB > SAMPLE 5 FROM C1 INTO C2
```

SAVE 'filename'

The current Minitab worksheet is permanently saved under the given filename. All entries in any column or constant box are thereby saved in the file. A SAVEd file can be RETRIEVEd at a later time.

Example.
```
MTB > SAVE 'CARDIAC'
```

SET C

Allows the user to enter data into the specified column. The data must be numbers separated by either a space or a comma. Data are entered until the user specifies END.

Example.
```
MTB > SET C7
DATA> 3 7 11 2:6
DATA> 9, 17    143
DATA> END OF DATA
MTB > PRINT C7
```

Advice. PRINT and check after SETting up any column.

SINTERVAL [conf] C C

Constructs a sign interval (s-interval) at the [conf] specified level of confidence on the data in each of the given columns. If no [conf] confidence level is specified, Minitab uses 95% by default.

Example.
```
MTB > SINTERVAL 90 C1 C5-C8
```

SORT C INTO C

Orders the numbers in the first specified column from smallest to largest. The ordered data set is then put in the second specified column.

Examples.
```
MTB > SORT C4 INTO C17
MTB > SORT C1 INTO C1
```

SQRT(C)

Used in a LET statement to take the square root of each number in the specified column.

Example.
```
MTB > LET C2 = SQRT(C1)
```

STACK C − C INTO C;
SUBSCRIPTS C.

Stacks data from the first group of columns C − C into column C. The corresponding levels are carried in the column specified in the SUBSCRIPTS subcommand. The command is particularly helpful for using the MOOD and ONEWAY commands.

Example.
```
MTB > STACK C1 - C4 INTO C11;
SUBC> SUBSCRIPTS C12.
```

STANDARD DEVIATION C

Computes the standard deviation of the specified column.

Example.
```
MTB > STANDARD DEVIATION C1
```

Example.
```
MTB > LET K1 = STDEV(C1)
MTB > PRINT K1
```

STEM-AND-LEAF C C

Constructs a stem-and-leaf diagram for the data in each specified column.

Examples.
```
MTB > STEM-AND-LEAF C1
MTB > STEM-AND-LEAF C1 - C3
```

STEST refno C;
ALTERNATE K.

Performs a signs test (s-test) for comparing the median against the given reference number "refno" for the data in column C. *K* denotes the test alternate.

Example.
```
MTB > STEST 27.2 C1;
SUBC> ALTERNATE -1.
```

STOP

Exits Minitab and returns the user to the computer's operating system.

Example.
```
MTB > STOP
```

STORE 'programname'

Creates a program file of Minitab commands. The file is labeled with the specified 'programname'.

The commands in the file are not executed until directed by an EXECUTE command. Once a STOREd program is created, it can be EXECUTEd anytime during the current or future Minitab sessions. Warning: Do not RETRIEVE a STOREd program; merely EXECUTE it.

A STOREd program's 'programname' must be enclosed in single quotes. Use only alphanumeric characters, that is, letters of the alphabet or digits. Do not use any special characters like :, ., $, etc.

The sequence of commands to be placed in the STOREd program is terminated by END (or END OF PROGRAM).

Example.
```
MTB > STORE 'FREQTAB'
STOR> NOTE Relative Frequency Table
```

```
STOR> NAME C1 'FREQ', C2 'RELFREQ'
STOR> SET C1
STOR> 645 32 93 371
STOR> LET C2 = C1/SUM(C1)
STOR> PRINT C1 C2
STOR> END
```

Warning: If you SET a column within a STOREd program, do *not* use the END OF DATA command to signal the end of data entry. Minitab interprets just the END and will think that it is the END OF PROGRAM.

SUM

Determines the sum of the specified column and displays the resulting sum on the screen.

Examples.
```
MTB > SUM C3
MTB > LET K1 = SUM(C3)
MTB > PRINT K1
```

TABLE C C

Constructs a two-factor frequency distribution table for the data given in columns C C. The marginal sums for the specified columns may be included with the subcommand ALL C C. Cell row percents and column percents may be included with the subcommands ROWPERCENTS and COLPERCENTS. A chisquared analysis on the resulting table can be obtained with the subcommand CHISQUARED.

Examples.
```
MTB > TABLE C1 C2

MTB > TABLE C1 C2;
      ALL C1 C2;
      ROWPERCENTS;
      COLPERCENTS;
      CHISQUARED.
```

TALLY C

Constructs a frequency distribution table for the numbers in the specified column. One may obtain a percent frequency distribution table with the subcommand PERCENTS.

Examples.
```
MTB > TALLY C1
MTB > TALLY C3;
SUBC>   PERCENTS.
```

TINTERVAL [confidence] C

Calculates a confidence interval [optional: at the specified level of confidence] for the data in the specified column.

Example.
```
MTB > TINTERVAL 90 C1
```

TTEST refno C;
    ALTERNATE code.

Conducts a t-test of hypothesis for the mean against the reference value specified by "refno." The test is conducted on the sample data contained in column C. The type of test (one-, two-tailed) is conducted according to the instruction provided in the subcommand ALTERNATE as follows:

Code	Test
−1	left-tailed test
0	two-tailed test
1	right-tailed test

Examples.

```
MTB > TTEST 16 C1;
SUBC>   ALTERNATE -1.

MTB > TTEST 0 C5;
SUBC > ALTERNATE 0.
```

TWOSAMPLE [confidence] C C;
    ALTERNATE code.

Conducts a test of hypothesis comparing the means of two populations based on the samples contained in the two specified columns. Optional: The user may specify a level of confidence for a confidence interval for the difference of the two means. If "confidence" is not specified, Minitab gives a default 95% confidence interval for the difference of the two means. A subcommand ALTERNATE must be given to indicate the type of test for comparison of means (one- or two-sided; same as with TTEST command). If the user wants a POOLed comparison of means, the subcommand POOLED is used.

Examples.

```
MTB > TWOSAMPLE C1 C2;
SUBC>   ALTERNATE 1;
SUBC>   POOLED.

MTB > TWOSAMPLE 90 C11 C12;
SUBC>   ALTERNATE 0.
```

TWOWAY C C C;
    MEANS C C.

Performs two-way analysis of variance on a balanced data set presented in a stacked format. The subcommand means provides a graphic for individual 95% confidence intervals for each level within each factor specified in the MEANS subcommand.

Example.

```
MTB > TWOWAY C11 C12 C13;
SUBC> MEANS C12 C13.
```

ZTEST refno stdev C;
    ALTERNATE code.

Conducts a large-samples z-test of hypothesis for the mean against the reference value specified by "refno." The standard deviation for the test must be specified. The test is conducted on the sample data contained in the specified column C. The type of test (one-, two-tailed) is conducted according to the instruction provided in the subcommand ALTERNATE as follows:

Code	Test
−1	left-tailed test
0	two-tailed test
1	right-tailed test

Examples.

```
MTB > LET K1 = STDEV(C1)
MTB > ZTEST 16 K1 C1;
SUBC>   ALTERNATE -1.

MTB > LET K5 = STDEV(C5)
MTB > ZTEST 0 K5 C5;
SUBC > ALTERNATE 0.
```

ZINTERVAL [conf] stdev C

Constructs a large-samples z-confidence interval [optional: at the specified level of confidence] on the data in the specified column. The standard deviation must be provided.

Examples.

```
MTB > LET K1 = STDEV(C1)
MTB > ZINTERVAL 95 K1 C1

MTB > LET K5 = STDEV(C5)
MTB > ZINTERVAL 90 K5 C5
```

SECTION 1.1

Warm-ups 1.1

1. Sample; **2.** 48; **3.** improved (I), unchanged (U), worse (W); **4.** 34, 5, 9; **5.** 48, yes; **6.** 34, 48, 34, 48, .71; **7.** 5, 48, .11; **8.** 9, 48, .19; **9.** yes; **10.** .71, 71, .10, 10, .19, 19; **11.** 100

12.

Clinical Outcome	Frequency	Relative Frequency
Improved (I)	34	.71
Unchanged (U)	5	.10
Worse (W)	9	.19
Total	48	1.00

Problems 1.1

1.a. Total number reporting: 45
Relative frequency: 0.33, 0.29, 0.20, 0.11, 0.07; sum = 1.00
Percent relative frequency: 33, 29, 20, 11, 7; sum = 100

b(iii). Pie chart degrees: 120, 104, 72, 40, 24 (sum = 360°)

3. 217, 458, 675, 410, 241, 410
Note: Frequencies are *whole* numbers. These frequencies add up to 2411. It is impossible, on the basis of the information given in the table, to determine where the 2412st hospital belongs in the table. This problem illustrates why a frequency distribution table should carry both the absolute and relative frequencies.

5.a.

Sex	Frequency	Percent
Female	7	23
Male	23	77
Total	30	100

b.

Grafts	Frequency	Percent
2	8	27
3	14	47
4	6	20
5	2	7
Total	30	101*

*Deviation from ideal of 100% is due to round-off error.

c.

Number of Grafts	Females		Males	
	Frequency	Percent	Frequency	Percent
2	1	14	7	30
3	4	57	10	43
4	2	29	4	17
5	0	0	2	9
Total	7	100	23	99*

*Deviation from ideal of 100 is due to round-off error.

7.

Episodes	Milking	Stripping
0	34	39
1	17	13
2	14	10
3	6	10
4	5	6
5	6	3
6	4	7
7	7	6
8	7	6
Total	100	100

9.a.

Cause	Frequency	Relative Frequency
Ventricular Perforation	9	.29
Severe Aortic Regurgitation	4	.13
Fatal Cardiac Arrest	13	.42
Cerebrovascular Accident	2	.06
Amputation	3	.10
Total	31	1.00

b.

c. Pie chart degrees: 105, 46, 151, 23, 35 (sum = 360°)
11. .59; **13.** .21; **15.** .28;
17.

Developed ARDS	Frequency	Relative Frequency
Yes	7	.24
No	21	.76
Total	29	1.00

19.

Risk Group	Frequency	Relative Frequency
Trauma	4	.57
Perforated Bowel	2	.29
Pancreatitis	1	.14
Total	7	1.00

21. .00566
23. .387

SECTION 1.2

Warm-ups 1.2

1. Hospitalized septic inpatients treated in part with parenteral nutrition in a surgical nutrition unit who are not receiving steroids or drugs known to affect metabolic rates; **2.** Categorical; **3.** 5; **4.** The sum of the x column is 214.4. The entries for the x^2 column are 2209.00, 1497.69, 1998.09, 1747.24, 1780.84; sum 9232.86; **5.** x; **6.** 214.4; **7.** 214.4/5 = 42.88; **8.** variance; **9.** 5, 214.4, 45967.36, 9232.86; [5(9232.86) − (45967.36)]/20 = 9.847; **10.** The square root of 9.847 is 3.14; **11.** 42.88 ± 3.14; **12.** 42.88, 3.14, 39.74, 46.02; the 1SD window extends from 39.74 to 46.02; **13.** 3, 60%; **14.** 36.60, 49.16, from 36.60 to 49.16, 5, 100; **15.** 41.8, 42.2, 44.7; **16.** $\bar{x}$; **17.** 42.2; **18.** 47.0, 38.7, 8.3

Problems 1.2

1.a. 38.86, 38.70, 6.5, 2.27
  b. 1SD window from 36.59 to 41.13; 2SD: 34.32 to 43.40; 3SD: 32.06 to 45.67
  c. 1SD window, 5 out of 8 (62.5%); 2SD window, 8 out of 8 (100%)
3. Group 1: **a.** 68.0, 69.0 19, 5.0
  b. 1SD window from 63.0 to 73.0; 2SD: 58.0 to 78.0; 3SD: 53.0 to 83.0
  c. 1SD window, 12 of 15 (80%); 2SD window, 14 of 15 (93%); 3SD window, 15 of 15 (100%).
  Group 2: **a.** 69.1, 70.0, 21, 6.0
  b. 1SD window from 63.1 to 75.0; 2SD: 57.2 to 81.0; 3SD: 51.2 to 86.9
  c. 1SD window, 11 of 15 (73.3%); 2SD: 14 of 15 (93.3%); 3SD: 15 of 15 (100%)

5.

	1st PaO_2	2nd PaO_2	Change
mean	80.3	78.5	1.8
median	86.0	84.0	2.0
range	49	49	9
stdev	16.1	15.3	2.4

Change Data:
1SD window from −0.6 to 4.3; 8 of 11 (73%)
2SD window −3.1 to 6.7; 10 of 11 (91%);
3SD window −5.5 to 9.1; 11 of 11 (100%)
7.a. 0.2 liters/min; **b.** yes; **c.** 4.2 liters/min (4.17 liters/min is also acceptable)
9.a. 3.46, 4.72, 4.56, 5.16, 5.14, 4.40, 5.14; **b.** .74, 1.43, 1.17, 1.15, 1.05, .81, .95

  c.

	Start	15 m	30 m	1 h	1.5 h	2 h	3 h
n	5	5	5	5	5	5	5
mean	3.46	4.72	4.56	5.16	5.14	4.40	5.14
SD	.74	1.43	1.17	1.15	1.05	.81	.95

d. Start: from 2.72 to 4.20; 15 minutes: from 3.29 to 6.15; 30 minutes: 3.37 to 5.75; 1 hour: 4.01 to 6.31; 1.5 hours: 4.09 to 6.19; 2 hours: 4.59 to 6.21; 3 hours: 4.19 to 6.09

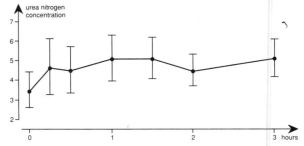

f. Urea nitrogen rises during the first hour, with most of the increase in the first 15 minutes, then levels out.

SECTION 2.1

Warm-ups 2.1

1. Nominal, ordinal, and interval; **2.a.** nominal, **b.** ordinal, **c.** interval; **3.** Patient is nominal, Gender is nominal, eye is nominal, age is interval, outcome is ordinal; **4.** numbers; **5.** patient identification number; **6.** worse, unchanged, improved; **7.** sort
8. 1 2789
   2 0011122345578889
   3 000111223355678
   4 00113799
   5 0256
   6 1

9. b; **10.** e; **11.** a; **12.** c; **13.** d; **14.** The age data are roughly symmetrical about the median (31) and range from 12 to 61. The data are bunched toward the middle and tail off toward the ends; **15.** Exploratory data analysis (EDA).

Problems 2.1

1.a. Ordinal; **b.** nominal; **c.** nominal; **d.** ordinal; **e.** (i) nominal, (ii) nominal, (iii) interval; **f.** interval; **g.** interval; **h.** interval; **i.** Subject is nominal, while the others (age, height, weight, and body mass index) are all interval.

3. Stem-and-leaf diagram for prefilled syringes, iced
```
2 247789
3 012234444455555778888889
4 0025678
5 037
6 27
7 2
```
Stem-and-leaf diagram for prefilled syringes, room
```
2 35557888
3 02222345556778888999
4 0112238
5 35
6 0179
```
The two distributions appear roughly the same.

5.
```
MTB > NAME C11 'Sorted'
MTB > SORT C1 INTO C11 #raw data set is in C1
MTB > PRINT C11 #The sorted data set.

Sorted
 2.2   2.4   2.7   2.7   2.8   2.9   3.0   3.1   3.2   3.2   3.3
 3.4   3.4   3.4   3.4   3.5   3.5   3.5   3.5   3.7   3.7   3.8
 3.8   3.8   3.8   3.8   3.8   3.9   4.0   4.0   4.2   4.5   4.6
 4.7   4.8   5.0   5.3   5.7   6.2   6.7   7.2

MTB > DOTPLOT C1
```

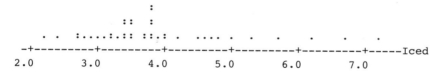

```
MTB > BOXPLOT C1
```

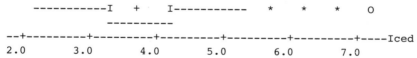

```
MTB > STEM-AND-LEAF C1

Stem-and-leaf of Iced   N  = 41
Leaf Unit = 0.10

     2     2 24
     6     2 7789
    15     3 012234444
   (13)    3 5555778888889
    13     4 002
    10     4 5678
     6     5 03
```

```
       4     5 7
       3     6 2
       2     6 7
       1     7 2

MTB > HISTOGRAM C1

Histogram of Iced    N = 41

Midpoint    Count
     2.0       1   *
     2.5       3   ***
     3.0       6   ******
     3.5      11   ***********
     4.0      10   **********
     4.5       3   ***
     5.0       2   **
     5.5       2   **
     6.0       1   *
     6.5       1   *
     7.0       1   *

MTB > GHISTOGRAM C1
```

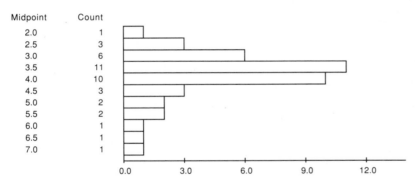

Iced PFS   N =   41

```
7. MTB > NOTE The Iced Co-Set data are in column C3
   NTB > NOTE the Room Co-Set data are in column C4.
   MTB > DOTPLOT C3
```

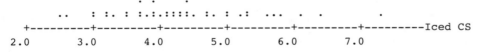

```
   MTB > DOTPLOT C4
```

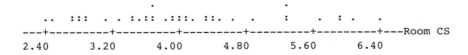

```
MTB > DOTPLOT C3 C4;
SUBC> SAME.


                             .  .       .
           ..    : :.  :  :.:.::::.  :.  :  .:   ...   .   .           .
         +---------+---------+---------+---------+---------+-------Iced CS
                       .                  .
           .. :::  .  .:.::.:::.::..   .   :    .  :  .  .
         +---------+---------+---------+---------+---------+-------Room CS
        2.0       3.0       4.0       5.0       6.0       7.0
```

9.
```
MTB > NOTE The Weight data are in column C4.
MTB > SORT C4 INTO C11
MTB > PRINT C11
Sorted
     61    62    63    63    65    67    67    68    69    69    69
     70    70    71    72    72    73    74    74    75    76    77
     78    80    80    82    84    86   111

MTB > DOTPLOT C4

                   .
           ..:  .  :.:.:.:.:.... :  .  .                          .
         -+---------+---------+---------+---------+---------+-----Weight
         60        70        80        90       100       110

MTB > BOXPLOT C4

                 ----------
           -------I   +   I---------                         O
                 ----------
         --+---------+---------+---------+---------+---------+----Weight
          60        70        80        90       100       110

MTB > STEM-AND-LEAF C4
Stem-and-leaf of Weight    N  = 29
Leaf Unit = 1.0

         4    6  1233
        11    6  5778999
        (8)   7  00122344
        10    7  5678
         6    8  0024
         2    8  6
         1    9
         1    9
         1   10
         1   10
         1   11 1

MTB > HISTOGRAM C4
Histogram of Weight   N = 29
Midpoint   Count
       60       2   **
       65       5   *****
```

```
        70           9   *********
        75           6   ******
        80           4   ****
        85           2   **
        90           0
        95           0
       100           0
       105           0
       110           1   *
```

```
MTB > GHISTOGRAM C4
  Weight      N =      29
```

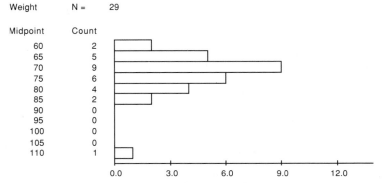

```
Midpoint    Count
     60        2
     65        5
     70        9
     75        6
     80        4
     85        2
     90        0
     95        0
    100        0
    105        0
    110        1

          0.0    3.0    6.0    9.0    12.0
```

11. A stem-and-leaf diagram for the body mass index data.

```
18 4
19 449
20 127
21
22 12455789
23 3599
24 177
25 7
26 08
27 77
28
29
30 4
31
32
33
34
35
36
37
38
39
40
41 3
```

The stem-and-leaf diagram indicates a nonsymmetrical distribution.

Warm-ups 2.2

1. 41; **2.** 6; **3.** c; **4.** b; **5.** 0.1; **6.** max = 7.2, min = 2.2, u = .1, uer = 5.1; **7.** uer = 5.1, k = 6, uer/k = 5.1/6 = .85, w = .9 (round answer to uer/k = .85 *up* at unit of measurement's position, which is the first place past the decimal point—recall u = .1); **8.** 6, .9, 5.4; **9.** 5.4, 5.1, .3, 3; **10.** 2.2, m = 2.2, 2.1, 2.0, 1.9; **11.** 4.7, 5.6, 6.5;

12–13.

Class Limits		Frequency	Relative Frequency
Lower	Upper		
2.0	2.8	5	.12
2.9	3.7	16	.39
3.8	4.6	12	.29
4.7	5.5	4	.10
5.6	6.4	2	.05
6.5	7.3	2	.05
	Total	41	1.00

Problems 2.2

1.a. n = 29; k = 5; u = .01; uer = 3.77; w = .76; ar = 3.80; ar − uer = .03 (three unit steps); m = 2.62, 2.61, 2.60, 2.59 (choose m = 2.60).

Frequency distribution table for the Daily and Mersch cardiac output study, ice-temperature injectates.

Class Limits	Frequency	Relative Frequency	% Relative Frequency
2.60–3.35	5	.17	17
3.36–4.11	6	.21	21
4.12–4.87	7	.24	24
4.88–5.63	7	.24	24
5.64–6.39	4	.14	14
Total	29	1.00	100

1.b.

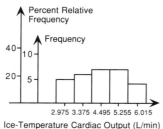

Bar Graph

Ice-Temperature Cardiac Output (L/min)

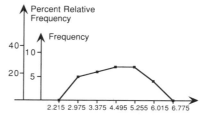

Polygon

3. n = 41; k = 6; u = .1; uer = 4.9; w = .9; ar = 5.4; ar − uer = .5 (five unit of measurement steps); m(options) = 2.5, 2.4, 2.3, 2.2, 2.1, 2.0 (choose 2.3 or 2.2) The frequency distribution table using m = 2.2 follows.

Frequency distribution table for the Barcelona et al cardiac data set, ice-temperature injectates (Co-Set).

Class Limits		Frequency	Relative Frequency
Lower	Upper		
2.2	3.0	4	.10
3.1	3.9	12	.29
4.0	4.8	14	.34
4.9	5.7	7	.17
5.8	6.6	3	.07
6.7	7.5	1	.02
	Total	41	.99*

*Deviation from ideal of 1.00 due to round-off error.

3.b.

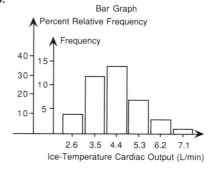

Bar Graph

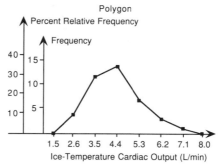

Polygon

5.a. $n = 29, k = 5, u = .01,$ uer $= .96 - (-1.87) + .01 = 2.84, w = 2.84/5 = .57$ (round *up* at u $= .01$ position), ar $= 2.85,$ ar $-$ uer $= .01, m$(options) $= -1.87, -1.88.$ The frequency distribution table using $m = -1.88$ follows.

Frequency distribution table for the Daily and Mersch cardiac output Study, Room $-$ Fick.

Class Limits	Frequency	% Relative Frequency
$-1.88 - -1.32$	3	10
$-1.31 - -.75$	3	10
$-.74 - -.18$	9	31
$-.17 - .39$	12	41
$.40 - .96$	2	7
Totals	29	99*

*Deviation from ideal of 1.00 due to round-off error.

5.b.

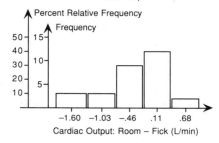

Bar Graph

Cardiac Output: Room $-$ Fick (L/min)

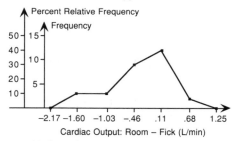

Polygon

Cardiac Output: Room $-$ Fick (L/min)

7.a. $n = 41; k = 6; u = .1;$ uer $= 4.7; w = .8;$ ar $= 4.8;$ ar $-$ uer $= .1$ (one unit step); m(options) $= 2.3, 2.2.$
The frequency distribution table using $m = 2.2$ follows.

Frequency distribution table for the Barcelona et al data, prefilled syringes, room-temperature injectates.

Class Limits		Frequency	Relative Frequency
Lower	Upper		
2.2	2.9	8	.20
3.0	3.7	13	.32
3.8	4.5	13	.32
4.6	5.3	2	.05
5.4	6.1	3	.07
6.2	6.9	2	.05
	Total	41	1.01*

*Deviation from ideal of 1.00 due to round-off error.

7.b.

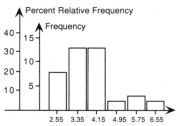

Bar Graph

Room-Temperature Cardiac Output Prefilled Syringes (L/min)

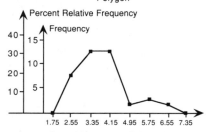

Polygon

Room-Temperature Cardiac Output Prefilled Syringes (L/min)

9.a. $n = 29, k = 5, u = 1,$ uer $= 16, w = 4,$ ar $= 20,$ ar $-$ uer $= 4, m$(options) $= 18, 17, 16, 15, 14$ (choose $m = 16$).

Frequency distribution table for age.

Class Limits		Frequency	Relative Frequency
Lower	Upper		
16	19	3	.10
20	23	8	.28
24	27	14	.48
28	31	3	.10
32	35	1	.03
	Total	29	.99*

*Deviation from ideal of 1.00 due to round-off error.

9.b.

Bar Graph

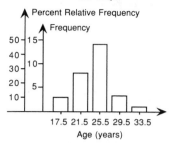

Polygon

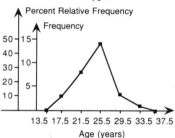

11.a. $n = 29, k = 5, u = 1,$ uer $= 51, w = 4,$ ar $= 55,$
ar $-$ uer $= 4, m$(options) $= 61, 60, 59, 58, 57$
(choose $m = 59$).

Frequency distribution table for weight.

| Class Limits | | Frequency | Relative Frequency |
Lower	Upper		
59	69	11	.38
70	80	14	.48
81	91	3	.10
92	102	0	.00
103	113	1	.03
	Total	29	.99*

*Deviation from ideal of 1.00 due to round-off error.

11.b.

Bar Graph

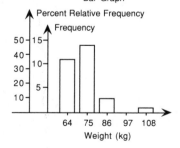

Polygon

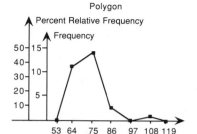

13.a. $n = 51,$ so $k = 6$ (yes)

b. Yes, they are exhaustive, mutually exclusive, and easy to understand.

c. .35, .22, .24, .12, .06, .02 (sum of 1.01 due to round-off error)

13.d.

(i) Bar Graph

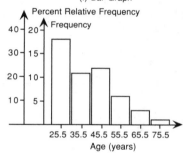

(ii) Polygon

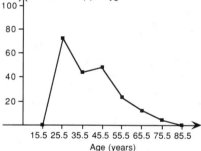

14.a. 32.9, 31.0, 49, 11.3

b. 1SD (21.6, 44.2) 67%
2SD (10.3, 55.5) 96%
3SD ($-1.0, 66.8$) 100%

c. $n = 48; k = 6; u = 1;$ uer $= 50; w = 9;$ ar $= 54;$
ar $-$ uer $= 4$ (four unit steps); $m = 12, 11, 10, 9,$
8 (choose $m = 10$).

Frequency distribution table for age

Class Limits		Frequency	Relative Frequency
Lower	Upper		
10	18	3	.06
19	27	12	.25
28	36	18	.38
37	45	7	.15
46	54	5	.10
55	63	3	.06
	Total	48	1.00

SECTION 2.3

Warm-ups 2.3

1. .122, .390, .293, .098, .049, .049; **2.** 0.1; **3.** $u/2 = .1/2 = .05$; **4.** lower class boundary: 1.95, 2.85, 3.75, 4.65, 5.55, 6.45; upper class boundary: 2.85, 3.75, 4.65, 5.55, 6.45, 7.35

5.

Class Boundaries		Frequency	Relative Frequency
Lower	Upper		
1.95	2.85	5	.12
2.85	3.75	16	.39
3.75	4.65	12	.29
4.65	5.55	4	.10
5.55	6.45	2	.05
6.45	7.35	2	.05
	Total	41	1.00

6. c; **7.** e; **8.** c;
9. class 2 mark $= (2.85 + 3.75)/2 = 6.60/2 = 3.30$
class 3 mark $= (3.75 + 4.65)/2 = 8.40/2 = 4.20$
class 4 mark $= (4.65 + 5.55)/2 = 10.20/2 = 5.10$
class 5 mark $= (5.55 + 6.45)/2 = 12.20/2 = 6.00$
class 6 mark $= (6.45 + 7.35)/2 = 13.80/2 = 6.90$
10. d; **11.** horizontal: 3.30, 4.20, 5.10, 6.00, 6.90; vertical: 10, 20, 30, 40
12.

Class Boundary		Freq	Cumul Freq	Rel Freq	Cumul Rel Freq	% Rel Freq	Cumul % RF
Lower	Upper						
1.95	2.85	5	5	.12	.12	12	12
2.85	3.75	16	21	.39	.51	39	51
3.75	4.65	12	33	.29	.80	29	80
4.65	5.55	4	37	.10	.90	10	90
5.55	6.45	2	39	.05	.95	5	95
6.45	7.35	2	41	.05	1.00	5	100

13. a; **14.** a; **15.** e.

Problems 2.3

1.a. Frequency distribution table for the Daily and Mersch cardiac output study, ice-temperature injectates.

Class Boundaries	Frequency	Relative Frequency	% Relative Frequency
2.595–3.355	5	.17	17
3.355–4.115	6	.21	21
4.115–4.875	7	.24	24
4.875–5.635	7	.24	24
5.635–6.395	4	.14	14
Total	29	1.00	100

1.b.

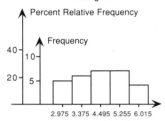

Histogram

Ice-Temperature Cardiac Output (L/min)

1.c. Cumulative frequency distribution table for the Daily and Mersch cardiac output study, ice-temperature injectates.

Class Boundaries	Frequency	Cumulative Frequency	% Cumulative Frequency
2.595–3.355	5	5	17
3.355–4.115	6	11	38
4.115–4.875	7	18	62
4.875–5.635	7	25	86
5.635–6.395	4	29	100
Total	29		

1.d.

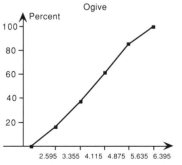

Ogive

Ice-Temperature Cardiac Output (L/min)

3.a. Frequency distribution table for the Barcelona et al cardiac data set, ice-temperature injectates (Co-Set).

Class Boundaries Lower	Upper	Frequency	Relative Frequency
2.15	3.05	4	.10
3.05	3.95	12	.29
3.95	4.85	14	.34
4.85	5.75	7	.17
5.75	6.65	3	.07
6.65	7.55	1	.02
	Total	41	.99*

*Deviation from ideal of 1.00 due to round-off error.

3.b.

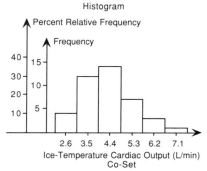

Histogram

3.c. Cumulative frequency distribution table for the Barcelona et al cardiac output study, ice-temperature injectates (Co-Set).

Class Boundaries	Frequency	Cumulative Frequency	% Cumulative Frequency
2.15–3.05	4	4	10
3.05–3.95	12	16	39
3.95–4.85	14	30	73
4.85–5.75	7	37	90
5.75–6.65	3	40	98
6.65–7.55	1	41	100
Totals	41		

3.d.

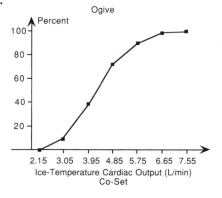

Ogive

5.a. Frequency distribution table for the Daily and Mersch cardiac output study, room − Fick.

Class Boundaries	Frequency	% Relative Frequency
−1.885−−1.315	3	10
−1.315−−.745	3	10
−.745−−.175	9	31
−.175−.395	12	41
395−.965	2	7
Total	29	99*

*Deviation from ideal of 1.00 due to round-off error.

5.b.

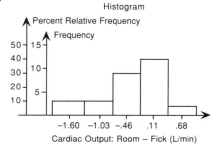

Histogram

5.c. Cumulative frequency distribution table for the Daily and Mersch cardiac output study, room − Fick.

Class Boundaries	Frequency	Cumulative Frequency	% Cumulative Frequency
−1.885−−1.315	3	3	10
−1.315−−.745	3	6	21
−.745−−.175	9	15	52
−.175−.395	12	27	93
395−.965	2	29	100
Total	29		

5.d.

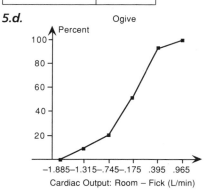

Ogive

7.a. Frequency distribution table for the Barcelona et al data, prefilled syringes, room-temperature injectates.

Class Boundaries Lower	Upper	Frequency	Relative Frequency
2.15	2.95	8	.20
2.95	3.75	13	.32
3.75	4.55	13	.32
4.55	5.35	2	.05
5.35	6.15	3	.07
6.15	6.95	2	.05
Total		41	1.01*

*Deviation from ideal of 1.00 due to round-off error.

7.b.

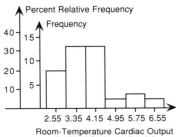

Histogram

Room-Temperature Cardiac Output Prefilled Syringes (L/min)

7.c. Cumulative frequency distribution table for the Barcelona et al data, prefilled syringes, room-temperature injectates.

Class Boundaries	Frequency	Cumulative Frequency	% Cumulative Frequency
2.15–2.95	8	8	20
2.95–3.75	13	21	51
3.75–4.55	13	34	83
4.55–5.35	2	36	88
5.35–6.15	3	39	95
6.15–6.95	2	41	100
Total	41		

7.d.

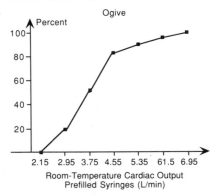

Ogive

Room-Temperature Cardiac Output Prefilled Syringes (L/min)

9.a. Frequency distribution table for age.

Class Boundaries Lower	Upper	Frequency	Relative Frequency
15.5	19.5	3	.10
19.5	23.5	8	.28
23.5	27.5	14	.48
27.5	31.5	3	.10
31.5	35.5	1	.03
Total		29	.99*

*Deviation from ideal of 1.00 due to round-off error.

9.b.

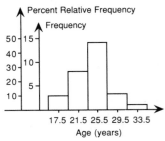

Histogram

Age (years)

9.c. Cumulative frequency distribution table for the Daily and Mersch cardiac output study, ice-temperature injectates.

Class Boundaries	Frequency	Cumulative Frequency	% Cumulative Frequency
15.5–19.5	3	3	10
19.5–23.5	8	11	38
23.5–27.5	14	25	86
27.5–31.5	3	28	97
31.5–35.5	1	29	100
Total	29		

9.d.

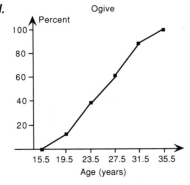

Ogive

Age (years)

11.a. Frequency distribution table for weight.

Class Boundaries Lower	Upper	Frequency	Relative Frequency
58.5	69.5	11	.38
69.5	80.5	14	.48
80.5	91.5	3	.10
91.5	102.5	0	.00
102.5	113.5	1	.03
Total		29	.99*

*Deviation from ideal of 1.00 is due to round-off error.

11.b.

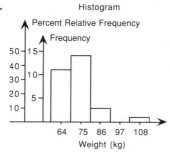

Histogram

11.c. Cumulative frequency distribution table for weight.

Class Boundaries	Frequency	Cumulative Frequency	% Cumulative Frequency
58.5–69.5	11	11	38
69.5–80.5	14	25	86
80.5–91.5	3	28	97
91.5–102.5	0	289	7
102.5–113.5	1	29	100
Total	29		

11.d.

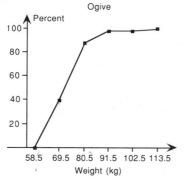

Ogive

13.a. Frequency distribution table for the Macey and Bouman age data.

Age (yr)	Frequency	Percent
20.5–30.5	18	35
30.5–40.5	11	22
40.5–50.5	12	24
50.5–60.5	6	12
60.5–70.5	3	6
70.5–80.5	1	2
Total	51	101*

*Deviation from the ideal of 100 is due to round-off error.

13.b.

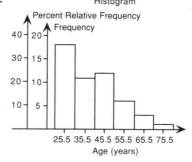

Histogram

13.c. Cumulative frequency distribution table for the Macey and Bouman age data.

Class Boundaries	Frequency	Cumulative Frequency	% Cumulative Frequency
20.5–30.5	18	18	35
30.5–40.5	11	29	57
40.5–50.5	12	41	80
50.5–60.5	6	47	92
60.5–70.5	3	50	98
70.5–80.5	1	51	100
Total	51		

13.d.

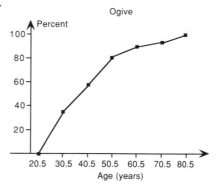

Ogive

SECTION 3.1

Warm-ups 3.1

1. c; **2.** b; **3.** d; **4.** e; **5.** a; **6.** VVV, VVF, VFV, VFF, FVV, FVF, FFV, FFF; **7.** b; **8.** *(a)* VVV; *(b)* FFF; *(c)* VVV, VVF, VFV, FVV; *(d)* VVF, VFV, VFF, FVV, FVF, FFV, FFF (i.e., all except VVV); *(e)* VVF, VFV, FVV; **9.** {VVV, VVF, VFV, FVV, FFF}; **10.** b; **11.** $2^5 = 32$

Problems 3.1

1. 214,656
3.a.

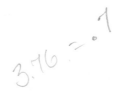

$3.76 = .7$

3.b. $n = 4 \times 2 = 8$
5.a(i). $101/492 = .205$
a(ii). $31/492 = .063$
b. $31/101 = .307$
7. 2,160

SECTION 3.2

Warm-ups 3.2

1. c; **2.** b; **3.** 720, 5040; **4.** b; **5.** 7, 1, 1, 7; **6.** d; **7.** a; **8.** 56, 56; **9.** c; **10.** c; **11.** c; **12.** d.

Problems 3.2

1. 21, 120, 1, 1, 9, 9
3. A + .3485, A − .0615, B + .0765, B − .0135, AB + .0340, AB − .0060, O + .3910, O − .0690
5. 18,564
7. 720
9.a. .5625; **b.** .0625; **c.** .1875; **d.** .1875; **e.** .0625

c. .173; **d.** .085; **e.** .053; **f.** .048
13.b. .01; **c.** .0125; **e.** .31
15.a. 3.535316×10^{18} (calculator answer); **b.** .25; **c.(i)** 3160, **(ii)** 1200/3160 ≈ .38, **(iii)** 190/3160 ≈ .06; **d.(i)** 1581580, **(ii)** .433, **(iii)** .2126, **(iv)** .0432, **(v)** .0031, **(vi)** .2589

SECTION 4.1

Warm-ups 4.1

1. Disease status and cootie test; **2.** 70, 80; **3.** 65, 85; **4.** .9; **5.** .1; **6.** 78/80, .975; **7.** SC absent, SC absent, 2/80, .025; **8.** 63/65, .969; **9.** ≤5, 78/85, .918; **10.** .94; **11.** 70/150, .467; **12.** prevalence = 46.7%, Sn = 90%, F − R = 10%, Sn + (F − R) = 100%, Sp = 97.5%, F + R = 2.5%, Sp + (F + R) = 100%, PV+ = 96.9%, PV− = 91.8%; **13.** d.

Problems 4.1

1.a. Sn = .682, F − R = .318, Sp = .474, F + R = .526, PV+ = .633, PV− = .529, accuracy = .593; **b.** .615, .570; **c.** no, little change in PVs.
3.a. .5; **b.** Sn = 1, F − R = 0, Sp = .647, F + R = .353, accuracy = .824, PV+ = .739, PV− = 1; **c.** Yes, PV− = 100%.

5.a. Bladder cancer; **b.** new: AMF urine test, old: biopsy; **c.** population: 46,000 new cases each year, study: 22/49 = .45; **d.**

Bladder Cancer

		Yes	No	
AMF Test	Positive	22	2	24
	Negative	0	25	25
		22	27	49

Sn = 22/22 = 100%, F − R = 0/22 = 0%, Sp = 25/27 = 93%, F + R = 2/27 = 7%, PV + = 22/24 = .92%, PV − = 25/25 = 100%, accuracy = 47/49 = 96%; **e.** Yes, PV − = 100% (good test to rule out bladder cancer). Biopsy only those patients who receive a positive test.

7.a. A. Beta strep pharyngitis; **b.** scorecard, throat culture; **c.** no, 54/285 = 18.9%; **d.**

Beta Strep

		Yes	No	
Scorecard	Positive	16	39	55
	Negative	38	192	230
		54	231	285

Sn = 16/54 = 29.6% (29% given); F − R = 38/54 = 70.4%; Sp = 192/231 = 83.1% (83% given); F + R = 39/231 = 16.9%; PV + = 16/55 = 29.1%; PV − = 192/230 = 83.5%; accuracy = 208/285 = 73.0%; no. Sn is too low, resulting in too many undiagnosed contagious children. Sp is too low, resulting in too many children unnecessarily being sent home.

9.a.

Substernal Pain

		Yes	No	Total
MI	Yes	68	5	73
	No	102	25	127
	Total	170	30	200

b. Sn = .93, F − R = .07, Sp = .20, F + R = .80, PV + = .40, PV − = .83, accuracy = .465

11.a.

Severe Pain

		Yes	No	Total
MI	Yes	54	19	73
	No	35	92	127
	Total	89	111	200

b. Sn = .74, F − R = .26, Sp = .72, F + R = .28, PV + = .61, PV − = .83, accuracy = .73

13.a.

Perspiration

		Yes	No	Total
MI	Yes	41	32	73
	No	22	105	127
	Total	63	137	200

b. Sn = .56, F − R = .44, Sp = .83, F + R = .17, PV + = .65, PV − = .77, accuracy = .73

15.a.

Referred to

		CCU	Ward	Total
MI	Yes	375	47	422
	No	298	230	528
	Total	673	277	950

Sn = .89, F − R = .11, Sp = .44, F + R = .56, PV + = .56, PV − = .83, accuracy = .64

17. Sn = .98, F − R = .02, Sp = .77, F + R = .23, PV + = .88, PV − = .95, Accuracy = .90

19. Sn = .60, F − R = .40, Sp = .83, F + R = .17, PV + = .82, PV − = .62, Accuracy = .70

SECTION 5.1

Warm-ups 5.1

1. b; **2.** d; **3.** a; **4.** e; **5.** The first column lists the possible values for X, the second column lists the respective probabilities; **6.** b; **7.** b; **8.** d; **9.** d;

10.

x	f(x)	xf(x)	x^2	$x^2f(x)$
1	.32	.32	1	.32
2	.48	.96	4	1.92
3	.14	.42	9	1.26
4	.06	.24	16	.96
	1.00	1.94		4.46

11. c; **12.** 4.46, 1.94, 0.696; **13.** 0.6964, 0.835; **14.** .19, .79, .60, .21, .40; **15.** .27, .60, .67, .33, .40

Problems 5.1

1. QC, QD, QC, QD, QD, C, QD, QD, C, C, QC, C
3.a. F(g): .03125, .18750, .50000, .81250, .96875, 1.00000
b. (i) P[G = 5] = .03125; (ii) P[G = 0] = .03125; (iii) P[G ≥ 1] = .96875; (iv) P[G < 5] = .96875; (v) P[G ≥ 3] = .5; (vi) P[G ≤ 2] = .5
c. 2.5, 1.25, 1.12
5.a. numerical discrete; **b.** .905; **c.** .752896, .868
7. Mean = 2.5, standard deviation = $\sqrt{3584/3080}$ = 1.1

9.a. .25, .75; **b.** .25; **c.** .43; **d.** The "typical" number of children in a family of one child whose parents carry the CF gene is .25 ± .43. About one child in four born to CF carrier parents will have CF.

11.a. .76; **b.** .76; The "typical" number of children with CF in a family of three children born to CF carrier parents is .76 ± .76 (from 0 to 1.52 children).

13.a. $f(0) = .99710$

b. The PDF:

x	f(x)
0	0.999710
20	0.000286
100	0.000003
500	0.000001
1000	0.000000
5000	0.000000
10000	0.000000
100000	0.000000
2000000	0.000000

c. The expected value is .035413, between 3 and 4 cents.

SECTION 5.2

Warm-ups 5.2

1. e; **2.** c; **3.** 3, .75; **4.** c; **5.** 3, .75; **6.** b; **7.** c; **8.** d; **9.** e; **10.** d; **11.** b; **12.** b; **13.** d; **14.** a; **15.** e

Problems 5.2

1.a. PDF for $X = $ Bino(3, .9):

x	f(x)
0	.001
1	.027
2	.243
3	.729

b. 2.7; **c.** .27; **d.** .52; **e.(i)** .729, **(ii)** .001, **(iii)** .271, **(iv)** .999

3.a. PDF for $X = $ Bino(4, .78). Obtain from Minitab as follows:

MTB > PDF;
MTB > BINO 4 0.78.

x	f(x)
0	.0023
1	.0332
2	.1767
3	.4176
4	.3702

b. 3.12; **c.** .6864, .83; **d.**(i) .3702, **(ii)** .0023, **(iii)** .9977, **(iv)** .6298, **(v)** .7878

5.a. Punnet Square.

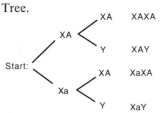

Tree.

b. **(i)** .5; **(ii)** .25; **(iii)** 0; **(iv)** .25; **(v)** .75; **(vi)** .25

c. Let $X = $ #color perceptives, so $X = $ Bino(3, .75) **(i)** $P[X = 3] = .422$; **(ii)** $P[X < 3] = .578$; **(iii)** $P[X = 0] = .016$; **(iv)** 2.25

d. $X = $ Bino(5, .75) **(i)** $P[X = 5] = .237$; **(ii)** $P[X < 5] = .763$; **(iii)** $P[X = 0] = .001$; 3.75

7. $X = $ #die, $X = $ Bino(100, .05) **a.** $E[X] = 5$; **b.** 4.75, 2.18; **c. (i)** .006; **(ii)** .180; **(iii)** .616; **(iv)** .384; **d.** $P[X = 6] = .150$ (not unlikely).

9.a. $n = 20, p = .95$; **c.** .358; **d.** .642; **e.** .736; **f.** .925; **g.** .984; **h.** They must have used a coin. $Prob[X \leq 15] < .0026$.

SECTION 6.1

Warm-ups 6.1

1. 0, 1; **2.** Z; **3.** c; **4.** .054799, .052616, .049471, .045514; **5.** e; **6.** 1; **7.** a; **8.** .052616, .947384; **9.** .052616; **10.** .241964, .194894, .008198, .006387; **11.** .006387, .993613; **12.** 3, .102042, 4, .264347; **13.** a; **14.** .366389, .633611, .633611; **15.** 1.5; **16.** 1.5, .067; **17.** −1.8, .035930; **18.** −1.8, .5, −1.8, .5, .035930, .308538, .344468, .655532; **19.** 11.3, 111.3; **20.** .67; **21.** 106.7

Problems 6.1

1.a. .069437; **b.** .994915; **c.** .261086; **d.** .340933; **e.** .044565; **f.** .786561; **g.** .231737; **h.** .682690; **i.** .954500; **j.** .997300; **k.** .749189; **l.** .319336

3. (i) a. 0 **b.** 1; **c.** −2; **d.** −1/3; **e.** −.933; **f.** −1.433 **(ii) a.** 20.26; **b.** 22; **c.** 13.99; **d.** 12.07; **e.** 16

5.a. 96.8 percentile; **b. (i)** 100, **(ii)** 105.6, **(iii)** 108.8, **(iv)** 116.7, **(v)** 121.4, **(vi)** 130.2

7.a. ≥ 544; **b.** ≥ 665, 604–664, 553–603, 448–552, ≤ 447
9.a. .9949, Sn = 99.49%, F − R = 0.51%
b. .0109, Sp = 98.91%, F + R = 1.09%
11.a. 19.0%; **b.** 33.0%; **c.** 66.8%
13. 58.9%
15. 41.2%

SECTION 6.2

Warm-ups 6.2

1. 14; **2.** 10, 15; **3.** .8804, .9910; **4.** 0, .8804, .9110, 1;
5. nonnormal, normal; **6.** .959; **7.** e; **8.** F; **9.** F;
10. T; **11.** T.

Problems 6.2

1. RTCO: .984; ITCO .993; Fick .990; all consistent with normal
3. All normal except arterial 1.6, venous 1.6, and difference (arterial − venous) 4.8-mL discard. The critical correlation for a sample of size $n = 20$ is .929. The sample nscore correlations are:
a. 1.6-mL discard: .697, .674, .939;
b. 3.2-mL discard: .921, .946, .986;
c. 4.8-mL discard: .951, .965, .910
5. Age normal, sample nscores correlation .980
Height normal, sample nscores correlation .994
Weight nonnormal, sample nscores correlation .905
BMI nonnormal, sample nscores correlation .852
Critical correlation ambiguous zone: .9408–.9490

Review I

1.a. $n = 24$, $\Sigma x = 136$, $\Sigma x^2 = 850$; **b.** 5.7, 5.5, 6;
c. 3.45; **d.** 1.9
e.

Tests	Freq	Rel F	% Rel F	C Freq	C Rel F	% CRF
3	3	.13	13	3	.13	13
4	5	.21	21	8	.33	33
5	4	.17	17	12	.50	50
6	3	.13	13	15	.63	63
7	5	.21	21	20	.83	83
8	2	.08	8	22	.92	92
9	2	.08	8	24	1.00	100
Total	24	1.01*	101*			

*Deviation from ideal 1.00 (100%) is due to roundoff error.

2.a. 51; **b.** 1; **c.** 10
d.

Class Boundaries Lower	Upper	Relative Frequency	Cumulative Relative Frequency
49.5	59.5	.04	.04
59.5	69.5	.20	.24
69.5	79.5	.45	.69
79.5	89.5	.29	.98
89.5	99.5	.02	1.00
Total		1.00	

e.

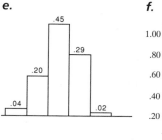

f.

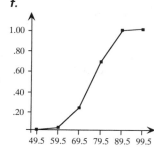

3.a. .27; **b.** .03; **c.** .29; **d.** 2.14, 2.14, 1.46
4.a. Sn = .73, F − R = .27, Sp = .95, F + R = .05, PV+ = .79, PV− = .93, accuracy = .90
b. .21
c. .04
d. to detect LBC, no; to rule out LBC, yes (PV+ = .999 in general population)
5.a. .328; **b.** .672; **c.** 4
6.a. **(i)** P[ectopic serum progesterone < 20] > .99995 (Minitab); Sn > .99995, F − R < .00005
(ii) P[nonectopic serum progesterone > 20] = .942 (Minitab: .941814); Sp = .942, F + R = .058
b. 14.1; **b.** 14.8

SECTION 7.1

Warm-ups 7.1

1. Baseline heart rate 4 hours after CABG surgery is (approximately) normally distributed; **2.** 26, 93.0, 18.0;
3. 25, 2.0595; **4.** 85.7; **5.** 93.0, 2.0595, 18.0, 26, 93.0, 7.3, 100.3; **6.** 100.3; **7.** c; **8.** 51, 1332, 598; **9.** 50, 2.0085; **10.** 1332, 168.2, 1163.8, 1332, 2.0085, 598, 51, 1332, 168.2, 1500.2; **11.** 1163.8, 1500.2; **12.** 1.960; **13.** 1332, 1.960, 598, 51, 1332, 164.2, 1167.9, 1332, 1.960, 598, 51, 1332, 164.2, 1496.1; **14.** 1167.9, 1496.1.

Problems 7.1

1. A sample mean is a mean of a small data set drawn from the population at large. A population mean is the mean value of the random variable of interest with respect to the entire population.

3. A 95% confidence interval for the mean is an interval estimate for the mean obtained by a procedure that produces an interval that actually contains the population mean for 95% of all possible samples.

5.a. The sample is consistent with normal: the sample nscores correlation is .992, the critical correlation for $n = 15$ is .9110; **b.** 90% (15.0, 16.1), 95% (14.9, 16.2), 99% (14.6, 16.5); **c.** the CI widens.

7.a. V_T group, control (109.8, 156.2), time 0 (149.1, 240.9), time 30 (120.5, 171.5), time 60 (120.1, 159.9), time 120 (114.6, 161.4), time 180 (110.4, 159.6), time 300 (108.6, 157.4)

7.b.

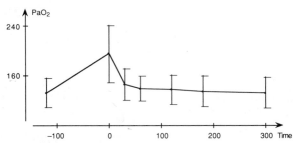

9.a. 0 min (138.3, 173.7), 1 min (225.4, 234.6), 2 min (224.1, 277.9), 3 min (161.9, 200.1), 4 min (152.3, 187.7)

9.b.

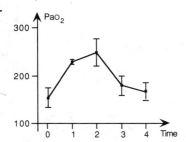

11. (z-intervals) **a.** bell (110.87, 116.77), diaphragm (109.18, 115.40)
b. bell (71.46, 76.46), diaphragm (72.46, 76.54)
c. bell (62.32, 67.32), diaphragm (64.30, 68.56)

13. experimental (29.2, 40.8), control (38.6, 49.8). The CIs overlap; hence, the population means could be equal. There is no perceptible difference in the population means from these CIs.

15.a.

	Start	End	1 min	5 min
size	6	6	6	6
mean	79.8	74.0	78.12	82.3
SD	11.1	11.0	14.3	17.1

b. start (68, 92), end (62, 86), 1 min (63, 94), 5 min (64, 101)

Warm-ups 7.2

1. before and after, method A versus method B;
2. d; **3.** An RV is measured at two points in time. The first point in time is called "before," the second point, "after." Example: Measure weight "before" and "after" for each person in a weight reduction program; **4.** An RV is measured by two methods, A and B. Example: cardiac output with (A) an ice-temperature injectate and (B) a room-temperature injectate. Each method is to be applied to each subject in a study; **5.** **(a)** with (iii), **(b)** with (i), **(c)** with (ii); **6.** **(a)** with (ii), **(b)** with (iii), **(c)** with (i); **7.** a; **8.** b; **9.** D is normally distributed; **10.** 2.0930; **11.** 13.1, 2.9030, 2.7, 20, 13.1, 1.3; **12.** (11.8, 14.4)

Problems 7.2

1. The sample is consistent with normality. The t-CIs are: **a.** (36.57, 37.63); **b.** (36.40, 37,80); **c.** (36.22, 37.98); **d.** (35.80, 38.40)

3.a. method A versus method B
b. 1.6-mL discard (.7, 3.5), 3.2-mL discard (-0.4, 2.2), 4.8-mL discard, t-interval not justified since the sample data are inconsistent with normal

5.a. **(i)** normal, (-0.07, 0.18), **(ii)** inconsistent with normal
b. **(i)** ($-.08$, .18), **(ii)** (.05, .54)
c. the z-interval for the mean difference iced $-$ room for the prefilled syringes group is slightly shorter than the corresponding t-interval, but they are approximately equal.
d. 0 is in the CI for the prefilled syringes group, indicating that, on average, there is no perceptible difference between the ice- and room-temperature methods. For the Co-Set group, the CI is positive

$(+, +)$, indicating that, on average, the ice-temperature method gives a higher reading by at least .05 liters/minute and perhaps as much as .54 liters/minute. The clinical application is that, based on the given data, use the prefilled syringes method with room-temperature injectates.
7.a. $(-0.40, -0.24)$; **b.** $(-, -)$. On average, with 95% confidence, total cholesterol among fasting people measured by screening is less than total cholesterol measured by the labororatory by at least 0.25 mmol/liter and perhaps as much as 0.39 mmol/liter.
9.a. $(0.07, 0.21)$; **b.** $(+, +)$. On average, with 95% confidence, serum triglycerides among fasting people were measured greater by screening than serum triglycerides measured by the laboratory by at least 0.07 mmol/liter and perhaps as much as 0.21 mmol/liter.
11.a. $(-0.14, 0.03)$; **b.** $(-, +)$. On average, with 95% confidence, LDL cholesterol measured by screening and by the laboratory are basically the same.

SECTION 8.1

Warm-ups 8.1

1. c; **2.** a; **3.** b; **4.** >30; **5.** d; **6.** e; **7.** 95%; **8.** (3.480, 3.800); **9.** (3.4, 3.8); **10.** (3.624, 4.186); **11.** (3.6, 4.2); **12.** The s-interval is for the median, η; the z-interval, for the mean, μ. Because of outliers, the s-interval is probably the better confidence interval for the average cardiac output.

Problems 8.1

1. Age normal, t-interval (23, 26) years
Height normal, t-interval (175, 181) cm
Weight nonnormal, s-interval (69, 76) kg
BMI nonnormal, s-interval (22.3, 24.0) kg/m^2
3. Arterial 1.6-mL discard, nonnormal, 95% s-CI (30.5, 36.0)
Venous 1.6-mL discard, nonnormal, 95% s-CI (29.8, 34.1)
Difference = arterial − venous, normal, 95% t-CI (0.7, 3.5)
5. (8.7, 9.7); **7.** (8.8, 9.6); **9.** (2.07, 2.58); **11.** (2.00, 2.72)

SECTION 8.2

Warm-ups 8.2

1. Asymptomatic women with acquired bacteriuria treated with single-dose therapy; **2.** resolved infection (yes or no); **3.** categorical; **4.** 30, 37, .81; **5.** 81; **6.** 1.960; **7.** .65 or 65%; **8.** .97 or 97%; **9.** d; **10.** 1.960, .20, 96.04, 97; **11.** 385.

Problems 8.2

1.a. .215; **b.** (.199, .231), (.195, .235), (.189, .241)
3.a. .62; **b.** (.50, .74); **c.** yes
5. 1028, 1692, 2401, 3382, 4148
7.a. .00755; **b.** (.0046, .0104), (.0041, .0109), (.0030, .0120)
9.a. proportion of women whose catheter-acquired urinary tract infection resolved within 14 days without therapy for the infection; **b.** .36 or 36%; **c.** (.20, .51)
11.a. .89, (.76, 1.00); **b.** .62, (.45, .78)
13.a. yes, (.68, .94); **b.** yes, (.21, .51); **c.** yes, (.64, .93); **d.** yes, (.81, .97); **e.** yes, (46, .77)

SECTION 9.1

Warm-ups 9.1

1. a(ii), b(iii), c(iv), d(i), e(v); **2.** c; **3.** d; **4.** d; **5.** d; **6.** b; **7.** a; **8.** c; **9.** e; **10.** b.

Problems 9.1

1.a. neonates in the community
b. birth weight
c. quantitative, interval, continuous
d. average
e. location
f–h. not applicable
3.a. neonates in the community
b. low birth weight (yes or no)
c. categorical
d. proportion
e. comparison
f. $H_0: p \le .10$ versus $H_a: p > .10$
g. The health care worker believes that the proportion of low-birth-weight neonates in the community is greater than 10% when in reality the proportion

weight neonates is $\leq 10\%$. The health care worker will seek to remedy a problem that doesn't exist.

h. The health care worker believes that the proportion of low-birth-weight neonates in the community is $\leq 10\%$ when in reality the proportion exceeds 10%. The health care worker believes no problem exists when in reality a low-birth-weight problem does exist in the community.

5.a. ventilator-dependent patients

b. D (change in PaO_2) = start PaO_2 − end PaO_2

c. quantitative, interval, continuous

d. average (mean)

e. comparison

f. $H_0: \mu_D \leq 0$ versus $H_a: \mu_D > 0$

g. Researchers believe a drop in PaO_2 occurs during the suctioning period when in fact no drop in PaO_2 occurs.

h. Researchers believe no drop in PaO_2 occurs during the suctioning period when in fact a drop in PaO_2 does occur.

7.a. families with six children

b. majority of girls (yes or no)

c. categorical

d. proportion (of families with six children having a majority of girls)

e. comparison

f. $H_0: p = .3438$ versus $H_0: p \neq .3438$

g. Researchrs believe that the proportion of families with six children having a majority of girls is other than .3438 when in reality the proportion is .3438.

h. Researchers believe that the proportion of families with six children having a majority of girls is .3438 when the proportion in reality is otherwise.

9.a. post–myocardial infarction patients not prone to ventricular tachycardia (VT)

b. less than 25 microvolts in the last 40 milliseconds of the QRS waveform (yes or no)

c. categorical

d. proportion (of post-MI patients not prone to VT who answer "no")

e. location

f–h. not applicable

11.a. post-MI patients with ≥ 25 microvolts in the last 40 milliseconds of the QRS waveform

b. same as 9b

c. categorical

d. proportion (of patients described in (a) who are not prone to VT)

e. location

f–h. not applicable

13.a. women

b. packed cell volume (PCV)

c. quantitative, interval, continuous

d. average

e. location

f–h. not applicable

15.a. men

b. PCV

c. quantitaive, interval, continous

d. average

e. comparison

f. $H_0: \mu = .443$ versus $H_a: \mu \neq .433$

g. Researchers believe that the mean PCV for men as determined by the new system deviates from .433 when in fact it doesn't.

h. Researchers believe that the mean PCV for men as determined by the new system is consistent with the value of .433 as reported in the literature when in fact the new system yields a significantly different mean PCV for men.

17.a. critically ill patients with heart failure

b. D = cardiac output (TEB) − cardiac output (thermodilution)

c. quantitaive, interval, continous

d. average

e. comparison

f. $H_0: \mu_D \geq .5$ versus $H_a: \mu_D < .5$

g. Researchers believe that, in general, cardiac outputs taken by TEB and thermodilution are within .5 liters/minute of each other when in fact they are not.

h. Researchers believe that cardiac outputs taken by TEB and thermodilution are in general inconsistent with each other when in fact the readings are usually within .5 liters/minute of each other.

SECTION 10.1

Warm-ups 10.1

1. b; **2.** a; **3.** d; **4.** d; **5.** d; **6.** yes; **7.** no; **8.** $H_0: p \leq .5$; **9.** $H_a: p > .5$; **10.** .5; **11.** 496, .5, 248, yes; **12.** one-tailed; **13.** (c); **14.** 1.645; **15.** (c);

16.

Do Not Reject H_0 | Reject H_0
————————————————→ Z
1.645

17. .044354839/.022450663 (calculator display) = 1.976; **18.** reject H_0 zone; **19.** confirms; **20.** The majority of patients admitted to an adult trauma center are transferred to an intensive care unit.

Problems 10.1

1.a. (.507, .582)

   b. $H_0: p \geq .7$ versus $H_a: p < .7$, critical z (LOS .05) $= 1.645$, sample $z = -7.564$, reject H_0

   c. $H_0: p = .55$ versus $H_a: p \neq .55$, critical z (LOS .05) $= 1.960$, sample $z = -.253$, retain H_0

3.a. .63

   b. (.53, .73)

   c. $H_0: p \leq .5$ versus $H_a: p > .5$, critical z (LOS .05) $= 1.645$, sample $z = 2.333$, reject H_0

   d. $H_0: p = 2/3$ versus $H_a: p \neq 2/3$, critical z (LOS .05) $= 1.960$, sample $z = -.707$, retain H_0

5.a. (.364, .410)

   b. $H_0: p \leq .5$ versus $H_a: p > .5$, critical z (LOS .05) $= 1.645$, sample $z = -9.920$, do not reject H_0

   c. $H_0: p = .4$ versus $H_a: p \neq .4$, critical z (LOS .05) $= 1.960$, sample $z = -1.230$, retain H_0

7.a. $79/375 = .211$ or 21.1%

   b. (.160, .262)

   c. $H_0: p \leq .05$ versus $H_a: p > .05$, critical $z = 1.645$, sample $z = 14.276$, reject H_0

   d. $32/79 = .41$, (.29, .52)

   e. $32/375 = .085$, (.034, .136)

   f. $H_0: p \leq .05$ versus $H_a: p > .05$, critical z (LOS .05) $= 1.645$, sample $z = 11.195$, reject H_0

9. $H_0: p \leq .10$ versus $H_a: p > .10$, critical z (LOS .05) $= 1.645$, sample $z = 8.343$, reject H_0

11.a. $H_0: p = .004936$ versus $H_a: p \neq .004936$, critical z (LOS .05) $= 1.960$, sample $z = -1.1155$, retain H_0.

   b. 46.6, no

   c. same

13.a. $H_0: p = .02421$ versus $H_a: p \neq .02421$, critical z (LOS .05) $= 1.960$, sample $z = -3.451$, reject H_0.

   b. 228, yes

   c. greater; that is, 228/9440 is statistically significantly greater than 177/9440 under $H_0: p = .02421$.

15.a. $H_0: p = .02279$ versus $H_a: p \neq .02279$, critical z (LOS .05) $= 1.960$, sample $z = -1.393$, do not reject H_0.

   b. 239.3, no

   c. the same as since we retain $H_0: p = .02279$

17.a. $H_0: p = .00752$ versus $H_a: p \neq .000752$, critical z (LOS .05) $= 1.960$, sample $z = -1.916$, do not reject H_0.

   b. 79.0, no.

   c. the same as since we retain $H_0: p = .00752$

19. $H_0: p \leq .055$ versus $H_a: p > .055$, critical z (LOS .05) is 1.645, sample $z = 5.038$, reject $H_0: p \leq .055$.

21.a. .124; **b.** at least (.081, .167), approximately (.096, .152) see Problem 8.2.13, exact (.095, .155) see Problem 8.2.14.

23. $H_0: p \leq .5$ versus $H_a: p > .5$, critical $z = 1.645$, sample $z = 2.944$, reject H_0.

SECTION 10.2

Warm-ups 10.2

1. d; **2.** erythrocyte cell vitamin E level; **3.** b; **4.** d; **5.** a; **6.** yes; **7.** a; **8.** b; **9.** c; **10.** b; **11.** (b); **12.** one; **13.** 10, 9; **14.** 1.83313; **15.** (b);

16.

Reject H_0	Do Not Reject H_0
	-1.83313 T_9 →

17. 2.270, 4.5, .991, 10, -7.116; **18.** reject H_0;

19. Children with cystic fibrosis present an overnight cell vitamin E deficiency; **20.** The formal write-up for the test of hypothesis follows:

Preliminary Test for Normality. The critical nscores correlation for a sample of size 10 is .8804. Since the sample nscores correlation is .969, which is greater than .8804, then the sample is consistent with an assumption of normality. Hence, we assume that overnight cell vitamin E levels in cystic fibrosis children is (approximately) normally distributed.

Main Test of Hypothesis.

   1. Hypothesis. $H_0: \mu \geq 4.5$ one-tailed test; $H_a: \mu < 4.5$ test alternate (b)

   2. LOS. .05

   3. Test Statistic. $\frac{\mu - 4.5}{s/\sqrt{n}}$

   4. Critical Value. 1.83313 (Table 9, $df = 9$)

   5. Decision Line.

Reject H_0	Do Not Reject H_0
	-1.83313 T_9 →

   6. Sample Value. $\frac{\mu - 4.5}{s/\sqrt{n}} = \frac{2.270 - 4.5}{.991/\sqrt{10}} = -7.116$

   7. Conclusion. Based on the given data, at the 5% level of significance, reject $H_0: \mu \leq 4.5$ and accept $H_a: \mu > 4.5$. Children with cystic fibrosis present an overnight fasting cell vitamin E deficiency.

Problems 10.2

1.a. Normality OK; $H_0: \mu = 15.25$ versus $H_a: \mu \neq 15.25$, critical t (LOS .05, $df = 14$) is 2.1448, sample $t = 1.03$, retain H_0.

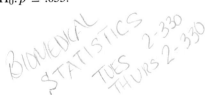

BIOMEDICAL STATISTICS   2-330   TUES 2-330   THURS 2-330

b. Normality OK; H_0: $\mu = .397$ versus H_a: $\mu \neq .397$, critical t (LOS .05, $df = 13$) is 2.1604, sample $t = 2.49$, reject H_0.

c. Normality OK; H_0: $\mu = .443$ versus H_a: $\mu \neq .433$, critical t (LOS .05, $df = 14$) is 2.1448, sample $t = .79$, retain H_0.

d. Normality OK, (13.0, 14.9)

e. Yes. The CI interval from (d) overlaps 13.45 ± 1.07. Further, testing H_0: $\mu = 13.45$ results in retaining H_0.

3.a. Yes; **b.** $n = 8, \bar{x} = 37.10, s = 1.04$; **c.** (36.2, 38.0);

d. H_0: $\mu = 37.0$ versus $\mu \neq 37.0$, critical t (LOS .05, $df = 7$) is 2.3646; sample $t = .27$; do not reject H_0.

5.a. Nonormal, conduct s-test. H_0: $\eta \leq 80$ versus H_a: $\eta > 80, p = .0002$, reject H_0: $\eta \leq 80$ and accept H_a: $\eta > 80$ at LOS .05.

b. One possible "curved" grading system is to construct a histogram based on six classes where the middle two classes define a C. This yields F(36–46), D(47–57), C(58–79), B(80–90), A(91–100).

7. Normality OK; H_0: $\mu \leq 4.5$ versus H_a: $\mu > 4.5$, critical t (LOS .05, $df = 9$) is 1.83313, sample $t = 1.97$, reject H_0: $\mu \leq 4.5$. Cell vitamin E level shows recovery in 9 hours.

9.a. Normality OK; hence, t-test. H_0: $\mu \geq 20.9$ versus H_a: $\mu < 20.9$, critical t (LOS .05, $df = 9$) is 1.83313, sample $t = -7.79$, reject H_0: $\mu \geq 20.9$.

b. Normality OK; hence, t-test. H_0: $\mu \geq 20.9$ versus H_a: $\mu < 20.9$, critical t (LOS .05, $df = 9$) is 1.83313, sample $t = -7.81$, reject H_0: $\mu \geq 20.9$.

c. Normality OK; hence, t-test. H_0: $\mu \geq 20.9$ versus H_a: $\mu < 20.9$, critical t (LOS .05, $df = 9$) is 1.83313, sample $t = -1.94$, reject H_0: $\mu \geq 20.9$.

11. Normality OK; hence, t-test. H_0: $\mu = 20.9$ versus H_a: $\mu \neq 20.9$, critical t (LOS .05, $df = 9$) is 2.2622, sample $t = 0.76$, do not reject H_0: $\mu = 20.9$.

13. Normality OK; hence, t-test. The sample t value is -1.89.

a. Reject region > 1.83313; do not reject H_0: $\mu \leq 20.9$.

b. Reject region between -2.2622 and 2.2622; do not reject H_0: $\mu = 20.9$.

c. Reject region < -1.83313; reject H_0: $\mu \geq 20.9$.

d. H_0 is what you assume to be the state of affairs until presented evidence to the contrary; *(i)* c; *(ii)* a; *(iii)* b.

15. Normality OK; hence t-test. H_0: $\mu \geq 4.5$ versus H_a: $\mu < 4.5$, critical t (LOS .05, $df = 4$) is 2.1319

a. Sample $t = -6.32$, reject H_0.

b. Sample $t = -2.12$, do not reject H_0.

c. Sample $t = -1.05$, do not reject H_0.

17. Normality OK; hence, t-test. H_0: $\mu \geq 20.9$ versus H_a: $\mu < 20.9$, critical t (LOS .05, $df = 4$) is 2.1319, sample $t = -5.48$, reject H_0.

19. Normality OK; hence t-test. H_0: $\mu \leq 20.9$ versus H_a: $\mu > 20.9$, critical t (LOS .05, $df = 4$) is 2.1319

a. Sample $t = 1.40$, do not reject H_0.

b. Sample $t = 2.24$, reject H_0.

21. Normality OK; hence t-test. H_0: $\mu \geq 20.9$ versus H_a: $\mu < 20.9$, critical t (LOS .05, $df = 4$) is 2.1319, sample $t = -.55$, do not reject H_0

SECTION 10.3

Warm-ups 10.3

1. Yes, each patient is measured for a before and an after weight; **2.** before and after; **3.** d; **4.** before − after; **5.** c; **6.** a; **7.** b; **8.** b; **9.** we may assume that the difference D is normally distributed; **10.** d; **11.** 1.7959; **12.** 9.07, 3.69, 12, 8.515; **13.** reject H_0: $\mu_D \leq 0$; **14.** they lose weight.

Problems 10.3

1.a. D = RTCO − Fick, normality OK; hence, t-test. H_0: $\mu_D = 0$ versus H_a: $\mu_D \neq 0$, critical t (LOS .10, $df = 28$) = 1.70112, sample $t = -2.81$, reject H_0: $\mu_D = 0$.

b. D = ITCO − Fick, normality OK; hence, t-test. H_0: $\mu_D = 0$ versus H_a: $\mu_D \neq 0$, critical t (LOS .10, $df = 28$) = 1.70112, sample $t = -2.21$, reject H_0: $\mu_D = 0$.

3.a. D = arterial − venous (1.6 mL), normality OK; hence, t-test. H_0: $\mu_D = 0$ versus H_a: $\mu_D \neq 0$, critical t (LOS .05, $df = 19$) = 2.0930, sample $t = 3.17$, reject H_0: $\mu_D = 0$.

b. D = arterial − venous (3.2 mL), normality OK; hence, t-test. H_0: $\mu_D = 0$ versus H_a: $\mu_D \neq 0$, critical t (LOS .05, $df = 19$) = 2.0930, sample $t = 1.56$, do not reject H_0: $\mu_D = 0$.

c. D = arterial − venous (4.8 mL), normality not OK; hence, s-test. H_0: $\eta_D = 0$ versus H_a: $\eta_D \neq 0$, $p = .8238$, do not reject H_0: $\eta_D = 0$.

5. S1: assume D = bell − diaphragm is (approximately) normally distributed.
H_0: $\mu_D \leq 0$ versus H_a: $\mu_D > 0$, critical t (LOS .05, $df = 55$) = 1.67589 (using Table 9, $df = 50$) [or critical t at LOS .05, $df = 55$ = 1.6730 from Minitab], sample $t = 2.31$, reject H_0: $\mu_D \leq 0$.
D4: assume D = bell − diaphragm is (approximately) normally distributed.

$H_0: \mu_D \leq 0$ versus $H_a: \mu_D > 0$, critical t (LOS .05, df = 55) = 1.67589 (Table 9, df = 50) [or critical t at LOS .05, df = 55 = 1.6730 from Minitab], sample t = 0.60, do not reject $H_0: \mu_D \leq 0$.

D5: assume D = bell − diaphragm is (approximately) normally distributed.

$H_0: \mu_D \geq 0$ versus $H_a: \mu_D < 0$, critical t (LOS .05, df = 55) = 1.67589 (Table 9, df = 50) [or critical t at LOS .05, df = 55 = 1.6730 from Minitab], sample t = −1.91, reject $H_0: \mu_D \geq 0$.

Hence, the research hypothesis about S1 and D5 is supported, but the research hypothesis about D4 is not supported by the given data.

7.a. Normality OK; critical t (LOS .05, df = 21) is 1.7208, sample t = 4.95, reject H_0.
   b. Normality OK; critical t (LOS .05, df = 21) = 1.7208, sample t = 5.69, reject H_0.
   c. Normality OK; critical t (LOS .05, df = 21, two-tailed) is 2.0796, sample t = −2.92, reject H_0.
   d. Seated (92.7, 96.9), standing (94.7, 100.3).
   e. Sample mean difference is −2.7, sample standard deviation is 4.3, a 95% CI for μ_D is (−4.6, −0.7). The CI for the mean value of D = seated − standing is of the form (−, −), indicating that the seated DBP is significantly less than the standing DBP. This CI interval result is consistent with the test of hypothesis, which indicated that the mean difference is statistically significantly different from 0.

9. Normality OK; D = before − after, $H_0: \mu_D \leq 0$ versus $H_a: \mu_D > 0$, critical t (LOS .05, df = 11) is 1.7959, sample t = 6.46, reject $H_0: \mu_D \leq 0$.

SECTION 10.4

Warm-ups 10.4

1. Reject H_0 | Do Not Reject H_0 | Reject H_0 at −2.567 and 2.567, Z

2. Reject H_0 | Do Not Reject H_0 | Reject H_0 at −1.960 and 1.960, Z

3. Reject H_0 | Do Not Reject H_0 | Reject H_0 at −1.645 and 1.645, Z

4. Reject H_0 | Do Not Reject H_0 | Reject H_0 at −1.282 and 1.282, Z

5. a; **6.** less; **7.** d; **8.** 1.960 and 2.326; **9.** .05 and .02; **10.** .02 < p-value < .05; **11.** .20; **12.** .00001; **13.** .001 < p-value < .005.

Problems 10.4

The following p-values were obtained using Table 9, Appendix:
1. .005 < p-value < .01
3. p-value > .10
5. p-value > .20
7. .0001 < p-value < .001
9. .98 < p-value < .99
11. .02 < p-value < .05
13. p-value > .20
15. p-value > .10
17. p-value < .0005
19. .005 < p-value < .01
21. p-value > .10
23. p-value > .9995
25. .99 < p-value < .995
27. p-values for the odd-numbered problems in Section 10.2 are based on Table 9.
1.a. p-value > .20; **b.** .02 < p-value < .05; **c.** p-value > .20
3.d. p-value > .20
5.a. p-value = .0002
7. .025 < p-value < .05
9.a. p-value < .0005; **b.** p-value < .0005; **c.** .025 < p-value < .05
11. p-value > .20
13.a. .95 < p-value < .975; **b.** .05 < p-value < .10; **c.** .025 < p-value < .05
15.a. .0005 < p-value < .005; **b.** .05 < p-value < .10; **c.** p-value > .10
17. .005 < p-value < .0005
19.a. p-value > .10; **b.** .025 < p-value < .05

SECTION 11.1

Warm-ups 11.1

1. d; **2.** a; **3.** 30-mg group (1555, 228), 280-mg group (1576, 240); **4.** .147, 240, 1576, .152; **5.** $H_0: p_{30\,mg} = p_{283\,mg}$ versus $H_a: p_{30\,mg} \neq p_{283\,mg}$; **6.** 468/3131; **7.** 2663/3131; **8.** 232.4, 2898.6, 235.6, 1340.4, yes; **9.** 1.960;

10. Reject H_0 | Do Not Reject H_0 | Reject H_0 at −1.960 and 1.960, Z

11. −.566; **12.** retain; **13.** $p > .20$; **14.** There is no significant difference in the proportion of vascular events between the two groups.

Problems 11.1

1. Group 1 = enalapril group. **a.** z-test OK. $H_0: p_1 = p_2$ versus $H_a: p_1 \neq p_2$, critical z (LOS .05, two-tailed test) is 1.960, sample $z = 5.756$, reject $H_0: p_1 = p_2$, p-value < .00001.

b. $H_0: p_1 \leq p_2$ versus $H_a: p_1 > p_2$, critical z (LOS .05, one-tailed test) is 1.645, sample $z = 5.756$, reject $H_0: p_1 \leq p_2$, p-value < .000005.

3. Group 1 = terazosin group. z-test OK. $H_0: p_1 \leq p_2$ versus $H_a: p_1 > p_2$, critical z (LOS .05, one-tailed test) is 1.645, sample $z = 0.1805$, do not reject $H_0: p_1 \leq p_2$, p-value > .10; hence, no warning for general body ailments is needed (the proportion of patients with general body ailments on terazosin does not exceed the proportion of patients with general body ailments on placebo).

5. Group 1 = ibuprofen group. z-test OK. $H_0: p_1 = p_2$ versus $H_a: p_1 \neq p_2$, critical z (LOS .05, two-tailed test) is 1.960, sample $z = 0.478$, do not reject $H_0: p_1 = p_2$, p-value > .20; hence, there is no statistically significant difference between ibuprofen and placebo in the proportion of patients who report upset stomach.

7.a. Group 1 = female. z-test OK. $H_0: p_1 = p_2$ versus $H_a: p_1 \neq p_2$, critical z (LOS .05, two-tailed test) is 1.960, sample $z = 1.091$, do not reject $H_0: p_1 = p_2$, p-value > .20.

b. Group 1 = previous MI. z-test OK. $H_0: p_1 \leq p_2$ versus $H_a: p_1 > p_2$, critical z (LOS .05, one-tailed test) is 1.645, sample $z = 2.408$, reject $H_0: p_1 \leq p_2$, .005 < p-value < .01.

c. Group 1 = previous stroke. z-test OK. $H_0: p_1 \leq p_2$ versus $H_a: p_1 > p_2$, critical z (LOS .05, one-tailed test) is 1.645, sample $z = 6.762$, reject $H_0: p_1 \leq p_2$, p-value < .000005.

d. Group 1 = previous drug therapy. z-test OK. $H_0: p_1 = p_2$ versus $H_a: p_1 \neq p_2$, critical z (LOS .05, two-tailed test) is 1.960, sample $z = -.233$, do not reject $H_0: p_1 = p_2$, p-value > .20.

9. Group 1 = control. **a.** z-test OK. $H_0: p_1 \geq p_2$ versus $H_a: p_1 < p_2$, critical z (LOS .05, one-tailed test) is 1.645, sample $z = -4.710$, reject $H_0: p_1 \geq p_2$, p-value < .000005.

b. z-test OK. $H_0: p_1 = p_2$ versus $H_a: p_1 \neq p_2$, critical z (LOS .05, two-tailed test) is 1.960, sample $z = .239$, do not reject $H_0: p_1 = p_2$, p-value > .20.

11. Group 1 = 30-mg group. z-test OK. $H_0: p_1 = p_2$ versus $H_a: p_1 \neq p_2$, critical z (LOS .05, two-tailed test) is 1.960, sample $z = -1.303$, do not reject $H_0: p_1 = p_2$, .10 < p-value < .20.

13. Group 1 = 30-mg group. z-test OK. $H_0: p_1 = p_2$ versus $H_a: p_1 \neq p_2$, critical z (LOS .05, two-tailed test) is 1.960, sample $z = -2.611$, reject $H_0: p_1 = p_2$, .002 < p-value < .01.

15. Group 1 = treatment. z-test OK. $H_0: p_1 \geq p_2$ versus $H_a: p_1 < p_2$, critical z (LOS .05, one-tailed test) is 1.960, sample $z = -4.7$, reject $H_0: p_1 \geq p_2$, p-value < .000005.

17. Group 1 = complied. z-test OK. $H_0: p_1 \geq p_2$ versus $H_a: p_1 < p_2$, critical z (LOS .05, one-tailed test) is 1.960, sample $z = -1.73$, reject $H_0: p_1 \geq p_2$, .025 < p-value < .05.

19. The proportion of patients presenting a complete response to radiation therapy following surgery for head or neck cancer is significantly greater among nonsmokers than smokers ($z = 3.167, p = .0008$).

SECTION 11.2

Warm-ups 11.2

1. yes; **2.** raw data set; **3.** female: $n = 14$, mean = 13.93, SD = 1.56, male: $n = 15$, mean = 15.55, SD = 1.14; **4.** yes; **5.** yes; **6.** b; **7.** c; **8.** 1.557, 1.139, 1.86792; **9.** 1.557, 14; **10.** 1.139, 15; **11.** 13, 14, 3.7452; **12.** 1, 3.7452, $F_{13, 14}$; **13.** with pooling; **14.** (a); **15.** two; **16.** 27; **17.** 2.0519; **18.** top boxes: Reject H_0, Do Not Reject H_0, Reject H_0, bottom boxes: -2.0519, 2.0519, T_{27}; **19.** -3.22; **20.** reject; **21.** on average, Hb for females is different than Hb for males; **22.** .0033; **23.** c.

Problems 11.2

1.a. Apply large-samples z-test (Chart 5C). $H_0: \mu_1 = \mu_2$ versus $H_a: \mu_1 \neq \mu_2$, critical z (LOS .05, two-tailed test) 1.960, sample $z = -2.267$. The mean active labor time between the two groups is significantly different ($z = -2.267, .02 < p < .05$).

3. Assume amount of Buprenex used is (approximately) normally distributed. Apply pooled t-test for comparison of means (sample $f = 1.515$). $H_0: \mu_{PCA} \geq \mu_{control}$ versus $H_a: \mu_{PCA} < \mu_{control}$, critical t (LOS .05, $df = 14$) is 1.76133, sample $t = -2.50388$. The mean amount of Buprenex used by the PCA group is less than the mean amount of Buprenex used by the control group ($t = -2.50, df = 14, .01 < p < .025$).

5.a. (i) (15.208, 16.326), **(ii)** (14.744, 15.922), **(iii)** pooled $(-7.523, 1.157)$
  b. No, CI for the difference between means is of the form $(-, +)$.
  c. Pooled t-test, no significance difference between means $(t = 1.375, df = 10, p = .199)$.
7.a. No; normality OK, pooled t-test $(t = -.53, df = 28, p = .6)$.
  b. Yes. Consider the change D = baseline $- 15$ minutes. Normality OK, paired data t-test of $H_0: \mu_D = 0$ versus $H_a: \mu_D \neq 0$, $(t = -5.63, df = 14, p = .0001)$.
9.a. Paired-difference t-test (from the df); **b.** $p > .20$ (Table 9).
11. Test $H_0: \mu_{SE} = \mu_{LE}$ versus $H_a: \mu_{SE} \neq \mu_{LE}$. Energy intake is significantly different in the two groups $(z = -9.587, p < .00001)$.
13. Assume "index neurological score" is (approximately) normally distributed in both groups; homoscedastic (sample f-value 1.082, critical f 2.116), apply pooled t-test for comparison of means. The mean index neurological score for the neuropsychiatric group is significantly less than the mean index neurological score for the neurological-only group $(t = 3.0, df = 82, p = .02)$.
15.a. Assume "hospital stay" is (approximately) normally distributed in both groups; homoscedastic (sample f-value 7.84, critical f 2.37), apply Smith-Satterthwaite t-test for comparison of means. The mean hospital stay for the neuropsychiatric group is significantly greater than for the neurological-only group $(t = 2.29, df = 79, p = .01)$.
  b. 95% CI for the mean difference $\mu_1 - \mu_2$ is (2.5, 35.7) days. Hence, with 95% confidence, the neuropsychiatric patients in general have a hospital stay of 2.5 to 35.7 days longer then the neurological-only patients.
17.a. Assume normality, heteroscedastic (sample f 256, critical f 3.03), apply Smith-Satterthwaite t-test. The mean number of days to persistent negative stool culture is significantly greater in the ampicillin group than in the ceftriaxone group $(t = 4.6, df = 19, p = .0001)$.
19.a. Large-samples z-test, no $(z = .094, p = .9)$.
  b. Large-samples z-test, no $(z = .974, p = .3)$.
  c. IMV (20.6, 210.4), T-piece (47.9, 86.9). T-piece CI is a subset of the IMV CI.
  d. Heteroscedastic $(f = 22.95, df = (97, 101), p < .01)$
  e. Individual variation for IMV is significantly greater than for T-piece.

21.a. Apply Smith-Satterthwaite test, no $(t = -1.005, df = 21, p = .33)$
  b. Apply Smith-Satterthwaite test, no $(t = 1.543, df = 18, p = .14)$
23.a. Data are not independent.
  b. Paired-data t-test since both methods applied to same group of patients.
  c. No. One cannot obtain the standard deviation of the differences from the presentation of the data.
25.a. Group 1 = smoking mothers, group 2 = non-smoking mothers. Normality OK (sample nscores correlations .970, .956), homoscedastic (sample f = 2.10), apply pooled t-test to resolve $H_0: \mu_1 = \mu_2$ versus $H_a: \mu_1 \neq \mu_2$. There is no significant difference in the weight of the babies at the start of the study $(t = -1.12, df = 18, p = .28)$.
  b. No. Normality OK (sample nscores correlations are .962, .953; critical nscores correlation .8804); homoscedastic (sample f = 2.236, critical f = 5.351); apply pooled t-test for comparison of means. There is no statistically significant difference in the weight of the infants at the end $(t = -2.08, df = 18, p = .052)$.
  c. Yes. Normality OK (sample nscores correlations 985 .976; critical nscores correlation .8804); homoscedasticity OK (sample f = 1.886, critical f = 5.351); apply pooled t-test for comparison of means. Babies nursed by nonsmoking mothers have a significantly greater weight gain than babies nursed by smoking mothers $(t = 3.11, df = 18, p = .003)$.

Review II

1. No, pooled t-test, $t = .6096, df = 20, p = .55$
3. reject $H_0: \mu_{IVIG} = \mu_{placebo}, t = 2.36685, df = 10, p = .039$
5. The IVIG start to 24-hour data is paired data; that is, the samples are not independent. Hence, the appropriate test is the paired-difference t-test. To conduct the paired t-test, we would need the mean difference and the standard deviation of the differences. It is impossible to determine the stdev of the differences from the given information.
7. .609, (.495, .578)
9. no significant difference $(z = -1.048, p = .24)$
11. normality OK, reject $H_0: \mu > 150, t = 2.64, df = 21, p = .0077$
13. (156, 172), (152, 168)

15. 1.864, .113
17. normality OK, t-interval (1.79, 1.94)
19. 1.067, .113
21. normality OK, paired t-test: $t = 32.84, df = 11, p \approx 0$
23. assume normality, homoscedasticity OK, pooled t-test: $t = -5.075, df = 35, p = .00001$
25. assume normality, homoscedasticity fails, Smith-Satterthwaite t-test: $t = -.487, df = 34, p = .63$
27. no, pooled t-test: $t = .31, df = 10, p = .76$

Warm-ups 12.1

1. fixed treatments model, independent random samples, normal distributions, homoscedasticity; **2.** yes ($.8804 <$ critical $r < .9110$); **3.** .4861; **4.** .2732; **5.** 3.1658; **6.** yes ($5.5 <$ critical $f_{max} < 8.6$); **7.** yes; **8.** $H_0: \mu_{controls} = \mu_{first} = \mu_{second} = \mu_{third}$; **9.** The distribution for level 4 (third trimester) is clearly shifted to the right. The distributions for levels 1, 2, 3 appear similar; **10.** $p < .0005$; **11.** rejected; **12.** 16.13; **13.** 3, 48; **14.** $f = 16.13, df = 3, 48, p < .0005$; **15.** The mean daytime energy expenditure during the third trimester is significantly greater than the mean daytime energy expenditure at any of the other three time periods; **16.** yes; **17.** There is a 5% risk that at least one of the intervals does not contain the difference of the given means; **18.** .523, 1.320; **19.** 98% (.9807); **20.** $(+, +)$; **21.** 98, .523, 1.320; **22.** $H_0: \eta_{control} = \eta_{first} = \eta_{second} = \eta_{third}$ (i.e, the *medians* are all equal); **23.** .001; **24.** rejected; **25.** 16.83, 3, .001; **26.** ANOVA; **27.** The p-value for ANOVA is smaller than the p-value for the Mood test.

Problems 12.1

1. The samples are not independent. The same patients are used for all four methods.

3. No, the samples are not independent. The same patients are used to obtain the venous and arterial samples at each of the three discard volumes.

5. Assumptions for ANOVA are met. For the control suctioning period, the mean baseline (start) PaO_2 measurements are not significantly different between the three treatment groups ($f = 1.71, df = 2, 13, p = .2$).

7. Normality fails for all three groups. Appealing to robustness, the ANOVA result is to retain $H_0: \mu_1 = \mu_2 = \mu_3$; that is, there is no signficant difference in the mean change in PaO_2 between the three groups using the control suctioning method ($f = .27, df = 2, 13, p \approx .77$). The Mood test yields a similar result: retain $H_0: \eta_1 = \eta_2 = \eta_3$; that is, there is no significant difference in the median change in PaO_2 between the three groups using the control suctioning method (chisquare $= 3.20, df = 2, p = .20$).

9. There is insufficient evidence to assert that there is a statistically significant difference in the change in PaO_2 levels between the three groups. For ANOVA, normality fails; however, appealing to robustness yields no significant difference in the mean changes for the three groups ($f = 3.76, df = 2, 13, p \approx .05$). The Mood test result is that there is no significant difference in the median changes for the three groups (chisquare $= 4.33, df = 2, p = .115$).

11. It would be inappropriate for the researcher to randomly assign a study subject to be a member of either the anorexic, bulimic, or control group.

13. ANOVA justified. The mean total energy intake during lunch in a high-energy preload setting is not statistically significantly different between the three groups ($f = 2.82, df = 2, 24, p = .079$).

15. Assumptions for ANOVA are met except for homoscedasticity (sample f_{max} 11.3, critical f_{max} 9.9). Appeal to the robustness of ANOVA. There is a statistically significant difference in the mean energy intake during a lunch with no preload among the three given groups ($f = 4.81, df = 2, 24, p \approx .02$). In particular, energy intake during a lunch with no preload is greater among bulimics than among anorexics.

17. Assumptions for ANOVA are met. There is a statistically significant difference in mean weight between the four groups ($f = 7.18, df = 3, 50, p < .0005$). In particular, pregnant Gambian women weigh significantly more during their third trimester than at any other time during their pregnancy.

19. ANOVA justified (sample nscores correlations: .978, .953, .949, .960; sample f_{max} value 3.17). The mean fat-free mass among the given classes of pregnant Gambian women is significantly different ($f = 11.83, df = 3, 50, p < .0005$). In particular, the mean fat-free mass of pregnant Gambian women in their third trimester is significantly greater than at other times.

21. ANOVA justified (sample nscores correlations: .963, .980, .983, .980; sample f_{max} value 2.86). There is no statistically significant difference in the mean weight-adjusted 24-hour energy expenditure among the given classes of pregnant Gambian women ($f = .27, df = 3, 50, p = .8$).

23. Normality fails for plants A and C. Since the other assumptions for ANOVA hold, appeal to robustness of ANOVA. There is no significant difference in the baseline serum triglyceride level between the three plants ($f = 1.35, df = 2, 50, p \approx .27$).

Warm-ups 12.2

1. Normality; **2.** assume normality if the random variable of interest is continuous; **3.** normality and homoscedasticity; **4.** yes; **5.** 3.32935; **6.** 2,451; **7.** .0366993 (report .037); **8.** $H_0: \mu_1 = \mu_2 = \mu_3$ versus H_a: means otherwise; **9.** reject; **10.** In the Rovner et al study, ADL scores are not the same between the depression groups ($f = 3.23, df = 2, 451, p = .037$); **11.** yes; **12.** ANOVA is a powerful test for comparison of means. The confidence interval picture is not nearly as powerful at determining which level means are different as ANOVA is in determining that a difference of some kind does indeed occur; **13.** The confidence intervals for the mean ADL score between the depression symptoms group and no depression group overlap only slightly. One may suspect a significant difference between the mean ADL scores between these two groups. This inference may be tested by pooled t-test for comparison of means between these two groups.

Problems 12.2

1.a. Assume BMI is (approximately) normal in each of the three groups; assume homoscedasticity (sample $f_{max} = 1.56$); there is a significant difference in mean BMI between the three groups ($f = 11.6, df = 2,708, p = .00001$).

b. Assume voltage is (approximately) normal in each of the three groups; heteroscedasticity fails (sample $f_{max} = 5.975$). Appeal to robustness of ANOVA; there is a significant difference in mean voltage between the three groups ($f = 139.7, df = 2,708, p < .05$).

3. Assume diameter of largest gallstone fragment is (approximately) normally distributed in each of the three groups; heteroscedasticity fails (sample $f_{max} = 4.46$). Appeal to robustness of ANOVA; there is a significant difference in mean diameter of the largest gallstone fragment between the three groups. The confidence intervals show that the mean is significantly different among all three groups.

5. Assume total number of claims among hypertensive employees is (approximately) normally distributed in each of the four sites; heteroscedasticity fails (sample $f_{max} = 6.4$). Appeal to robustness of ANOVA; there is a significant difference in mean total claims among hypertensive employees between the four sites ($f = 3.936, df = 3,1052, p = .08$). The confidence intervals show that the mean total claims are significantly lower at site 4 compared with either site 1 or site 2.

7. Assume total number of claims among nonhypertensive employees is (approximately) normally distributed in each of the four sites; heteroscedasticity fails (sample $f_{max} = 3.2$). Appeal to robustness of ANOVA; there is no significant difference in mean total claims among nonhypertensive employees between the four sites ($f = 1.775, df = 3,1023, p \approx .15$).

9. Assume plasma vitamin A concentration is (approximately) normally distributed in each of the four groups; heteroscedasticity fails (sample $f_{max} = 2.6$). Appeal to robustness of ANOVA; there is no significant difference in mean plasma vitamin A concentration between the four groups ($f = 1.9, df = 3,2263, p \approx .13$).

11. Yes; for example, plasma concentration of β-carotene is significantly higher in survivors than in those who died with bronchus or stomach cancer. However, there appears to be no significant relationship between cancer mortality and plasma vitamin A level or plasma vitamin C level.

13. Assume weight is (approximately) normally distributed in each of the four groups; homoscedasticity appears reasonable (sample $f_{max} = 1.43$). There is a significant difference in mean weight between the four groups ($f = 17.66, df = 3,210, p < .05$). From the confidence intervals, the mean weight between young and elderly males is not significantly different, young and elderly females are not significantly different, and both female groups are significantly less than either male group.

15. Assume obesity index (OI) is (approximately) normally distributed in each of the four groups; homoscedasticity appears reasonable (sample $f_{max} = 1.99$). There is a significant difference in mean OI between the four groups ($f = 8.19, df = 3,210, p = .000035$). From the confidence intervals, the OI for elderly females is significantly greater than the OI for either male group.

17. Assume body mass index (BMI) is (approximately) normally distributed in each of the two male groups; homoscedasticity appears reasonable (sample f_{max} = 1.417). There is a significant difference in mean BMI between the two male groups (f = 11.096, df = 1, 98, p = .001). From the confidence intervals, the BMI for young males is significantly less than the BMI for elderly males.

19. Assume weight is (approximately) normally distributed in each of the two female groups; homoscedasticity appears reasonable (sample f_{max} = 1.44). There is no significant difference in mean weight between the two female groups (f = .328, df = 1,112, p = .57).

21. Assume obesity index (OI) is (approximately) normally distributed in each of the two female groups; assume homoscedasticity (sample f_{max} = 1.00). There is a significant difference in mean OI between the two female groups (f = 16.4, df = 1,112, p = .0001). From the confidence intervals, the OI for young females is significantly less than the OI for elderly females.

23. Yes (f = 39.4, df = 3, 7313, $p \approx 0$). From the CIs, the mean BMI for American Chinese women is significantly less than the mean BMI for American Filipino and other American Asian women.

25. Yes (f = 17.4, df = 3, 7313, $p \approx 0$). American Filipino women have a significantly higher mean diastolic blood pressure.

27. No (f = .69, df = 3, 7313, p = .56).

29. Yes (f = 13.02, df = 3, 5710, p < .05). American Filipino men have a significantly higher mean diastolic blood pressure.

31. Yes (f = 5.03, df = 3, 5710, p = .002). American Japanese men have a significantly higher cholesterol level than American Chinese or other American Asian males, and other American Asian men have a lower cholesterol level than Filipino or Japanese men.

33. Yes (f = 10.066, df = 2, 87, p = .0001). The cholesterol level is significantly higher in the panic disorder group compared with the other two groups.

SECTION 12.3

Warm-ups 12.3

1. d; **2.** start, end, 1 minute, 5 minutes; **3.** fixed;
4. patients 1 through 6; **5.** random; **6.** k = 4, n = 6;
7. (3, 15); **8.** (1, 5); **9.** 3.2874; **10.** 6.6079; **11.** 0.73;
12. rejected; **13.** no; **14.** yes.

Problems 12.3

1. One-way repeated measures ANOVA: sample f = 4.81, conservative critical f = 4.0848; hence, significant difference between method means.

3. One-way repeated measures ANOVA: sample f = .68, liberal critical f = 3.8625; hence, no significant difference between time means.

5. One-way repeated measures ANOVA: sample f = 1.22, liberal critical f = 3.2874; hence, no significant difference between time means.

7. One-way repeated measures ANOVA: sample f = 2.35, liberal critical f = 3.2874; hence, no significant difference between time means.

9. One-way repeated measures ANOVA: sample f = 35.28, conservative critical f = 4.6001; hence, significant difference between RL position means in group 1.

11. One-way repeated measures ANOVA: sample f = 13.02, conservative critical f = 4.6001; hence, significant difference between position means in group 2.

13. One-way repeated measures ANOVA: sample f = 12.53, conservative critical f = 4.6001; hence, significant difference between supine position means in group 2.

15. One-way repeated measures ANOVA: sample f = 21.04, conservative critical f = 5.1174; hence, significant difference between time means in erythrocyte vitamin E for CF children.

17. One-way repeated measures ANOVA: sample f = 12.41, conservative critical f = 7.7086; hence, significant difference between time means in erythrocyte vitamin E for CF children with no CDL.

19. One-way repeated measures ANOVA: sample f = 25.41, conservative critical f = 7.7086; hence, significant difference between time means in serum vitamin E for CF children with CDL.

21. Two-way ANOVA: no interaction ($f \approx 0$, df = (1, 13), p = .964). Using GLM with no interaction term, there is no significant difference in mean heart weight between genders (f = 1.32, df = (1, 13), p = .270) or between races (f = 1.86, df = (1, 13), p = .195).

SECTION 13.1

Warm-ups 13.1

1. Goodness of fit and independence of attributes;
2. c; **3.** b; **4.** d; **5.** b; **6.** .50, .25; **7.** .50, 100, 200, .25, 50; **8.** 99, 100, 100, .01, 47, 50, 50, .18; **9.** observed: 54,

99, expected: 50, 100, 50, 200, chisquared: .32, .01, .18, .51; **10.** c; **11.** yes; **12.** $H_0: p_{red} = .25, p_{pink} = .50,$ $p_{white} = .25$ versus H_a: the proportions are otherwise; **13.** 2; **14.** 5.9915;

15.

Do Not Reject H_0 Reject H_0

0   5.9915 χ_2^2

16. .51; **17.** retained; **18.** $.25 < p < .50$; **19.** .51, 2, $.25 < p < .50$; **20.** flower color is consistent with simple dominant-recessive Mendelian genetics.

Problems 13.1

1.a. $H_0: p_{females} = .5$ versus $H_a: p_{females} \neq .5, z = 11.639, p < .000005$ (Table 8); the ratio of women to men admitted to nursing homes in the Rovner et al study is not one to one.
  b. Sample chisquared 135.4, $df = 1, p < .005$ (Table 12).
  c. $z^2 = 135.4 =$ sample chisquared.
3. Sample chisquared $= 2.496, df = 3, p = .48$.
5. $H_0: p_{heads} = .5, p_{tails} = .5$ versus H_a: proportions otherwise, sample chisquared $= .64, df = 1, p = .42$
7.a. No (sample chisquared 13.2, $df = 5, p = .02$).
  b. No (sample chisquared 77.1, $df = 5, p < .005$).
9. The distribution of MIs is not uniform over the days of the week (sample chisquared 13.18, $df = 6, p = .04$). There are more heart attacks on Monday than expected, and fewer on Tuesdays.
11. The distribution of MIs for women is uniform over the days of the week (sample chisquared 4.356, $df = 6, p = .628$).
13. Glove perforation is not equally likely at the given sites (sample chisquared $= 38, df = 5$, p $= .0000004$).

Warm-ups 13.2

1. Cancer site and smoking history; **2.** The attributes for the cancer site factor are lung, oral-bladder, other cancer, no cancer. The attributes for the smoking history factor are never, light, medium, heavy; **3.** row marginal totals: lung, 181; oral-bladder, 152; other cancer, 726; no cancer, 4639; column marginal totals: never, 2344; light, 1204; medium, 1148; heavy, 1002; **4.** 41.1%; **5.** 18.6%; **6.** The factors of cancer site and smoking history are independent (the cancer attributes are distributed the same way in each of the smoking categories); **7.** 42; **8.** 1148, 5698, 30.6241; **9.** 30.62; **10.** tough call; **11.** 4.226; **12.** 218.584; **13.** 9; **14.** $< .005$ (Table 12); **15.** 16.9190; **16.** heavy smokers among lung cancers; **17.** never smoked among

lung cancers; **18.** No question about it. By habitual smoking, one increases the chance of cancer. It isn't worth it.

Problems 13.2

1.a. **(i)** 82; **(ii)** 35; **(iii)** 45; **(iv)** 72; **(v)** 117
  b.

		Sex		
		Male	Female	Total
Gallstone	Yes	28 31.54	17 13.46	45
Disease	No	54 50.46	18 21.54	72
	Total	82	35	117

  c. Gallstone disease and sex are independent (sample chisquared 2.157, $df = 1, p = .14$).
3. Gallstone disease and age class in men are independent factors (sample chisquared .697, $df = 1, p = .40$).
5. Duration of dialysis and race are independent factors (sample chisquared 5.736, $df = 4, p = .22$).
7.a. There is no significant difference in the proportion of patients contracting infection between the two hospitals ($z = 1.313, p = .19$).
  b. There is no significant difference in the proportion of patients contracting infection between the two hospitals (sample chisquared 1.725, $df = 1, p = .19$).
9.a. The proportion of patients with infiltrations does not significantly differ from the type of flush (saline versus heparin) used ($z = 1.584, p = .11$).
  b.

Type of Flush	Infiltration		
	Yes	No	Total
Heparin	8	17	25
Saline	5	29	34
Total	13	46	59

  c. Flush factor: heparin, saline; infiltration factor: yes, no.
  d.

Type of Flush	Infiltration		
	Yes	No	Total
Heparin	8 5.51	17 19.49	25
Saline	5 7.49	29 26.51	34
Total	13	46	59

  e. Infiltration and flush are independent (sample chisquared 2.508, $df = 1, p = .11$).
11. Stop: chisquared test not justified since 2 of 6 cells (33% > 20%) have expected frequencies less than 5.
13. Depression and dementia are dependent (sample chisquared 9.927, $df = 2, p = .007$).

15. Depression and 1-year survivorship are dependent (sample chisquared 9.002, $df = 2, p = .01$).

17. Treatment modality and change in offset potential are dependent (sample chisquared 21.724, $df = 3, p = .00007$).

19. Primary cancer site and county are dependent (sample chisquare 35.568, $df = 10, p = .0001$).

21. Coronary classification and coffee consumption are dependent (sample chisquared 145.564, $df = 8, p < .005$ (Table 12)).

23. Coronary classification and alcohol consumption are dependent (sample chisquared 117.659, $df = 6, p < .005$ (Table 12)).

25. Episiotomy and activity group are dependent (sample chisquared 10.731, $df = 1, p = .001$).

27.a. Yes total: 116; no: 104, 127, 115, 68 45, 35, total 494.
 b. Age and dementia are dependent (sample chisquared 24.078, $df = 5, p = .0002$).

29. The groups (method of shock wave treatment) and number of stones (single/multiple stones) are independent (sample chisquared 15.957, $df = 2, p = .0003$).

SECTION 14.1

Warm-ups 14.1

1. Yes; **2.** yes; **3.** yes; **4.** yes; **5.** we assume so; **7.** 4.496 liters/minute; **8.** 4.838 liters/minute; **9.** (4.496, 4.838); **13.** .842; **14.** .842; **15.** unknown; **16.** d; **17.** to determine whether the sample data are consistent with an assumption of linear correlation between the variates RTCO and Fick cardiac outputs; **18.** .471 (Table 13)

19.

Negative Linear Correlation	No Linear Correlation	Positive Linear Correlation
-1	$-.471$ .471	1

20. The sample is consistent with an assumption of positive linear correlation from RTCO to Fick cardiac output.

Problems 14.1

1. Graph (e), graph (c), graph (a), graph (b), graph (d)
3. Normality fails.
5. Normality fails.
7. Normality OK; **c.** $r = .987$; **d.** critical $r = .561$, positive linear correlation.
9. Normality OK; **c.** $r = .109$; **d.** critical $r = .917$, no linear correlation.
11. Normality OK; **c.** $r = .277$; **d.** critical $r = .917$, no linear correlation.

13. Normality OK; **c.** $r = .896$; **d.** critical $r = .917$, no linear correlation.
15. Normality OK; **c.** $r = .823$; **d.** critical $r = .917$, no linear correlation.
17. Normality OK; **c.** $r = .651$; **d.** critical $r = .641$, positive linear correlation.
19. Normality OK; **c.** $r = .807$; **d.** critical $r = .641$, positive linear correlation.
21. Normality OK; **c.** $r = -.145$; **d.** no linear correlation.
23. Normality fails.
25. Normality fails.

SECTION 14.2

Warm-ups 14.2

1. .471;

2.

Negative Linear Correlation	No Linear Correlation	Positive Linear Correlation
-1	$-.471$ .471	1

3. .748; **4.** yes; **5.** yes; **6.** Fick $= 1.01 + .850$ ITCO; **7.** enhanced (nondata) points; **8.** 3.78 liters/minute; **9.** 5.26 liters/minute; **10.** .802 liters/minute; **11.** No. Clinically, one would like cardiac output within .5 liters/minute. The error between ITCO and Fick exceeds .5 liters/minute in the sample in 13 patients out of 29 (45%). The standard deviation $s = .8499$ confirms that the amount of deviation between Fick and ITCO on a patient-to-patient basis is too great.

Problems 14.2

1. Regression equations for appropriate exercises in Problems 14.1:
  14.1.7. venous $= -.13 + 1.01$ arterial
  14.1.9. 5 min $= 64.3 + .332$ start
  14.1.11. end $= -5 + .942$ start
  14.1.13. end $= 3.23 + .8864$ start
  14.1.15. end $= 14.35 + .8869$ start
  14.1.17. for group 1, RL 1 hr $= 35.26 + .5548$ RL0
  14.1.19. for group 2, RL 2 hr $= 41.226 + .44462$ RL0
  14.1.21. height $= 185.088 - .280$ age
3.a. The critical correlation for $n = 50$ is .361; hence, evidence for positive linear correlation.
 b. 7666
5. age 32.0 ± 9.5 years, height 160.3 ± 5.8 cm, weight 59.3 ± 15.8 kg
7. Normality OK, sample correlation $r = .277$, no linear correlation.

9. Normality fails.

11. Systolic 127.5 ± 14.5 mm Hg, diastolic 78.6 ± 11.4 mm Hg.

13. Normality OK (sample nscores correlation for SBP .991, DBP .988); positive linear correlation (sample $r = .649$, critical r ($n = 18$) .590); regression equation: DBP $= 13.74 + .5088$ SBP.

15. Normality OK (sample nscore correlations: injectate lumen .968, infusion lumen .963); positive linear correlation (sample correlation .963, critical correlation .549); regression equation: injectate lumen cardiac output $= -.0789 + 1.01758$ infusion. Yes, the proximal infusion lumen may act as a suitable substitute for the proximal injectate lumen for the purpose of approximate cardiac output determinations. The correlation is high between the two variates.

Review III

1.

Infection	Frequency	Percent
MSF	248	54
Typhoid	149	33
Meningitis	61	13
Total	458	100

MSF Mediterranean spotted fever

3. The proportion of G6PD cases among boys with bacterial infections is consistent with the proportion of G6PD-deficient males in the general population ($z = .087, p > .20$).

5. Do not reject $H_0: p_1 \le p_2$. The proportion of girls with bacterial infections who have G6PD deficiency is not statistically significantly greater than the proportion of boys with bacterial infections who have G6PD deficiency ($z = -1.634, p = .51$).

7. The sample size is adequate ($< 20\%$ of the expected values are < 5). The factors of disease and G6PD deficiency are independent in girls ($\chi^2 = .202, df = 2, p = .90$).

9. normality OK: sample nscores correlation .988

11. Sample legend: size 7, mean 29.3, standard deviation 8.7

13. (21, 38)

15. Both samples consistent with normality; hence, confidence t-intervals are justified. The t-intervals overlap. Hence, the sample means are not statistically significantly different.

17. The sample correlation is .944, the critical correlation for $n = 7$ is .875. Hence, the sample provides evidence for positive linear correlation.

19. Because of the large sample size, we appeal to the robustness of ANOVA. The mean hemoglobin levels differ significantly between the four groups ($f = 57.5$, $df = 3,890, p \approx 0$). In particular, the mean hemoglobin level for infants fed with unfortified cow's milk was significantly smaller than with human milk, which was smaller than either iron group. There was no significant difference between iron-fortified cow's milk formula and iron dextrose injection.

21. Because of the large sample size, we appeal to the robustness of ANOVA. The mean transferrin saturation levels differ significantly between the four groups ($f = 61.4, df = 3,890, p \approx 0$). In particular, the mean transferrin saturation level for infants fed with unfortified cow's milk was significantly smaller than with human milk, which was smaller than with iron-fortified cow's milk formula, which was smaller than iron dextrose injection.

23. 60

25. The sample size is adequate ($< 20\%$ of the expected values are < 5). The factors of ABO blood type and MIA reactivity are independent ($\chi^2 = 5.697, df = 3, p = .13$).

27.a. There is a significant difference in the 5-year survival rate between the two groups ($z = -4.692, p = .000003$).

   b. There is a significant difference in the 5-year survival rate between the two groups ($\chi^2 = 22.017, p = .000003$).

   c. The general conclusions are identical.

29.a. There is an association between the factors of smoking history and PID ($\chi^2 = 15.397, df = 3, p = .0015$).

   b. There are significantly more PID cases in the < 10 category than expected and significantly fewer PID cases among the never-smoked category. The relationship between smoking history and PID is somewhat puzzling from this chi-squared analysis. At first glance, heavier smoking (≥ 10) seems to have no effect on PID. A chi-squared analysis that lumps the two smoking categories together shows smoking is a significant factor in PID ($\chi^2 = 10.7, df = 2, p = .005$). In particular, smokers display more PID cases than expected, while those who have never smoked display few PID cases than expected.

α 229 level of significance (Greek alpha)
ANOVA 320 analysis of variance
ar 58 adjusted range

β 229 power of a statistical test (Greek beta)
b(x; n, p) 145 binomial probability
bino(n, p) 144 binomial random variable

χ^2 335, 374 chisquared (Greek chi)
C(n, k) 87 combination
CDF 129 cumulative density function
CI 186 confidence interval

D 197 difference
df 189 degrees of freedom

E' 78 complement of an event
EDA 46 exploratory data analysis
E[X] 132 expected value of X

f(x) 127, 129 function value
$F(x) = Prob[X \leq x]$ 130 cumulative function
F + R 105 false positive rate
F − R 104 false negative rate

GLM 363 general linear model

η 27, 206 population median
H_a 171, 224 alternate hypothesis
H_0 171, 224 null hypothesis

k 57 number of classes

LOS 229 level of significance

μ 26, 132, 156 population mean
$\hat{\mu}$ 185 point estimate for the population mean
μ_X 131 mean of the random variable X
m 58 data set minimum, adjusted minimum

n 10 size of a data set
n! 86 n-factorial

p 10, 211 proportion
p 142 probability of success

$\hat{p}$ 211 point estimate for a population proportion
p-value 308 probability value
PDF 126 probability density function
Prob[X = x] 127 probability
PV + 105 predictive value of a positive test result
PV − 105 predictive value of a negative test result
$P[a < X \leq b]$ 157 probability X is between a and b
P[occurrence] 74 probability of occurrence

q 142 probability of failiure

ρ 403 population correlation
r 172, 403 sample correlation
RV 24 random variable

Σ 26 summation
σ 157, 289 population standard deviation
s 30, 133 sample standard deviation
s^2 30 sample variance
SD 31 standard deviation
SEM 195 standard error of the mean
Sn 104 sensitivity of a diagnostic test
Sp 105 specificity of a diagnostic test

TOH 227 test of hypothesis

u 57 unit of measurement
uer 58 unit extended range

V[X] 132 variance of the random variable X

w 58 class width

x 10 outcome
$\{x_1, x_2, \ldots, x_n\}$ 25 generic data set
$\bar{x}$ 26 sample mean
$\tilde{x}$ 27 sample median

$Y = a + bX$ 415 equation of a linear regression line

Z 158 standard normal random variable